AF663480

MANUAL OF PRACTICAL PHYSIOLOGY FOR MBBS

Books for MBBS Students

1. Textbook of Physiology Vol. I by Prof. A.K. Jain
2. Textbook of Physiology Vol. II by Prof. A.K. Jain
3. Comprehensive MCQs in Human Physiology by Prof. A.K. Jain
4. Human Physiology in Nutshell by Prof. A.K. Jain
5. Manual of Practical Biochemistry for MBBS by Dr. S.K. Gupta, Dr. Veena Singh Ghalaut & Dr. Anju Jain
6. Essentials of Immunology by Prof. S.K. Gupta
7. Textbook of Microbiology by Prof. C.P. Baveja
8. Practical Microbiology for MBBS by Prof. C.P. Baveja
9. Medical Parasitology by Prof. C.P. Baveja & Dr. V. Baveja
10. Concise Microbiology by Prof. C.P. Baveja & Dr. V. Baveja
11. Textbook of Pathology for MBBS Vol I by Dr. A.K. Mandal & Dr. Shramana Choudhury
12. Textbook of Pathology for MBBS Vol II by Dr. A.K. Mandal & Dr. Shramana Choudhury
13. Practical Pathology by Dr. K. Uma Chaturvedi & Dr. Tejinder Singh
14. Text and Practical of Haematology for MBBS by Dr. Tejinder Singh
15. MCQs in Pathology by Prof. K. Uma & Prof. T. Singh
16. MCQs in Advanced Medical Pharmacology by Dr. K.V. Ramesh
17. Textbook of Medicine for MBBS by Dr. S.N. Chugh
18. Fundamentals of ECG by Dr. Vipin Gupta
19. Textbook of ENT by Dr. Sharad Maheshwari & Dr. Subirendra Kumar
20. MCQs in Respiratory Medicine by Dr. B.L. Bhardwaj, Dr. Kanchan Bhardwaj & Dr. Aastha Miranpuri
21. Concise Radiology for Undergraduates by Dr. Bhushan N. Lakhkar, Dr. Chandra Kant & M. Shetty
22. Concise Psychiatry for Undergraduates by Dr. P.D. Garg & Dr. Aseem Garg

MANUAL OF PRACTICAL PHYSIOLOGY

For MBBS

Dr. A K Jain
M.D., MNAMS
Director Professor,
Department of Physiology
Maulana Azad Medical College
New Delhi

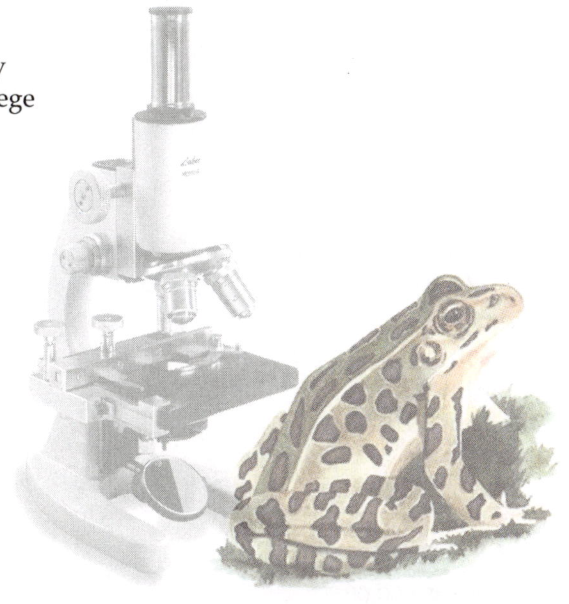

ARYA PUBLICATIONS
(AVICHAL PUBLISHING COMPANY)
Industrial Area, Kala Amb-173030, Distt. Sirmour (H.P.)
Delhi Office: **1002 Faiz Road (opp. Hanuman Murti), Karol Bagh, New Delhi 110 005**

The book has been published in good faith that the material provided by the author is original.

All rights reserved. No part of this publication may be reproduced or transmitted in any form or by any means [graphic, electronic or mechanical, including photocopying, recording, taping or information retrieval system] without the written permission of the copyright holder, application for which should be addressed to the publisher. Such written permission must also be obtained before any part of this publication is stored in a retrieval system of any nature. Breach of this condition is liable for legal action.

Exhaustive efforts have been made to ensure accuracy and correctness of contents of the book at the time of going to press. However, in view of possibility of human error or changes in medical science, neither the author, publisher nor any other person who has been involved in preparation of this work accepts any responsibility for any errors or omissions or results obtained from use of information given in the book.

The publisher shall not be liable for any direct, consequential, or incidental damages arising out of the use of the book.

In case of binding mistake, misprints, or missing pages etc, the publisher's entire liability, and your exclusive remedy, is replacement of the book within one month of purchase by similar edition/reprint of the book. In case of any dispute, all legal matters are to be settled under Delhi Jurisdiction only.

Published by:
ARYA PUBLICATIONS
(Avichal Publishing Company)
Industrial Area, Trilokpur Road
Kala Amb-173030, Distt. Sirmour (H.P.)
Ph. : 01702-238688, 238832

Delhi Office:
1002 Faiz Road (opp. Hanuman Murti)
Karol Bagh, New Delhi 110 005 (India)
Phones : 011-28752745, 28752604, 28755383
Fax : 011-28756921
E-mail : medical@apcbooks.co.in, info@apcbooks.co.in
Website : www.apcbooks.co.in

© Author

ISBN-978-81-7855-315-5

First Edition : 2003
Second Edition : 2007
Third Edition : 2008
Reprint : 2009, 2010
Fourth Edition : 2012
Reprint : 2013
Reprint : 2014

Price : ₹ 400.00

Typeset & Designed at:
Laser Tech Prints

Printed at:
Prince Print Process
Delhi

Dedicated to

My parents

(Late) Shri M.C. Jain

and

(Late) Shrimati Lajwanti Jain

(whose blessings and love have always been with me throughout my endeavour)

My wife Shalu, sons Ashish-Avnish and daughter-in-law Latika

(whose support enabled me to complete it)

My teachers, colleagues and friends

(who have made me capable of what I am today)

My students

(who have been my teachers and suggested me to start the project)

PREFACE

I would like to thank all the readers for an overwhelming response and appreciation given to all my Books of Physiology written till date. The purpose of this *"Manual of Practical Physiology"* for MBBS is to emphasise the need for quantitative improvement in human physiology experiments with its clinical correlates. This is in line with the new curriculum policy of the Medical Council of India (MCI) for first MBBS students. The implementation of MCI policy made it necessary to bring out a revised ***Manual of Practical Physiology*** on the basis of curriculum prepared by them which could bring uniformity of practicals in all medical colleges.

This Textbook is meant for anyone who wishes to acquire the skill of learning through cause-effect relationship. Thus it should be visualised as a medium to train a student to think logically and analyse the things accordingly. I have left no stone unturned in furnishing text material of high quality. Also, the teaching of practical physiology is suitably redesigned to bring it in line with modern technological devices. The important topics covered in this manual are grouped under four units as:

I. **Haematology experiments**

II. **Nerve and muscle experiments (*Frog*)**

III. **Human experiments**

IV. **Mammalian (*Dog/Rabbit*) experiments**

Some of the salient features of this Textbook are:

1. It furnishes basic information about physiology experiments giving emphasis on every aspect evenly.
2. All the experiments in the Textbook are classified as student exercises; working steps are so framed that any experiment can be handled by a beginner.
3. More number of practicals on human physiology have been included and their application to clinical medicine stressed.
4. Well-labelled diagrams, pictures and graphs/records depicting analysis and reasoning is one of the salient features of this Textbook.
5. Some of the *important viva-voce questions with answers* are given at the end of each practical. This will give an idea to the students of the type of questions asked in the examination.
6. New concepts have been introduced along with suitable examples.
7. *Objective Structured Practical Examination* (OSPE), a tool to assess practical skills, has been placed in a separate box (wherever necessary) at the end of the practical.
8. *Spotting:* List of frequently asked spots in the examination has been placed at the end of the Textbook in a separate appendix.
9. The matter on Human Experiments has been furnished with its clinical correlates. This will be of great 'help' to the students during their clinical posting subsequently.
10. The Textbook contains 556 diagrams and pictures. These will help the students in easy reproducibility and understanding of the subject better.

I am thankful to Dr. Vipin Gupta who inspired me to initiate this project and invited me to join this national endeavour for the improvement of practical knowledge in Physiology. He took a lot of interest in this project and greatly helped me bring out this Textbook.

I express my sincere thanks and deep appreciation to all my colleagues in the department of Physiology, Maulana Azad Medical College, New Delhi. All of them with utmost interest not only spared their valuable time for me but also provided me with original graphs and records collected over the years for preparing this ***Manual of Practical Physiology***. Special thanks are due to Dr (Mrs.) Rashmi Babbar, Head of the department of Physiology, for enabling me to complete this project.

I extend my heartfelt thanks to Shri V.K. Manchanda, Shri Rajiv Manchanda, Ms Harsha and to the whole staff of M/s. Laser Tech Prints, New Delhi, who took a lot of pains in shaping the manuscript in the press-worthy form and seeing it through the press.

I shall be doing injustice if I do not thank the members of my family—my wife, Mrs Shailesh Jain; sons, Ashish and Avnish; and daughter-in law, Latika, who throughout this project supported me patiently, provided me with appropriate environment to give my best and made my life so much more enjoyable.

Curriculum development is a dynamic and continuous process. No one can claim to have developed a perfect curriculum material. There will always be some scope for further improvement, so I request all those who will be using this textbook to evaluate the material with an open mind and offer their valuable suggestions for improving the quality in future.

A.K. Jain

CONTENTS

INTRODUCTION

It is most important for students to realise that *laboratory teaching* in physiology is designed to give an opportunity for the practice of principles involved in observing. Memorising the methods and results is of no advantage in comparison with an understanding of the correct method of approach in obtaining the results. This, in fact, is true and can be realised from the following famous Chinese proverbs:

If I hear, I forget;
If I see, I remember; and
If I do, I understand.

Laboratory teaching fascination, therefore, lies in learning by doing. Its main objectives are:

1. Introducing, developing and reinforcing theoretical concepts;
2. Developing practical skills, for example, doing blood counts, handling of live tissues, etc.;
3. Introducing and developing the skills of scientific approach to a problem; and
4. Building confidence to handle unexpected events and observations scientifically.

The following advice would, therefore, be of some value to a student beginning the course.

(A) General Guidelines

1. Read the instructions carefully regarding the objective of the experiment.
2. Acquaint yourself thoroughly with the apparatus before starting the experiment.
3. When you have obtained and analysed your results, discuss them with your table teacher.
4. Summarize your results as briefly and concisely as possible, in your laboratory manual.

> **Important Note:** Approach each experiment without any pre-formed idea regarding the probable results.

(B) Guidelines for Laboratory Procedure

1. Student must wear white coats (overalls/aprons) in the laboratories, and should bring the following instruments to the practical classes:
   (i) disposable injection needle (24 gauge)
   (ii) a piece of clean cloth
   (iii) dissection box containing pithing needle, scalpal, scissors (large/fine), a seeker and forceps (toothed/fine)
   (iv) Stethoscope (Littman type)
   (v) Patellar hammer
   (vi) pencil torch
2. Bring your laboratory instruction manual/textbook to the laboratory.
3. Check the laboratory schedule at least one day in advance. Read the assigned experiment paying attention to any special instruction since these may require advance preparation.
4. Equipment/apparatus required in each day's experiment may be checked out at the distribution table. Each student would be required to sign for the apparatus taken. At the completion of the experiment, the equipment must be returned in the same condition in which it was received.
5. Maintain neatness at all times during the experiments. All cotton, gauze or paper, whether dry or wet, must be placed in the dustbin.
6. Before leaving the laboratory:
   (i) all equipment must be left in the proper order;
   (ii) all switches should be turned off; and
   (iii) table tops must be cleaned.
7. For certain experiments, students may work in pair or in a group of 3 or more. Therefore, when graphs or records are made during the experiment, the record must, if possible, be duplicated so that each student may have a copy.
8. Study your records carefully, attempt to account for any discrepancy which may occur between the experimental results and the results which your textbooks indicate that should have occurred.
9. **OSPE (Objective Structured Practical Examination):** OSPE is a recently introduced tool to assess practical skills (and *not the knowledge*) of students on a more reliable and uniform basis. Here, the student is asked to perform a part of practical with clearly outline objectives within a given time-frame. The examiner silently observes the *stepwise* procedure of the practical being performed by the students

as per *checklist* provided. Each step of the practical carries marks and is evaluated accordingly. Thus, the students should practise the procedure of each practical carefully as described in the manual/ textbook.

Note: In the examination, the students are usually assessed for five practicals by going through five ***OSPE stations*** spending two minutes at each station.

(C) Guidelines for Writing Records

1. Every student has to maintain a record of the exercises performed and demonstrations attended. The records are evaluated at the time of terminal and university examinations.
2. A record should be neatly written as follows:
   (i) Write the date of experiment on the top left-hand side of the experiment;
   (ii) The results should be presented in the form of tables and graphs and conclusions drawn.
   (iii) Answer the questions given at the end of each practical/demonstration.
3. The practical records should be checked by the teaching staff at regular intervals.

Important Note: A student will be admitted for the practical class only if his work is up-to-date and if he has completed the previous experiments unless there is justification for not doing so. As per MCI guidelines, a student will be permitted to appear at the annual University examination only after satisfactorily obtaining 80% attendance and a minimum of 35% marks in day-to-day assessment.

Unit I
Haematology

Date: ....

1 Study of a Compound Microscope

I. Parts of the microscope
II. Formation of the image
III. Focussing of an object
IV. Precautions

I. PARTS OF THE MICROSCOPE

The microscope was invented by *Antony van Leeuwen-Hoeck*. It is an instrument by which very small things can be seen which are not seen by the naked eye. A compound microscope essentially consists of the following parts: (Fig. 1.1.1)

1. The stand

It comprises a heavy **foot**, often shapes like a horse shoe, to provide stability; and the **limb** which bears the optical system.The limb is attached to the foot by a **hinged joint** so that the microscope may be set at a comfortable angle for the observer.

2. The optical system

It is mounted on the tube which is usually in two parts:

(i) an **external tube** which bears at its lower end a revolving **nose piece** in which inter-changeable three **objective lenses** of various magnifications are fitted:

(a) low power: X10
(b) high power: X40
(c) oil immersion: X100

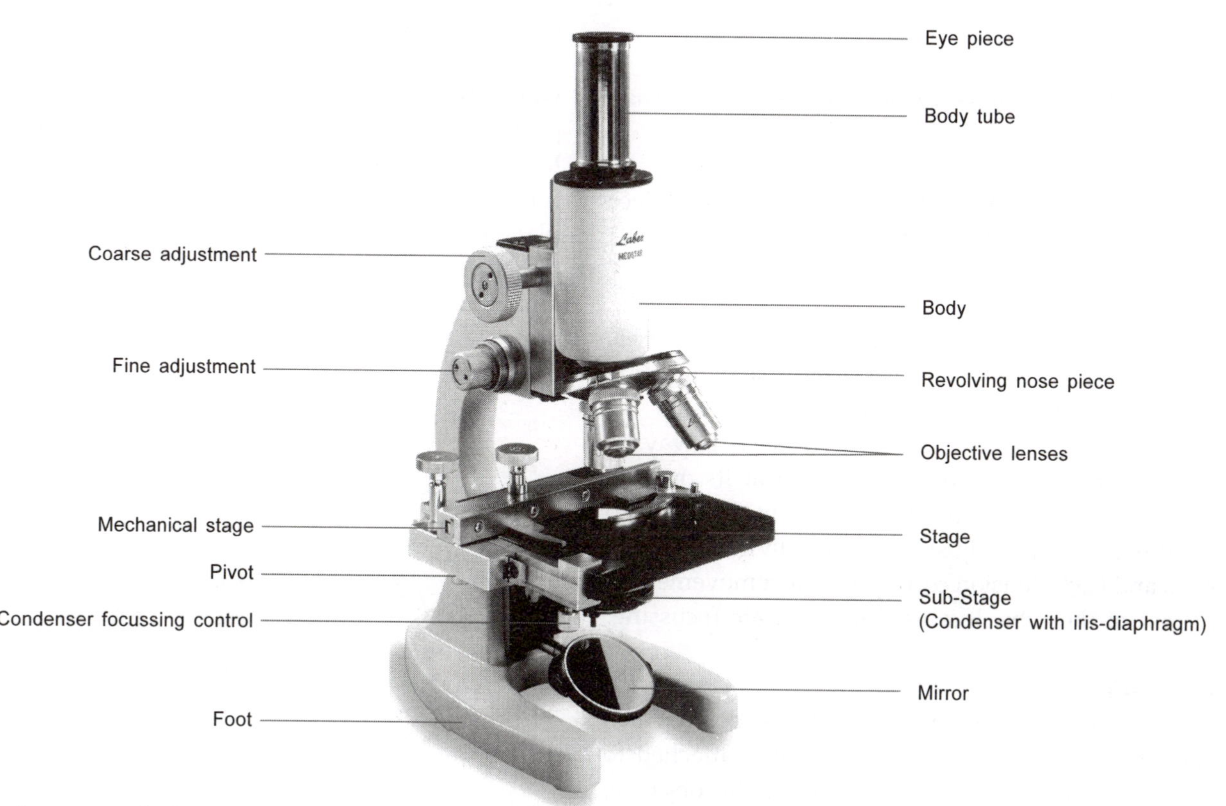

Fig. 1.1.1 A compound microscope

Note: The objective lenses can be identified by magnification imprinted on them. In addition, oil-immersion lens has a black rim around its lower end. It has become customary for the objective lenses to be marked with their magnifying power rather than their focal length (Fig. 1.1.2). The approximate equivalents are as follows:

Focal length (mm)	*Magnification*
2	X100
4	X40
16	X10
40	X4

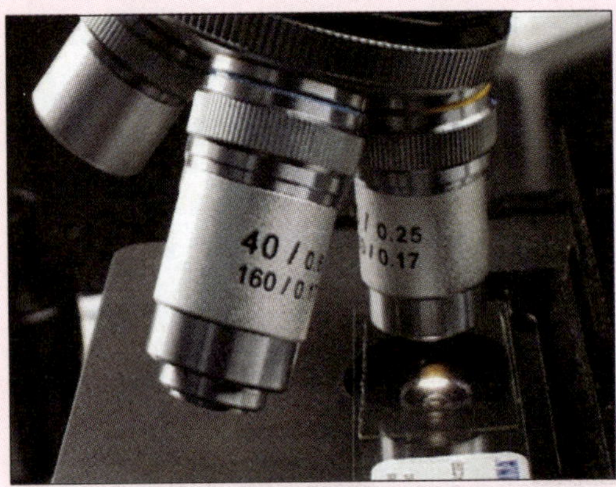

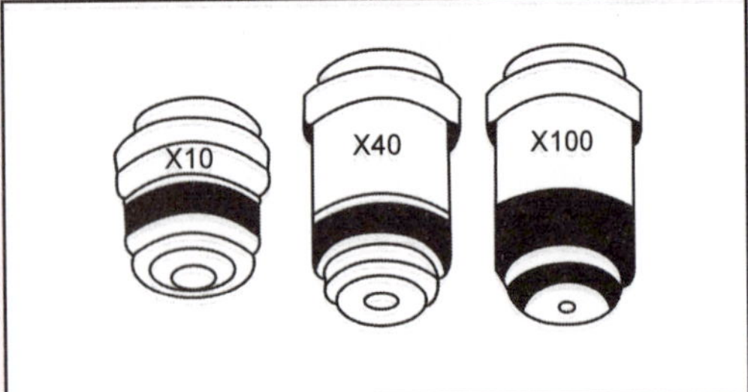

Fig. 1.1.2 Objective lenses—low, high and oil-immersion lens

(ii) an **inner draw tube** that carries the eye piece (magnification X10) at its upper end

3. The body

The whole assembly is held in position by the *body* which consists of two mechanisms: the **coarse** and **fine adjustments**. With the help of these adjustments the height of the tube can be adjusted in such a way so that the objective lens can be positioned at its optimal working distance (*i.e.* its focal length) from the object to be examined. The fine adjustment is usually graduated in 1/50ths and each division corresponds to a movement of 0.002 mm of the tube. It is used for accurate focussing.

4. The stage

It is a platform that accommodates a glass slide on which the object to be examined is mounted. It is attached to the limb immediately below the level of the objective lens and has an aperture in the centre to permit light to reach the object.

A **mechanical stage** is fitted to the fixed stage so that the object may be moved from side to side and before backwards.

5. The substage

It lies beneath the stage which can be lowered or raised by means of a screw. The stage is fitted with a **condenser** and **iris diaphragm**.

(i) The **condenser** consists of two lenses, it serves to condense the rays of light and to focus them on the object. The height of condenser and, therefore, the focus of light can be varied.

(ii) Immediately below the condenser is the **iris diaphragm** that can control the amount of light reaching the object.

6. The mirror

Fitted to the tail piece below the condenser is a hinged **double reflecting mirror** which is *plane* on one side and *concave* on the other. The plane side of the mirror is used when the condenser is used. The mirror can be tilted and rotated in all directions.

II. FORMATION OF THE IMAGE

It is the lenses composing the objective which initiate the magnifying process. An objective operates at a distance from the object that is roughly equal to its focal length, and admits rays that are to form a **real, an inverted, enlarged image** in the upper part of the tube. At this point, there is interposed another lens, the **field lens** whose function is to collect the diverging rays of the primary image so that they may pass through the **eye lens** of the eye piece which magnifies the image still further. The field lens is accommodated in the lower plane of the eye piece. Rays, as they leave the eye piece to reach the observer's eye, are once more divergent and thus the image seen by the retina is virtual, appearing to be about 25 cm (10 inches) in front of the eyes (Fig. 1.1.3).

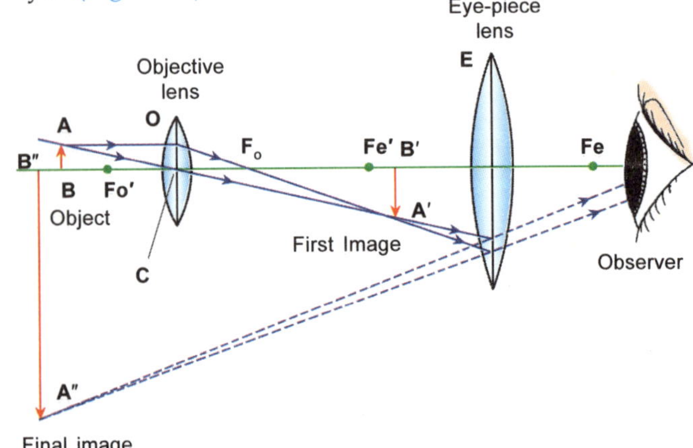

Fig. 1.1.3 Image formation in a compound microscope

A. Magnification

The magnification of the object is determined by multiplying the power of the eye piece with that of the objective (X inscribed on the objective or eye piece denotes the unit of the magnification). For example, if the eye piece magnification is X10 and that of objective lens is X100, then a given object gets magnified by 1,000 times.

B. Resolution

The limit of useful magnification is set by the resolving power of the lens *i.e.* its ability to reveal closely the adjacent structural details as separate and distinct. It is this power which determines the amount of structural details that can be observed.

C. Oil Immersion Objective

Oil immersion objective is most frequently used in haematology because of its greater magnification and resolution.

It has been seen that any factor which reduces the amount of rays falling on the objective, impairs the quality of the image. In case of oil immersion objective, the space between the object and the objective lens is filled with some transparent fluid (such as *liquid paraffin, glycerine or transparent oil*) with the same refractive index as glass (= 1.515) then the rays of light do not undergo refraction and pass directly into the objective. The most commonly used fluid is the ***cedar wood oil***.

III. FOCUSSING OF AN OBJECT

A. Under Low Power

1. Place the slide to be focussed on the stage and fit it into the mechanical stage. By means of the screw of the mechanical stage bring the object on the central aperture in the stage.
2. Using the light source and by adjusting the plane mirror, focus the light on the object. Partially close the iris diaphragm and lower the objective (X10) with coarse adjustment near the slide.
3. The position of the slide is so adjusted that the aperture of the objective lens is just above the point to be focussed on the slide.

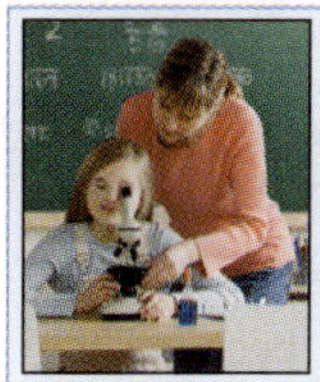

Important Note: *Always keep looking from the side of the microscope as you are lowering the optical tube, otherwise you are liable to damage the slide.*

4. Now look into the eye-piece; the optical tube is moved upwards (again using coarse adjustment) slowly and confidently, till the object comes under view. Once this is achieved, the coarse adjustment should ***not*** be used.
5. Lower the condenser from the top position till the object is properly illuminated. ***The condenser usually occupies a low position.***
6. Next, using the fine adjustment only, the slide can be brought to a sharp focus.

B. Under High Power

1. For focussing under high power (X40), simply rotate the nose-piece so that the high power objective lens may come to lie above the slide to a sharp focus.
2. The iris diaphragm is fully opened and concave mirror is used to condense the light on the object.
3. The condenser is kept in the beginning at the top and is then gradually lowered till the object is properly illuminated. The ***condenser usually occupies a higher position*** than that for focussing under the low power.
4. With the fine adjustment screw, attempt the final focussing.

C. Under Oil Immersion Lens

1. For focussing under oil immersion lens (X100), a drop of cedar-wood oil is placed on the slide. Then turn the nose piece further so that the oil immersion lens may be in use. It will automatically dip into the drop of oil.
2. As the slide is moved, the drop of oil will also get moved on its own. Thus any part of the slide can be observed.
3. The iris diaphragm is kept fully opened and *the condenser is kept in the top position.* Use only the fine adjustment to focus the necessary area.

Important Note: While putting the stained slide, care should be taken so that the stained smear may be facing the objective.

Important Points to Remember

1. ***Position of condenser***. The desired position of the condenser is as follows:

Objective lens power	Condenser position
(i) Low power (X10)	(i) Lowest
(ii) High power (X40)	(ii) Higher (in between i and iii)
(iii) Oil immersion (X100)	(iii) Highest

2. ***Type of mirror to be used***
   (i) The Plane side of the mirror is used when:
      (a) a condenser is used;
      (b) The source of light is diffuse such as daylight.

(ii) Concave mirror is used when source of light is from a point source such as bulb, as used in labs.

3. The higher the magnification, the smaller the area that can be examined at a time. Therefore, to start with, irrespective of what is being examined, **it is always advisable to focus a slide under low power (X10) first**. Obtain a general view of the object and choose the field you would like to examine in detail. Bring this field in the central portion. Then switch over to the next high power. Now use only the fine adjustment for focussing. If necessary, select the field further and bring it in the centre again.

IV. PRECAUTIONS

1. A clear image can never be seen through dirty lenses. Make sure that the eye piece as well as all the objectives is clean.
   While cleaning microscope lenses, do not rub them with dry cotton or rough cloth which might leave permanent scratch marks on the lenses. Apply *xylene* to the lenses (to dissolve the grease) and then wipe dry gently with a piece of silk cloth or softest material available.

> **Note:** Always clean the microscope lenses before and after the use.

2. Do not clean the objective with alcohol, as it may dissolve the cement which unites the component lenses.
3. Never lower the optical tube while you are looking through the eye piece.
4. Make minimal and careful use of ONLY the fine adjustment while using the high power and oil immersion lenses.
5. If the microscope has to be moved, it should be held upright by the limb keeping a hand below its foot.

OSPE

Aim: Focus the given slide under low power/high power/oil immersion lens of the microscope provided.

Procedure steps: Refer to page 5.

Checklist

1. Uses screw of the mechanical stage to bring the slide on the central aperture. **(Yes/No)**
2. Uses the light source. **(Yes/No)**
3. Correctly uses the objective lens power
   (i) low power (X 10);
   (ii) high power (X 40)
   (iii) Oil immersion lens (X 100) **(Yes/No)**
4. Correctly adjusts the condenser position
   (i) low power (X 10)
   (ii) high power (X 40)
   (iii) oil immersion lens (X 100) **(Yes/No)**
5. Whether or not looks from the side of the microscope while lowering the optical tube. **(Yes/No)**

IMPORTANT VIVA-VOCE QUESTIONS

Q.1. *Which type of image do you observe under the compound microscope?*

Ans. The image seen in a compound microscope is a virtual image of the primary image; latter being a real image of the object (page 4).

Q.2. *The optical tube is generally of a standard length. How much is it and why?*

Ans. The optical tube length is 250-260 mm; this is so because a X10 lens will furnish an image 10 times the diameter of the object as it naturally appears when held at 255 mm, *i.e.* 25 cm (10") from the eye.

Q.3. *How will you identify the oil immersion objective lens?*

Ans. Page 4.

Q.4. *What precautions must you take while using the oil immersion lens?*

Ans. Pages 5 and 6.

Q.5. *How would you calculate the magnification of an object you are observing under the microscope?*

Ans. Page 5.

Q.6. *Why has the oil immersion objective lens only a pin-hole aperture?*

Ans. The oil immersion lens has a very short focal length and if the aperture was more than a pin-hole then spherical and chromatic abberation would distort the image.

Q.7. *Why should the condenser position be low for low power lens and highest for oil immersion lens?*

Ans. The aperture of the low power lens is largest. Therefore, it will permit the largest amount of light. If the condenser position is raised too high, the clarity of the image will be lost because of excessive brightness.

Q.8. *Name the fluids which can be used for viewing the object under oil immersion lens.*

Ans. Page 5.

Q.9. *What is the function of the condenser and what should be its position while using the oil immersion lens?*

Ans. The intensity of illumination can be controlled by raising or lowering the condenser and amount of light can be regulated by varying the aperture size of the iris-diaphragm fixed at the base of the condenser.

While using the oil immersion lens, condenser should be raised right up to the stage to intensify the illumination and the aperture of the iris-diaphragm should be widely opened to allow the maximum light.

Q.10. *Give the different arrangement available for varying the illumination of the object.*

Ans. By using a plane or a concave mirror, the condenser and the iris-diaphragm, the illumination of the object can be varied (refer to page 5).

Maximum illumination is obtained by using the concave mirror with the condenser up and the iris-diaphragm open. Minimum illumination results from the opposite combination.

In general, we need less illumination while viewing a clear preparation under low power; maximum illumination is required while viewing a stained preparation under oil-immersion lens.

STUDY NOTES

OBSERVATIONS AND COMMENTS

....

....

....

....

....

....

....

....

....

....

....

....

....

....

....

....

....

....

....

....

Date: ....

2 An Introduction to Experiments on Blood

I. Collection of a blood sample
II. Commonly used anticoagulants
III. Haematological values for normal individuals
IV. Haemocytometer: RBC and WBC pipettes; improved Neubauer's counting chamber

Blood has an intimate give-and-take relationship with all parts of the body. Therefore, experiments on blood are the most clinically related experiments. Since it is possible to obtain a sample of blood with minimal pain and trauma at no risk, blood tests are done routinely in a clinical setup.

I. COLLECTION OF A BLOOD SAMPLE

For most haematological examinations done routinely in clinical setting, two types of blood samples are commonly used: *capillary (peripheral) blood* and *venous blood.*

A. Capillary (Peripheral) Blood

Capillary blood can be obtained from an **ear-lobe** or a **finger** of an adult or from the **heel** of an infant. A *free flow* of blood is essential, and only the very gentlest squeezing is permissible. Ideally speaking, a large drop of blood should come out slowly and spontaneously.

1. Pricking the finger (Fig. 1.2.1)

Use a sterilized disposable needle (24 gauge) or sterilize it by heating over flame. Heat kills the hepatitis virus while spirit does not. However, the sharpness of the needle is adversely affected by heat but not by spirit.

(i) Distal digit of the 3rd or 4th finger on its palmer surface, about 3-5 mm lateral from the nail bed is used for pricking purpose.

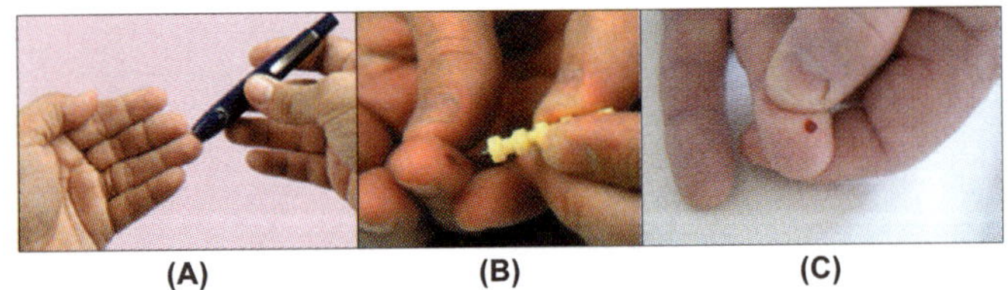

(A) (B) (C)

Fig. 1.2.1 Pricking the finger by (A) Lancet; (B) Needle and (C) An optimal blood drop size

(ii) Apply spirit to the finger with a cotton swab. Do not prick till the spirit dries up because:
  (a) sterilization by spirit is effective only after it has dried up, and
  (b) the blood gets hemolysed if it comes in contact with spirit.

(iii) Then prick the finger by a single stabbing action just deep enough (about 5 mm) to give free flowing blood.

(iv) Wipe away the first few drops and collect the sample when the blood is flowing spontaneously.

Note: *If blood has to be obtained by squeezing the finger, it gets diluted by the tissue fluids, thereby giving low values and the results are unreliable.*

2. Pricking the ear-lobe (Fig. 1.2.2)

Rub the ear in between the fingers gently until warm. Then prick it to a depth of 2-3 mm with a sterile needle (24 gauge) on the ear-lobe by a single stabbing action. Wipe away the first few drops and collect the sample when the blood is flowing spontaneously.

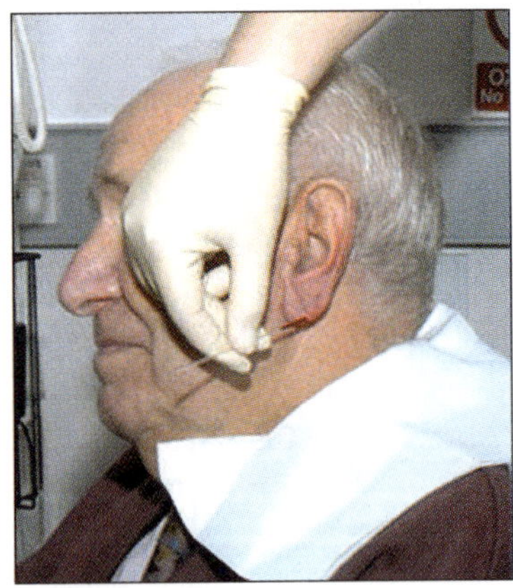

Fig. 1.2.2 Pricking the ear-lobe

3. Pricking the heel (Fig. 1.2.3)

This is a satisfactory method to obtain the sample of blood in infants. Make sure that the heel is really warm. Then a deep prick is made on the lateral or medial parts of the plantar surface of the heel.

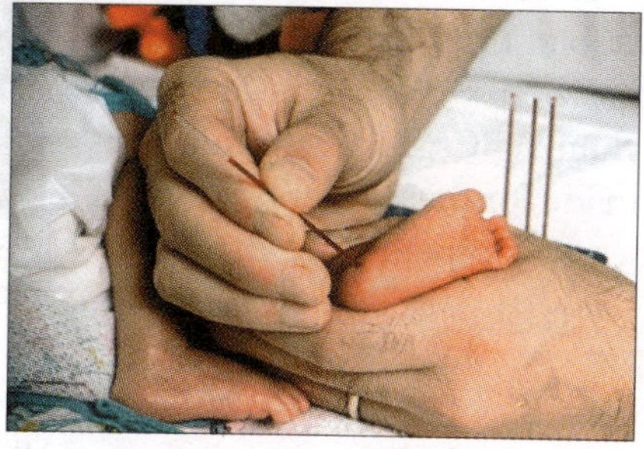

Fig. 1.2.3 Pricking the heel

Note: The central plantar area and the posterior curvature should not be punctured in infants to avoid the risk of injury to the underlying tarsal bones.

B. Venous Blood

Venous blood is preferred for most haematological examinations. It is best withdrawn from an *antecubital vein* by means of a dry, disposable plastic syringe (Fig. 1.2.4). In obese patients, it may be easier to use a vein on the dorsum of the hand.

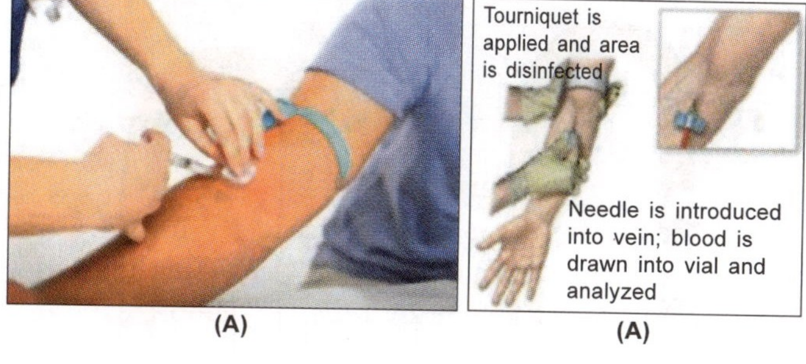

Fig. 1.2.4 (A) Right arm showing application of tourniquet and (B) Steps for collection of blood by vene puncture

1. Apply a sphygmomanometer cuff kept at diastolic BP or a tourniquet to the upper arm; clean the skin with spirit over the selected vein and allow it to dry, veins suitable for puncture will usually become apparent.
2. Place the thumb of the left hand about 5 cm below the vein and exert traction on the skin towards the digits. This fixes the vein and prevents it from sliding about during the insertion of the needle.
3. By means of a dry disposable plastic syringe, a needle (23 or 24 gauge) is inserted into the vein. When the needle enters the vein all resistance is felt to cease; blood will also be seen to enter the barrel of the syringe. The piston of the syringe should be withdrawn slowly and no attempt should be made to withdraw blood faster than the vein is filling.
4. Loosen the tourniquet, withdraw the needle and apply pressure for several minutes over the vein.
5. After detaching the needle, deliver the blood carefully from the syringe into a container (the differences between capillary and venous blood are given in Table 1.2.1).

Table 1.2.1 Differences between capillary and venous blood

Capillary (peripheral) blood	Venous blood
1. It can be obtained by skin puncture from the finger or ear-lobe or heel.	1. It can be obtained by vene puncture from any convenient vein.
2. There is greater likelihood of contamination and risk of transmission of diseases.	2. There is lesser risk of transmitting diseases.
3. It is liable to give erroneous results even if it is free flowing as it is more nearly arteriolar in composition. Therefore, PCV, Hb content and RBC and platelet count are significantly less.	3. PCV, Hb content and RBC and platelet count are significantly higher.

II. COMMONLY USED ANTICOAGULANTS

For the purpose of routine haematological work, a number of different anticoagulants are available.

A. Ethylenediamine tetra-acetic acid (EDTA)

1. The sodium and potassium salts of EDTA are powerful anticoagulants. They act by **chelating effect** on the calcium molecules in blood. This requires a concentration of 1.2 mg of the anhydrous salt per ml of blood.
2. The *anticoagulant of choice* is the dipotassium salt as it is very soluble. It is preferred over disodium salt which is considerably less soluble. The tripotassium salt produces some *shrinkage of RBCs* which results in a 2-3% decrease in PCV.
3. Excess of EDTA (>2 mg/ml of blood):
   (i) affects both RBCs and WBCs, causing shrinkage and degenerative changes;
   (ii) decreases PCV and MCHC; and
   (iii) causes platelets to swell and then disintegrate, resulting in high platelet count (as the fragments are large enough to be counted as normal platelets).
4. EDTA is not suitable for use in the investigation of coagulation studies such as in the estimation of prothrombin time (PT).

5. It is the anticoagulant used in Wintrobe's method for the estimation of ESR.

B. Trisodium Citrate

1. It is the *anticoagulant of choice* in coagulation studies; for this nine volumes of blood are added to 1 volume of the sodium citrate solution.
2. It is most widely used in the estimation of ESR (Westergren's method); for this 4 volumes of venous blood are diluted with 1 volume of the sodium citrate solution.
3. It acts by its chelating effect, *i.e.* by forming insoluble salt with calcium molecules.

C. Heparin

1. It is an effective anticoagulant at a concentration of 10-20 I.U./ml of blood, and does not alter the size of RBCs.
2. It reduces the chances of lysis of RBCs occurring after blood has been withdrawn.
3. It should **not** be used for making blood films as it gives a faint blue colouration to the background when the films are stained. This is specially marked in the presence of abnormal proteins.
4. It is the *best anticoagulant to be used for osmotic fragility tests.*
5. It should not be used for WBC count as it tends to cause the WBCs to clump.
6. It acts by facilitating the action of antithrombin III, thereby inhibiting the active form of clotting factors, IX, X, XI and XII.

Effects of anticoagulation on blood cell morphology

1. Striking changes occur in film made from anticoagulated blood which has been standing for more than 1-3 hours at room temperature (18-25°C); small vacoules appear in the cytoplasm and the nuclear lobes become separated with ill-defined margins.

   All these changes can be avoided if anticoagulated blood is kept at 4°C.
2. In fresh blood films, the platelets usually clump. Such films are of particular value in investigating patients suspected of suffering from purpura as the absence of platelet clumping is a useful indicator to the diagnosis of purpura.

III. HAEMATOLOGICAL VALUES FOR NORMAL INDIVIDUALS

Refer to Appendix II.

IV. HAEMOCYTOMETER

A haemocytometer is an apparatus used for the counting of blood cells. It consists of two pipettes (RBC and WBC) and a ruled slide called the **Improved Neubauer's counting chamber**.

A. Pipette

The pipette is used to dilute the blood with a suitable fluid in an accurately known proportion. Since RBCs are more numerous than WBCs, different dilutions have to be made for the RBC and the WBC count. Hence two pipettes are provided.

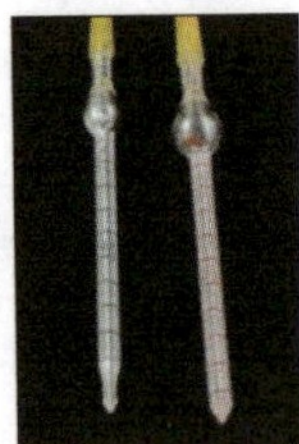

WBC and RBC pipettes

1. RBC pipette

(i) This consists of a capillary tube, the **stem** which widens into a **bulb** containing a small **red glass bead** (Fig. 1.2.5).

(ii) The pipette is calibrated in 10 divisions between the bulb and tip, the centre calibration being marked 0.5 and the nearest the bulb 1.0.

(iii) On the opposite side of the bulb is another calibration labelled 101. *These markings refer to relative rather than absolute volumes.*

(iv) The pipette is supplied with a **rubber tube** and **mouthpiece** (or rubber teat) to facilitate filling by suction. This rubber tubing is sufficiently long to enable the observer to read the pipette calibrations comfortably during the process of filling.

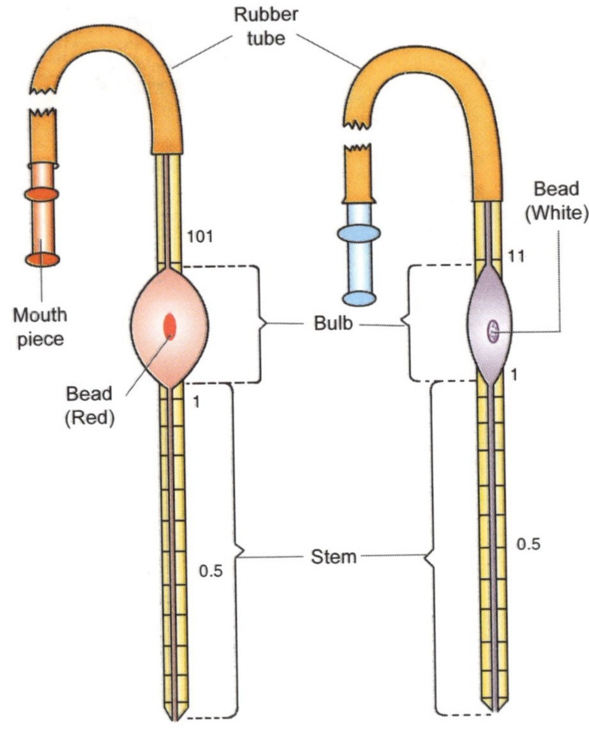

Fig. 1.2.5 RBC and WBC pipette compared

2. WBC pipette

It is similar to the RBC pipette but has a *smaller bulb* with a *white glass bead*. The graduations are 0.5 and 1 on the stem and 11 above the bulb (Fig. 1.2.5).

B. Improved Neubauer's Counting Chamber

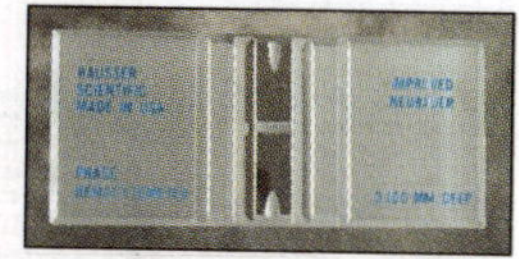

The counting chamber was originally invented by *Crammer* in 1885 and was later modified by *Neubauer*.

1. It is used to obtain a very thin film of the fluid of the known volume for cellular counts. It consists of a **thick glass slide** with a polished **central platform** divided by a short **transverse gutter** into two portions; each portion of which is ruled with a counting **grid** (Fig. 1.2.6).
2. On either side, the central platform is bounded by a groove called as **moat**. Each moat, in turn, is bounded on its outer side by another platform, which is slightly higher than the central platform.
3. A perfectly ground cover slip rests upon the two lateral platforms, thus bridging the moats and covering the central platform. The chamber is so constructed that there is a space of 0.1 mm between the ruled platform and the cover slip.
4. The counting grid is made up of a ruled area measuring 3 mm × 3 mm. This area is divided by **triple lines** into 9 large equal squares each having an area of 1 sq. mm. (1 mm × 1 mm). Of these the 4 large squares at the corners are used for WBC counting while the large square in the centre is used for RBC counting (Fig. 1.2.6.).
5. Each of the 4 large squares at the corners of the ruled area is used for WBC counting and is called ***WBC square***. Each square is further divided into 16 smaller squares each having an area of 1/16 sq. mm (1/4 mm × 1/4 mm).

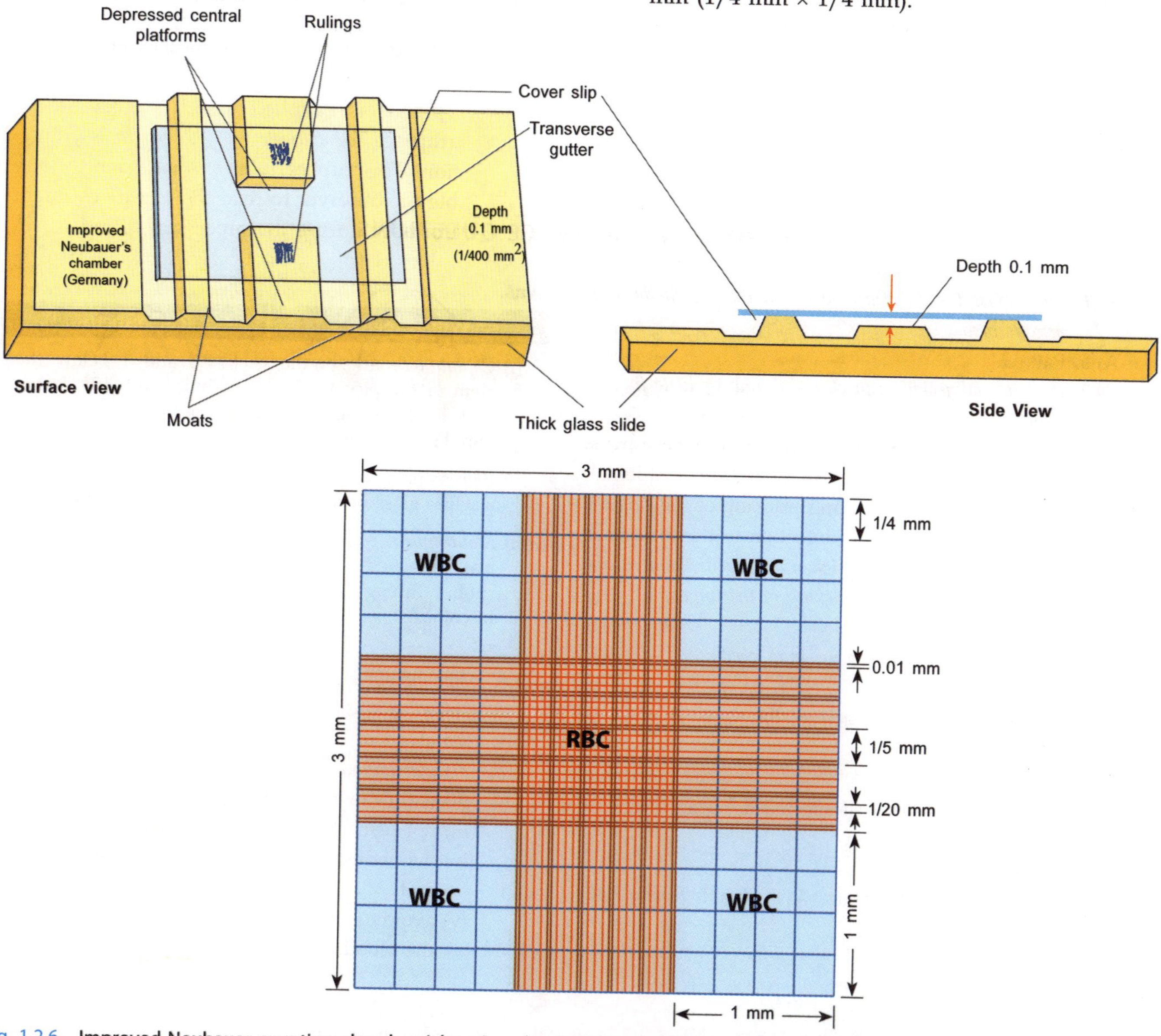

Fig. 1.2.6 Improved Neubauer counting chamber (above) and as it is seen under low power objective of X10 (below)

6. The central large square is for the RBC counting and is called as ***RBC square***. It has an area of 1 sq. mm (1 mm × 1 mm). It is further divided by means of *triple lines* (width 0.01 mm) into 25 medium-sized squares, each with an area of 1/25 sq. mm (1/5 mm × 1/5 mm). Each medium-sized square is further divided into 16 small squares, each with an area of 1/400 square mm (1/20 mm × 1/20 mm).

Important Note: With a X10 eye piece lens and X10 objective, one large square (area 1 sq. mm) usually occupies the microscope field. (Fig. 1.2.7)

7. For the total RBC count, the central square containing 400 *smallest* squares is used. Each smallest square has an area of 1/400 sq. mm. If a cover slip is placed, the depth of the chamber is 1/10 mm making the total volume over each of the smallest squares as 1/4000 µL.
8. For total leucocyte count (TLC), four corner squares are used. Each of these corner squares has a side of 1 mm and the depth of 1/10 mm, so that the volume of fluid over one square is 1/10 µL.

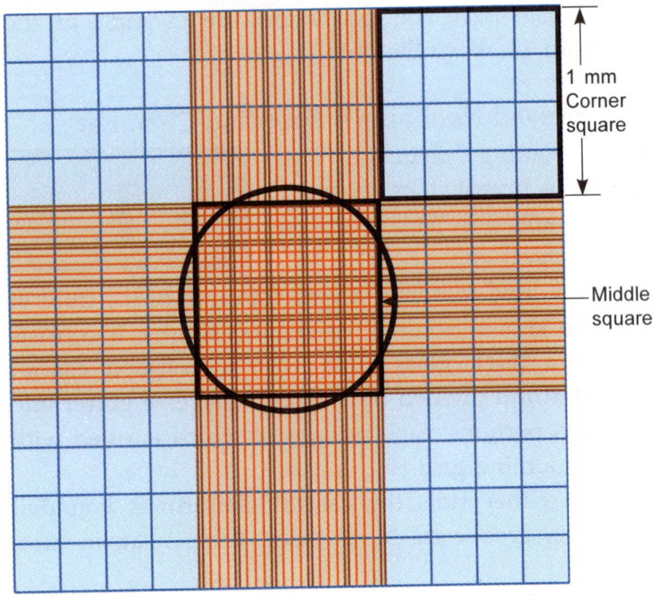

Fig. 1.2.7 Microscopic field with X 100 magnification

IMPORTANT VIVA-VOCE QUESTIONS

Q.1. *Enumerate the differences between the peripheral and venous blood.*

Ans. Page 9.

Q.2. *It is not advisable to prick the thumb or little finger. Why?*

Ans. Since the underlying palmer fascia from these areas extends up to the forearm, therefore, accidental injury to this fascia during pricking of the fingers results in the spread of infection to the forearm.

Q.3. *What measures should be taken to prevent the hepatitis infection following the pricking of the finger?*

Ans. Page 8.

Q.4. *How will you sterilize a pricking needle?*

Ans. Page 8.

Q.5. *It is not advisable to squeeze the finger in order to obtain blood. Why?*

Ans. Page 8.

Q.6. *Name the appropriate sites to obtain a blood sample in infants.*

Ans. Page 8.

Q.7. *How will you differentiate a WBC pipette from a RBC pipette?*

Ans.

WBC pipette	RBC pipette
(i) *Calibration* marks on the stem of the pipette: 0.5 and 1 below the bulb, and 11 above the bulb.	(i) 0.5 and 1 below the bulb and 101 above the bulb.
(ii) *Bulb* is smaller containing a white glass bead.	(ii) Bulb is larger containing a red glass bead.
(iii) *Mouth piece* : a rubber teat attached to the rubber tubing is white in colour.	(iii) Mouth piece : a rubber teat attached to the rubber tubing is red in colour.

Q.8. *What measures should you take to prevent hemolysis of blood obtained following a vene puncture?*

Ans. Hemolysis of blood can be avoided by:

(i) using clean apparatus;
(ii) withdrawing the blood slowly;
(iii) not using too fine a needle;
(iv) delivering the blood gently into the receiver, and
(v) avoiding frothing during the withdrawal of the blood.

Q.9. *Give* the mode of action of various anticoagulants.

Ans. Page 9.

Q.10. *Give the differences between films made of fresh blood and anticoagulated blood.*

Ans. Page 10.

Q.11. *How does the Neubauer counting chamber differ from the Improved Neubauer counting chamber? Or What modification has been done in the improved Neubauer counting chamber?*

Ans.

Neubauer counting chamber	Improved Neubauer counting chamber
The total ruled area is 3 mm × 3 mm; the central ruled area is 1 mm × 1 mm. In the *central area 16 groups of 16 small squares* are separated by triple rulings. (Fig. 1.2.8)	The total ruled area is 3 mm × 3 mm; the central ruled area (1 mm × 1 mm) consists of 25 groups of 16 small squares separated by triple rulings. (Fig. 1.2.6, page 11)

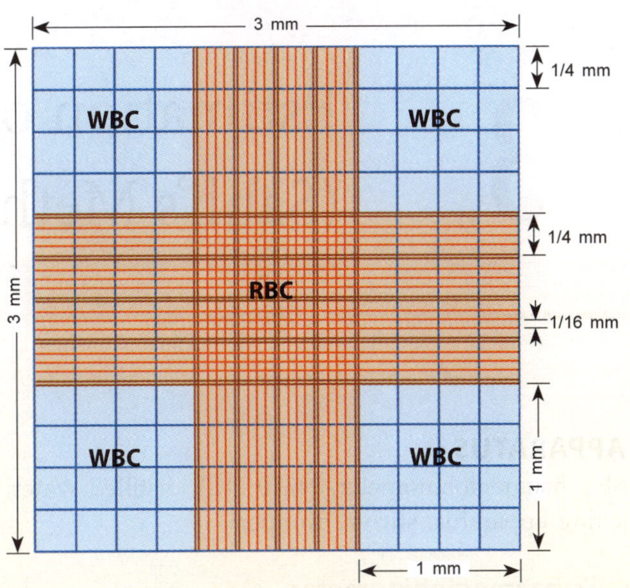

Fig. 1.2.8 Neubauer counting chamber

Note: In the central area, 16 groups of 16 small squares are separated by triple rulings.

STUDY NOTES

OBSERVATIONS AND COMMENTS

....

....

....

....

....

....

....

....

....

....

....

....

....

....

Date: ....

3 Estimation of Haemoglobin (Sahli's Method)

I. APPARATUS

Sahli's haemoglobinometer, N/10 HCl, distilled water, pricking apparatus, stirrer, dropper

Sahli's haemoglobinometer

It consists of: (Fig. 1.3.1.)

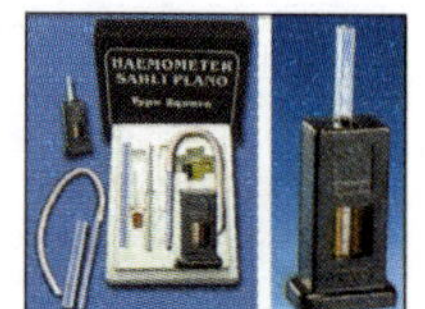

1. A single mark **pipette** (**haemoglobinometer pipette**) for measuring 20 μL (0.02 ml) of blood.
2. A round or square **haemoglobinometer tube** graduated in percentage (10 to 140) and gram per cent (2 to 22)
3. A glass rod, used as a **stirrer**
4. A rectangular box, **comparator** fixed with two solid **standard coloured glass rods**. The opaque **white background** provides the necessary contrast for easy comparison.

II. PRINCIPLE

The amount of haemoglobin can be estimated by the conversion of the known volume of blood into **acid-haematin** by the addition of dilute HCl and subsequent calorimetric comparison with a suitable *standard*.

III. PROCEDURE

1. With the help of a dropper, take N/10 HCl in the graduated haemoglobinometer tube up to its lowest mark (usually 10% or 2 gm/dL).
2. Prick the finger under aseptic precautions. When a drop of reasonable size has collected, hold the pipette horizontally, apply its tip to the drop and draw exactly 20 μL of blood into the pipette, taking care that there should be no air bubbles. Take the pipette away and wipe off any blood adhering to the tip.

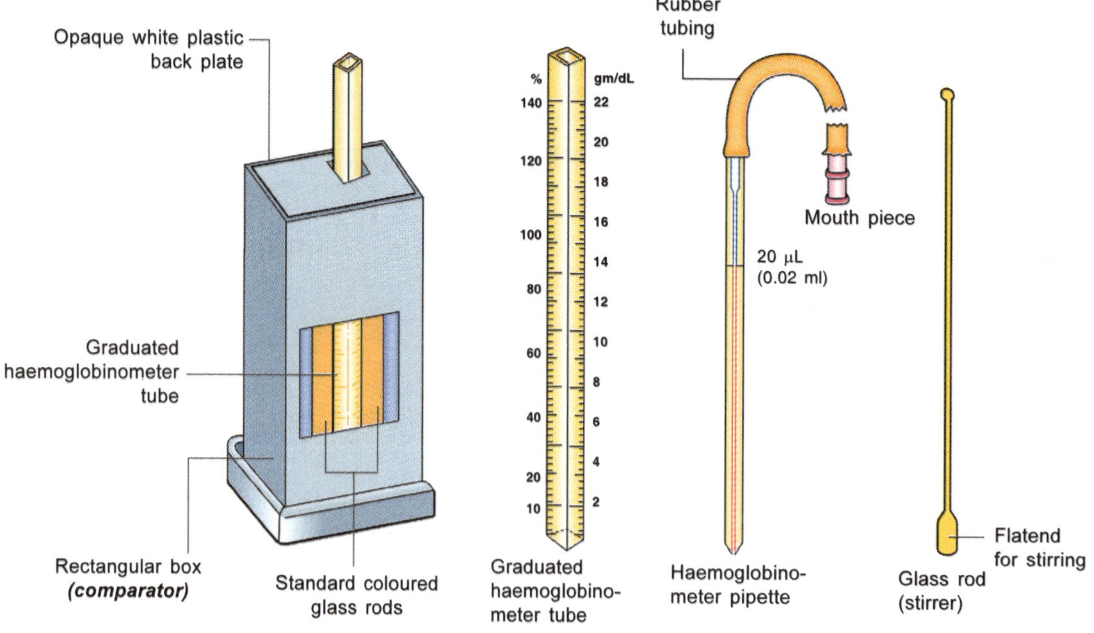

Fig. 1.3.1 Components of Sahli's haemoglobinometer

3. Immediately transfer the blood from the pipette into the N/10 HCl in the graduated haemoglobinometer tube and rinse the pipette several times by drawing the N/10 HCl used for mixing the blood. Avoid foaming.
4. Mix the contents thoroughly and leave the solution to stand for about 10 minutes for the maximum conversion of haemoglobin in blood to **acid haematin** (*brown in colour*).
5. Dilute the acid haematin by adding distilled water in drops. Keep mixing it with the stirrer thoroughly.

> **Important Note:** *At no stage the stirrer should be completely taken out of the tube.*

6. Continue dilution till its colour matches with that of the *standard*. Before comparing the colour, the stirrer should be lifted above the solution only.
7. Note the reading of the meniscus from the scale provided on the haemoglobinometer tube and express the haemoglobin content as gm per 100 ml of blood.

> **Note:** *For coloured transparent fluids, lower meniscus needs to be read.*

> **Important Note:** Since the colours may seem to match over a wide range of dilutions, it is advisable to take the average of two readings during the course of dilution; the first when it is *just* discernably darker and the second when it *just* gets a shade lighter than the *standard*. (Fig 1.3.2)

IV. PRECAUTIONS

1. The finger should not be squeezed to take out the blood, otherwise tissue fluid might come out, thus giving the lower estimation of haemoglobin.
2. Blood from the pipette should be transferred quickly into the tube containing N/10 HCl to prevent the clotting of blood in the pipette.

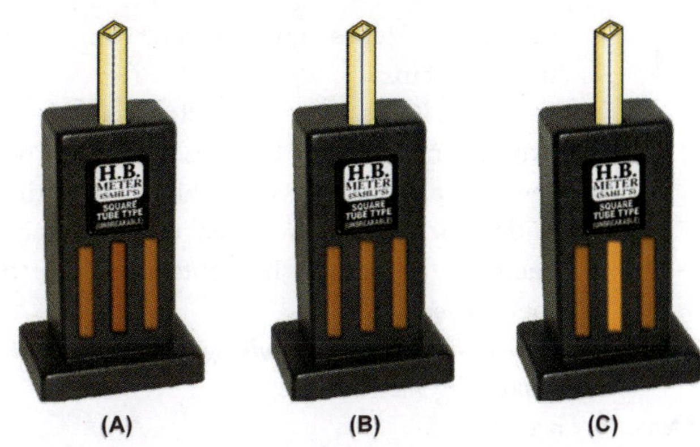

Fig. 1.3.2 Diluted acid haematin colour (A) darker (B) standard and (C) lighter

3. Blood, after mixing with N/10 HCl, should be left for at least 8-10 minutes for the complete formation of acid haematin.
4. Distilled water should be added drop by drop to dilute the acid haematin, otherwise over dilution will occur.
5. The matching of colours should be done only against the natural source of light.

OSPE

Aim: Convert a known volume of blood (of a given sample) into acid haematin with the help of the apparatus provided.

Procedure steps: Refer to page 14.

Checklist

1. Checks for the cleanliness of the apparatus provided. **(Yes/No)**
2. Takes N/10 HCl in haemoglobinometer tube up to its lowest mark (10% or 2 gm/dL). **(Yes/No)**
3. Draws correctly 20 μL of blood sample into the pipette without any air bubbles. **(Yes/No)**
4. Wipes off any blood adhering to the tip of the pipette. **(Yes/No)**
5. Rinses the pipettle several times by drawing the N/10 HCl into the tube. **(Yes/No)**

IMPORTANT VIVA-VOCE QUESTIONS

Q.1. *What is the underlying principle of the experiment?*

Ans. Page 14.

Q.2. *Why is Sahli's method most commonly employed for the estimation of haemoglobin?*

Ans. The advantage of Sahli's method is the relative ease with which the brown colour of acid haematin may be matched optically. In contrast, the red tint of oxyhaemoglobin is notoriously difficult to match with precision.

Q.3. *Define 'normality' of a solution or what is 'normal' solution?*

Ans. In a normal solution, 1 gm equivalent weight of a substance is dissolved in 1 litre of the solvent.

Q.4. *How will the experiment be affected if more or less than the required amount of N/10 HCl is taken in the tube?*

Ans. (i) If less than the required amount of HCl is taken, then it may not be enough to convert all haemoglobin in 20 μL of blood to acid haematin. Hence give lower values for haemoglobin.

(ii) If more HCl is taken, it will *not* affect the experiment as long as the subject is not severely anaemic (haemoglobin <5 gm/dL); under such conditions even undiluted acid haematin colour will be lighter than that of the *standard*.

Q.5. *Can we use N-HCl or any strong agent (acid or alkali) for haemolysing the RBCs?*

Ans. *No,* because:

(i) all these agents will cause the destruction of protein present in the haemoglobin and thus interfere with its estimation;

(ii) 'standard' colour of acid haematin needed for comparison corresponds to the N/10 HCl.

Q.6. *Can we use N/10 HCl instead of distilled water for dilution purposes?*

Ans. *Yes,* but it is *not* used in practice because of economic reasons.

Q.7. *Why is it necessary to allow the solution to stand for 10 minutes before dilution?*

Ans. Because this much of time is necessary for the complete hemolysis of RBCs and maximum conversion of haemoglobin in blood to form acid haematin.

Q.8. *Can tap water be used for dilution purposes instead of the distilled water?*

Ans. *No,* because distilled water is free from impurities and other salts. If tap water is used for dilution purposes, it might alter the colour of the acid haematin solution and thus interfere with the colour matching.

Q.9. *During colour matching, why is it important to lift the stirrer above the solution but not completely out of the tube?*

Ans. If the stirrer remains within the solution, it will lighten the colour of the solution. If the stirrer is taken out of the tube, there will be loss of fluid and this will give lower value for haemoglobin.

Q.10. *For comparing the colours, why is it necessary to convert haemoglobin into acid haematin?*

Ans. If we do not convert haemoglobin to acid haematin, we get the colour of oxyhaemoglobin which has a wide spectrum of colours, and it is not possible to standardize the procedure.

Q.11. *Out of the two scales provided on the graduation haemoglobinometer tube, which one is preferred and why?*

Ans. Gram per cent (gm/dL) scale is preferred over percentage scale, because there is not a single standard value of haemoglobin which is taken as 100%.

Q.12. *Give the normal range of the values of haemoglobin.*

Ans. (i) At birth: 23 gm/dL, because RBC count is more.

(ii) At the end of 3 months: 10.5 gm/dL (as an infant is totally on milk feed which is devoid of iron).

(iii) After 3 months haemoglobin increases and at the end of one year it becomes 12.5 gm/dL.

(iv) Adults: (a) Males: 14-18 gm/dL (average: 15.5 gm/dL).

(b) Females: 12-15.5 gm/dL (average: 14 gm/dL).

(*Clinically,* 14.8 gm/dL haemoglobin, irrespective of sex, is regarded as 100% haemoglobin.)

Q.13. *What is the oxygen carrying capacity of the blood? Give its significance.*

Ans. 1 gm/dL haemoglobin, when fully saturated, combines with 1.34 ml of oxygen, therefore, haemoglobin concentration is an index of ***oxygen carrying capacity*** of blood.

Normal values: Males: 21 ml/dL

Females: 18 ml/dL

Q.14. *What do you understand by 100% saturation of haemoglobin with oxygen?*

Ans. When blood gets equilibrated with 100% oxygen (pO_2 120 mmHg), the haemoglobin becomes 100% saturated.

Q.15. *How much is the iron-content in 1 gm of haemoglobin?*

Ans. The iron-content of haemoglobin is 0.33%; therefore, 100 ml of blood containing 15 gm of haemoglobin contains 15 × 0.33/100 = approx. 50 mg of iron. Hence, in 1 gm of haemoglobin, the iron-content is 50/15 = 3.34 mg.

Q.16. *Mention the other methods of the estimation of haemoglobin.*

Ans. (i) **Talliquist's method**. Touch a drop of blood with a piece of white filter paper, and allow the blood to diffuse through the paper so as to produce an even stain. As soon as the stain loses its gloss, and before drying is evident, match the colour against a printed colour scale representing the various concentrations of haemoglobin expressed in percentage.

(ii) **Photoelectric Calorimetric method (Spectrophotometry)**. This involves the use of photo-electric calorimeter that measures the amount of light absorbed by a solution. The light used in these instruments is of limited wave band and this band is chosen to correspond with the part of the spectrum that is maximally absorbed by the solution being tested.

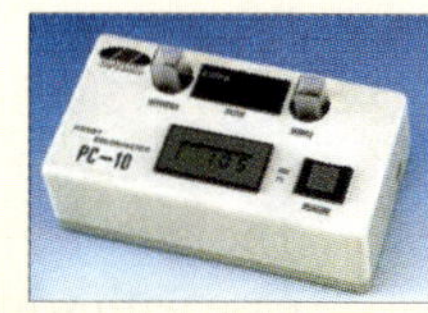

The one that is commonly used is the **cyanmethaemoglobin** method. Here haemoglobin is converted into cyanmethaemoglobin by *Drabkin's reagent* ($NaHCO_3$ 1 gm; potassium cyanide 50 mg; potassium ferri-cyanide 200 mg and distilled water 1 litre). The absorbance of the solution is measured in a photoelectric calorimeter provided with yellow green filters (at a wavelength of 540 nm). The standard solution of cyanmethaemoglobin is available as such.

(iii) By finding the oxygen carrying capacity of blood. (see above)

(iv) By determining the iron-content. (see above)

(v) **Haldane's method**. This involves the haemolysis of RBCs in hypotonic solution (distilled water) and carbon monoxide is added to the solution. The colour developed is compared with that of standard.

(vi) **Alkaline haematin method**. This is done to estimate the HbF content in the blood. Here, to 50 μL of blood, 4.95 ml of N/10 NaOH is added. Keep the mixture in water bath at 37°C for 4-5 minutes, then cool rapidly in cold bath and watch against the standard in a photoelectric calorimeter at a wavelength of 540 nm (or yellow green filter). This method is unsuitable for routine use.

Q.17. *What are the different types of haemoglobins?*

Ans. Different types of haemoglobins are:

(i) *Adult haemoglobin*

(a) HbA ($\alpha_2\beta_2$)

(b) HbA_2 ($\alpha_2\delta_2$)

(ii) *Foetal haemoglobin* – HbF ($\alpha_2\gamma_2$)

(iii) *Oxyhaemoglobin* – HbO_2. Haemoglobin combined with oxygen.

(iv) *Reduced (deoxygenated) haemoglobin*– Hb. Haemoglobin from where oxygen has been removed.

(v) *Carboxyhaemoglobin* or carbon monoxyhaemoglobin. Haemoglobin combined with carbon monoxide.

(vi) *Carbaminohaemoglobin* – HbNHCOOH. Haemoglobin combined with carbon dioxide.

(vii) *Methaemoglobin* – HbOH. Haemoglobin in which the ferrous (Fe^{2+}) is oxidised to ferric (Fe^{3+}) iron.

(viii) *HbS* – Sickle cell disease.

Q.18. *Define anaemia. How will you grade its severity based on the estimation of the haemoglobin-content?*

Ans. Reduction in the number of RBCs less than 4 million/μL or their content of haemoglobin less than 12 gm/dL or both.

Grading of severity of anaemia

(i) Mild anaemia:
Haemoglobin 8-12 gm/dL

(ii) Moderate anaemia:
Haemoglobin 5-8 gm/dL

(iii) Severe anaemia:
Haemoglobin <5 gm/dL

Q.19. *Give some common causes of increase and decrease in haemoglobin values.*

Ans. *(A) Causes of increase in the Haemoglobin-content*

(1) *Experimental errors*

(i) Blood taken is more than the required quantity of 20 μL.

(ii) Fading of the colour of solid standard rods in the comparator (rare cause).

(2) *Due to increase in RBC count*

(i) Physiological causes: new-born; adult males, high altitude.

(ii) Pathological causes: chronic hypoxia of bone marrow due to exercise or any cardio-respiratory disorders; polycythemia vera.

(B) Causes of decrease in the haemoglobin-content

(1) *Experimental errors*

(i) Blood sample obtained by squeezing the finger.

(ii) Blood taken is <20 μL.

(iii) Less than the required quantity of N/10 HCl is taken for hemolysis purposes.

(iv) Fail to wait for 8-10 minutes after mixing the blood with the N/10 HCl.

(2) *Due to decrease in RBC count*

(i) Physiological causes: after birth 0-3 months, adult females.

(ii) All pathological causes of anaemia (refer to the textbook).

Q.20. *How does the HbA differ from HbF?*

Ans. Refer to the textbook.

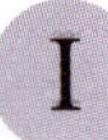

STUDY NOTES

OBSERVATIONS AND COMMENTS

Table 1.3.1 Reading of diluted acid haematin as compared to the standard coloured glass rods

Sl. No.	When just darker (gm/dL)	When just lighter (gm/dL)	Average (gm/dL)
1.			
2.			

Important Note: Ideally, the difference between the reading of diluted acid haematin when it is first darker or lighter as compared to the standard colour should not be more than 0.4gm/dL.

RESULTS

The Haemoglobin content of my blood is……

COMMENTS AND DISCUSSION

State whether it is within the normal range or not. If not, comment on the posssible causes.

....

....

....

....

....

....

....

....

....

....

....

....

....

....

....

....

....

....

Date: ....

4 Determination of Total Erythrocyte (*Red Blood Cell*) Count

I. APPARATUS

Improved Neubauer's counting chamber, RBC pipette, RBC diluting fluid (**Hayem's Fluid**); compound microscope, cover-slips, pricking apparatus

RBC Diluting Fluid (Hayem's Fluid)

Composition: Each100 ml of fluid contains:

1. Sodium Sulphate (Na_2SO_4): 2.5 gm (to prevent the aggregation of RBCs, *i.e.* rouleaux formation).
2. Sodium Chloride (NaCl): 0.5 gm (to maintain the isotonicity of the fluid. Therefore, RBCs remain suspended in the solution)
3. Mercuric Chloride ($HgCl_2$): 0.25 gm (preservative: antibacterial and antifungal)
4. Distilled Water: 100 ml (solvent)

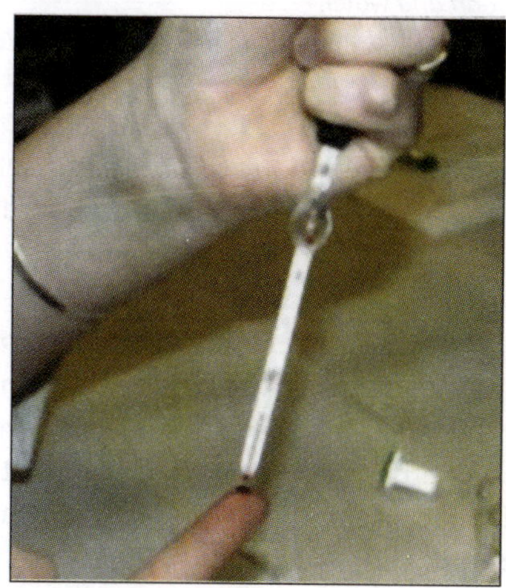

Fig. 1.4.1 Filling of RBC pipette

II. PRINCIPLE

Since the normal RBC count runs in millions, the count is made possible by diluting the sample of blood before counting and subsequently multiplying the count by the **dilution factor**.

III. PROCEDURE

1. Ensure that the improved Neubauer's chamber, cover-slips and the lenses of the microscope are absolutely clean and the RBC pipette is dry and patent.
2. Take adequate RBC diluting fluid in a watch glass.
3. Prick the finger taking the necessary precautions (page 8).
4. Wipe off the first drop of blood. Suck the next drop of blood in RBC pipette exactly up to 0.5 mark, taking care that there should be no air bubbles. (Any excess of blood drawn in can be removed by tapping the tip of the pipette against the palm of your hand.) (Fig. 1.4.1)
5. Wipe off the blood sticking to the tip of the pipette.
6. Immediately, thereafter, holding the pipette in a nearly horizontal position, Hayem's fluid is sucked into the pipette exactly up to 101 mark, just above the bulb.
7. The pipette is then kept horizontally between the palms and rolled gently for about a minute to ensure the thorough mixing of the blood and the fluid. This will give a suspension of RBCs in the bulb of the pipette (dilution: 1/200).
8. A clean cover-slip is placed in the Neubauer's chamber so as to cover the ruled area on both sides.
9. Focus the RBCs squares of Neubauer's ruling under the low power objective (X10) of the microscope (page 11). The chamber is then removed from the microscope and placed on the table. The focus of the microscope is not disturbed.
10. Discard the first few drops of fluid from the RBC pipette. They constitute the unmixed Hayem's fluid present in the stem of the pipette.
11. ***Charging the Neubauer's Chamber***
    (i) A small drop of fluid is allowed to form at the tip of the pipette and this drop is gently brought in contact with the edge of the cover-slip. The fluid is drawn into the chamber by *capillary action*. Both sides of the Neubauer's chamber are charged.

(ii) **An ideally charged chamber** is one which has been charged with a single adequate-sized drop which just fills the chamber without leaving any air bubbles. This is learnt by practice.

(iii) If the fluid overflows into the gutters, it is called **over-charging**. If it is insufficient to fill the chamber or having air bubbles, it is said to be **under-charged**.

Important Notes

1. *Should the chamber be over or under-charged, the procedure is repeated after thoroughly cleaning the chamber and the cover-slip with soap and water.*
2. *The chamber should not be charged in parts by two or more smaller drops.*

12. Allow some time (about 1 minute) for cells to settle down in the counting chamber so that all the cells present may be in the same plane.
13. The charged Neubauer's chamber is now kept under the low power of the microscope (already in focus). Using only the fine adjustments, the cell along the ruled area is brought into focus.
14. Check whether cells are uniformly distributed or not. If not, clean the Neubauer's chamber and recharge it. (Fig. 1.4.2)

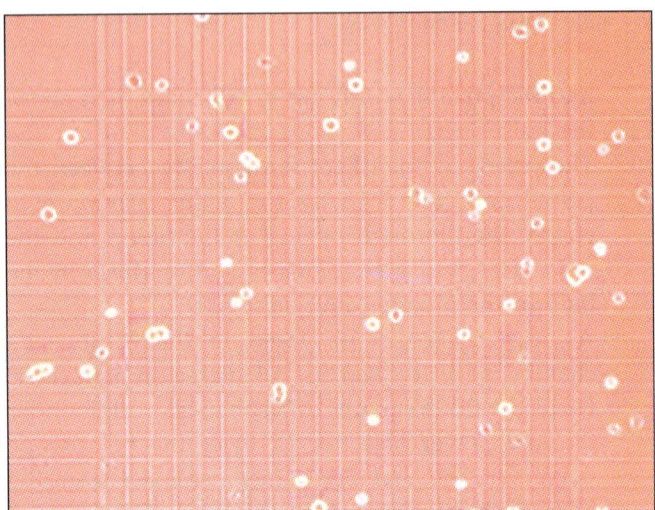

Fig. 1.4.2 Uniform cells distribution under the microscope

Note: If the difference in total count of RBCs in different medium-sized squares is more than 20, it indicates an uneven distribution of cells.

15. Focus the RBC squares (central square of Neubauer's chamber) under high power objective (X40) and count the RBCs in 4 medium-sized corner squares and one medium-sized central square (1/5 mm side), *i.e.* in 80 small squares (1/20 mm side) (see Fig. 1.2.6, page 11).
16. ***Rules for the counting of cells***. In order to avoid counting the same cell twice, the following rules need to be observed: (Fig. 1.4.3.)
    (i) any cell which is lying on the upper or left border of a square is counted in that particular square; and
    (ii) omit the cells lying on the lower or right border of a square.Vice-versa, if any one may desire, the cells lying on the right or upper border of a square can be counted in that particular square. Omit the cells lying on the left or lower border of the square.

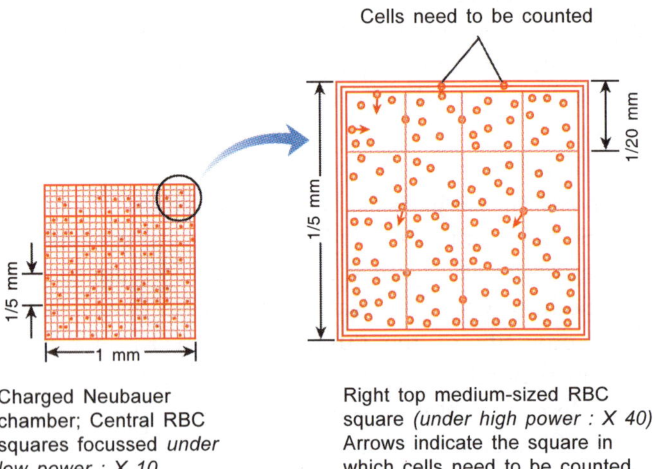

Fig. 1.4.3 Rules for counting the cells

Important Note: *In squares bordered by triple lines, the middle of the triple lines is assumed to be the boundary of the square and the same rules outlined above are followed.*

(iii) Count the RBCs in 4 medium-sized corner squares and one medium-sized central square. Enter your observations in the corresponding squares (Fig. 1.4.4.).

IV. CALCULATIONS

A. Calculation of Dilution Factor

0.5 part of blood and 100.5 parts of RBC diluting fluid are present in the pipette. As blood gets mixed up with the diluting fluid only in the bulb of the pipette; therefore, 1 part of diluting fluid which remains in the stem of the pipette, does not mix with the blood. Thus 0.5 part of the blood mixes with 99.5 parts of the diluting fluid in the bulb of the pipette to form 100 (0.5 + 99.5) parts of the solution. Hence, dilution factor is:

$$\frac{\text{Final volume achieved (100 parts)}}{\text{Original volume taken (0.5 parts)}} = 200$$

B. Calculation of volume of fluid examined

Area of 5 medium sized RBC squares
= 5 × 1/5 mm × 1/5 mm = 1/5 sq.mm.
Depth of the chamber
= 1/10 mm
Hence, volume of fluid in 5 RBC squares
= 1/5 sq.mm × 1/10 mm
= 1/50 μL

C. Calculation of total RBC count

Let 'N' be the total number of RBCs counted in 5 medium-sized squares *i.e.* in 1/50 μL of the *diluted blood.*

Therefore, number of RBCs in 1 μL of *undiluted blood* = N × 50 × Dilution factor (200) = N × 10,000.

Important Note: In spite of the utmost precautions, the error in count is ±20% because of the following factors:

1. *Pipette error.* The marks on the pipette may not be accurate.
2. *Chamber error.* The depth of the chamber may not be accurate.
3. *Statistical error.* As the multiplication factor is 10000, therefore, error in the counting of even one RBC will cause the variation of total RBC count by 10000/μL of blood. This can be reduced by counting more number of cells ($E = 1/\sqrt{n}$).
4. *Field error.* After charging, the cells may not get distributed uniformly throughout the chamber.
   The error in counting RBCs can be reduced to 5% if double the number of cells is counted.

V. PRECAUTIONS

1. Prick should be bold enough to give free flowing blood. At no stage the finger should be squeezed to take out the blood. (Why? See page 8)
2. Both haemocytometer and cover slip must be dry and free of grease.
3. Use only dry pipette.
4. Never use a broken cover-slip.
5. Before charging the chamber, the fluid in the stem of the pipette has to be discarded.
6. The cover-slip should be placed symmetrically so as to cover the ruled area completely.
7. There should be no under-or over-charging of the chamber (count will be low in both cases).
8. After charging the chamber, allow some time for cells to settle down but the count should be made before the fluid in the chamber starts drying up.
9. While counting the cells, the stage of the microscope should not be tilted.

OSPE-I

Aim: Dilute the given sample of blood to 200 times with the help of diluting fluid and RBC pipette provided to you.

Procedure steps: Refer to page 19.

Checklist

1. Checks that the pipette is absolutely clean, dry and patent. **(Yes/No)**
2. Takes adequate diluting fluid in a watch glass. **(Yes/No)**
3. Sucks the blood into the pipette exactly up to 0.5 mark and there are no air bubbles. **(Yes/No)**
4. Wipes off the blood sticking to the tip of pipette. **(Yes/No)**
5. Sucks diluting fluid into the pipette exactly up to 101 mark, just above the bulb. **(Yes/No)**
6. Immediately holds the pipette in a nearly horizontal position between the palms and rolls gently. **(Yes/No)**

OSPE-II

Aim: Charge the improved Neubauer's chamber with diluted blood sample provided to you in a pipette.

Procedure steps: Refer to page 19.

Checklist

1. Ensures that the improved Neubauer's chamber and cover-slip are clean. **(Yes/No)**
2. Properly mixes the diluted blood sample by horizontally holding the pipette between the palms. **(Yes/No)**
3. Places the cover-slip on the Neubauer's chamber so as to cover the ruled area on both sides. **(Yes/No)**
4. Discards the first few drops of the fluid from the pipette. **(Yes/No)**
5. Charges the chamber with a single adequate-sized drop which just fills the chamber without leaving any air bubbles or fluid flowing into the gutters. **(Yes/No)**

IMPORTANT VIVA-VOCE QUESTIONS

Q.1. *How will you identify the RBC pipette?*
Ans. RBC pipette has:
(i) Red bead in the bulb.
(ii) Bulb is larger as compared to the WBC pipette bulb.
(iii) Marking on the pipette: 0.5 and 1.0 below the bulb; 101 above the bulb.

Q.2. *How will you clean the pipette?*
Ans. The Pipette can be cleaned by sucking up and blowing out distilled water several times, then sucking up and blowing out acetone for drying it.

Q.3. *How will you clean the chamber and cover slips?*
Ans. These can be cleaned by first washing them with soap and water and then with alcohol.

Q.4. *How will you clean the pipette blocked by a blood clot?*

Ans. Wash the pipette first either with strong acid or alkali or with H_2O_2 to remove the blood clot; then rinse with distilled water to clean the acid or alkali. Finally, rinse with alcohol or ether to dry it.

Q.5. *What are the functions of the bead in the bulb of the pipette?*

Ans. (i) Helps in mix the blood thoroughly with the diluting fluid.

(ii) Indicates whether the bulb is dry or not. If it is dry, bead will roll freely with no tendency to adhere to the side of the bulb.

(iii) Helps to identify whether it is RBC or WBC pipette.

Q.6. *What are the units of the marking on the pipette?*

Ans. There are no units of markings on the pipette.

Q.7. *How is a dilution of 1:200 achieved?*

Ans. Page 20.

Q.8. *What are the factors which determine the degree of dilution?*

Ans. Page 20.

Q.9. *Why is there need to dilute the blood for counting the RBCs?*

Ans. Page 19.

Q.10. *List the uses of RBC pipette other than counting the RBCs.*

Ans. RBC pipette can be used for:

(i) sperm count

(ii) platelets count

(iii) WBC count (when WBCs increases tremendously as in leukaemias).

Q.11. *Why should any small excess of blood drawn into the pipette not be removed by a piece of cotton?*

Ans. Small excess of blood into the pipette should be removed by tapping against the palm. A piece of cotton should not be used because cotton absorbs fluid portion only and not the cellular portion. This will result in higher RBC count.

Q.12. *Can any other fluid be used instead of Hayem's fluid for counting the RBCs?*

Ans. Isotonic saline can be used in place of Hayem's fluid but then counting of cells must be performed immediately. However, Hayem's fluid is always preferred, as Na_2SO_4 in it prevents rouleaux formation; moreover, a stock solution can be prepared because of anti-bacterial and anti-fungal actions of $HgCl_2$.

Q.13. *Why is it important to discard the first few drops of fluid from the pipette before charging?*

Ans. The first few drops of fluid are discarded because they constitute the unmixed Hayem's fluid present in the stem of the pipette.

Q.14. *How is the RBC count affected when the chamber is under-or over-charged?*

Ans. (i) When the chamber is over-charged, the count decreases because the RBCs being heavier than the fluid flow into the gutters.

(ii) When the chamber is under-charged, obviously the count decreases.

Q.15. *How will you differentiate RBCs from dust particles?*

Ans. RBCs are of regular size and shape and are seen as bright rounded bodies, while dust particles are of irregular size and shape; moreover, they disappear with the change of the focus or if they are sticking to the eye piece, they move by rotating it.

Q.16. *Why should you charge both sides of the chamber?*

Ans. Both sides of the chamber need to be charged and RBCs are counted on both sides; then the average is taken to reduce the error in counting (page 21).

Q.17. *Why is it sometimes difficult to get the cells and the rulings of the chamber under the same focus of the microscope?*

Ans. As a depth of 0.1 mm exists between the cells and the rulings of the chamber, therefore, at times it is difficult to focus them together; especially if the illumination is not proper or if the RBC diluting fluid is not freshly prepared.

Q.18. *Why is it important to observe the rules of counting?*

Ans. It is important to avoid the recounting of cells.

Q.19. *What is the fate of WBCs while doing the RBC count? How does it affect the RBC count?*

Ans. WBCs can be seen during the RBC count. They can be distinguished by their large size, uneven outline and halo around them. In humans, the ratio of RBCs:WBCs is 700:1. As the total number of RBCs counted in 5 medium-sized RBCs squares will be approx. 550, therefore, hardly one WBC will come across in the field of counting. However, if counted, it will increase the RBC count by 10000/μL of blood (because multiplication factor is 10,000 - page 21).

Q.20. *What is the function of the cover-slip?*

Ans. The cover-slip is used to control the volume of fluid. It also helps in the uniform distribution of cells by preventing the flow of fluid into the gutters.

Q.21. *Why should a broken cover-slip not be used?*

Ans. A broken cover-slip will be placed assymetrically and thus may cause the uneven distribution of the cells.

Q.22. *Do you know any other accurate method for the determination of RBC count?*

Ans. An accurate and more reliable method for counting the RBCs is by way of electronic cell counter in which error is only about 2%.

Q.23. *Enumerate the sources of error in this method.*

Ans. This method is subject to many errors. Briefly, these are:

(i) *Pipette error:*

(a) inaccuracy in the calibration;

(b) inaccuracy in measuring the blood sample and the diluting fluid.

(ii) *Field error:* Unequal distribution of cells over the grid caused by:

(a) under or over-charging of the chamber;

(b) presence of grease on slide or cover-slip.

(iii) *Personal error:* counting fewer cells than are actually present (due to inexperience).

(iv) *Statistical error:* It is inversely proportional to the square root of the number counted.

Q.24. *What are the physiological variations in RBC count?*

Ans. Normal RBC count:

(i) At birth: 6-7 million/μL.

(ii) Adults:

(a) Males: 5-6 million/μL (average 5.5 million/μL);

(b) Females: 4.5-5.5 million/μL (average 4.8million/μL). (Clinically, 5 million/μL is taken as 100% count.)

For physiological variations, see page 17.

Q.25. *Define anaemia.*

Ans. Page 17.

Q.26. *What is Polycythemia? How does it differ from polycythemia vera?*

Ans. Polycythemia is a condition in which RBC count increases above 6 million/μL. Polycythemia vera is a cancerous condition of bone marrow which causes marked increase in the RBC count.

Q.27. *Give the normal life-span of a RBC.*

Ans. 120 days.

Q.28. *Name the sites of formation and destruction of RBCs.*

Ans. The site of formation of RBCs is the red bone marrow; the site of destruction is the tissue macrophage system (for details, see the textbook).

STUDY NOTES

OBSERVATIONS

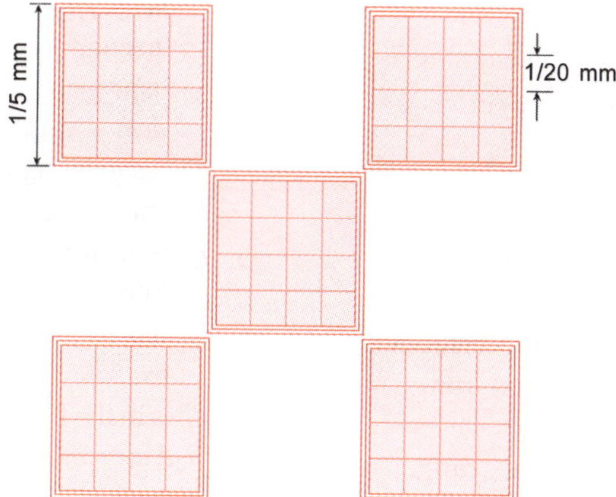

Fig. 1.4.4 Enter the observations after counting the RBCs in the corresponding squares

CALCULATIONS

....

RESULTS, COMMENTS AND DISCUSSION

State whether it is within the normal range or not. If not, comment on the posssible causes.

....

....

Date: ....

5 Determination of RBC Indices (Blood Standards)

I. APPARATUS

As for the estimation of haemoglobin (page 14), RBC count (page 19) and packed cell volume - PCV (page 50).

II. PRINCIPLE

The values for RBC count, haemoglobin content and packed cell volume (PCV) can be used to obtain certain RBC indices (also called **Absolute Values of Blood Index**). These indices indicate the size and haemoglobin concentration within the RBC and thus help diagnos the type of anaemia. The various blood indices are given as under.

A. ***Mean Corpuscular Volume (MCV),*** *i.e.* volume of a single RBC in cubic microns (μm^3). It can be derived from the formula as:

$$MCV\ (\mu m^3) = \frac{\text{PCV per 100 ml blood}}{\text{RBC count in million}/\mu L} \times 10$$

$$= 45/5 \times 10$$

$$= 90 \text{ (average)}$$

Normal range = 78-94 μm^3 (86 ± 8 μm^3).

1. RBCs with normal MCV are called **Normocytes**;
2. RBCs whose MCV exceed normal range are **Macrocytes**, and
3. RBCs with MCV below normal range are **Microcytes**.

B. ***Mean Corpuscular Haemoglobin (MCH),*** *i.e.* average amount of haemoglobin in a single RBC in picogram (10^{-12} gm) or micro-micro gram (μμgm-γγ). It can be derived from the formula as:

$$MCH\ (pg) = \frac{\text{Haemoglobin in gm/dL}}{\text{RBC count in million}/\mu L} \times 10$$

$$= 15/5 \times 10$$

$$= 30 \text{ (average)}$$

Normal range = 28-32 pg (29.5 ± 2.5 pg).

Note: *This blood index is not used clinically.*

C. ***Mean Corpuscular Haemoglobin Concentration (MCHC),*** *i.e.* amount of haemoglobin expressed as percentage of the volume of a RBC *or* it is the haemoglobin concentration in a single RBC.

$$MCHC = \frac{\text{Haemoglobin in gm/dL}}{\text{PCV per 100 ml blood}} \times 100$$

$$= 15/45 \times 100$$

$$= 33 \text{ (average)}$$

Normal range = 32% - 38% (35 ± 3%).

1. If the MCHC is within normal range, the RBC is **Normochromic**.
2. If the MCHC value is below the normal range, the RBC is **Hypochromic**. This usually indicates that an individual is suffering from iron deficiency anaemia.
3. MCHC values *never* exceed 38% because RBCs cannot hold haemoglobin beyond its saturation point, *i.e.* metabolic limit of the cells haemoglobin forming mechanism, therefore, **anaemia can never be hyperchromic**.

D. ***Colour Index (CI).*** It denotes the ratio of haemoglobin to RBC.

$$CI = \frac{\text{Haemoglobin percentage*}}{\text{RBC percentage**}}$$

$$= 100/100$$

$$= 1 \text{ (average)}$$

Normal range = 0.85 - 1.15 (1 ± 0.15).

* 14.8 gm/dL haemoglobin = 100%.

** 5 million/μL RBC count = 100%

Note: It is an insignificant index, because the normal range of RBC is very wide; hence clinically not in use.

III. PHYSIO-CLINICAL SIGNIFICANCE

Based on the size and haemoglobin concentration within a RBC, an important morphological classification of anaemias can be given as described in Table 1.5.1.

Table 1.5.1 Morphological classification of anaemias

	Normochromic	Hypochromic
1. *Normocytic*	(i) After acute haemorrhage (ii) All haemolytic anaemias except thalassaemia (iii) Aplastic anaemia	After chronic haemorrhage
2. *Macrocytic*	All megaloblastic anaemias due to deficiency of vitamin B_{12}, folic acid or intrinsic factor	Secondary to liver diseases
3. *Microcytic*	Chronic infections	(i) Iron deficiency anaemia (ii) Thalassaemia

Note: Iron deficiency anaemia is **microcytic hypochromic.**

IMPORTANT VIVA-VOCE QUESTIONS

Q.1. *Derive the formulae given above for MCV, MCH and MCHC.*

Ans. (i) MCV $= \dfrac{\text{PCV of 1 μL blood}}{\text{RBC count per μL blood}}$

$$= \frac{0.45\ \mu\text{L (As normal PCV = 45\%)}}{5 \times 10^6}$$

$$= \frac{0.45 \times 10^3\ \mu\text{m} \times 10^3\ \mu\text{m} \times 10^3\ \mu\text{m}}{5 \times 10^6}$$

(Since 1 mm = 10^3 μm)

$$= \frac{45 \times 10^7}{5 \times 10^6}$$

$$= \frac{45}{5}$$

Therefore, MCV in μm^3

$$= \frac{\text{PCV of 100 ml blood}}{\text{RBC count in million/μL}} \times 10$$

(ii) MCH $= \dfrac{\text{Haemoglobin content per 100 ml blood}}{\text{RBC count per 100 ml blood}}$

$$= \frac{15\ \text{gm/dL}}{5 \times 10^6 \times 10^3 \times 100}$$

(As 1 cc or 1 ml = 10^3 μL)

$$= \frac{15 \times 10^{12}\ \text{pg (1 gm} = 10^{12}\text{) pg}}{5 \times 10^{11}}$$

$$= \frac{15}{5} \times 10\ \text{pg}$$

Therefore, MCH in pg

$$= \frac{\text{Haemoglobin in gm/dL}}{\text{RBC count in million /μL}} \times 10$$

(iii) MCHC $= \dfrac{\text{Haemoglobin content in a single RBC, i.e. MCH}}{\text{Volume of a single RBC, i.e. MCV}} \times 100$

$$= \frac{\text{Haemoglobin content per 100 ml blood}}{\text{Volume of RBCs per 100 ml blood}} \times 100$$

$$= \frac{\text{Haemoglobin in gm/dL}}{\text{PCV per 100 ml blood}} \times 100$$

(As > 99% of PCV is due to presence of RBCs alone)

Q.2. *Which blood index is the most reliable and why?*

Ans. Of all the blood indices, MCHC is the most reliable, because:

(i) MCH and MCV are dependent on RBC count, which, if done by visual method, (page 19) is subjected to ±20% of error; hence inaccurate.

(ii) MCHC does not involve RBC count; moreover, if MCH increases, MCV also increases but the ratio of MCH to MCV remains unaltered. Hence, MCHC is most reliable and accurate blood index.

Q.3. *Why can MCHC not exceed the normal value of 38%? Explain.*

Ans. Page 24.

Q.4. *Enumerate the conditions in which RBC indices are of value.*

Ans. Refer to the table above.

Q.5. *Why is colour index not an appropriate index of haemoglobin content of RBC?*

Ans. Page 24.

Q.6. *Classify anaemias on the basis of MCV and MCHC.*

Ans. Refer to Page 24.

Q.7. *Calculate all blood indices from the following data: PCV = 40%; RBC count = 4 million/μL and haemoglobin = 10 gm/dL.*

Ans. (i) MCV ....

....

(ii) MCH ....

....

(iii) MCHC ....

....

(iv) Colour index (CI) ....

....

Q.8. *Give the etiological (causative) classification of anaemias.*

Ans. (i) **Haemorrhagic** anaemias due to blood loss

(ii) **Dietary deficiency** anaemias due to lack of iron, vitamins in the diet

(iii) **Dyshaemopoiesis** or **Aplastic** anaemias due to the destruction of bone marrow

(iv) **Haemolytic** anaemia due to the excessive destruction of RBCs

(for details, refer to the textbook)

STUDY NOTES

CALCULATIONS AND RESULTS

1. MCV

2. MCH

3. MCHC

4. Colour Index (CI)

COMMENTS AND DISCUSSION

....

....

....

....

Date: ....

6 Determination of Total Leucocyte (*White Blood Cell*) Count: *TLC*

I. APPARATUS

Improved Neubauer's counting chamber, WBC pipette, WBC diluting fluid (**Turk's Fluid**), compound microscope, cover-slips, pricking apparatus.

WBC diluting fluid (Turk's fluid)

Composition: Each 100 ml of fluid contains:

1. Glacial acetic acid: 3 ml (to lyse/destroy the membrane of WBCs, RBCs and platelets).
2. Gentian violet (1%): 1 ml (to stain the nuclei of WBCs deep violet-black so that they may be identified easily).
3. Distilled water: to make 100 ml (solvent).

II. PRINCIPLE

Same as in RBC count (page 19). However, as the WBC count is much lower than the RBC count, much lesser dilution (1:20) is employed.

III. PROCEDURE

1. Take WBC diluting fluid (Turk's fluid) in a watch glass.
2. After pricking the finger, suck the second drop of blood into the WBC pipette exactly up to 0.5 mark and dilute it with WBC diluting fluid by sucking the fluid up to 11 mark (dilution 1 in 20).

Note: Take the necessary precautions as given under procedure for the determination of total RBC count, page 19.

3. Gently rotate the pipette at least 3-4 minutes (as described on page 19).
4. Discard the first few drops of WBC fluid in the stem of the pipette, charge the counting chamber as done during RBC counting (page 19) and allow the time for the settling of cells.
5. Under low power objective, identify and check the distribution of WBCs in the four-corner WBC squares (page 11). Recharge the chamber if distribution is not uniform.

Important Note: *WBCs are seen as regular nucleated, rounded bodies with a clear refractility around them.*

6. Count the number of WBCs in each WBC square preferably under low power objective as per rules observed for counting the cells (page 20).
7. Count the WBCs in 4-corner WBC squares. Enter your observations in the corresponding squares. (Fig. 1.6.1.)

IV. CALCULATIONS

A. Calculation of dilution factor

Dilution factor:

$$\frac{\text{Final volume achieved (10 parts)}}{\text{Original volume taken (0.5 parts)}} = 20$$

(for details, refer to page 21).

B. Calculation of volume of fluid examined

Area of 4 WBC squares = 4 × 1 mm × 1 mm

= 4 sq.mm.

Depth of the chamber = 0.1 mm

Therefore, volume of fluid in the 4 WBC squares

= 4 sq.mm × 0.1 mm

= 0.4 μL

C. Calculation of total leucocyte count (TLC)

Let 'N' be the total number of WBCs in 4 WBC squares, *i.e.* in 0.4 μL of *diluted blood.*

Then total number of WBCs in 1 μL of *undiluted blood:*

$$= \frac{N \times \text{Dilution factor (20)}}{0.4}$$

$$= N \times 50$$

V. PRECAUTIONS

The same as in RBC count (refer to page 21).

OSPE

Aim: Dilute the given sample of blood to 20 times with the help of diluting fluid and WBC pipette provided to you.

Procedure steps: Refer above.

Checklist

1. Checks for pipette cleanliness, dryness and patency. **(Yes/No)**
2. Takes sufficient diluting fluid in a watch glass. **(Yes/No)**
3. Sucks the blood into the pipette exactly up to the 0.5 mark and there is no air bubble. **(Yes/No)**
4. Wipes off the blood sticking to the tip of the pipette. **(Yes/No)**
5. Sucks diluting fluid with the pipette exactly up to 11 mark, just above the bulb. **(Yes/No)**
6. Immediately holds the pipette in a horizontal position between the palms and rolls it gently. **(Yes/No)**

IMPORTANT VIVA-VOCE QUESTIONS

Q.1. *Enumerate the differences between a WBC and RBC pipette.*

Ans. Page 12.

Q.2. *Why is the bulb of WBC pipette smaller than RBC pipette bulb?*

Ans. Normal RBC count runs in millions for which a greater dilution of blood is required (dilution factor 1 in 200 - page 21); therefore, the bulb of WBC pipette is smaller than that of RBC pipette.

Q.3. *What are the functions of the bead in the bulb?*

Ans. Page 22.

Q.4. *List the other uses of the WBC pipette.*

Ans. WBC pipette can also be used for doing RBC count in severe anaemic patients.

Q.5. *Give the composition and functions of each component of Turk's fluid.*

Ans. Page 27.

Q.6. *What do you understand by the term 'Glacial'? Why should acetic acid used in Turk's fluid be glacial?*

Ans. 'Glacial' means pure; the acetic acid, if used pure, can only provide a clear refractility around the WBCs; thus, it helps in the better identification of the cells.

Q.7. *Can any other agent be used to lyse the RBCs?*

Ans. No, because any weak hemolytic agent will take a lot of time to lyse the RBCs; on the other hand, any strong agent will lyse the WBC nuclear membrane as well.

Q.8. *How long will an ideally charged chamber preparation last?*

Ans. Usually, it lasts for 90 minutes; however, the WBC count is stable for about 40 minutes. Thereafter, the smear starts receding and cell count decreases.

Q.9. *What is the error in counting WBCs by this method? Give some causes responsible for it.*

Ans. The percentage of error and factors causing it are the same as in counting RBCs (Refer to page 21).

Q.10. *How can the error in counting WBCs be reduced?*

Ans. The error can be reduced by counting more cells. If double the number of cell is counted, the error is reduced to 5%.

Q.11. *Give the normal range of WBC count and list* physiological *variations in the TLC.*

Ans.
- Normal TLC (i) At birth: 20000/µL
  (ii) Adults: 4000-11000/µL
- TLC increases in: newborn, in the evening, after exercise, after injection of epinephrine, stress, pregnancy, menstruation, lactation, etc.
- TLC decreases in: Refer to Q. No. 13.

Q.12. *Differentiate between leucocytosis and leukaemia.*

Ans. Leucocytosis means increase in TLC above 11000 per µL. Besides physiological cause (as given above) it also increases in any pyogenic (pus forming) or pyrogenic (fever producing) conditions.

Leukaemia is a *cancerous condition* of blood in which TLC is usually more than 50,000/µL and is associated with the presence of immature WBCs in the peripheral smear.

Q.13. *What is leucopenia? Give some causes responsible for it.*

Ans. Leucopenia means decrease in TLC below 4000 per µL.

Common causes are: starvation, typhoid fever, viral or protozoal infections, bone marrow depression.

Q.14. *Give the clinical significance of this experiment.*

Ans. TLC is a simple haematological investigation which helps to diagnose many diseases (see above, causes of variations in TLC).

Q.15. *Name a disease in which there can either be a marked leucocytosis or marked leucopenia.*

Ans. Leukaemia.

STUDY NOTES

OBSERVATIONS

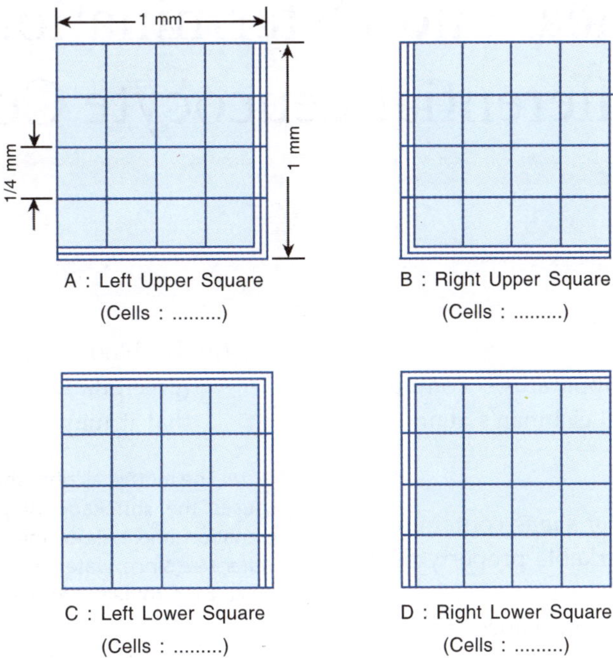

Fig. 1.6.1 Enter the observations after counting the WBCs in the corresponding squares

CALCULATIONS

RESULTS

Total leucocyte (WBC) count of my blood is

....

....

COMMENTS AND DISCUSSION

(State whether TLC is within the normal range or not; if not, explain.)

....

....

....

....

....

....

Date: ....

7 Preparation of a Peripheral Blood Smear and Determination of Differential Leucocyte Count (DLC)

I. APPARATUS

4-5 glass slides, pricking apparatus, compound microscope, cedar-wood oil and Leishman's stain

Leishman's stain

It belongs to *Romanowsky group of stains* containing an acidic and a basic dye. The remarkable property of this group of stain is:

(i) of making clear distinction in shades of staining; and

(ii) of staining granules differentially.

1. **Eosin**. It is an acidic dye (negatively charged) and stains positively charged (basic) particles viz., RBCs and granules of eosinophils.
2. **Methylene blue**. It is a basic dye (positively charged) and stains negatively charged (acidic) particles viz., the cytoplasm, nuclei of WBCs and granules of basophils.
3. **Acetone free methyl alcohol**. It is a *Fixative i.e.*

   (i) it preserves the cells in whatever chemical and metabolic state they are at the time of staining;

   (ii) the blood smear also gets fixed to the slide (precipitation of protein in it, by alcohol) so that it may not be washed off.

Note: The methyl alcohol should be acetone-free since acetone causes the shrinkage of the cells and may even produce crenation and lysis of the cells. It should also be completely *water-free* since water may affect the appearance of the film by causing rouleaux formation.

II. PROCEDURE

A. Preparation of a Blood Smear

1. Take 4 or 5 clean, grease-free glass slides with smooth edges; 3-4 to be covered with the blood film and one to be used as a ***spreader***.
2. Lay 3-4 glass slides on a table, prick the finger, touch the bleeding point lightly in the centre line about 1 or 2 cm from one end of the slides to obtain a small drop of blood on each.
3. Place the narrow edge of the *spreader* on the surface of slide just in front of the drop of the blood at an angle of 45° (Fig. 1.7.1). Draw the spreader

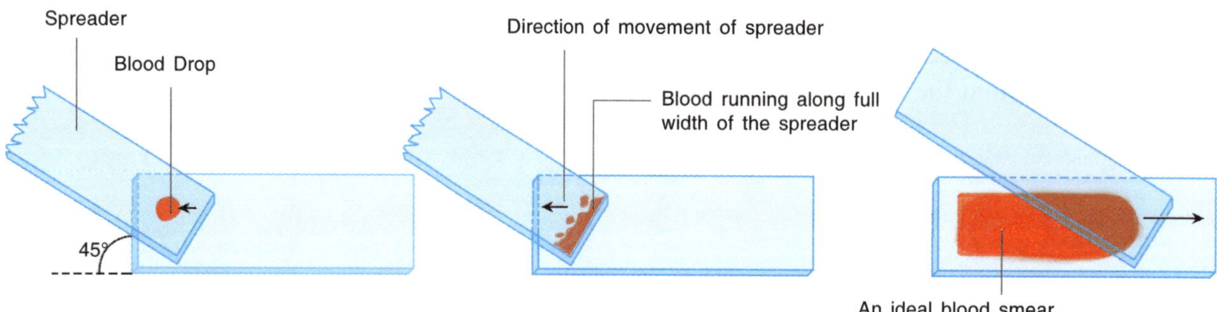

Fig. 1.7.1 Steps in preparation of a blood smear

backwards so as to touch the drop and hold there till the blood runs along the full width of the *spreader* at the line of junction.

4. The *spreader* is then moved slowly and smoothly to the other end of the slide maintaining an angle of 45°.

Note: A properly made blood film will be fairly uniform without uneven streaks or spots/vacoules in it and neither too thick nor too thin.

5. Allow the film to dry in air. Repeat the procedure with the other slides.

Note: Rouleaux formation is usually seen in varying degrees in the *wet* preparations of whole blood.

Criteria of a good blood smear (Fig. 1.7.2)

1. It should cover almost the entire width and about 3-4 cm length of the slide.
2. It is tongue-shaped with no tails at the end.
3. It is of uniform thickness *i.e.* it is neither too thin nor too thick. (A thick smear, when placed on a white background, appears red.)
4. There are no longitudinal/cross striations or air-gaps in the smear.

B. Fixing and staining of the blood smear

1. **Fixing the blood smear**
   (i) Place the blood smears across two of the parallel supports on the glass rods, so that the slides may be horizontal.
   (ii) Pour 8-12 drops of Leishman's stain on each slide, just enough to cover the smear. *Note the time.* Leave it for about 2 minutes (**fixation time**).

Important Notes
1. Note the number of Leishman's stain drops poured.
2. In hot weather, the stain should be watched to see that it does not become thick from the evaporation of the alcohol. If this occurs, the stain will precipitate on the film. This can be avoided by adding more stain to the one already on the slide.

2. **Staining the smear**
   (i) At the end of 2 minutes, add an equal number of drops of *buffered water* (pH 6.8) over the stain, taking care that the water is not spilled over.

Note: Double the number of drops of distilled water may be used in case of non-availability of buffered water.

   (ii) Mix the stain and water evenly by gently blowing air intermittently with the help of a dropper.
   (iii) If the dilution of the stain is correct, the fluid will be covered by a thin greenish scum. Leave the stain to act for 10 minutes (**staining time**).

Important Note: Depending on the strength of the Leishman's stain, the fixation time and staining time are variable; they are accordingly specified before the experiment.

3. At the end of 10 minutes, pour off the stain, hold the slide in a slanting position below the tap and the water is allowed to flow over the smear.
4. Wash the slide (up to 2 minutes) with tap water gently and thoroughly till the film gets a *pinkish* tinge. Make sure that:
   (i) none of the greenish scum settles on the surface of the blood film; and
   (ii) water stream should not strike the blood smear directly or else it may be washed off.

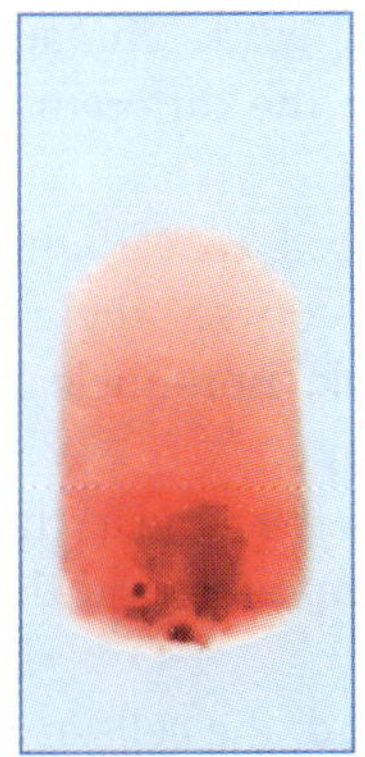

1. An ideal blood smear

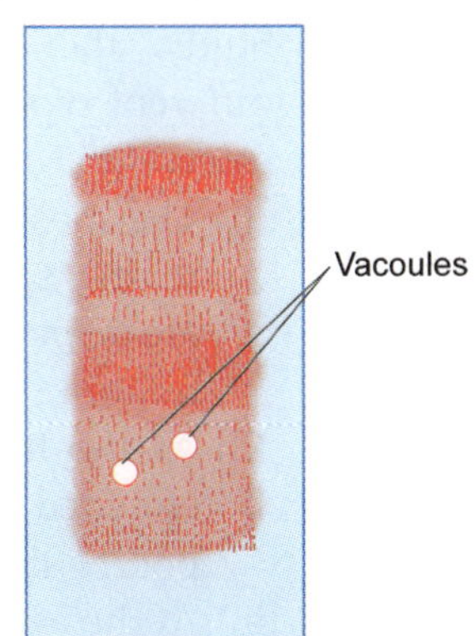

2. A film too long, too wide, grossly irregular in thickness made on a greasy slide

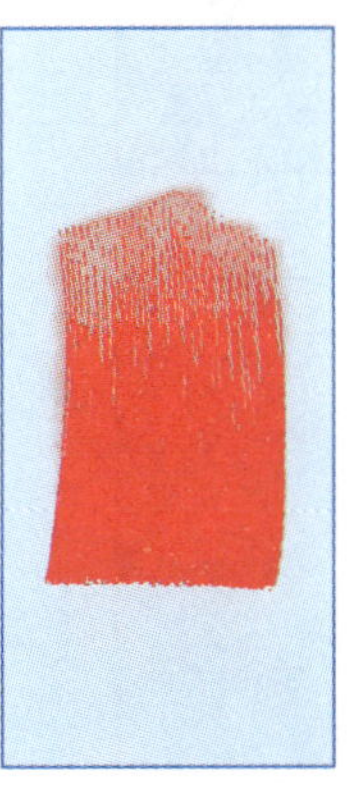

3. A film too thick

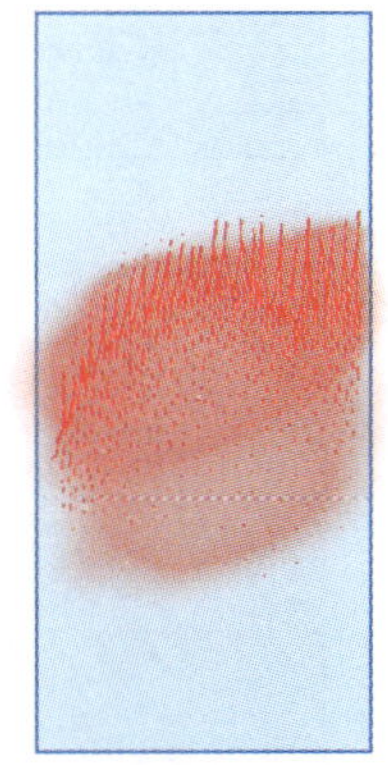

4. A film which has been spread with an irregular edged spreader; it also shows long tails.

Fig. 1.7.2 Blood films made on glass slides

5. Wipe clean the back of the slide and set it upright to dry.

C. Assessment of the quality of the stained smear

Check the staining and thickness of the blood smear by examining it *first* under low power objective and then under high power objective (Fig. 1.7.3). A well-stained blood smear has the following characteristics:

1. The smear is single-cell thick, with not much overlapping of the cells and the cells are uniformly distributed.
2. At least one WBC is seen per high power field (X100).
3. The RBCs are stained light pink.
4. In an **understained** smear, RBCs appear very pale and WBCs look almost colourless (Fig. 1.7.4 A).
5. In an **overstained** smear, RBCs look bluish-black and WBCs will take up more methylene blue, hence look totally purple (Fig. 1.7.4 B).

(A)

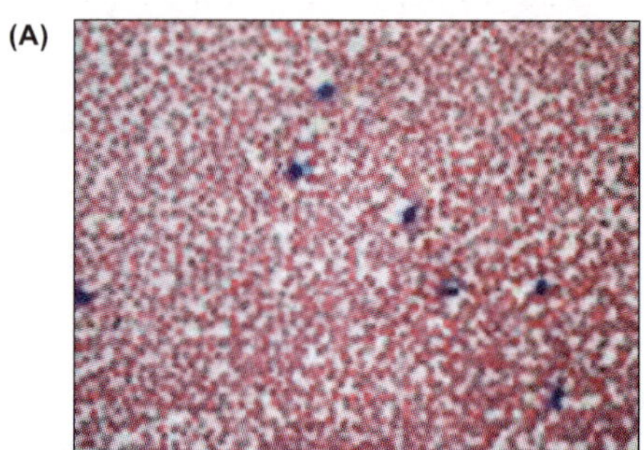

(B)

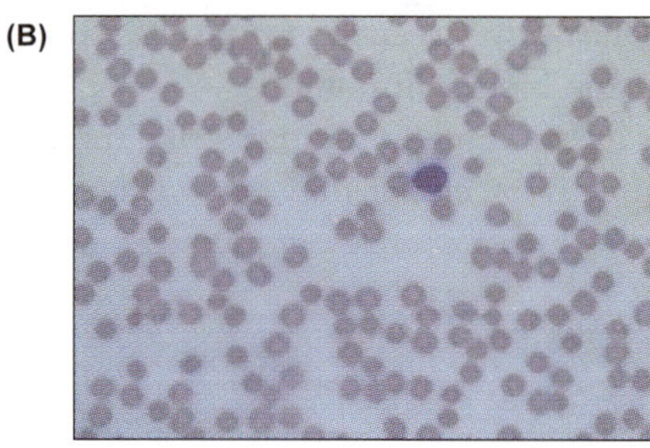

(C)

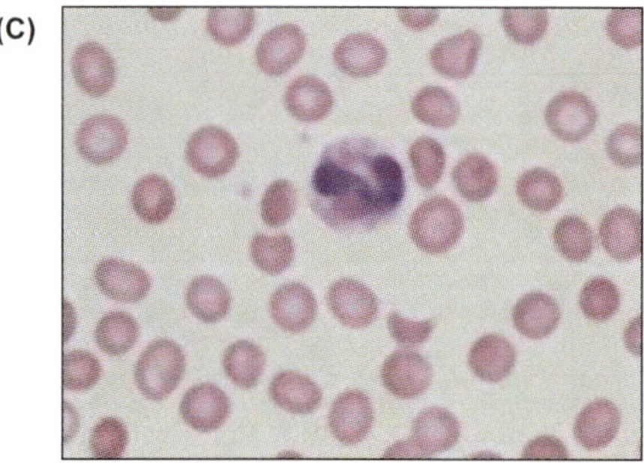

Fig. 1.7.3 An ideal Peripheral blood smear as seen under : (A) low power, (B) High power and (C) Oil immersion

Note: If smear is understained, add the stain and repeat the process for a few minutes. If it is overstained, wash the slide for a few minutes.

(A)

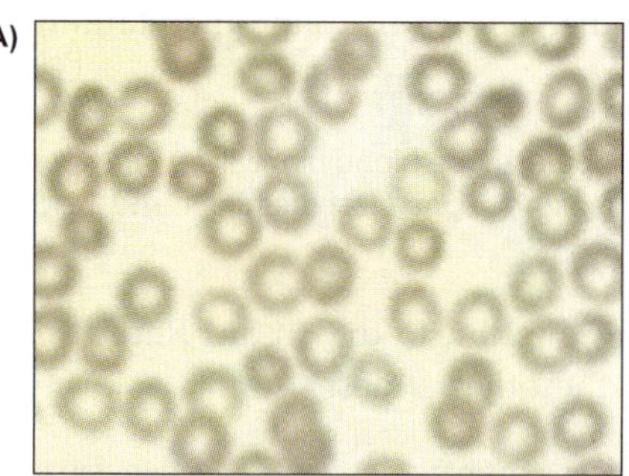

(B)

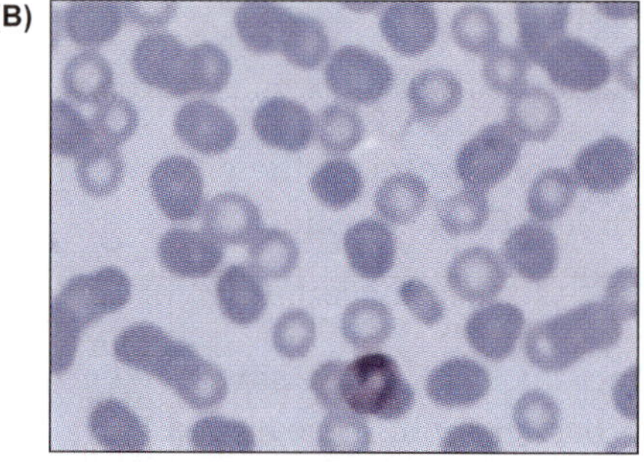

Fig. 1.7.4 (A) Understained and (B) Overstained peripheral blood smear

D. Examination of the stained smear under oil immersion

The identification of different types of blood cells is done under oil immersion. How?

1. Place a drop of cedar-wood oil on the blood film. Swing the oil-immersion objective into position. Carefully lower the objective until it just touches the drop oil. Now slightly raise the objective and focus the cells using fine adjustment only.
2. Study the distribution and characteristics of different types of cells in the different parts of the smear.
   (i) The most abundant cell type found anywhere in the smear is, of course, the RBCs. These are seen as light pink, non-nucleated discs of uniform size and shape.
   (ii) At the **head end** of the smear the RBCs are crowded and superimposed, and the WBCs are poorly stained.
   (iii) At the extreme **tail end**, the cells are wide apart and the WBCs are distorted.
   (iv) At the **upper and lower edges** of the smear, the WBCs are found in plenty but are poorly stained and abnormally rich in granulocytes.

Note: Irregularity in the distribution of WBCs is the rule; neutrophils and monocytes predominate at the margins and the tail, and lymphocytes in the middle of the film (Fig. 1.7.5).

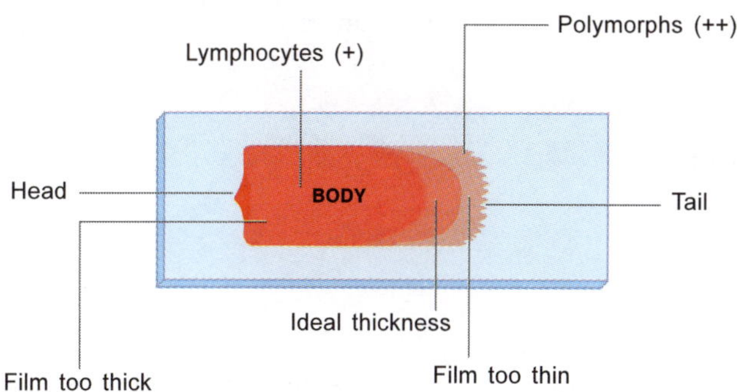

Fig. 1.7.5 Characteristic distribution of leucocytes in the different parts of a blood smear

E. Identification of different types of leucocytes

The identification and counting of different types of leucocytes is done under oil-immersion objective (Fig. 1.7.6) and Table 1.7.1. The WBCs can be differentiated from RBCs by the presence of nucleus and large size. While identifying the WBCs, keep four factors in mind:

1. *Size of the cells* (compare with the surrounding RBCs which are of uniform size, 7.2 µm);

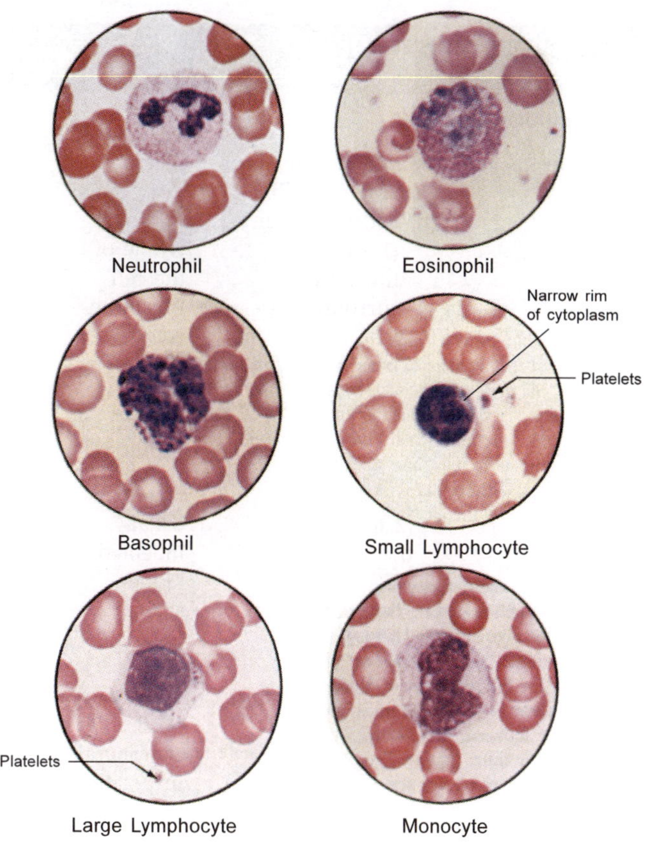

Fig. 1.7.6 Peripheral Smear showing different types of blood cells (Leishman's stain) at a magnification 400X

Table 1.7.1 Characteristic features of the different types of leucocytes (Also refer to Fig. 1.7.6)

Cell type	Cell size (diameter)	Nucleus	Cytoplasm	Granules	Functions
Granulocytes					
1. Neutrophil (50-70%)	10-14 µm (1.5 to 2 times the size of surrounding RBCs)	Multilobed (1-6 lobes), purple in colour	Slight bluish	• Very fine like sand particles • Numerous red brown or purplish in colour	1. *Phagocytosis* (First line of defence against bacterial infections) 2. Contain *endogenous pyrogen* (mediator of febrile response)
2. Eosinophil (1-4%)	-do-	• Usually bilobed (*spectacles shape*) • Purple in colour	Eosinophilic (acidic)- light pink, granular	• Large • Coarse • Brick red in colour • Do not cover the nucleus	1. Mild phagocytosis 2. Limit allergic reactions by degrading inflammatory mediator effects (*e.g.* histamine, bradykinin) 3. Provide local mucosal immunity
3. Basophil (<1%)	-do-	• Usually bilobed • Purple in colour	Basophilic (basic) appears blue, granular	• Large • Coarse • Purple or blue • Overlying the nucleus	1. Mild phagocytosis 2. Liberate histamine and *Eosinophil chemotactic factor of anaphylaxis* (ECF-A) → Allergic manifestations *e.g.* skin reactions to anaphylactic shock. 3. Contain heparin (an anticoagulant)

Cell type	Cell size (diameter)	Nucleus	Cytoplasm	Granules	Functions
Agranulocytes					
1. Lymphocyte (20-40%)	(i) Small: 7-10 μm (size of a RBC) (ii) Large: 10-14 μm (1.5 to 2 times the surrounding RBCs); irregular outline	• Single • Very big, occupying whole of the cell • Purple in colour • Oval or rounded • Central in position	• Scanty • Sky blue colour • Amount: less than the amount of nucleus	Absent	Produce antibodies, *i.e.* immune substances
2. Monocyte (2-8%)	• 10-18 μm (2 to 2.5 times the size of a RBC) • Irregular outline	• Single; usually indented kidney shape • Pale in colour • May be oval or circular • Peripheral in position	• Abundant (amount more than the nucleus amount) • Pale blue in colour	Absent	1. Active phagocytosis (*second line of defence*) 2. Enter the tissues to become *tissue macrophages* 3. Kill tumour cells

2. *Features of the nucleus* (colour, number of lobes);
3. *Features of the cytoplasmic granules* (pink or blue; fine or coarse); and
4. *Nuclear/cytoplasmic ratio*

F. Counting of the different types of leucocytes

A minimum of 100 WBCs are identified in a systematic manner (Fig. 1.7.7) and counting is made using the ***tally-bar method.**** Ideally, all the cells should be counted in a single strip running the length of the smear, proceeding from base to apex. Use the mechanical stage to traverse the full length of the film. Move the slide along vertically by a distance equivalent to 2 mm and again traverse the full length of the film, this time in the opposite direction. This method ensures that cells are counted no more than once.

> **Note:** In practice a 200-cell count is recommended as a routine procedure.

{*Keep putting a vertical bar (|) against a cell identified, the 5th bar should be marked obliquely so as to cut all the previous 4 vertical bars (卌). This will leave you with a bundle of five for easy calculation at the end.}

Alternatively the cell can also be counted by making an entry of each identified WBC in a preframed box containing 100 squares (Fig. 1.7.8).

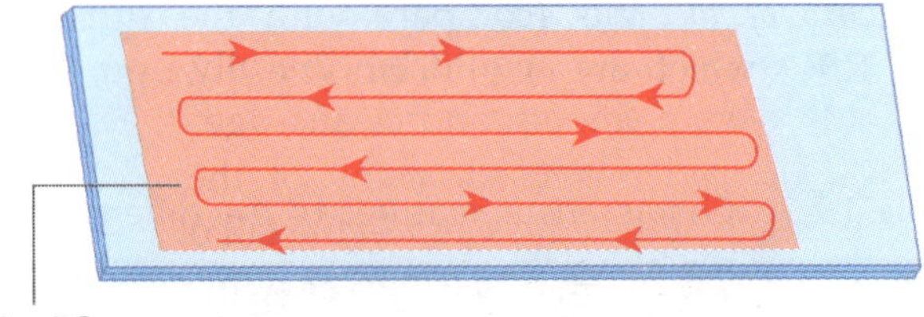

Fig. 1.7.7 Rules for counting the leucocytes. Arrows indicate the directions of movement of the slide.
Note: *The field moves to right/down when the slide is moved to left/up.*

N	E	N	N	N					

Fig. 1.7.6 Box with 100 squares showing entry of five identified WBCs, N: Neutrophil, E: Eosinophils.

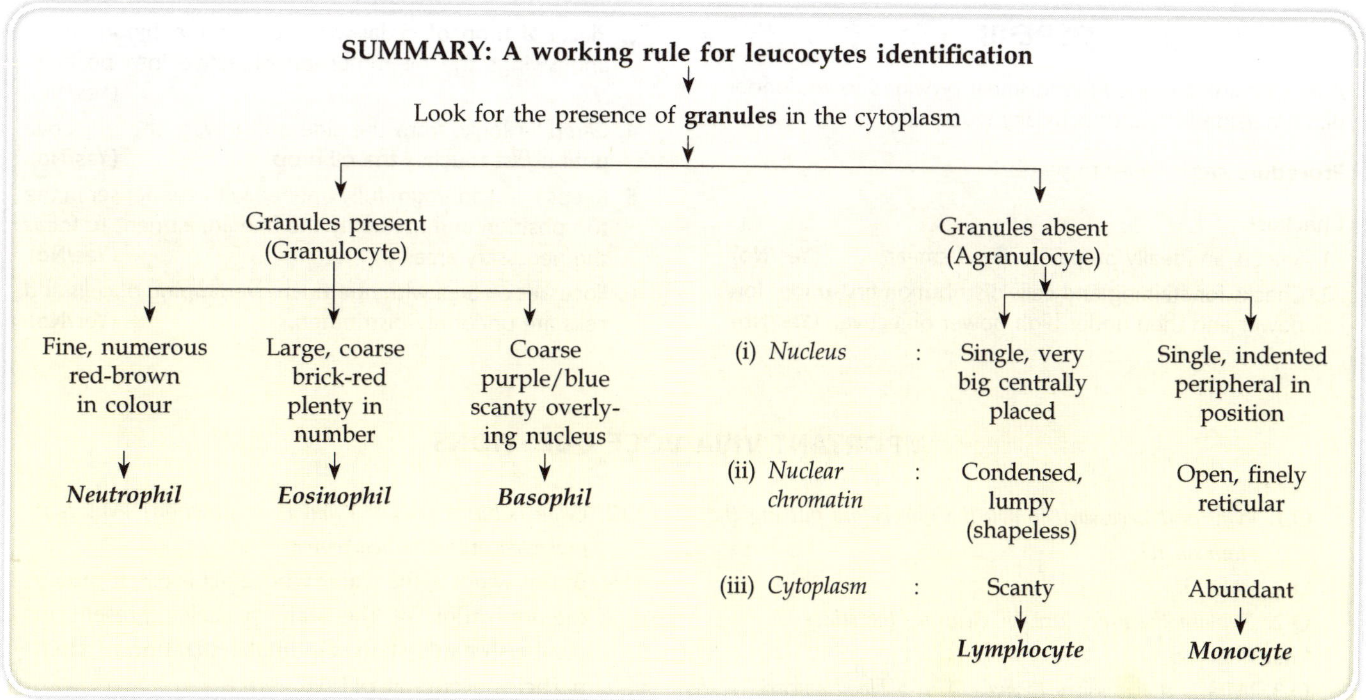

III. PRECAUTIONS

1. The slides should be clean and grease-free, therefore, these should be cleaned thoroughly with soap and water immediately before use.
2. The glass-spreader should be carefully selected. It should have a smooth and clean edge. If a rough-edged spreader is used, many of the leucocytes accumulate at the edges and in the tail of the smear. Also, a gross qualitative irregularity in distribution of cells will occur.
3. Make about 4-5 blood films so that at least one may be satisfactory.
4. Mark the smeared surface with a glass marking pencil.
5. Do not heat dry or blot dry the smear.
6. Stored blood should not be used for making smear (Why? See to page 10).
7. The smear should be stained not later than two hours after it has been prepared.
8. Assess the quality of the smear, both grossly and microscopically (under low power) before staining it.
9. Only a properly well-stained slide should be examined under the oil-immersion lens.

OSPE-I

Aim: Prepare a smear from a given sample of blood.

Procedure steps: Refer to page 30.

Checklist

1. Selects 4 or 5 clean, grease-free glass slides. **(Yes/No)**
2. Takes a small drop of blood on each about 1–2 cm from one end of the slide. **(Yes/No)**
3. Puts the spreader on the surface of slide just in front of the blood drop at an angle of 45°. **(Yes/No)**
4. Draws the spreader gently backwards and allows the blood to run along its full width. **(Yes/No)**
5. Moves the spreader slowly and smoothly to the other end of the slide maintaining an angle of 45°. **(Yes/No)**
6. Selects a smear of fairly uniform thickness without striations or vacoules in it. **(Yes/No)**

OSPE-II

Aim: Stain the given peripheral blood smear for the determination of differential leucocyte count (DLC).

Procedure steps: Refer to page 31.

Checklist

1. Selects 1 or 2 ideal smears and places them horizontally on parallel glass rods. **(Yes/No)**
2. Pours Leishman's stain on each slide, just enough to cover the smear and notes the number of stain drops poured. **(Yes/No)**
3. Adds an equal number of drops of buffer water over the stain and takes care that the water is not spilled over. **(Yes/No)**
4. Mixes the stain and water evenly by gently blowing air intermittently with the help of a dropper. **(Yes/No)**
5. Sees that at no stage stain becomes dry by adding more stain and buffer water. **(Yes/No)**

OSPE-III

Aim: Examine a stained blood smear provided to you under oil-immersion lens and focus any leucocyte.

Procedure steps: Refer to page 32

Checklist

1. Selects an ideally prepared blood smear. **(Yes/No)**
2. Checks for staining and cells distribution first under low power and then under high power objective. **(Yes/No)**
3. Places a drop of cedar-wood oil on the blood smear and swings the oil-immersion objective into position. **(Yes/No)**
4. Carefully looks from the side and lowers the objective until it just touches the oil drop. **(Yes/No)**
5. Keeps iris-diaphragm fully opened with condenser in the top position and uses only the fine adjustment to focus the necessary area. **(Yes/No)**
6. Focusses an area with not much overlapping of cells and cells are uniformly distributed. **(Yes/No)**

IMPORTANT VIVA-VOCE QUESTIONS

Q.1. *Why is it necessary to dry the film before putting the stain on it?*

Ans. Page 31.

Q.2. *Explain the procedure for cleaning the slides.*

Ans. Page 35.

Q.3. *Why is it necessary to make 4 or 5 blood smears?*

Ans. Page 35.

Q.4. *Enumerate the criteria of a good blood smear.*

Ans. Page 31.

Q.5. *Why must a blood film not be too thin?*

Ans. If the film is made too thin, neutrophils and monocytes accumulate at the edges and in the tail; this will give irregularity in the distribution of WBCs.

Q.6. *What are the functions of various constituents of Leishman's stain?*

Ans. Page 30.

Q.7. *Do you notice any other cells besides WBCs and RBCs in the smear? How do you distinguish them?*

Ans. Besides WBCs and RBCs, *platelets* are also seen. These are seen in clumps as faint blue cytoplasmic small oval or rounded bodies with reddish purple granules; nucleus is not present.

Q.8. *What all did you find most difficult to identify?*

Ans. Basophils, because:

(i) they are less numerous (<1%); and

(ii) close resemblance with eosinophil.

Q.9. *Why do the cells not get stained in the first two minutes of the staining procedure?*

Ans. This is because the Leishman's stain particles cannot enter the cells in the non-ionized form. They enter only after ionization which occurs on the addition of buffer water.

Q.10. *Why should the Leishman's stain be acetone-free?*

Ans. Page 30.

Q.11. *Is there any other way to fix the blood smear if Leishman's stain is not available?*

Ans. Yes. The smear can also be fixed by putting-few drops of methylated spirit on it.

Q.12. *What is buffer water? What is its function? Why is it preferred over distilled water?*

Ans. Buffer water is the water whose pH is 6.8. It causes the ionization of the stain particles present in the Leishman's stain. Optimal ionization of stain particles occurs at pH 6.8.

Q.13. *Can tap water ever be used for dilution purposes? If not, why?*

Ans. Tap water should never be used for dilution purposes as impurities present in it will give false appearance of granules; hence if interferes with proper identification of WBCs.

Q.14. *Which part of the smear should be avoided for counting the cells and why?*

Ans. The head end should always be avoided for counting the WBCs. Why? (Page 33).

Q.15. *Is it necessary to study the whole length of the smear for cell counting purposes and why?*

Ans. Page 34.

Q.16. *Draw a well-labelled diagram showing different types of leucocytes.*

Ans. Draw..... (You can take the help of Fig. 1.7.6).

Q.17. *How can we estimate approximate size of the WBCs under the microscope?*

Ans. Page 33.

Q.18. *What all informations can one gather from a peripheral smear?*

Ans. Other uses of a peripheral smear are:

(i) in the diagnosis of malaria as the organism can be seen within the RBCs;

(ii) it is used to comment on the type of anaemia;

(iii) a diagnosis of leukaemia can be made considering the number of blast cells;

(iv) toxic granules within the neutrophils indicate bacterial infection;

(v) a sex differentiation can be made but special staining technique is required.

Q.19. *How does the DLC of a child differ from that of an adult?*

Ans. A child has lymphocytes rather than the granulocytes as the predominant cells. Lymphocytes form 40-60% of total leucocytic population.

Q.20. *Name the different types of leucocytes. Give the identification feature of each type.*

Ans. Refer to page 33.

Q.21. *Mention the functions of each type of the leucocyte.*

Ans. Refer to page 32.

Q.22. *Give the causes of variations in different types of leucocytes.*

Ans. A. Neutrophilia means increase in neutrophils. Causes are:
- (i) After injection of epinephrine
- (ii) Exercise
- (iii) Pregnancy, menstruation and lactation
- (iv) Any pyogenic (pus forming) infection
- (v) Following tissue destruction e.g. burns, haemorrhage, after surgery, etc.

B. Neutropenia means decrease in neutrophils. Causes are:
- (i) In children (normal count: 40%)
- (ii) Typhoid fever
- (iii) Viral infections
- (iv) Bone marrow depression

C. Eosinophilia, *i.e.* increase in eosinophils. Causes are:
- (i) Allergic conditions like bronchial asthma
- (ii) Parasitic infestation e.g. worms
- (iii) Skin diseases

D. Eosinopenia, *i.e.* decrease in eosinophils - seen after injection of ACTH or corticosteroids; Cushing's syndrome

E. Lymphocytosis, *i.e.* increase in lymphocytes. Causes are:
- (i) Children - (normal count 40-60%) - called as *Relative Lymphocytosis*
- (ii) Chronic infections like tuberculosis
- (iii) Lymphocytic leukaemia
- (iv) Viral infections

F. Lymphopenia, *i.e.* decrease in lymphocytes. Causes are:
- (i) Hypoplastic bone marrow
- (ii) AIDS (acquired immuno-deficiency syndrome).

G. Monocytosis, *i.e.* increase in monocytes. Causes are:
- (i) Tuberculosis
- (ii) Syphilis
- (iii) Some leukaemias

H. Monocytopenia, *i.e.* decrease in monocytes, seen in hypoplastic bone marrow.

STUDY NOTES

OBSERVATIONS

....

....

RESULTS

....

....

....

COMMENTS AND DISCUSSION

....

....

....

....

Date: ....

8 Determination of Arneth Count

I. APPARATUS

The same as for DLC (Page 30).

II. THEORY

The segmentation of neutrophil is a normal phenomenon. It enables the cell to pass through the small spaces in the blood vessels. Neutrophil count based on the lobes of its nucleus is called ***Arneth Count***. It indicates the state of development (*i.e.* maturity) of the neutrophils.

1. A newly formed neutrophil in the bone marrow is single-lobed (stage 1). Its cells are typically U-shaped and are called **stabs** or **schafs**.
2. As the age increases the number of lobes in the nucleus increases and the most mature neutrophils have ≥ 6 lobes in the nucleus, called as **senile neutrophils** (Fig. 1.8.1).
3. ***Normal Arneth count*** *i.e.* distribution of neutrophils based on the number of lobes of their nuclei. N_1 means one-lobed neutrophils (stage 1). $N_{5\&6}$ means 5- and 6-lobed neutrophils, both are stage 5.

   N_1 - Stage 1 : 5%
   N_2 - Stage 2 : 30%
   N_3 - Stage 3 : 45% (maximum in number; fully mature and functionally most efficient)
   N_4 - Stage 4 : 18%
   $N_{5\&6}$ - Stage 5 : 2% (less motile, scanty granules, poorly stained, cells break up readily while making smear, functionally less active)

4. *Clinical significance*
   (i) If $N_1 + N_2 + N_3$ exceeds 80%, it is called **shift to left** or **regenerative shift**. This indicates *hyperactive* functioning of the bone marrow. The common causes are: pyogenic infection, haemorrhage, repeated exposure to X-rays.
   (ii) If $N_4 + N_5 + N_6$ exceeds 20%, it is called **shift to right** or **degenerative shift** and is indicative of *hypoactive* bone marrow. Its common causes are: pernicious anaemia, vitamin deficiencies, aplasia of the bone marrow.

Arneth count thus reflects the state of the bone marrow activity. This can be assessed simply with the help of peripheral blood smear without puncturing the bone marrow.

III. PROCEDURE

1. Prepare and stain a blood smear, the same as for doing DLC (page 30).
2. The stained smear is examined under oil-immersion (X100) objective. The neutrophils are identified and the number of lobes of the nucleus in each cell is observed.

> **Note:** For two lobes to be called separate from each other, they should be connected only by a band of chromatin and no nucleoplasmic connection should exist between them.

3. Count at least 100 neutrophils each with its nuclear lobes. Follow the same rules for counting the cells as already described under DLC (page 34).

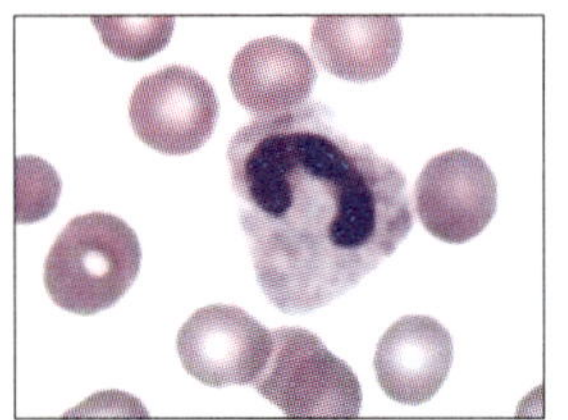

Single Lobe : Stab/Schaf Cell
N_1 : 5%

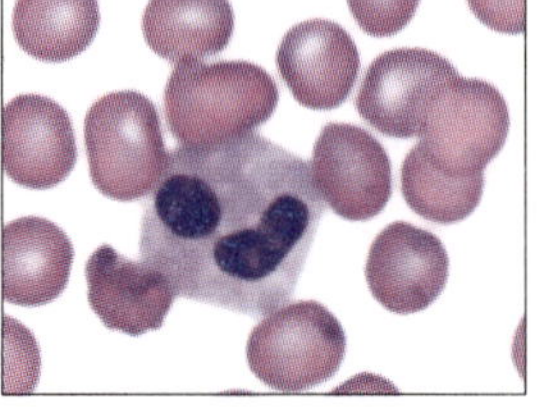

2 Lobed
N_2 : 30%

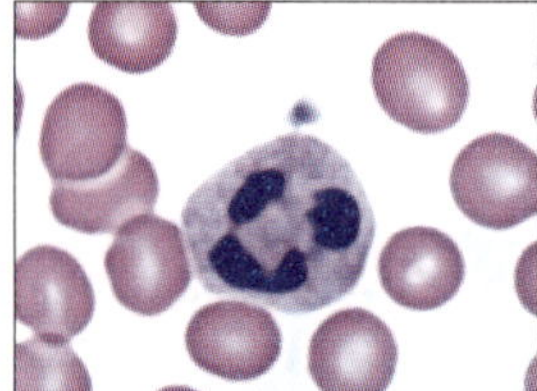

3 Lobed
N_3 : 45%

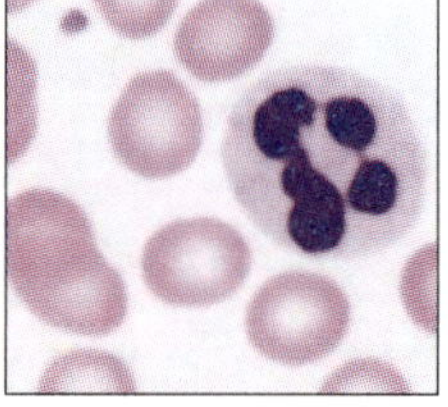

4 Lobed
N_4 : 18%

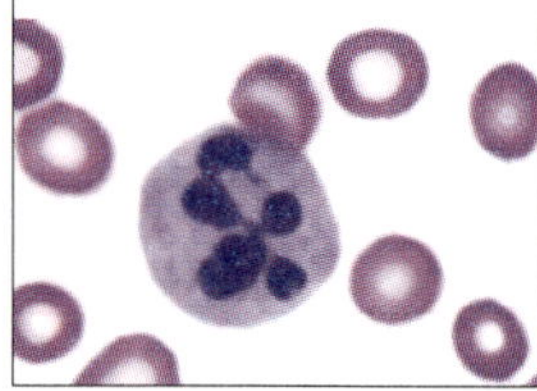

5 or more lobed (*senile*)
$N_{5\&6}$: 2%

Fig. 1.8.1 Distribution of neutrophils based on the number of lobes in their nucleus

4. The tally-bar method is used (page 34) for tabulating observations.
5. Express the results as the percentage of the total neutrophils counted.

N_1 : Single-lobed (Stage 1)
N_2 : Two-lobed (Stage 2)
N_3 : Three-lobed (Stage 3)
N_4 : Four-lobed (Stage 4)
$N_{5\&6}$: Five or more lobed (Stage 5)

IV. PRECAUTIONS

The same as for DLC (Page 35).

IMPORTANT VIVA-VOCE QUESTIONS

Q.1. *How has Arneth count derived its name?*
Ans. It has derived its name after Mr Arneth, a German physiologist.

Q.2. *Explain the relationship of the nuclear lobes with the age of the neutrophils.*
Ans. Page 38.

Q.3. *Enumerate the additional features for differentiating old from young neutrophils.*
Ans. Page 38.

Q.4. *Plot a graph of your observed values with neutrophil types on X-axis and the number of cells on Y-axis. Compare it with a normal Arneth count graph and interpret your observations.*
Ans.

Q.5. *If the TLC of a person is within the normal range, but towards a higher side, say 10,500/µL, how will you exclude the possibility of an early leucocytosis?*
Ans. Under given circumstances, it can be proved that leucocytosis has occurred by doing the Arneth count for the person. It would indicate a large increase in the number of young cells (stage I and II).

Q.6. *Give the characteristic features of a senile neutrophil.*
Ans. Page 38.

Q.7. *Enumerate the conditions in which bone marrow is hypo and hyper-functioning.*
Ans. Page 38.

Q.8. *Although Arneth count provides such an important information about the functioning/activity of the bone marrow yet it is not used as an important clinical tool for diagnosing diseases. Why?*
Ans. With the advancement of technology in the field of medical science, better, more accurate and reliable techniques have come up to assess the condition of the bone marrow. Arneth count thus has become an obsolete method.

STUDY NOTES

OBSERVATIONS AND CALCULATIONS

....

....

RESULTS

....

....

....

COMMENTS AND DISCUSSION

....

....

....

....

Date: ....

9 Determination of Bleeding Time (*BT*) and Clotting Time (*CT*)

I. APPARATUS

Pricking apparatus, filter paper, thin capillary tubes, stop watch

II. THEORY

A. **Bleeding Time**. It is the time taken from the puncture of the blood vessel to the stoppage of bleeding.

B. **Clotting Time**. It is the time taken from the puncture of the blood vessel to the formation of a fibrin thread.

There are many ways of determining the bleeding time (BT) and clotting time (CT). The results of different methods are not strictly comparable since they depend very much on the exact details of the technique.

> **Important Note:** Assessment of bleeding time is more important than the clotting time; the latter concerns the blood only *i.e.* how firm the clot is formed, whereas the bleeding time involves the interaction of blood with the injured tissues.

III. PROCEDURE

Bleeding Time (BT). The two methods commonly used for determining the BT are: *Duke's method* and *Ivy's method.*

A. Duke's method (Fig. 1.9.1)

It is convenient and commonly used method in practice.

1. Set the stop watch at 'zero'.
2. The tip of a finger is cleaned thoroughly with spirit and allowed to dry. Make a puncture deep enough (about 3-4 mm) to ensure free flow of blood without squeezing.
3. Immediately start the stop watch or note the time. The time of puncture of the finger is referred as **Zero Time**.
4. Thirty seconds later escaping blood is dried on the edge of a clean piece of filter paper.

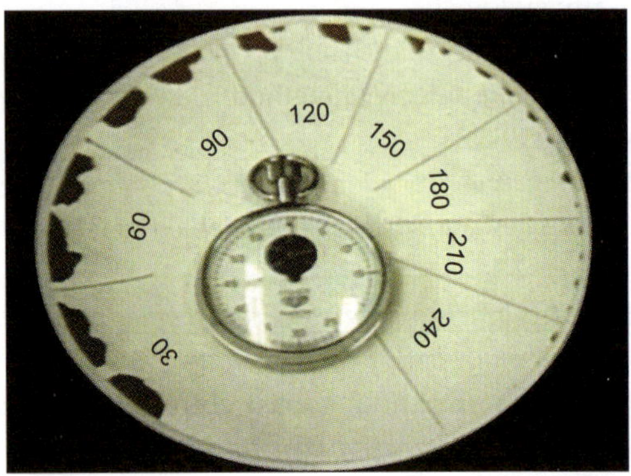

Fig. 1.9.1 Bleeding time: Duke's method

5. Repeat the procedure in every 30 seconds using a fresh area of the paper on each occasion until bleeding ceases and no further blood spot appears on the filter paper. Therefore, each blot of blood on the filter paper represents 30 seconds flow of blood.

> **Important Notes**
> 1. Usually the blood flow is maximum between first 2-1/2 minutes after pricking; thereafter, the rate is abruptly slowed, but may not cease for a further 2 or 3 minutes.
> 2. *Do not* apply pressure or squeeze the finger at any stage to take out the blood.

6. Count the total number of blood spots on the filter paper and multiply this by 1/2. This will give the BT in minutes. *Normal bleeding time by this method is 2-6 minutes.*

B. Ivy's method (Fig. 1.9.2)

1. Clean the anterior surface of the forearm with spirit.
2. Apply pressure of 40 mmHg to the upper arm with a sphygmomanometer and maintain this pressure till the end of the experiment.
3. Sterilize the needle (page 8) and make a puncture deep into the skin on the anterior surface of the forearm. Remove the drop of blood on filter paper as described above.

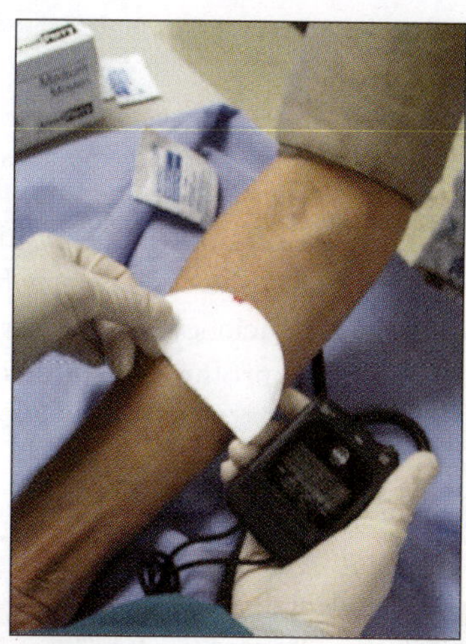

Fig. 1.9.2 Bleeding time: Ivy's method

4. *Normal bleeding time by this method is 3–6 minutes at 37°C.*

Clotting Time (CT)

Here also two methods are commonly used for determining the CT: *capillary glass tube method and Lee and White method.*

A. Capillary glass tube method

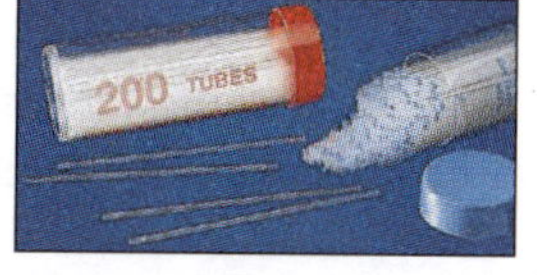

This is the most convenient and commonly used method in practice. (Fig. 1.9.3)

1-3. These are the same steps as described above in Duke's method.

4. When a large drop of blood has collected, introduce the end of the *capillary tube* into the drop holding the tube such that its other end will be at a lower level. Blood flows rapidly into the capillary tube.
5. Hold the capillary tube filled with blood in the palm of the hand so as to maintain it at body temperature.
6. At the end of one minute, break off about 1 cm of the tube from one end and notice if a thread of fibrin connects the broken ends of the tube. If there is no fibrin thread, repeat the procedure every 30 secs till a fibrin thread appears. The appearance of *fibrin thread* of about 5 mm length indicates that the blood has clotted.

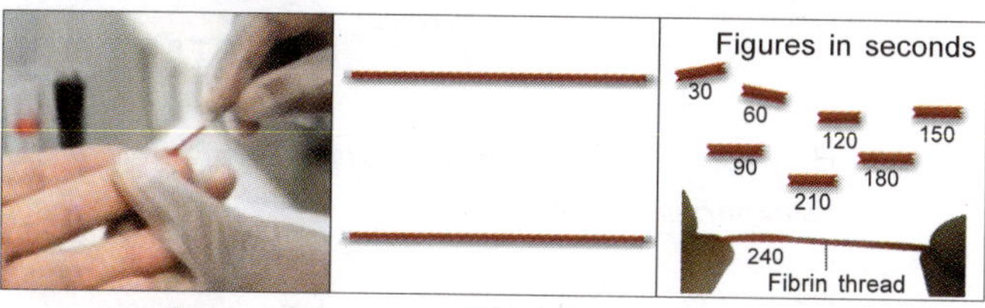

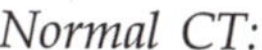

Fig. 1.9.3 Steps to determine clotting time by capillary glass tube method. (A) Capillary filling (B) Capillary filled with blood (C) Breaking the capillary every 30 secs till a fibrin thread appears

7. The total time taken from the time of puncture (**zero time**) till the formation of a fibrin thread is the CT. *Normal value of CT by this method is 3-8 minutes at 37°C.*

B. Lee and White method (Fig. 1.9.4)

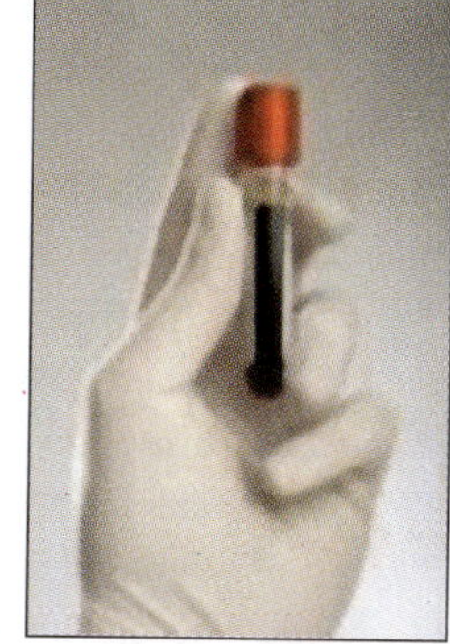

Fig. 1.9.4 Clotting time: Lee and White method

1 ml of venous blood drawn via vene puncture is delivered into a small tube, diameter 11 mm. Rock gently in a water bath at 37°C. Note the time from the time of vene puncture till the blood stops flowing.

Normal CT:

(i) in glass tube : 6-12 minutes.
(ii) in silicon tube : 20-60 minutes

IV. PRECAUTIONS

1. The finger should be pricked by a single stabbing action to give free flowing blood. At no stage it should be squeezed to obtain the blood.
2. Be alert and carefully note the 'zero time' (page 40).
3. Glass capillary tube should never be filled with blood by means of sucking at the other end of the tube.
4. Strictly follow the procedure steps and preferably experiment should be carried out at normal body temperature of 37°C.

IMPORTANT VIVA-VOCE QUESTIONS

Q.1. *How does bleeding time differ from clotting time? Give their normal values.*

Ans. Page 40.

Q.2. *What do you understand by the term Haemostasis?*

Ans. Spontaneous arrest or prevention of bleeding by physiological process is called haemostasis.

Q.3. *How does the bleeding get arrested? or Enumerate the series of events involved in haemostasis.*

Ans. Three major events which get involved during the arrest of bleeding are:

(i) Constriction of injured blood vessel due to release of 5-HT from the damaged platelets
(ii) Formation of a haemostatic plug of platelets
(iii) Seal of damaged blood vessel by the blood clot

Q.4. *How is the coagulation of blood brought about?*

Ans. The clotting mechanism responsible for the formation of fibrin involves a complex series/cascade of reactions. Here inactive enzymes are activated which, in turn, activate other inactive enzymes. The ultimate step is the conversion of prothrombin to thrombin (an enzyme) by a substance thromboplastin. Thrombin then converts fibrinogen into fibrin.

Q.5. *Name the clotting mechanism by which the clotting of blood is brought about in the capillary glass tube mechanism.*

Ans. The clotting mechanism involved is the intrinsic system/pathway since it is brought by exposing the blood to electronegatively charged wettable surface, glass.

Q.6. *Name the factors on which BT and CT depend.*

Ans. (i) Factors on which BT depends are:

(a) condition of the vessel wall;
(b) formation of temporary haemostatic plug, and
(c) temperature

(ii) Factors on which CT depends are:

(a) presence of all clotting factors; and
(b) temperature

Q.7. *Name the conditions where BT and CT are altered.*

Ans. (i) BT gets prolonged when there is:

(a) decreased platelet count as in thrombocytopenic purpura;
(b) abnormality/weakness in the walls of the capillaries, as in purpura haemorrhagica; and
(c) when temperature increases, it delays the contraction of vessel wall; conversely, BT decreases with decrease in temperature.

(ii) CT gets prolonged when there is:

(a) deficiency of clotting factors; *hemophilia* being the commonest condition seen, which is due to the deficiency of factor VIII;
(b) vitamin K deficiency; it is required for the synthesis of prothrombin (factor II) and factors VII, IX and X in the liver;
(c) anticoagulant overdose

Q.8. *Define purpura.*

Ans. Purpura is a condition with various manifestations and different causes, characterized by capillary abnormality resulting in haemorrhages into the skin, mucous membranes, internal organs and other tissues.

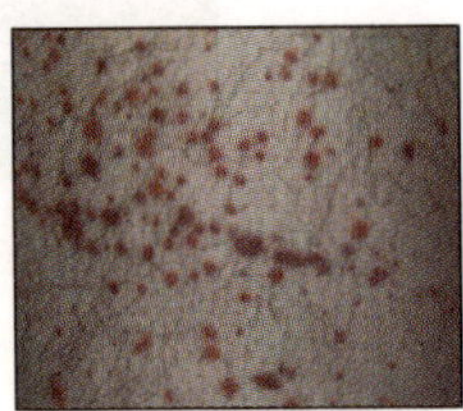
Petechial haemorrhages over forearm

Q.9. *What happens to BT and CT in hemophilia and purpura?*

Ans. (i) *In purpura,* BT increases to 10-20 minutes or more whereas CT is normal.

(ii) *In hemophilia,* CT increases markedly whereas the BT is normal.

Q.10. *Calcium plays an important role in many stages of cascade reactions during clotting mechanism. However, calcium deficiencies do not produce coagulation disorders. Explain.*

Ans. This is because the traces of calcium are required for coagulation. Even if very severe calcium deficiency occurs, it may produce other symptoms like **tetany** before coagulation disorders develop.

Q.11. *What is* ***zero time****? What is its significance?*

Ans. Page 40.

Q.12. *What is the clinical significance of determining BT and CT?*

Ans. It is very important to know BT and CT in the following conditions:

(i) before surgery;
(ii) before any biopsy, especially liver or bone marrow biopsy; and
(iii) before putting any patient on anticoagulant therapy (ideally, prothrombin time should be assessed).

Q.13. *Name one method each for BT and CT which are not commonly in use.*

Ans. For determining BT, Ivy's method (page 40) and for CT, Lee and White method (page 41).

Q.14. *What is Athrombocytopenic purpura and thromboasthenic purpura?*

Ans. Purpura with normal platelet count is Athrombocytopenic purpura, while in thromboasthenic purpura, there are abnormal circulating platelets but platelet count is normal.

Q.15. *Give the physiological importance of coagulation.*

Ans. The physiological significance of coagulation is obvious from the following effects:

(i) prevention of further blood loss by sealing an injury;

(ii) drawing together of wound edges by shrinkage of the clot;

(iii) protection against injury and drying by scab formation; and

(iv) provision of a framework for tissue repair.

Coagulation is thus the initial step in the repair of tissue injury.

Q.16. *Give common causes of bleeding disorders.*

Ans. These can be grouped as

(i) Defective blood clotting due to:

(a) deficiency of clotting factors I, II, V, VIII, IX and X

(b) vitamin K deficiency

(c) anti-coagulant overdose

(ii) Defective capillary contractility - *purpura*

(iii) Combined defects

Q.17. *Name some tests to assess bleeding disorders.*

(i) BT (page 40)

(ii) CT (page 41)

(iii) Platelet count (page 59)

(iv) Prothrombin time: Normal 11-16 seconds

(v) Clot retraction time

(vi) Thromboplastin (prothrombin activator) generation test

(vii) Skin microscopy

(viii) Determination of capillary resistance or fragility

Q.18. *Describe the following tests: Clot retraction, thromboplastin (prothrombin activator) generation test; skin microscopy and capillary resistance or fragility.*

Ans. Refer to the textbook for the details of each test.

STUDY NOTES

OBSERVATIONS AND RESULTS

1. Bleeding time by Duke's method is

....

....

....

2. Clotting time by capillary glass tube method is

....

....

....

COMMENTS AND DISCUSSION

....

....

....

....

....

....

Date: ....

10 Determination of Blood Groups (*A, B, O and Rh System*)

I. APPARATUS

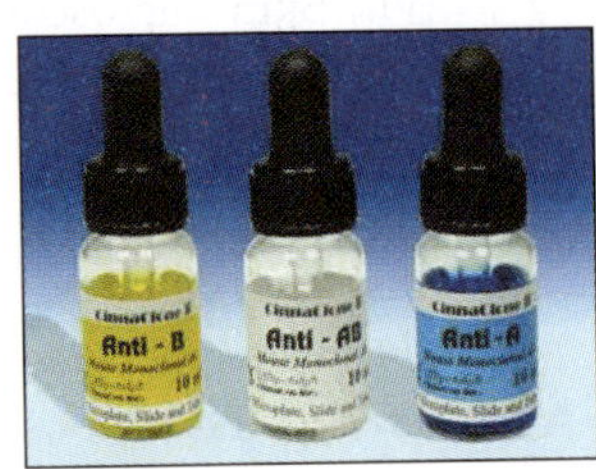

Anti-serum A, Anti-serum B, Anti-serum Rh, isotonic saline (0.9% NaCl), glass slides, applicator sticks, compound microscope, glass marking pencil and capillary dropper

II. THEORY

1. More than 30 blood group specific antigen (*i.e.* agglutinogens) can be recognized on the membrane of human RBCs. These antigens enable the blood group of different individuals to be differentiated. The chief blood groups are:
   (i) *Classical ABO blood groups, and*
   (ii) *Rhesus (Rh) blood group.*
   (iii) *M and N blood group*
2. The ABO blood group system was first discovered by Landsteiner in 1900. It is based on the presence or absence of blood group specific substances A, B and O in the RBCs. Accordingly, human beings can be divided into 4 main groups viz., **A, B, AB** and **O blood groups.**
3. The Rh blood group system was discovered by Landsteiner and Weinar in 1940. RBCs of Rhesus monkeys when injected into rabbits, the rabbits responded to the presene of an antigen in these cells by forming an antibody which agglutinated Rhesus RBCs. If the immunized rabbit's serum is tested against human RBCs, agglutination occurs in 85% of men, these people are called ***Rh '+' (positive)*** and their serum contains *no* Rh antibody. No agglutination occurs in 15%, these are called ***Rh '–' (negative)*** and their serum also contains *no* Rh antibody.
4. The procedure is based on the principle of **agglutination,** *i.e.* clumping of RBCs. The phenomenon of agglutination is due to the interaction between the factors - agglutinogen (antigen) present on the RBCs membrane and agglutinin (antibody) present in the plasma.
5. Normal human RBCs possessing a particular antigen will show agglutination in the presence of the corresponding antibody. This may occur quite soon but may not develop for several minutes, if the agglutinin titre of the serum is low.

III. PROCEDURE

A. Preparation of Red Cell Suspension

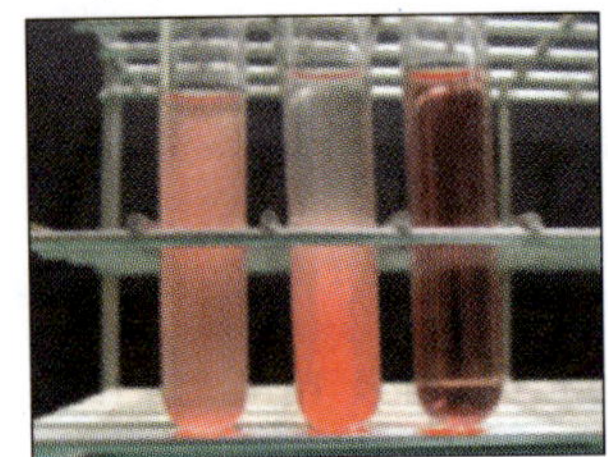

Take 3 ml of isotonic saline (0.9% NaCl) in a clean test tube. The finger is pricked under aseptic precautions so as to assure free flow of blood, the first drop of blood is wiped away with a clean piece of cloth and a drop of blood is added to the test tube. Alternatively, red cell suspension may be prepared simply by inverting the test tube over the finger pricked.

B. Determination of Blood Groups

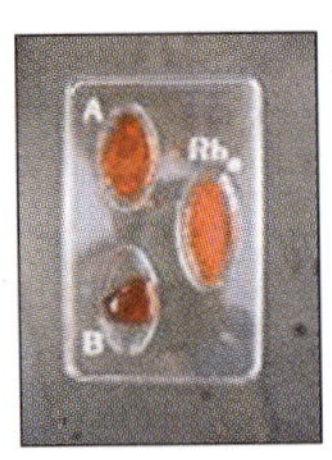

1. Take an ordinary grease-free, clean glass slide and one drop each of antiserum-A (*i.e.* serum containing α-antibodies), anti serum-B (*i.e.* serum containing β-antibodies) and anti-serum Rh (*i.e.* serum containing antibodies, anti-D) is placed thereon with the help of a dropper. In addition, one drop of isotonic saline (used as control) is also placed on the slide. The slide is accordingly *labelled as anti-A, anti-B, anti-D and control.*
2. The red cell suspension is drawn from the bottom of the test tube into **capillary dropper** and a drop of it is added to each of the drops on the slide. (Take utmost care that the nozzle of the dropper should not touch any of the drops.) The two are mixed with the help of *separate* application sticks.

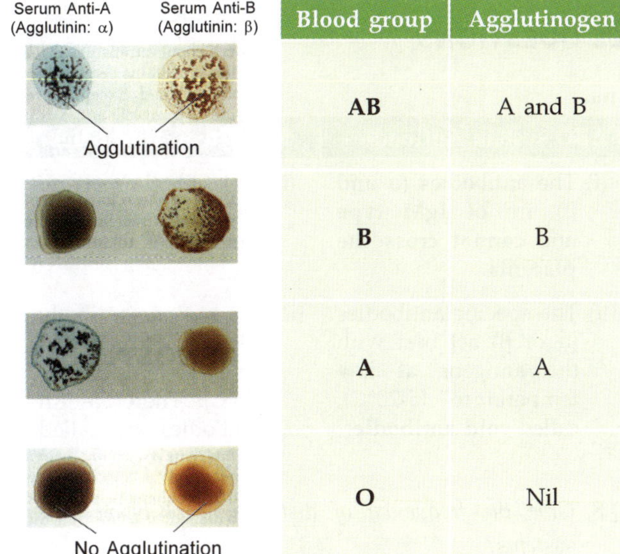

Blood group	Agglutinogen
AB	A and B
B	B
A	A
O	Nil

Fig. 1.10.1 Detemination of ABO blood types

3. Wait for 10 minutes; the slide is then gently rocked back and forth and examined for the presence of agglutination (clumping of RBCs). Confirm the findings under the low power of the microscope (Fig. 1.10.1):
   (i) if there is no agglutination, the RBCs remain separated and evenly distributed; and
   (ii) if agglutination occurs, the RBCs are massed together in clumps and lose their outline.
4. The blood group is determined as indicated in the table below and Fig. 1.10.2.

	Reaction with		
Blood Group	Serum-A i.e. (Antibody : β)	Serum-B i.e. (Antibody : α)	Anti serum-Rh (Anti-body : anti-D)
A	–	+	
B	+	–	
AB	+	+	
O	–	–	
Rh+			+
Rh–			–

'+' : **Agglutination,** *i.e.* RBCs are massed together in clumps and lose their outline.

'–' : **No agglutination,** *i.e.* RBCs remain separate and evenly distributed.

Important Notes

1. **False positive reaction** can occur due to the use of antisera contaminated with bacterial growth or infection of RBCs suspension by bacteria; and
2. **False negative reaction** occurs due to the loss of potency of the antisera because of improper storage.

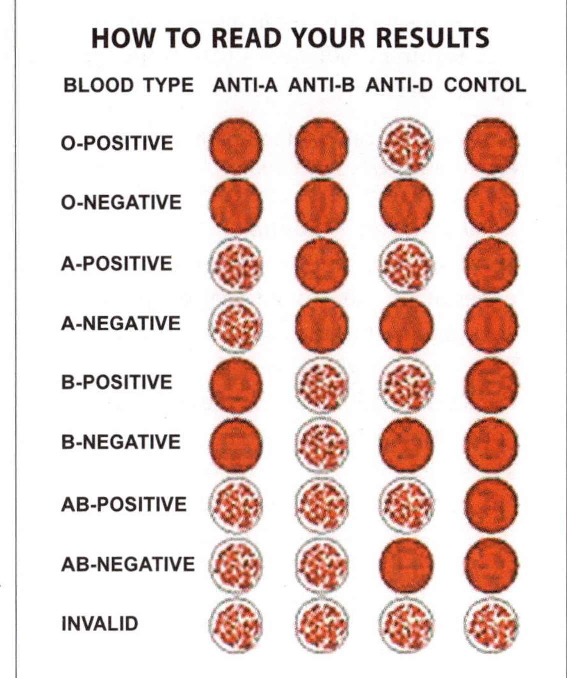

Fig. 1.10.2 How to read the blood group tests results

IV. PRECAUTIONS

1. The slides should be thoroughly cleaned with soap and water.
2. The slide should be labelled beforehand after placing the antisera A, B and Rh and isotonic saline.
3. There should not be any intermixing of the **four** drops placed on the slide.
4. The slide should be examined for agglutination before the solution dries up. Confirm the findings under the low power of the microscope.
5. Undiluted blood should never be mixed with the antisera directly, otherwise false positive reactions may develop.

IMPORTANT VIVA-VOCE QUESTIONS

Q.1. *How would you obtain antisera-A, B and Rh?*

Ans. (i) Antisera A, B or Rh can be obtained by injecting the respective antigen into a rabbit and collecting the antibodies from their serum.

(ii) Antisera A or B can also be obtained from the serum of individuals with blood group B or A respectively.

Note: If the blood is allowed to clot in a test tube, then the clot retracts and gives out serum.

Q.2. *What is the use of* **control**?

Ans. RBC suspension (*i.e.* control) is used for the experiment to avoid false positive results (see above) due to rouleaux formation.

Q.3. *What is 'Zone phenomenon'?*

Ans. For agglutination to occur the antigen and antibody concentration has to be the same. If it is not the same, then no reaction occurs. This is called *zone phenomenon.*

Q.4. *Why should we wait for 10 minutes before looking for agglutination?*

Ans. We should wait for 10 minutes to allow antigen-antibody reaction to occur.

Q.5. *Why should the preparation be examined before it starts getting dried up?*

Ans. The preparation should be examined before it starts getting dried up in order to avoid confusion due to rouleaux formation.

Q.6. *What is Landsteiner's Law? What is the exception to the law?*

Ans. Karl Landsteiner in 1900 framed a law; it has two major components:

(i) if an agglutinogen is present on the RBCs of an individual, the corresponding agglutinin must be absent from the plasma; and

(ii) if the agglutinogen is absent in the individual RBCs, the corresponding agglutinin must be present in the plasma.

Exception to the 2nd part is: absence of **Rh** agglutinogens from the RBCs which are not accompanied by presence in the plasma of anti-Rh agglutinins.

Q.7. *What are cold and warm antibodies?*

Or

How do the antibodies of ABO blood group system differ from those of Rh system?

Ans.

ABO system Antibodies	Rh system Antibodies
(i) The antibodies (α and β) are of **IgM type** and **cannot cross the placenta.**	(i) Rh antibodies are of **IgG type** and **can cross the placenta.**
(ii) The specific antibodies (α or β) act best with the antigens at low temperature (5-20°C), called **cold antibodies.**	(ii) The antigen-antibody reaction occurs best at the body temperature (37°C). Therefore Rh antibodies are called **warm antibodies.**

Q.8. *Give the frequency of distribution of blood group systems?*

Ans.

	ABO system				Rh system	
	A	*B*	*AB*	*O*	*Rh +ve*	*Rh −ve*
(i) Britain	42	9	3	46	85	15
(ii) India	21	39	9	31	94-95	5-6

Note: All values are in percentage.

Q.9. *Name the blood group systems.*

Ans. More than 30 blood group systems are known. The chief blood groups are:

(i) classical ABO blood group

(ii) Rhesus (Rh) blood group

(iii) M and N blood group

Q.10. *If a Rh negative mother carries a Rh positive foetus, what complications are likely to occur and why?*

Ans. If a mother is Rh negative and foetus is Rh positive, serious complications may occur. RBCs containing D-antigen may pass the placenta from the foetus to the mother, either during pregnancy or at the time of delivery. The mother responds by forming anti-D which returns to the foetal circulation and tends to destroy foetal RBCs, called **hemolytic disease of the newborn.**

Q.11. *Define the term* ***hemolytic disease*** *of the newborn. What are the forms in which it may manifest?*

Ans. Definition-see above Q.No. **10**. The various forms are:

(i) Hydrops foetalis.

(ii) Icterus gravis neonatorum (hemolytic jaundice).

(iii) Erythroblastosis foetalis.

(iv) Kernicterus.

Q.12. *What are the probability of hemolytic disease in a newborn child to a Rh positive father and Rh negative mother?*

Ans. Since the sensitization of a Rh negative mother by carrying a Rh positive foetus generally occurs at birth, the first child is usually normal. However, serious complications may occur in the 2nd or later pregnancies depending on the degree of sensitivity of the mother.

Q.13. *How can Rh hemolytic disease be prevented?*

Ans. Rh positive foetal cells in the mother's blood can be destroyed by administering a single dose of **anti-Rh antibodies** (to the mother) in the form of Rh-immune globulin soon after childbirth. This prevents active antibodies formation in the mother.

Q.14. *Explain why ABO incompatibilities rarely produce hemolytic disease of the newborn?*

Ans. ABO incompatibilities are rare because α and β antibodies are of IgM type and cannot cross the placenta.

Q.15. *If a Rh positive mother is carrying a Rh negative foetus, no complication occurs. Explain.*

Ans. This is because:

(i) RBCs containing 'D' antigen cannot cross the placenta from the mother to the foetus.

(ii) Even if a small amount of maternal blood leaks into foetal circulation due to placental insufficiency at any time during pregnancy, the foetus cannot respond by forming anti-D since the capacity to make an immunological response to foreign antigen develops after birth.

Q.16. *Enumerate the use of blood grouping tests.*

Ans. (i) In blood transfusion

(ii) In pregnancy, Rh incompatibility

(iii) Investigating a case of paternity dispute

(iv) Medico-legal value

(v) Help in cell recognition

(For details, refer to the textbook.)

Q.17. *What basic rules need to be observed before blood transfusion?*

Ans. (i) The plasma of the donor (which contains antibodies) can usually be ignored because it gets diluted by the much larger volume of recipient plasma.

(ii) No Rh negative female at any age before menopause should ever be given a Rh positive blood transfusion. Otherwise, the transfusion may make her permanently childless (if she gets married to a Rh positive person).

Q.18. *The classical terms, universal donor and universal recipient, are no longer valid. Explain.*

Ans. These terms are no longer valid as complications during blood transfusion can be produced by the existence of Rh and other factors.

Q.19. *What is the only safeguard procedure available against blood transfusion complication?*

Ans. **Direct cross matching** of the blood is the only safeguard against blood transfusion complication. It involves matching the serum of the recipient directly against the RBCs of the donor, and again matching the RBCs of the recipient against the serum of the donor.

Q.20. *What is the first effect of incompatible (mismatched) blood transfusion?*

Ans. After a little ml of incompatible blood has been introduced, the person complains of violent pain in the back or elsewhere and tightness in the chest, because agglutinated RBCs form clumps which blocks the capillaries.

STUDY NOTES

OBSERVATIONS

Reaction of the subject's cells

Control	*Antiserum-A*	*Antiserum-B*	*Antiserum-Rh*	*Blood Group*

'+' : Agglutination present

'–' : Agglutination absent

RESULTS

....

COMMENTS AND DISCUSSION

....

Date: ....

11 Determination of the Specific Gravity of Blood

I. PROCEDURE

To determine the specific gravity (S.G.) of the given sample of blood, the following methods are available.

A. Direct method

In this method, an equal volume of blood and water is taken in capillary tubes called **pyenometers** and weighed. The ratio of their weights gives the specific gravity of blood.

B. Indirect method

1. Hammer Schlag's method

In this, the specific gravity is determined by equalising the density of two miscible liquids like chloroform (specific gravity 1.470) and benzene (specific gravity 0.88) to that of blood.

2. Philips and Vanslyke's $CuSO_4$ method

Apparatus: Stock solution of copper sulphate ($CuSO_4$) of specific gravity 1.100, distilled water, test tubes, dropper

Principle: The specific gravity of blood is compared with the solutions of $CuSO_4$ of known specific gravities.

Procedure

(i) Prepare 10 ml of $CuSO_4$ solution of specific gravity (SG) ranging from 1.050 to 1.066 by mixing the distilled water with the stock solution of $CuSO_4$ as given in Table 1.11.1.

(ii) Mix each solution properly.

(iii) Deliver a drop of blood serially into each solution from a height of about 1 cm with the help of a pipette. Observe the behaviour of blood drop in the solution.

(iv) Blood drop will travel for some distance because of the momentum (Fig. 1.11.1)

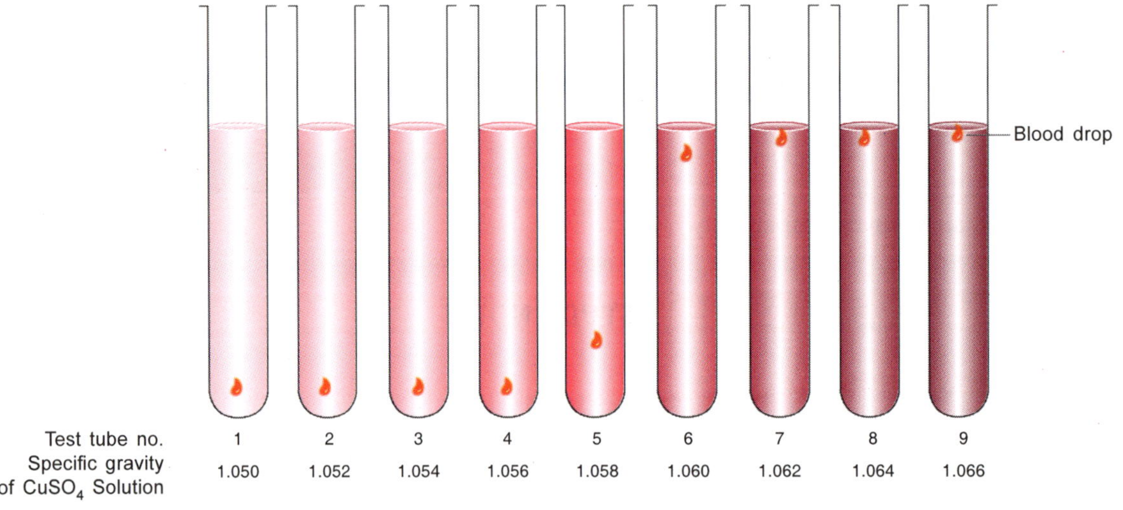

Fig. 1.11.1: Position of blood drop in $CuSO_4$ solution of SG ranging from 1.050 to 1.066

Table 1.11.1 Procedure for preparation of $CuSO_4$ solution of varying specific gravity (SG)

Test Tube Number	1	2	3	4	5	6	7	8	9
$CuSO_4$ solution (ml)	4.9	5.1	5.3	5.5	5.7	5.9	6.1	6.3	6.5
Distilled water (ml)	5.1	4.9	4.7	4.5	4.3	4.1	3.9	3.7	3.5
SG of solution	1.050	1.052	1.054	1.056	1.058	1.060	1.062	1.064	1.066

(a) if it is heavier than the solution, it will sink; and
(b) if it is lighter than the solution, it will float on the surface of the solution.

(v) Note the SG of the solution in which blood drop remains suspended for 15 to 20 seconds. This gives the SG of the blood sample. Blood drop remains discrete in the $CuSO_4$ solution due to the covering of *copper proteinate layer,* which is stable for about 15-20 seconds.

II. NORMAL VALUES

SG of blood : 1.048 - 1.066
SG of RBCs : 1.092 - 1.095
SG of plasma : 1.026 - 1.035

IMPORTANT VIVA-VOCE QUESTIONS

Q.1. *Define specific gravity.*

Ans. Specific gravity is defined as the mass of any volume of substance by mass of an equal volume of water at 4°C.

Note: At 4°C density of water is maximum.

Q.2. *Give normal values of SG of blood, RBC and plasma.*

Ans. See above.

Q.3. *What are the physiological and pathological conditions which alter the SG of blood?*

Ans. SG of blood is affected by:
(i) RBC count;
(ii) haemoglobin concentration;
(iii) plasma proteins, and
(iv) water content.

Physiological factors: SG of blood is low in females, in the afternoon, pregnancy and after high water-intake. It is comparatively high in males and at night.

Pathological factors: SG is high due to the loss of water such as vomiting and diarrhoea.

Q.4. *What is the significance of determining the SG of blood?*

Ans. It is used to measure the haemoglobin-content, PCV, blood proteins and degree of dehydration. For example:

(i) Haemoglobin content for 100 ml of blood

$$= \frac{33.9 \text{ (SG of blood - SG of plasma}}{\text{(1.097 - SG of plasma)}} \times 10$$

(ii) PCV

$$= \frac{100 \text{ (SG of blood - SG of plasma}}{\text{(1.097 - SG of plasma)}} \times 10$$

(iii) If the SG of blood is more than the specified range, the degree of dehydration is high and vice-versa.

STUDY NOTES

OBSERVATIONS AND RESULTS

....

....

....

....

COMMENTS AND DISCUSSION

....

....

....

....

....

Date: ....

12 Determination of Erythrocyte Sedimentation Rate (*ESR*) and Packed Cell Volume (*PCV*)

I. APPARATUS

Pricking apparatus, Wintrobe's haematocrit tube with rack, penicillin bottles, Westergren's pipette with rack, long-nozzled capillary pipette (Pasteur pipette), centrifuge machine, powdered mixture of ammonium and potassium oxalate, 3% solution of sodium citrate

Wintrobe's haematocrit tube

1. It is a thick-walled cylindrical tube, approximately 11 cm in length, with an internal bore of 2.5 mm (Fig. 1.12.1).

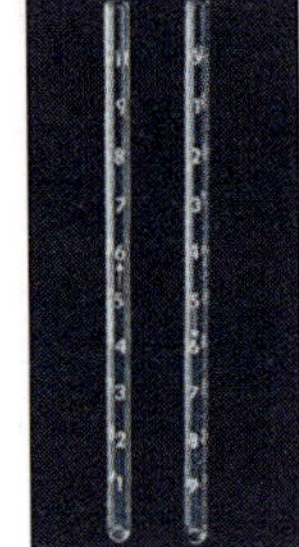

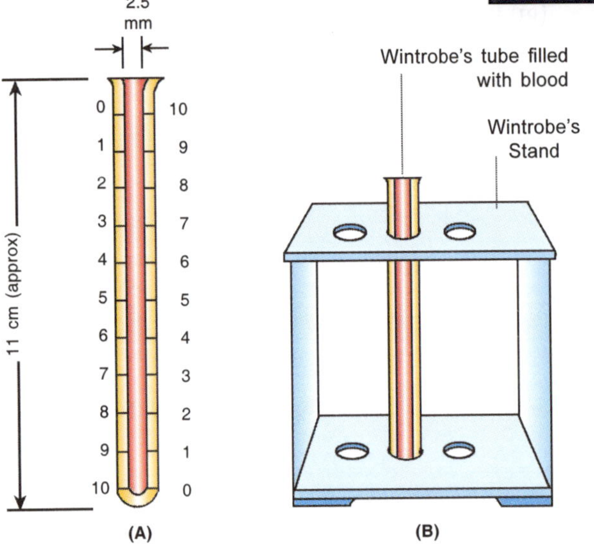

Fig. 1.12.1 Wintrobe's haematocrit tube (A) with its stand (B)

2. The tube is calibrated in both directions from 0-10 cm. Each cm has also been worked in millimetres (mm).
3. The markings, 0 to 10, from above downwards are used for reading ESR. Other graduations from below upwards are meant for PCV values.

Westergren's pipette

1. It is 300 mm (30 cm) long glass pipette (open from both ends) with internal bore of 2.5 mm (Fig. 1.12.2).

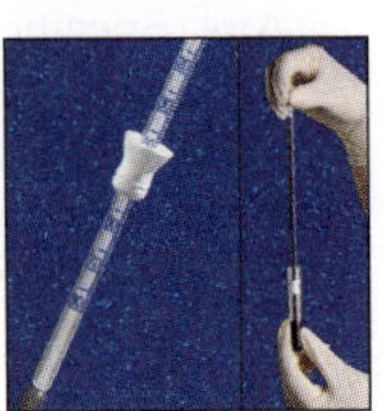

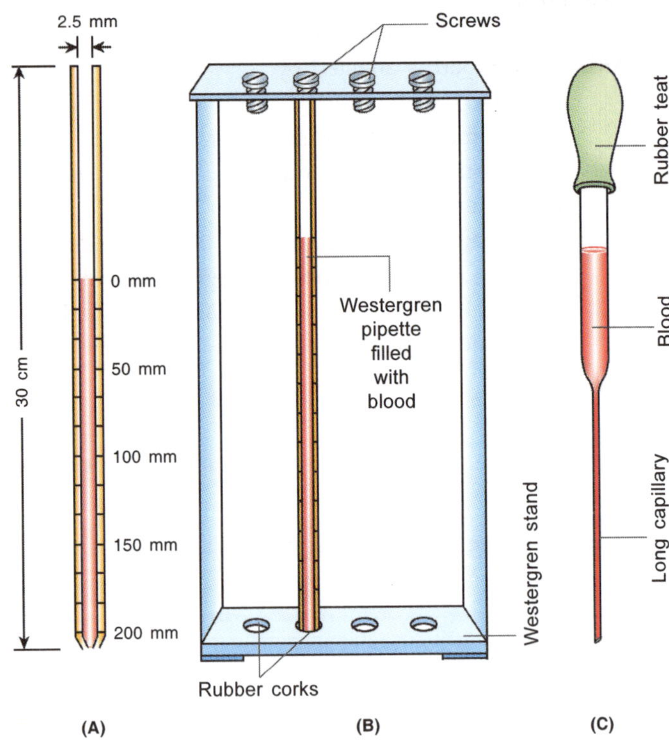

Fig. 1.12.2 Westergren's pipette (A) with its stand (B) and Pasteur pipette (C)

2. The pipette is graduated from 0 to 200 mm only along the lower 2/3rd of its length.
3. The tall rack (*Westergren's stand*) for holding the pipette vertically is provided with rubber corks (pads) at the lower end and clips or screws at the upper end.

II. THEORY

1. **ESR** is the rate at which RBCs settle down when blood, to which anticoagulant is added, is allowed to stand in a narrow tube for **one hour**. The ESR is expressed in mm of clear plasma at the end of the 1st hour.
2. **Mechanism of erythrocyte sedimentation**
   Sedimentation takes place in three stages:
   (i) Stage 1 of about 10 minutes during which time *rouleaux* formation (piling of RBCs) occurs and aggregation occurs;
   (ii) Stage 2 of approx. 40 minutes in which the sinking of the aggregates takes place at a constant speed.
   (iii) Stage 3 of 10 minutes during which aggregated cells pack at the bottom of the tube.

Note: The longer the tube used, the longer the second stage can last and the greater will be the ESR.

3. **PCV** is the volume of cellular elements per unit volume of whole blood. It is expressed as percentage or as number of ml per 100 ml of blood. It is determined by centrifuging oxalated blood in a graduated tube until no further reduction in the volume of cells is noted.

III. PROCEDURE

A. Determination of ESR

Two methods commonly used for ESR determination are: *Wintrobe's method* and *Westergren's method.*

Wintrobe's method

1. Draw 5 ml of venous blood from any convenient vein (antecubital vein is preferred) and gently mix it with powdered mixture of *Double Oxalate* (6 mg of ammonium oxalate and 4 mg of potassium oxalate) in a penicillin bottle.
2. Draw this anticoagulant mixed blood into the long-nozzled capillary pipette and pass the tip of the pipette right down the bottom of the Wintrobe's tube.
3. Applying pressure to the 'teat' of the pipette, force the blood slowly out of the pipette into the haematocrit tube. At the same time the pipette is gradually withdrawn out of the tube. This should be done at such a rate that air bubbles should not form in the tube. (Fig. 1.12.3 A)
4. Fill the tube up to '0' mark and keep it vertically in its rack. Note the time. Take the reading of the upper layer of RBCs (ESR) at the end of one hour. (Fig. 1.12.3 B)

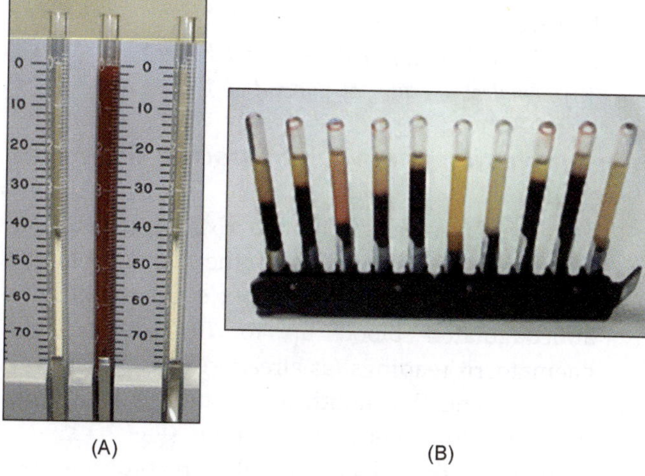

(A) (B)

Fig. 1.12.3 (A) Wintrobe's tube filled with blood and (B) Kept vertically in its rack

5. **Normal values** (Wintrobe's)
   (i) *Males: 0-9 mm at the end of one hour*
   (ii) *Females: 0-20 mm at the end of one hour*

Westergren's method

1. In a penicillin bottle, take 1 ml (or 1 part) of 3.8%, sodium citrate solution (anticoagulant) and mix it gently with 4 ml (or 4 parts) of blood taken after a vene puncture.
2. Suck the citrated blood in the Westergren's pipette up to '0' mark and immediately close its upper opening with the thumb to prevent blood from running down.
3. Then press the lower end tightly on a rubber pad (to prevent blood from escaping) and fix it in an exactly vertical position with levelling screws in the Westergren's stand. (Fig. 1.12.4)

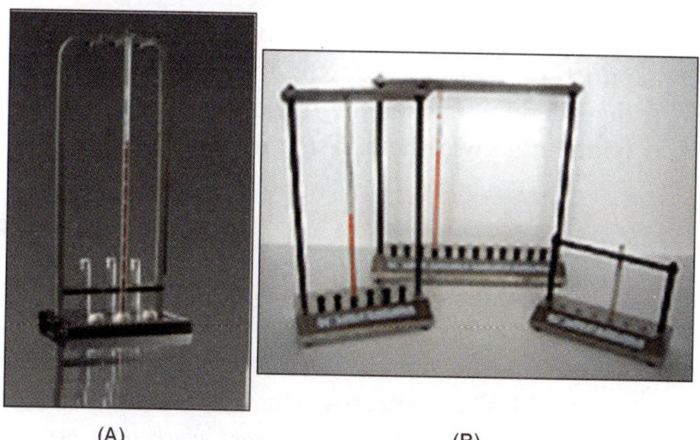

(A) (B)

Fig. 1.12.4 (A) Westergren pipette filled with blood and (B) Kept vertically in its rack

4. Note the time and take the reading for ESR (as above) at the end of one hour.

5. **Normal values** (Westergren's)
   (i) *Males: 3-5 mm at the end of 1 hour*
   (ii) *Females: 4-7 mm at the end of 1 hour*

B. Determination of PCV (Haematocrit): Wintrobe's method

1. Take the powder of double oxalate mixture in a penicillin bottle and add the blood obtained from a vein. Fill the Wintrobe's tube with this anticoagulated blood up to 10 mark of the haematocrit readings (as already explained above).
2. After closing the mouth of the tube with a cork, transfer it to a centrifuge machine. (Fig. 1.12.5 A)
3. Centrifuge the blood at 3,000 revolutions per minute for 30 minutes or more till all the cells have settled down by the centrifugal force. Three layers are formed:
   (i) Clear plasma above.
   (ii) Red layer below, of the RBCs
   (iii) **Buffy layer** in between (i) and (ii) of WBCs and platelets, seen as greyish-red layer. Its normal thickness is about 1 mm. (Fig. 1.12.4 B)
4. Take out the tube and read the PCV (haematocrit) value from the tube. The height of the column of cellular component is taken as PCV. Express the value as the percentage of the blood.
5. **Normal Values**
   (i) *Adult men: average 45% (range 40-50%).*
   (ii) *Adult women: average 42% (range 37-47%).*

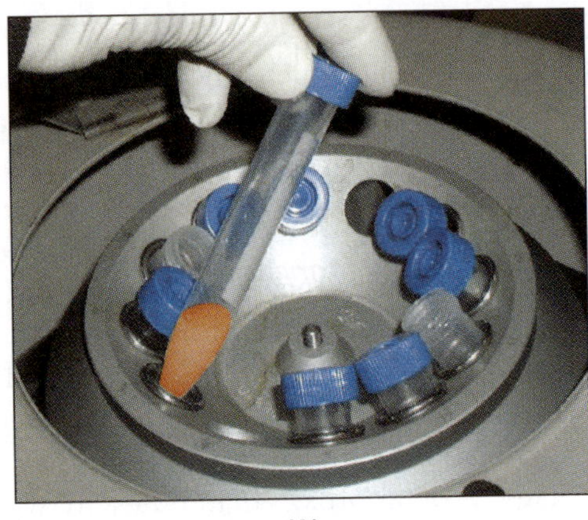

(A)

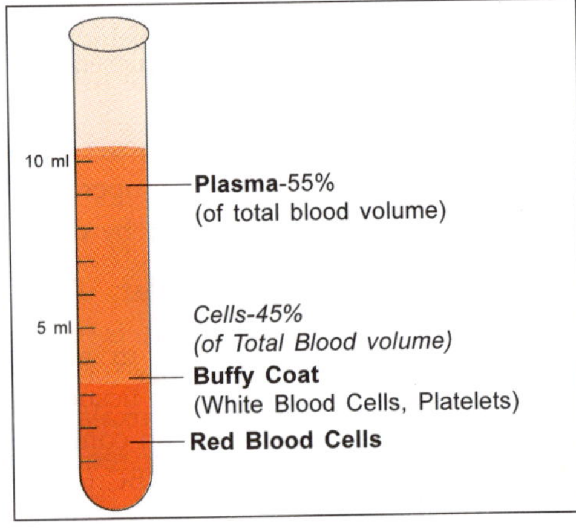

(B)

Fig. 1.12.5 (A) Centrifuge machine with blood filled test tubes (B) Formation of three layers after centrifugation

IV. PRECAUTIONS

1. Arrange and check all the apparatus before starting the experiment.
2. Ensure all glass apparatus like tubes, pipette, dropper, etc. are clear and absolutely dry.
3. Once the blood has been drawn after a vene puncture, detach the needle from the syringe and then gently transfer the blood into the penicillin bottle, otherwise hemolysis might occur.
4. Anticoagulant should be taken in the specific amount for a given method.
5. There should be no air bubble, while filling the Westergren's pipette or Wintrobe's tube with blood.
6. Note the time of fixing the tube/pipette and note the readings exactly after one hour.
7. Fill the pipette again in the event of escape of blood during fixing.

IMPORTANT VIVA-VOCE QUESTIONS

Q.1. *Why do the cells settle down in an anticoagulated sample of blood on standing?*

Ans. Cells settle down due to their greater density (SG 1.090) as compared to that of plasma (SG 1.030).

Q.2. *Explain the role of various factors which influence the process of sedimentation.*

Ans. Factors affecting sedimentation process are:
   (i) *Rouleaux formation* by increasing density and decreasing the surface area increases the settling of RBCs. Rouleaux formation is directly proportional to the concentration of fibrinogen and globulin (α_2, γ) in plasma. It is retarded by albumin.
   (ii) *Viscosity of plasma:* if increases, settling decreases (viscosity of water : plasma : blood :: 1 : 3 : 5).
   (iii) *Ratio of cells to plasma* (normal – 45:55), if alters as in anaemia, increases the rouleaux formation, hence settling of RBCs.

(iv) *Nature of anticoagulant used:* Liquid anticoagulants by altering cell-plasma ratio, increases the ESR.

Q.3. *Why is ESR reading taken normally after one hour?*

Ans. Because during the first hour, more than 95-98% of cells settle down (page 51).

Q.4. *Give the causes of variations in ESR value.*

Ans. *Physiological variations*

(i) Age: Lowest value in newborn (0.5 mm 1st hour – Westergren's method), because RBC count is more.

(ii) Sex: Higher value in females due to low RBCs count.

(iii) Pregnancy: ESR increases as fibrinogen increases during pregnancy (secondary to fall in albumin). This increases rouleaux formation.

(iv) Temperature: ESR values are directly proportional to the temperature within physiological limits. It acts by decreasing the blood viscosity.

Pathological Variations

A. Increase in ESR is seen in any condition which is associated with tissue damage or inflammation, the common conditions being:

(i) anaemia (as ratio of RBC to plasma gets altered);

(ii) any toxic or infective condition (acute or chronic; whether localised or generalised);

(iii) malignancies;

(iv) nephrosis, because it is associated with:

(a) increased fibrinogen and markedly decreased albumin,

(b) marked lipidaemia which increases the globulin.

(v) severe trauma.

B. Decrease in ESR value is found in:

(i) Polycythemia

(ii) Leukaemia

(iii) Pernicious anaemia

(iv) Congestive heart failure

(v) Protein shock e.g. burns, dehydration

(vi) Severe allergic reactions

Q.5. *Give the clinical significance of ESR.*

Ans. (i) ESR values are of no use in diagnosing a disease. It has only **prognostic** value. For example, if ESR increases, it indicates spread of some active disease process in the body.

Note: Estimation of ESR weekly, if shows increase in its value, is indicative of the worsening of condition.

(ii) ESR determination is useful in following the progress of patients suffering from chronic illness, such as pulmonary tuberculosis, rheumatoid arthritis, rheumatism, etc.

Q.6. *What is the advantage of using the double oxalate mixture in Wintrobe's method? Can we use any other anticoagulant?*

Ans. Double oxalate maintains the volume of RBCs constant (ammonium oxalate increases the size of RBCs, whereas potassium oxalate decreases it).

(i) Any anticoagulant like EDTA (1.5 mg/ml) or heparin (15-20 IU/ml) can be used provided it does not alter the plasma-cell ratio.

(ii) This method helps determine the PCV simultaneously.

Note: Liquid sodium citrate solution cannot be used in this method because beside causing the crenation of RBCs it also causes reduction in cell volume.

Q.7. *Give the significance of estimating PCV.*

Ans. (i) It is used as a simple screening test for anaemia.

(ii) It enables the calculation of *absolute values* (page 24).

Q.8. *List the conditions where PCV is increased and decreased.*

Ans. (i) Causes of increase in PCV: Polycythemia, congestive heart failure, protein shock such as burns, dehydration.

(ii) Causes of decrease in PCV: anaemia, bone marrow depression, severe leucopenia.

Q.9. *What contributes to the buffy coat? What is its normal thickness? When does it increase?*

Ans. Page 52. Causes of increase in thickness of buffy coat: Severe leucocytosis, leukaemia, marked increase in platelets.

Q.10. *What is the effect of increased PCV on circulation?*

Ans. Increase in PCV increases the viscosity of blood and hence circulation decreases.

Q.11. *Is there any difference in the PCV of arterial and venous blood?*

Ans. There are swollen RBCs in the venous blood due to the phenomenon of chloride shift; that is why PCV of venous blood is normally 3% greater than that of the arterial blood.

Q.12. *Why are the normal values of ESR more with Wintrobe's method as compared to Westergren's?*

Ans. Wintrobe's method gives higher values of ESR because:

(i) of the nature of powdered mixture of double oxalate anticoagulant used;

(ii) of the effect of atmospheric pressure over the blood column (tube is kept in its rack with top end open).

STUDY NOTES

OBSERVATIONS AND RESULTS

COMMENTS AND DISCUSSION

Date: ....

13 Determination of the Osmotic Fragility of Red Blood Cells

I. APPARATUS

Pricking apparatus, a set of clean test tubes, test tube rack, distilled water, freshly prepared 1% NaCl solution, pipette (2 ml) and dropper

II. THEORY

A. Definition

Ease with which the RBCs are broken down, *i.e.* **hemolysed** in hypotonic solution is called *osmotic fragility of RBCs.* It is expressed in terms of the concentration of hypotonic solution in which the cells are hemolysed.

B. Principle

1. When RBCs are placed in **isotonic solution,** *i.e.* solution with the same tonicity as that of plasma (e.g. 0.9% NaCl; 5% glucose; 10% mannitol and 20% urea solution), they remain suspended in it, *i.e.* neither swell nor shrink. This is because the osmotic pressure of the isotonic solution is equal to the osmotic pressure within the RBCs.
2. However, RBCs, when placed in **hypotonic solution** (e.g. <0.9% NaCl), they swell by absorbing water from outside and finally burst.
3. RBCs, when placed in **hypertonic solution** (e.g. >0.9% NaCl), fluid goes out of cells and they shrink.

C. Significance

1. In normal healthy individuals, osmotic fragility of RBCs **begins** in 0.48% NaCl and **ends** in 0.34% NaCl solution.
2. RBC's osmotic fragility increases when they become spherical e.g. in spherocytosis (independent of the cause). It **begins** in 0.7% NaCl and **ends** in 0.45% NaCl solution.
3. RBC's osmotic fragility is decreased when they become slender e.g. in iron deficiency anaemia and thalassaemia. It **begins** in 0.36% NaCl and **ends** in 0.24% NaCl solution.

III. PROCEDURE

1. Arrange the test tubes in the rack and number them serially from 1 to 12.
2. Prepare the solutions of increasing hypotonicity by mixing the required number of drops (volumes) of 1% NaCl solution and distilled water in serially numbered test tubes 1 to 12 as given in Table 1.13.1.
3. Note that the first tube contains normal saline which is nearly isotonic and the last tube is filled with distilled water (tonicity nil).
4. Shake tubes well and then add a drop of blood in each tube. Invert each tube gently only once to

Table 1.13.1 Procedure for the preparation of increasing hypotonicity of NaCl solution

Test Tube Number	1	2	3	4	5	6	7	8	9	10	11	12
Number of drops of distilled water	3	9	10	11	12	13	14	15	16	17	18	25
Number of drops of 1% NaCl	22	16	15	14	13	12	11	10	9	8	7	0
% saline solution	0.88	0.64	0.60	0.56	0.52	0.48	0.44	0.40	0.36	0.32	0.28	0

Important Note: Use the same dropper (after thorough rinsing) for saline and distilled water so that the volume of drops may be equal for all test tubes.

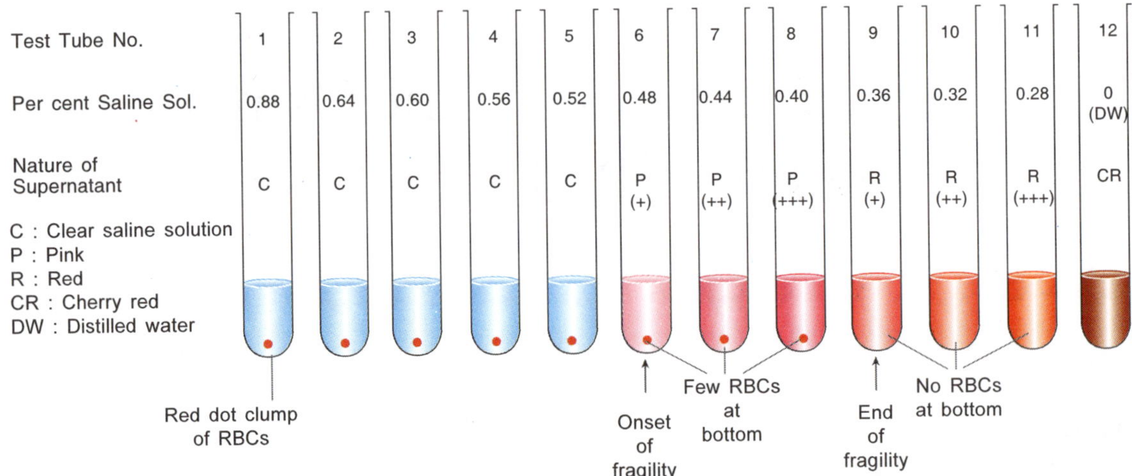

Fig. 1.13.1 Findings of RBC suspension after ONE HOUR in increasing hypotonity of NaCl solution and distilled water

mix the blood with saline. Let all tubes stand for an hour, in order that the unhemolysed RBCs may settle to the bottom. After one hour, observe the tube against white background without shaking.

Since at least 12 drops of blood are required for this test, it is advisable to take 1 ml (16 drops) of blood from a vein by means of syringe and put it into a bottle with anticoagulant such as calcium oxalate. Drops can then be placed in the test tubes by means of a pipette.

5. *Results* (Fig. 1.13.2)
   (i) Test tubes in which **no hemolysis** has occurred, RBCs will be seen forming a red dot at the bottom of the tube with clear saline solution above.

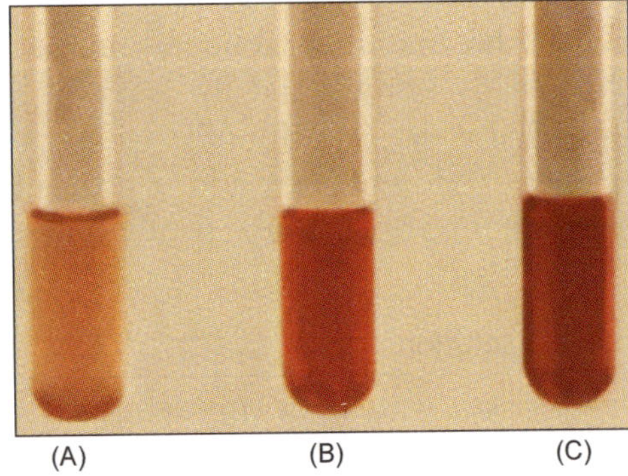

Fig. 1.13.2 (A) No hemolysis, (B) Some hemolysis, (C) Complete hemolysis

   (ii) Test tubes in which **some hemolysis** has occurred, the saline will be tinged red with haemoglobin and some RBCs will be seen as red dot at the bottom of the tube. This is called **onset of fragility**. Normally, this is seen in 0.48% NaCl solution.
   (iii) Test tubes in which **hemolysis is complete**, saline solution will be uniformly red with no red mass at the bottom of the tube, called **ending of fragility**. This usually occurs in 0.34% NaCl solution.

IV. PRECAUTIONS

1. Use the same dropper (after thorough rinsing each time) for saline, distilled water and the blood. (Why? Page 55)
2. After adding blood, the test tubes should be observed **exactly after one hour** without shaking them.

Note: If the test tubes are left as such and observed later, say 4-5 hours, complete hemolysis will occur in all tubes containing hypotonic saline.

3. After adding blood, the test tube should not be shaken vigorously for mixing purpose, otherwise mechanical hemolysis may occur.
4. Maintain the final pH of the blood in saline and the temperature at which the test is carried out.

IMPORTANT VIVA-VOCE QUESTIONS

Q.1. *Define the terms hemolysis and fragility.*

Ans. Hemolysis is defined as the breaking down of RBCs thereby releasing hemoglobin. Fragility is the susceptibility of the RBCs to be broken down.

Q.2. *Give the normal range of the osmotic fragility of RBCs.*

Ans. Page 55.

Q.3. *Give the conditions where osmotic fragility of RBCs is altered.*

Ans. Page 55.

Q.4. *Explain in brief the complications of the hemolysis of RBCs in the body.*

Ans. (i) Hemolysed RBCs cause an increased release of haemoglobin which gets metabolised to bilirubin producing **hemolytic jaundice**.

(ii) If urine is acidic and GFR is slow, the haemoglobin which passes through glomeruli is precipitated in the tubules as **acid haematin**. This obstructs the lumen of tubules producing renal tubular damage. Later **anuria** sets in resulting in renal failure.

(iii) Consequences of renal failure are:

(a) Uraemia (increased accumulation of nitrogenous substances in the body).

(b) Lethargy, coma and death

Q.5. *Name some hemolytic agents.*

Ans. (i) Hypotonic saline;

(ii) Incompatible blood group antigens;

(iii) Bacterial toxins;

(iv) Acids and alkalies;

(v) Snake venoms;

(vi) Hypersensitivity to drugs

Q.6. *What is the effect of the following on the RBCs: (i) 5% glucose, (ii) 10% glucose, (iii) urine, (iv) urea of any strength?*

Ans. (i) **5% glucose**, being isotonic, the RBCs which are suspended undergo no change.

(ii) **10% glucose**: Since it is hypertonic, the cells shrink. However, in vivo, when 10% or 25% glucose is administered into the circulation, initially RBCs shrink but later, after a few hours, glucose gets metabolised in the body and no harmful effects are seen.

(iii) **Urine**, being hypotonic, is able to diffuse into the RBCs, thereby resulting in the swelling of the cells.

(iv) **Urea of any strength**. Urea normally tries to diffuse in, thereby increasing its concentration inside the cell. The ultimate result is hemolysis.

Q.7. *Explain the mechanism ofhemolysis of RBCs in the body.*

Ans. If the surrounding plasma becomes hypotonic, the cell size increases due to end-osmosis; when the capacity of RBCs to accommodate water exceeds, RBCs undergo lysis, thereby releasing haemoglobin into the plasma.

Q.8. *Define terms isotonic and iso-osmotic in respect to solutions. Give examples.*

Ans. (i) Isotonic solutions are those which are said to have the same osmotic pressure as plasma, e.g. 0.9% solution of NaCl.

(ii) Iso-osmotic solutions are those which have the same osmotic pressure e.g. a solution of one mole of NaCl is iso-osmotic with another solution containing 2 moles of glucose.

Q.9. *Will there be any difference in the findings if the test tubes containing different strengths of saline and blood are observed after 5 hours of mixing?*

Ans. Page 56.

Q.10. *What concentration of saline is ideally suitable for diluting blood?*

Ans. Isotonic saline, *i.e.* 0.9% NaCl.

Q.11. *Will vigorous shaking of test tubes to mix the blood and saline solution make any difference in results?*

Ans. Page 56.

Q.12. *Do all the normal RBCs present in the given sample of blood have the same osmotic fragility to hypotonic solutions?*

Ans. Normal RBCs vary in their resistance to hypotonic solutions, the younger cells being the most resistant and the oldest cells the most fragile. This is due to the fact that old cells have a higher sodium-content and a decreased capacity to pump out sodium.

Q.13. *List the factors affecting osmotic-fragility test. Give reasons as well.*

Ans. Factors affecting are:

(i) The relative volume of blood and saline

(ii) The final pH of the blood in saline. The fragility of RBCs increased by a fall in pH. A shift of 0.1 of a pH unit is equivalent to altering saline concentration by 0.01 gm%.

(iii) Temperature - A rise in temperature decreases the fragility; a rise of 0.5°C being equivalent to an increase in saline concentration of 0.01 gm/dL.

Q.14. *What do you expect to osmotic fragility of RBCs in an individual after the removal of his spleen?*

Ans. After splenectomy, RBCs become unusually flattened in which the volume to surface area ratio is decreased and osmotic fragility decreases.

STUDY NOTES

OBSERVATIONS

Carefully observe each tube for the nature of supernatant liquid. Record when hemolysis starts and when it ends.

1. Beginning of hemolysis of RBCs is seen in ......% saline solution.

2. Complete hemolysis of RBCs is seen in ......% saline solution.

RESULT

Osmotic fragility of RBC in a given sample of blood ranges from ......% to ......% saline.

....

....

....

....

COMMENTS AND DISCUSSION

....

....

....

....

....

....

....

....

Date: ....

14 Determination of Platelet Count

I. APPARATUS

Improved Neubauer's counting chamber, RBC pipette, platelet diluting fluid (1% ammonium oxalate), compound microscope, cover-slips, pricking apparatus

Platelet diluting fluid

1% ammonium oxalate. It acts as:

(i) anticoagulant
(ii) preserves the platelets, and
(iii) destroys the RBCs

II. PRINCIPLE

The number of platelets in a sample of diluted blood is counted in a hemocytometer of known dimension. From the number of cells seen, the total platelet count of the undiluted sample is calculated.

III. PROCEDURE

1. Prick the finger under aseptic precautions and suck the blood up to 0.5 mark in the RBC pipette and then suck the platelet diluting fluid (1% ammonium oxalate) up to 101 mark (dilution factor is 1 : 200, refer to page 21).
2. Mix the solution and blood and wait for **10-15 minutes**. This is important for the complete hemolysis of RBCs, thus to get clear background at the time of counting the platelets.
3. Discard first a few drops and charge the improved Neubauer's chamber as explained earlier (page 19). Place the charged chamber in a moist petri dish (wet filter paper at the bottom). Wait for another **20-30 minutes** to allow the platelets to settle down.
4. Under high power objective (X40) of microscope, count the platelets in all the 25 RBC squares, *i.e.* central square (1 mm × 1 mm). Count the platelets on both sides of the chamber.

Note: The platelets can be seen as tiny (2-4 μm) diameter, well separated, highly refractile rounded bodies with silvery appearance. They can be recognised by carefully altering the focus of the microscope with fine adjustment and by reducing the illumination by closing iris diaphragm. (Fig. 1.14.1)

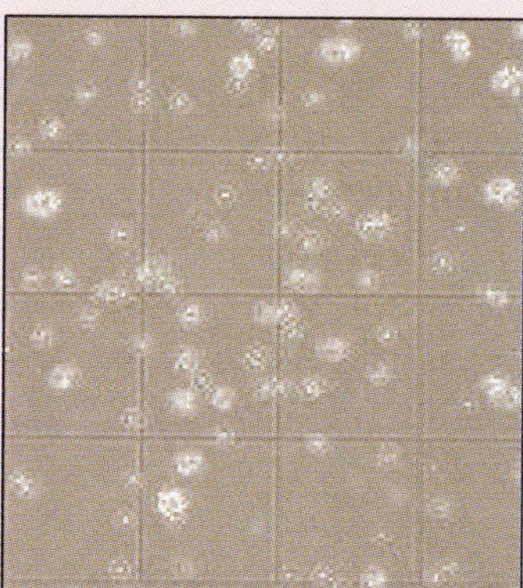

Fig. 1.14.1 Platelets under low power seen as refractile bodies

5. Count the platelets in all the 25 RBCs central squares under high power. (Fig. 1.14.2)

IV. CALCULATIONS

A. Dilution factor: 200 (page 21).

B. Volume of fluid examined in 25 RBC squares

$= 1 \text{ mm} \times 1 \text{ mm} \times 0.1 \text{ mm}$

$= 0.1 \ \mu L$

C. Total number of platelets per μL of blood:

Let 'N' be the total number of platelets in 25 RBC squares, *i.e.* 0.1 μL of diluted blood.

Then, the number of platelets in 1 μL of undiluted blood:

$$= \frac{N \times \text{dilution factor (200)}}{0.1}$$

$$= N \times 10 \times 200$$

$$= N \times 2000$$

V. PRECAUTIONS

1. The same as observed for RBC count (page 21).
2. Special care must be taken so that the apparatus and the diluting fluid may not get contaminated either with dust particles or bacteria, both of which may simulate platelets.

IMPORTANT VIVA-VOCE QUESTIONS

Q.1. *Name the other diluting fluids which may be used for platelet count.*

Ans. Direct REES-ECKER diluting fluid can be used for platelet count. Each 100 ml of fluid contains:

(i) Sodium citrate 3.8 gm (as anticoagulant).
(ii) Brilliant cresyl blue 0.1 gm (for staining purposes).
(iii) Formalin or formaldehyde - 2 ml (fixative for stain and for lysis of RBCs).
(iv) Distilled water: 100 ml (solvent)

Platelets are seen as bluish, tiny bodies, fairly regular in outline. The freshly prepared solution should be used, otherwise formaldehyde gets converted into formic acid which destroys the platelets.

Q.2. *Give the normal range of platelet count.*

Ans. The normal platelet count is 0.15 to 0.4 million/μL (1.5-4 lacs/μL). Average 2.59 lacs/μL. Its count is very much constant.

Q.3. *Enumerate the functions of platelets.*

Ans. Platelets play an important role in:

(i) Haemostasis, *i.e.* arrest of bleeding
(ii) Blood coagulation
(iii) Clot retraction
(iv) The phagocytosis of carbon particles, viruses and immune complexes
(v) The storage of 5 HT and histamine, which are released when the platelets disintegrate and act on the blood vessel (for details, refer to the textbook).

Q.4. *Give the life-span and site of the destruction of platelets.*

Ans. The average life-span of a platelet is 8-12 days. Platelets get destroyed mainly in spleen. That is why in hypersplenism they may almost disappear from circulation.

Q.5. *Define thrombocytosis and thrombocytopenia. Give their common causes.*

Ans. A. Thrombocytosis, *i.e.* increase in platelet count.

Causes:

(i) After the administration of epinephrine due to splenic contraction
(ii) After trauma e.g. surgery, injury, childbirth, etc.
(iii) Splenectomy, *i.e.* after the removal of spleen.
(iv) Stress, it causes increased epinephrine release.

B. Thrombocytopenia, *i.e.* decrease in platelet count. *Causes:*

(i) Bone marrow depression
(ii) Hypersplenism
(iii) Viral infections e.g. dengue fever, it particularly attacks platelets.
(iv) Drug hypersensitivity

Q.6. *What do the platelets look like in a peripheral blood smear, stained with Leishman's stain. Is it possible to make platelet count in stained smear?*

Ans. With Leishman staining platelets are seen in clumps as faint blue cytoplasm with distinct reddish purple granules, nucleus is not present. It is not possible to do platelet count because they are aggregated.

Q.7. *What is purpura?*

Ans. It is a clinical condition in which capillary abnormality results in bleeding. It is characterized by spontaneous haemorrhage beneath the skin, mucous membrane and in the internal organs.

Q.8. *Grade the severity of purpura based on platelet count.*

Ans. Purpura with low platelet count is called *thrombocytopenic purpura.* It can be graded as:

(i) Mild purpura - platelet count less than 50,000/μL.
(ii) Moderate purpura - platelet count less than 10,000/μL. It is associated with severe bleeding.
(iii) Fulminating purpura - platelet count less than 1000/μL.

STUDY NOTES

OBSERVATIONS AND CALCULATIONS

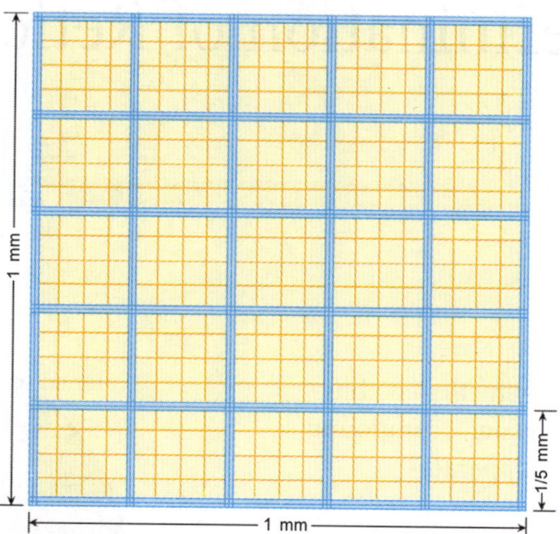

Fig. 1.14.2 Enter your observations in the central RBC square (dimension 1 mm × 1 mm)
Total number of platelets in 25 RBCs squares ....

RESULT

The total platelet count of my blood is

....

....

....

....

COMMENTS AND DISCUSSION

(State whether it is within the normal range or not. If not, comment on the possible causes.)

....

....

....

....

....

....

Date: ....

15 Determination of Reticulocyte Count

I. APPARATUS

Glass slides, brilliant cresyl blue or new methylene blue, incubator, anti-coagulant, distilled water, compound microscope, cedar-wood oil, pricking apparatus

II. THEORY

1. Reticulocytes (8 µm diameter) are ***juvenile RBCs***. They contain large amounts of the remnants of ribosomes and RNA. Chemically, the basophilic reticulum is RNA which is the remnant of the cytoplasm of the precursor cells.
2. Ribosomes have the property of reacting with certain dyes such as brilliant cresyl blue or new methylene blue to form a blue precipitate of granules or filaments. This reaction takes place only in **supravitally stained** unfixed preparations, *i.e.* staining cells in the living state at normal body temperature (37°C) before they have been killed by fixation, drying or lapse of time. They are used especially for blood cells. Only under these conditions, the ribosomal RNA takes up the stain.
3. The maturity of a reticulocyte is inversely related to the quantity of ribosomal material present. Therefore, the *most immature reticulocytes* are those with the largest amount of precipitable ribosomal material. On the contrary, in the *least immature*, only a few dots or short strands are seen (Fig. 1.15.1).
4. In pathological conditions e.g. lead poisoning, this stained material is sometimes present in clumps which appear as discrete particles. This is called **punctate basophilia**.

III. VITAL STAINS USED FOR DEMONSTRATION OF RETICULOCYTES

1. 1% brilliant cresyl blue in isotonic saline or methyl alcohol.

Or

2. 1 gm of ***new methylene blue*** is dissolved in 100 ml of iso-osmotic phosphate buffer, pH 7.4 (*i.e.* 24.3 gm/L of NaH_2PO_4 and 21.3 gm/L of Na_2HPO_4 for iso-osmotic buffer). It is *superior* to brilliant cresyl blue stain because it stains the reticulo-filamentous material in the reticulocytes more deeply and more uniformly.

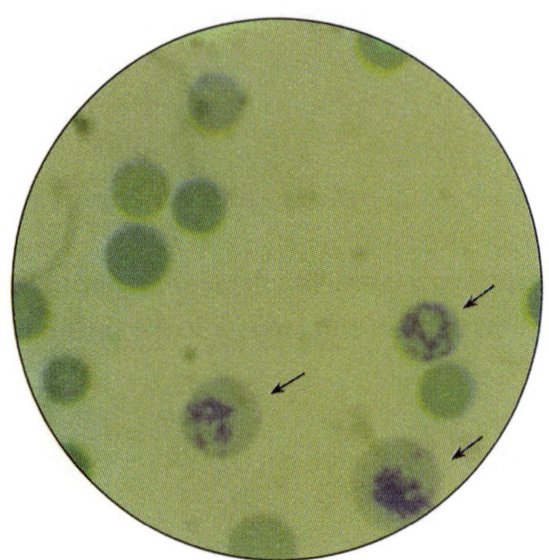

Fig. 1.15.1 Peripheral Blood Smear showing RBCs and Reticulocytes with fine reticular fibrils (arrows) – Supravital Staining

Important Note: New methylene blue is chemically different from methylene blue which is a poor reticulocyte stain and is prepared by dissolving 1 gm of methylene blue in 100 gm of citrate-saline buffer, pH 7.4 (3 gm/L sodium citrate + 9 gm/L NaCl + bicarbonate buffer, pH 7.4.

IV. PROCEDURE

1. Take 2 or 3 drops of vital stain in a test tube and add an equal number of drops of blood. Keep the test tube in an incubator at 37°C for 15-20 minutes. This is to simulate the living conditions so that the stain may go into the cells.
2. The RBCs are then re-suspended by gentle thorough mixing.
3. Make 4-5 moderately thick smear of this mixture on glass slides, dry and see under oil immersion without being fixed or counter-stained.

V. OBSERVATIONS

1. In a successful preparation, reticulocytes can be identified by their large size (diameter 8 µm, larger than surrounding RBCs) with reticulo-filamentous material in the cytoplasm stained deep blue. The RBCs and other non-reticulated cells are stained with the diffuse shades of pale-greenish-blue colour.
2. Put a small piece of paper with a hole in its centre below the eye piece lens. This will restrict the microscopic field. Use the mechanical stage to traverse the full length of the film.
3. For counting, an area of film should be chosen where the cells are undistorted and where the staining is good.
4. Count the RBCs under oil immersion in different microscopic fields (Fig. 1.7.7 page 34). Count 500 RBCs and record the number of reticulocytes encountered in this cell population as given below.

Field No.	Number of reticulocytes (1)	Number of RBCs (2)	Total Number of cells (1) + (2)
1			
2			
3			
⋮			
10			

4. Express the reticulocyte percentage as:

$$\frac{\text{No. of reticulocytes}}{\text{Total No. of RBCs counted}} \times 100$$

VI. NORMAL VALUES

1. Adults and children:
   (i) 0.2-2% (average 1%)
   (ii) Absolute count: 24000-84000/µL
2. Infants: 2-6%
3. Newborn: 30-50%, decreases to 1-2% in the first week of life.

Important Note: The percentage of reticulocytes in the blood is a fairly accurate reflection of the erythropoietic activity. Therefore, their number is increased whenever RBCs are being rapidly manufactured.

Reticulocytosis, *i.e.* increase in the reticulocyte count; it is seen in:

1. Recovery from anaemia. For example: the first blood change noticed when iron deficiency anaemia is treated with iron or when pernicious anaemia is treated with vitamin B_{12} injection. The increase in reticulocytes count following recovery from anaemia is called **Reticulocytic Response**.
2. After haemorrhage
3. Proliferation of bone marrow

IMPORTANT VIVA-VOCE QUESTIONS

Q.1. *What are the indications of doing a reticulocyte count?*

Ans. Indications are:
(i) In all conditions where reticulocytosis is suspected.
(ii) Haemolytic anaemia (reticulocytosis reflects haemolysis).
(iii) In jaundice to differentiate between pre-hepatic, hepatic and post-hepatic jaundice.

Q.2. *What is supravital staining? How does it differ from vital staining?*

Ans. Supravital staining - Definition (page 62).
Vital staining is the process where stains are used to colour living tissues by the injection of the dyes.

Q.3. *Why is it necessary to perform a supravital staining to demonstrate a reticulocyte?*

Ans. Because only under supravital conditions will a dye enter a cell.

Q.4. *What is the reticulum made up of clinically?*

Ans. Page 62.

Q.5. *Where does the ripening of the RBCs take place?*

Ans. The ripening of RBCs starts in the bone marrow and is completed in circulation, especially in spleen. It takes 2-3 days, out of which 24 hours are spent in circulation.

Q.6. *Give the normal values for reticulocyte count at different ages?*

Ans. See above.

Q.7. *Give the causes of reticulocytosis.*

Ans. (A) **Physiological**: Newborn, hypoxic conditions (high altitude), menstruation
(B) **Pathological**: Haemorrhage, haemolytic anaemia, hereditary spherocytosis, sickle cell anaemia, thalassaemia (any condition which causes the proliferation of bone marrow tissues).

Q.8. *What is reticulocytic response?*

Ans. See above.

Q.9. *List the differentiating features of reticulocyte from a erythrocyte.*

Ans. A reticulocyte:

(i) is a bit larger than a RBC;

(ii) contains a central core of RNA which takes up a basic stain.

Q.10. *Whether the exercise or smoking has any effect on reticulocyte count?*

Ans. Moderate to severe exercise and heavy smoking increases the reticulocyte count.

Q.11. *How does new methylene blue stain differ from methylene blue stain ?*

Ans. Page 62.

Q.12. *Why is it necessary to restrict the microscopic field to count the cells?*

Ans. Because this will allow the easy counting of cells and avoid the recounting of RBCs.

STUDY NOTES

OBSERVATIONS AND RESULTS

....

....

....

....

COMMENTS AND DISCUSSION

....

....

....

....

....

....

....

....

....

Date: ....

16 Determination of Absolute Eosinophil Count

I. APPARATUS

Improved Neubauer's counting chamber, WBC pipette, petridish, compound microscope, pricking apparatus, alcohol, filter paper, pilot's solution and diluting fluid

Composition of Pilot's solution

Each 100 ml of solution contains:

1. *Phloxine:*
   10 ml (stains only eosinophilic granules)
2. *Propylene glycol:*
   50 ml (solvent for stain and lyses RBCs)
3. *Sodium carbonate (1% aqueous solution):*
   1 ml (to enhance the staining of the eosinophil granules)
4. *Heparin:* 100 units (anticoagulant)
5. *Distilled water:*
   As required to make 100 ml. It lyses all WBCs except eosinophils which seems more resistant than other WBCs in this respect.

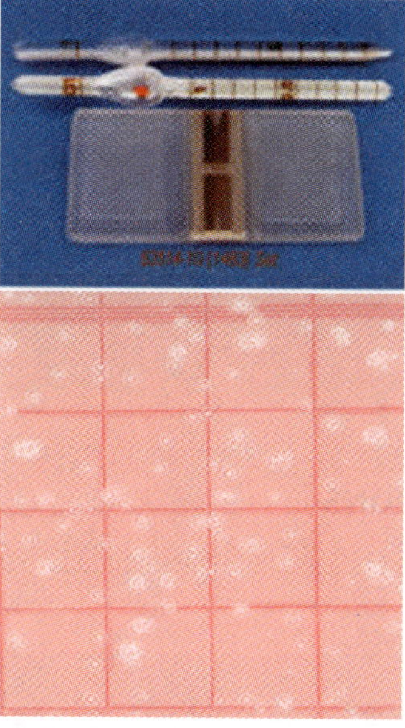

Fig. 1.16.1 (A) Haemocytometry for absolute eosinophil count (B) Eosinophils as seen under high power

II. PROCEDURE

1. With necessary precautions required for haemocytometry (page 19), suck the blood in WBC pipette exactly up to 0.5 mark and then suck Pilot's fluid up to mark 11 (dilution factor 1 : 20). (Fig. 1.16.1)
2. Gently shake the pipette well between the palms for 2-3 minutes.
3. Place a moistened filter paper in a petridish and keep the filled pipette on it.
4. Allow the pipette to remain in the moistened atmosphere for 15 minutes.
5. Remove the pipette from the petridish, shake it, discard first a few drops of fluid in its stem and charge the counting chamber.
6. Place the counting chamber in moist surroundings (as above, step 3). This allows the staining to occur without the evaporation of the fluid.
7. Count the eosinophils (seen as pink cells with nuclei) in the four WBC corner squares *preferably* under high power. Determine absolute eosinophils count per μL of blood (N × 50) (Refer to TLC, page 28) and (Fig. 1.16.2).

III. PRECAUTIONS

The same as followed for doing TLC, page 28.

IMPORTANT VIVA-VOCE QUESTIONS

Q.1. *Explain the clinical significance of absolute eosinophil count.*

Ans. This investigation helps diagnose the various diseases which especially alter the eosinophil count only.

Q.2. *Give the normal range of absolute eosinophil count.*

Ans. Normal value: 150-300/μL.

Q.3. *List the conditions which alter the eosinophil count.*

Ans. Page 37.

Q.4. *Mention any other diluting fluid used for this method.*

Ans. Dunger's fluid can also be used. It contains eosin instead of phloxine and acetone instead of propylene glycol.

Q.5. *Enumerate the functions of eosinophil.*

Ans. Eosinophil

(i) Phagocytose antigen-antibody reaction complex
(ii) Its granules are lysosomal in character.
(iii) It has a very high peroxidase-content.
(iv) It limits:
  (a) antigen-antibody reaction;
  (b) the effect of mediators such as histamine and bradykinin.

Q.6. *What is the advantage of determining absolute eosinophil count (AEC) over the eosinophils expressel as percentage of total leucocyte count (TLC)?*

Ans. The percentage of eosinophil remains unchanged with the proportionate increase or decrease in all types of the leucocytes (such as bone marrow hyper or hypoplasia). AEC changes exclusively with variations in eosinophils only.

STUDY NOTES

OBSERVATIONS

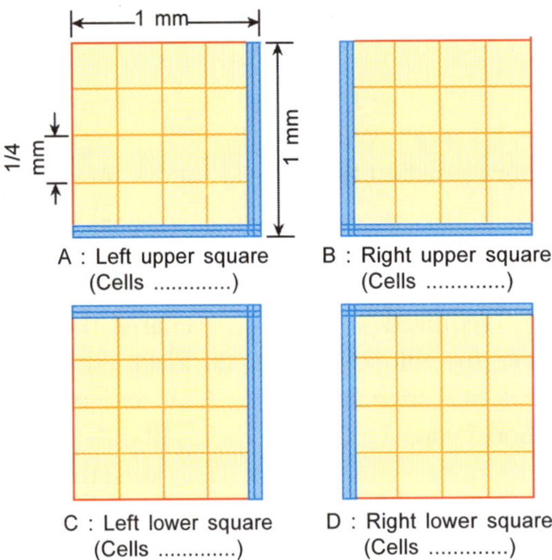

Fig. 1.16.2 Enter the observations after counting eosinophils in the corresponding WBCs squares.

CALCULATIONS

Calculate the number of eosinophils per cumm of blood (N × 50) (refer to total leucocyte count, page 22).

....

....

RESULTS, COMMENTS AND DISCUSSION

....

....

Date: ....

17 Study of the Haemopoietic Cells Present in the Bone Marrow

I. APPARATUS

Marrow biopsy aspiration needle: either **Salah's** or **Klima's** or **Jamshidi's biopsy needle**, glass slides, compound microscope, cedar-wood oil, Leishman's stain, Pasteur pipette

Marrow puncture needle

Most commonly used marrow puncture needles are *Salah's or Jamshidi's needles.* These are stout and made of hard stainless steel, about 7-8 cm in length, with a well-fitting **stilette** and provided with an **adjustable guard** (Fig. 1.17.1).

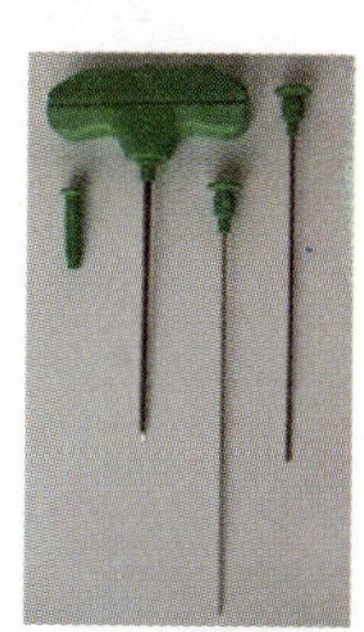

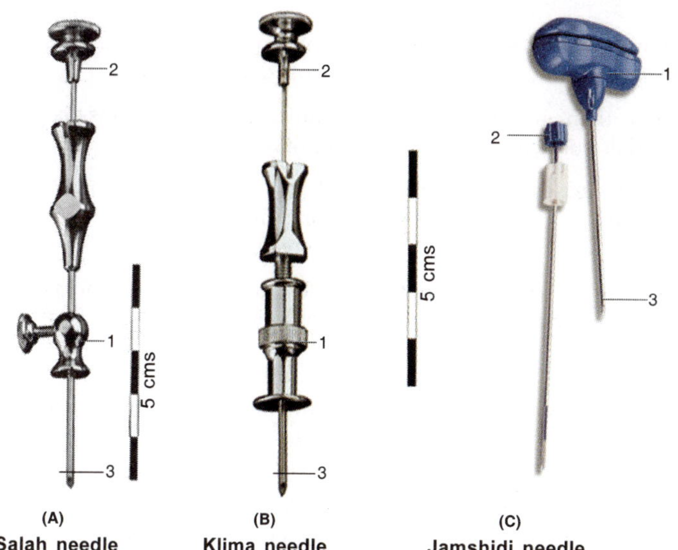

Fig. 1.17.1 Bone marrow puncture needles:
1. Adjustable guard, 2. Stilette, 3. Puncture needle

II. THEORY

A. Types of bone marrow

The bone marrow is of two types: Red and Yellow (*see* Table 1.17.1).

Table 1.17.1 Red bone marrow versus yellow bone marrow

Red bone marrow	Yellow bone marrow
1. It consists of numerous blood cells of all kinds and their precursors.	1. It consists of fat cells, blood vessels and a minimal framework of reticulum cells and fibres.
2. It is also called **active** marrow.	2. It is also called **inactive** marrow.
3. It includes the ends of long bones.	3. It includes the shaft of the bones.

Important Note: Up to the age of 20 years, all the bones contain active red marrow. After this age the red marrow is replaced by yellow inactive marrow in all the long bones of the body.

B. Biopsy of bone marrow

Bone marrow biopsy is an indispensable adjunct to the study of diseases of the blood. Marrow can be obtained by:

1. Needle aspiration (*needle or aspiration biopsy*);
2. Percutaneous trephine biopsy; and
3. Surgical biopsy

Needle (aspiration) biopsy

Advantages

1. It is simple and relatively painless and can be repeated many times.
2. It can be performed on out-patients.
3. It is safe in almost all circumstances, even in thrombocytopenic purpura.
4. Individual cells are perfectly preserved after staining. The difference between the cells can be recognised to a greater degree.

Disadvantages

1. The arrangement of the cells in the marrow and the relationship between one cell and another are more or less destroyed by the process of aspiration.

2. In fibrotic marrows, little or no blood may be aspirated (***Dry tap*** *or* ***blood tap***).

Contra-indication

It should never be attempted when there is a major disorder of coagulation as in haemophilia.

Indications

1. Absolute: megaloblastic anaemias; aleukaemic leukaemia
2. Diagnostic: aplastic anaemia, multiple myeloma
3. Confirmatory: all types of leukaemias; idopathic thrombocytopenic purpura; iron-deficiency anaemia
4. Transplantation: bone marrow grafting

C. Sites of Aspiration

1. In adults:
   - (i) Sternum: manubrium (preferred) or first or second piece of the body
   - (ii) Posterior superior iliac spine
   - (iii) Anterior iliac crest
2. In children (less than 2 years) – in addition to above sites:
   - (i) Tibia – medial aspect of upper end (site of choice)
   - (ii) Calcaneum

D. Myelogram

Cell count on aspirated normal bone marrow.

1. The percentage of haemopoietic cells (RBC, WBC and platelets series) in healthy adults is 50-80% in 0.25-0.5 ml bone marrow samples. The remaining are the fatty cells.
2. The degree of cellularity can be expressed as increased, normal or reduced. In general:
   - (i) if less than 25% of the particles is occupied by haemopoietic cells, it is **hypocellular**; and
   - (ii) if more than 75-80% are haemopoietic cells, it is **hypercellular**.
3. Physiological variations in the cell-content:
   - (i) In adults, a smaller proportion of the marrow cavity is occupied by haemopoietic marrow than in children and the proportion of fat cells to cellular marrow is increased.

E. Description of Cells Seen in Bone Marrow (refer to Fig. 1.17.2)

	Cell size	Nucleus	Cytoplasm
Erythrocyte Series, i.e. **RBCs and their precursors**			
1. Proerythroblast	15-20 μm	Very big, occupies 3/4 of cell volume; 2-3 nucleoli; chromatin open	Scanty, only a rim around the nucleus; deep basophilic
2. Early Normoblast	10-14 μm	Size decreases than its precursor; chromatin further condenses	Amount increases, remains deep basophilic
3. Intermediate Normoblast	10-14 μm	Size further decreases; chromatin further condenses	Marked; polychromatophilic staining due to the appearance of haemoglobin
4. Late Normoblast	7-10 μm	Very small with chromatin dot (*pyknotic*), uniformly deeply stained	Further increases, more acidic, less basophilic
Myeloid Series: **Granulocytes and their precursors**			
1. Myeloblast	16-20 μm	Large; occupying most of the cell; purple blue; many nucleoli; fine chromatin	Narrow blue rim all around the nucleus, no granules
2. Premyelocyte	14-18 μm	Size decreases, nucleoli disappears, chromatin condenses	Amount increases further; basophilic no granules
3. Myelocyte proper	12-16 μm	Size further decreases	Amount increases, less basophilic, *granules appear* (maximum in neutrophils)
4. Metamyelocyte	10-14 μm	Size further decreases; becomes indented and lobed	Amount further increases; granules take up specific staining and *show movements*
Megakaryocytes, i.e. **platelets and their precursors**			
These are giant cells with 35-160 μm diameter, multinucleated, *i.e.* contain irregular rings of lobed nuclei with dense purplish granular cytoplasm.			

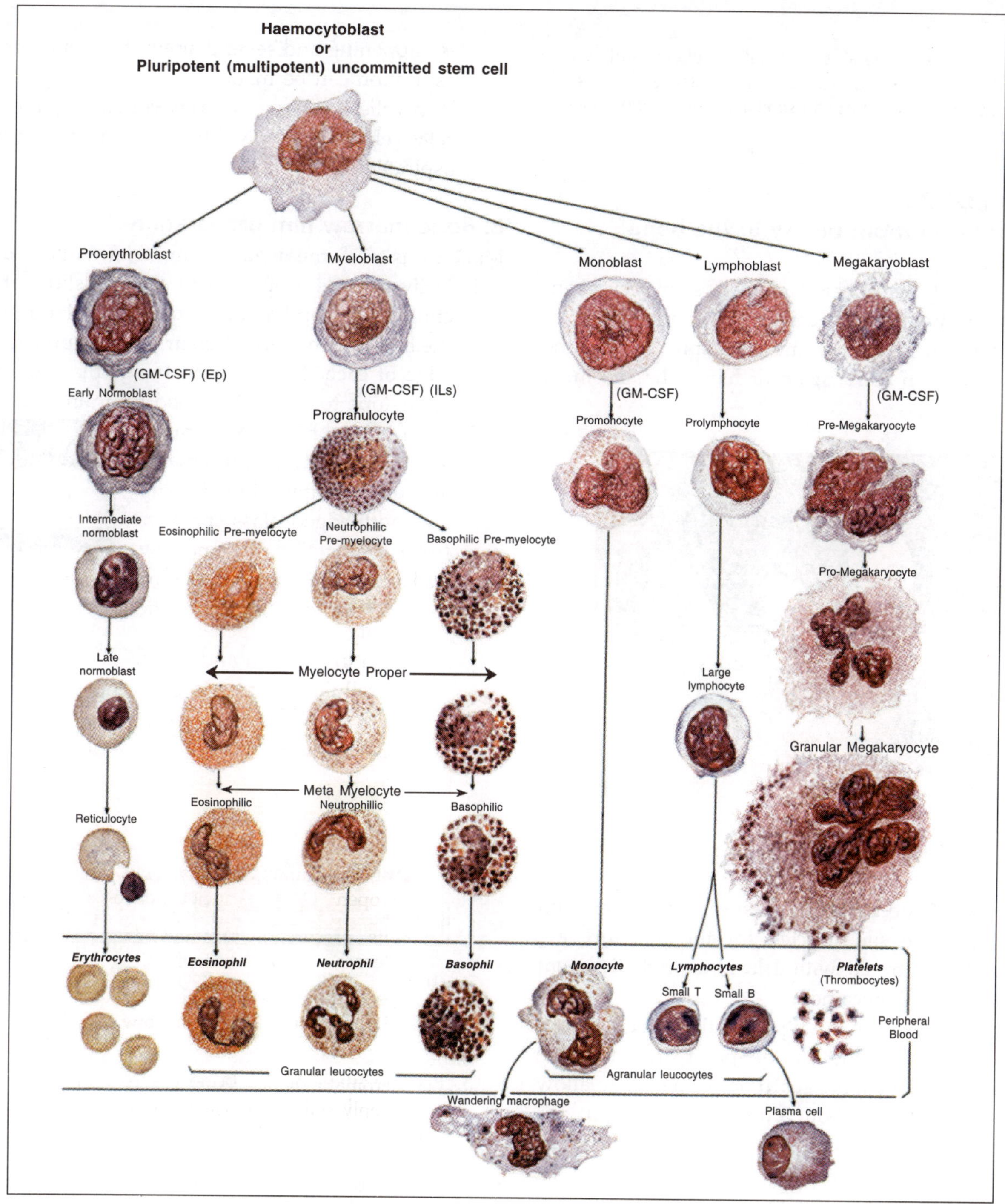

Fig. 1.17.2 Haemopoietic cells in the Bone Marrow
(IL: Interleukins; Ep: Erythropoietin; GM-CSF: Granulocyte macrophage colony stimulating factor)

(ii) The marrow undergoes slight to moderate hyperplasia in pregnancy; maximal in the third trimester.

4. *Ratios (normal range):*
   (i) Myeloid : erythroid ratio : : 2.5-15 : 1.
   (ii) Leuco : erythrogenic ratio : : 0.56-2.67 : 1.
   (iii) Myeloid : lymphoid ratio : : 1-1.7 : 1.
   (iv) Lymphoid : erythroid ratio : : 0.2-4.0 : 1.
5. *Normal values*
   (i) Percentage of erythroblasts: falls from birth, and at 2-3 weeks they form 10% of nucleated cells.
   (ii) Myeloid cells (granulocyte precursors): increase during first two weeks of life, then sharp fall occurs at the 3rd week, and by the end of the 1st month, 60% of the cells are myeloid.
   (iii) Lymphocytes:
   infants – 40% of nucleated cells
   at 2 years – 20% of nucleated cells
   afterwards – 15% of nucleated cells

Important Note: In general, the overall cellularity and type of maturity of haemopoiesis and the balance between erythropoiesis and leucopoiesis are similar of marrow withdrawn from different sites.

III. PROCEDURE

A. Needle (aspiration) biopsy of the bone marrow (Fig. 1.17.3)

1. The patient lies on his back in a semi-recumbent position and the skin covering the upper part of the sternum is cleaned first with spirit and iodine and then with spirit again (if hairy, the site must be shaved).

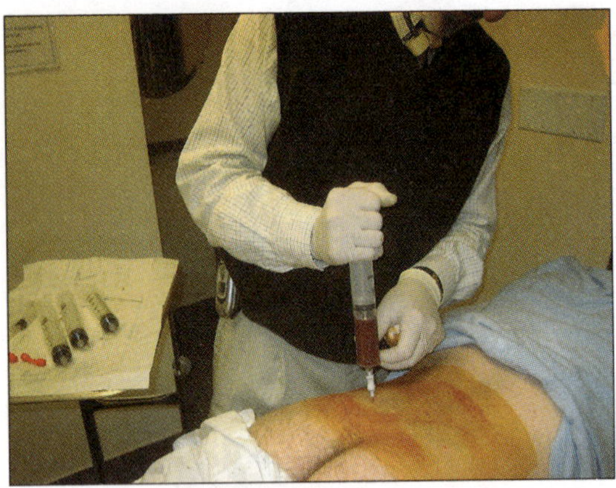

Fig. 1.17.3 Bone marrow biopsy procedure

2. The skin, subcutaneous tissue and periosteum overlying the site selected for the puncture are carefully infiltrated with a local anaesthetic agent (such as 2% lignocaine).
3. Puncture the skin and pierce the subcutaneous tissues. When the needle-point reaches the periosteum, adjust the guard on the needle to allow it to penetrate for about 5 mm further, and fix the guard tightly in position.
4. Then push the needle with a boring motion into the cavity of the bone. The amount of force required varies. It is usually easy to appreciate when the cavity of the bone has been entered; there is a **feeling of sudden loss of resistance**.
5. Remove the stilette and with a well-fitting 2 or 5 ml syringe suck up about 0.2 to 0.3 ml of marrow content (bone marrow diluted with a variable amount of blood).
6. If there has been a **dry tap** (or **blood tap**), repeat the whole procedure at some other appropriate site.

Puncture of the ilium

Advantage of puncturing the ilium is that:

1. The patient can lie on his side and cannot see what is happening and several attempts at puncture and aspiration can be made.
2. It overlies a large marrow-containing area and relatively a large volume of marrow can be aspirated from this site.

B. Bone marrow film preparation

Make films from the aspirated material without delay.

1. Deliver single drops of aspirate onto slides about 1 cm from one end and then quickly suck off most of the blood with a fine Pasteur pipette applied to the edge of each drop. (Alternatively, place the slides on a slope to allow the blood to drain away.)
2. Then make films, 3-5 cm in length, of the marrow fragments and the remaining blood using a smooth-edged glass spreader (refer to page 29). The marrow fragments are dragged behind the spreader and leave a trail of cells behind them (Fig. 1.17.4).

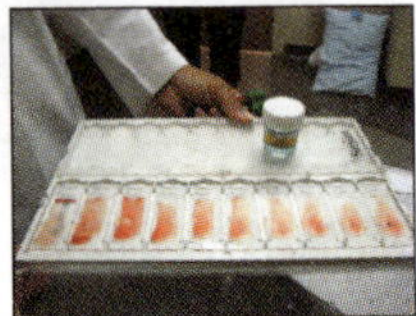

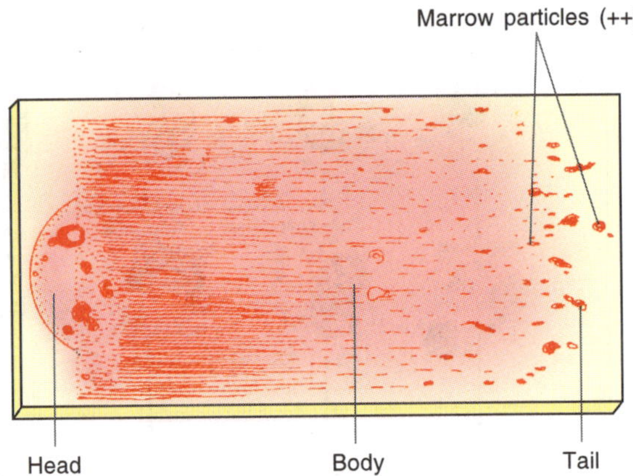

Fig. 1.17.4 Film of aspirated bone marrow

3. Fix the films of the bone marrow and stain them with Leishman's stain as for peripheral blood films (page 31).

Note: *A longer fixation time, at least 20 minutes, is needed in methanol for high-quality staining.*

IV. PRECAUTIONS

1. Follow all the precautions as already described on page 35 for preparation and staining of a peripheral blood smear.
2. All indications and contra-indications should be thoroughly kept in mind before starting the procedure (page [illegible]).
3. Reassure the patient beforehand and explain the procedure to overcome any anxiety or apprehension in him.
4. After the biopsy has been done, follow the patient

for any major bleeding from the site of puncture for at least half an hour.

5. Adhere strictly to all the aseptic precautions throughout the procedure including careful washing of the hands of the examiner.

Important Note

Reporting of the Results: The following format is usually adopted for reporting the results on bone marrow examination:

1. *Description of general cellularity of the marrow:* hypo; normo; or hyper-plastic.
2. *Description of the type of erythropoiesis:* megaloblastic or normoblastic.
3. *Description of the general maturity of the erythropoietic and leucopoietic cells.*
4. *Estimation of the ratios:*
   (i) myeloid : erythroid ratio
   (ii) leuco : erythrogenic ratio
   (iii) myeloid : lymphoid ratio
   (iv) lymphoid : erythroid ratio

IMPORTANT VIVA-VOCE QUESTIONS

Q.1. *Is there any variation in the component of cellular marrow withdrawn from diffrerent sites?*

Ans. No (refer to page 70).

Q.2. *Enumerate the indications of bone marrow examination.*

Ans. Page 68.

Q.3. *What are the other uses of studying the bone marrow?*

Ans. Bone marrow studies are also done:
(i) Kala-azar disease to see the Leishman Donovani bodies, *i.e.* to study the anti-bodies.
(ii) To diagnose glycogen storage disorders

Q.4. *Which is the single most important contra-indication of bone marrow aspiration?*

Ans. Page 68.

Q.5. *How does one know that the aspiration needle is in the marrow cavity?*

Ans. Page 70.

Q.6. *What is a* dry-tap (*or* blood tap)? *Mention a condition in which it is obtained?*

Ans. When we do not get any cellular marrow component or when blood alone is withdrawn after many attempts from bone marrow. Common conditions of dry tap are:
(i) hypoplastic or fibrosis of bone marrow
(ii) aplastic anaemia.

Q.7. *Do you know of any simpler method to assess the activity of the bone marrow without puncturing it?*

Ans. Yes. Arneth count determination (page 38).

Q.8. *Name the cells seen in the bone marrow aspiration. Also, give the characteristic feature of each type of cell.*

Ans. Page 68.

Q.9. *Although the RBCs in the peripheral circulation far outnumber the WBCs (700 : 1) yet the myeloid cells in the bone marrow outnumber the erythroid cells series (2.5 - 15 : 1). Comment.*

Ans. This is because the RBCs have a longer life-span (average 120 days) than WBCs (a few hours to a day) in the circulation.

STUDY NOTES

REPORTING OF THE RESULTS

The following format is usually adopted for reporting the results on bone marrow examination:

1. Description of general cellularity of the marrow: hypo-; normo-; or hyper-plastic.

....

....

....

2. Description of the type of erythropoiesis: megaloblastic or normoblastic.

....

....

....

3. Description of the general maturity of the erythropoietic and leucopoietic cells.

....

....

....

4. Estimation of the ratios:
   (i) myeloid : erythroid ratio

   ....

   ....

   ....

   (ii) leuco : erythrogenic ratio

   ....

   ....

   ....

   (iii) myeloid : lymphoid ratio

   ....

   ....

   ....

   (iv) lymphoid : erythroid ratio

   ....

   ....

   ....

COMMENTS AND DISCUSSION

....

....

....

....

....

....

....

Unit II
Amphibian (Frog) Experiments

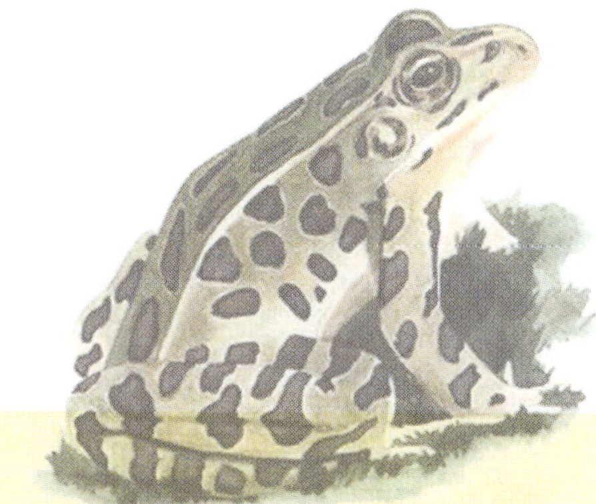

Date: ....

1 An Introduction to the Amphibian (Frog) Experiments

I. GENERAL INTRODUCTION

In order to study the response of a living tissue to a stimulus in the laboratory, we need a living tissue preparation, a stimulating device and a recording device.

1. A living tissue

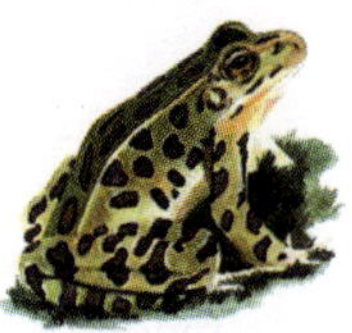

For studying the nerve-muscle physiology, ***frogs*** are the preferred animals because of the following reasons:

(i) Frogs are *cold-blooded animals.* Therefore, their nerve-muscle preparation survival under average experimental conditions is superior to that of warm-blooded animals.

(ii) They are easily available round the year and create no nuisance during storage or while handling (absolutely harmless).

(iii) Their tissues can survive for quite some time in vitro (outside the body) without oxygenation and temperature control. Their muscles can absorb oxygen directly from the atmosphere.

(iv) They are easy to handle during the experiment and can easily be disposed of afterwards.

2. A stimulating device

Of the various types of stimuli (mechanical, chemical, electrical, thermal, etc.) which can be used, electrical stimulus is usually employed because:

(i) its site, intensity, frequency, duration and timing can be accurately and easily controlled;

(ii) it is least injurious to the tissues;

(iii) it can be given either with a set of batteries and a pair of electrodes (**Galvanic current**) or by using an induction coil (**Faradic current** or **induced current**).

3. A recording device

The recording of the response is done by using a writing lever (provided with a capillary pen ink writer at its tip) which inscribes on the surface of a moving drum mounted on a kymograph. (Details page 78)

II. COMMON APPLIANCES USED IN AMPHIBIAN EXPERIMENTS

1. Low Voltage Mains

Low Voltage Mains or *2-pin plug point.* It is supplied with low voltage current, *6 volts DC* from a central rectifier, *i.e.* via a step-down transformer plugged to the high voltage mains.

2. High Voltage Mains

High Voltage Mains or *3-pin plug point.* It is supplied with high voltage current, *220 volts AC* and is meant exclusively for running the kymograph. (***Caution:*** No other electrical appliance used in amphibian experiment is to be connected to it, else it will get burnt completely.)

3. Simple Key or Primary Key (Fig. 2.1.1)

Simple Key or ***Primary Key*** (Fig. 2.1.1). It is used for opening or closing the primary circuit.

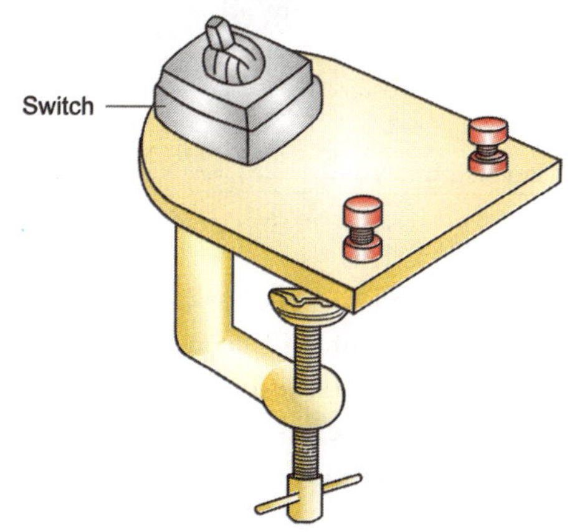

Fig. 2.1.1 Simple (primary) key

4. Short-Circuiting Key or Secondary Key

(i) It is connected in **parallel** in the secondary circuit and is *kept closed* for short circuiting the current, *i.e.* to prevent the accidental passage of the induced current flowing to the tissue (Fig. 2.1.2).

(ii) This key should be *opened only* when it is desired to stimulate the tissue.

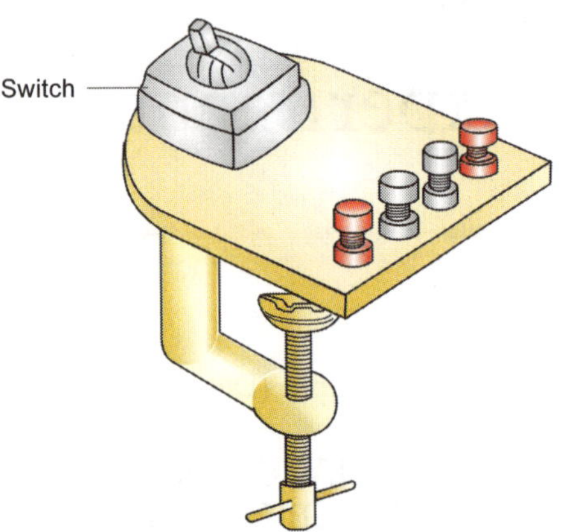

Fig. 2.1.2 Short circuiting (secondary) key

5. Reversing Key

This is used in experiments where two electrodes are required. It is employed for shunting the current from one electrode to the other (Fig. 2.1.3).

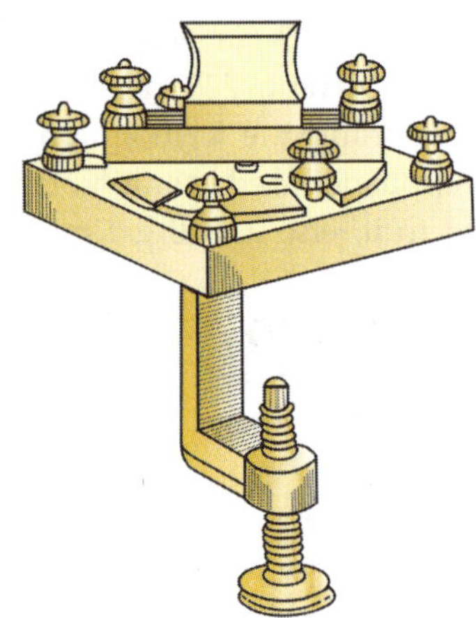

Fig. 2.1.3 Reversing key

6. Tap Key (Fig. 2.1.4)

(i) This key is used to make or break the circuit for a limited duration at will; to achieve this, press the key gently and release it suddenly.

(ii) It is connected in **series** with the low voltage mains in the primary circuit.

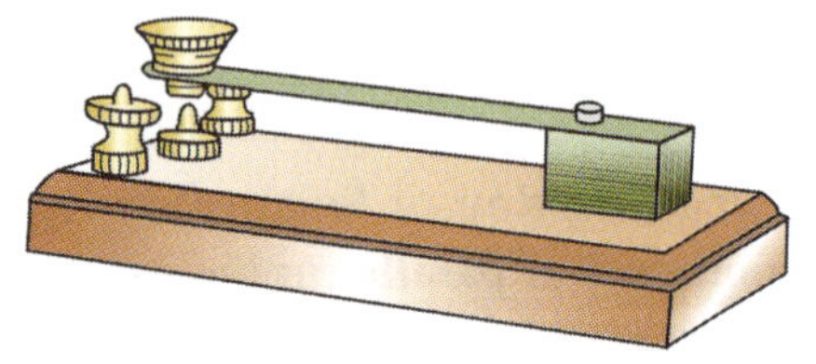

Fig. 2.1.4 Tap key

7. Dubois Raymond Induction Coil (Fig. 2.1.5)

(i) This is used for converting the available low voltage, high ampere, direct (continuous current) into induced current which is always of short duration. It is a high-voltage, low ampere, phasic current, *i.e.* voltage rises and falls rapidly.

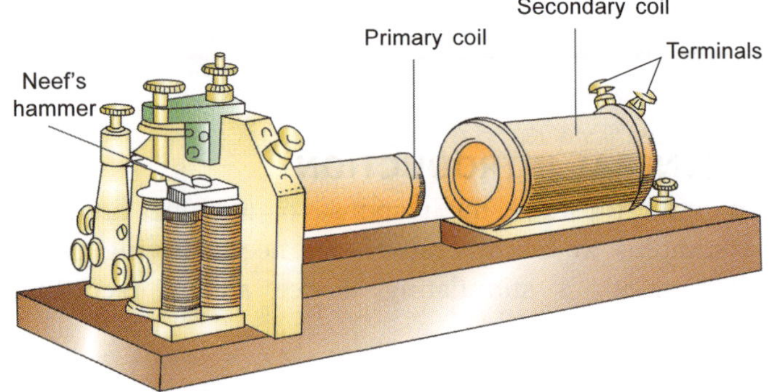

Fig. 2.1.5 Dubois Raymond induction coil with Neef's hammer

(ii) It consists of the **primary** and **secondary coils**, each made of well-insulated copper wire wound round a soft iron core. The secondary coil has a much larger number of turns (5,000) than the primary (3,000 turns) one.

(iii) The primary coil terminals are connected to the DC source while the secondary coil terminals are connected to the electrodes.

(iv) The secondary coil slides on two horizontal graduated metal slide rods. The graduation (in cm) gives the distance between the two coils.

(v) When the primary circuit is **closed**, the magnetic flux within the secondary increases *slowly* from Zero to maximum and an induced e.m.f. develops in the secondary circuit. Conversely, when the primary circuit is **broken**, the magnetic flux within the secondary drops very rapidly to Zero and a *strong* induced e.m.f. develops.

Thus the induced current is stronger at 'break' than at 'make'.

(vi) The closer the secondary coil is to the primary, the stronger is the magnetic field of the primary, and, therefore, the stronger the current induced in the secondary.

(vii) The induced current is strongest when the two coils are parallel, weaker when they are at an angle, and least or nil when they are at right angles.

8. Neef's Hammer

(i) It is a built-in automatic interrupter connected **in series** with the primary coil of the induction coil (Fig. 2.1.5).

(ii) It works on the principle of an electric bell.

(iii) It interrupts the primary circuit about 40 times per second, producing repeated induced currents of the same frequency in the secondary circuit.

9. Vibrating Variable Interrupter (Fig. 2.1.6)

(i) It is an electromagnetic interrupter which allows the vibration of a piece of metal on a brass rod, the frequency of which can be set with the help of an *adjusting screw*. When used, it is connected **in series** with the induction coil.

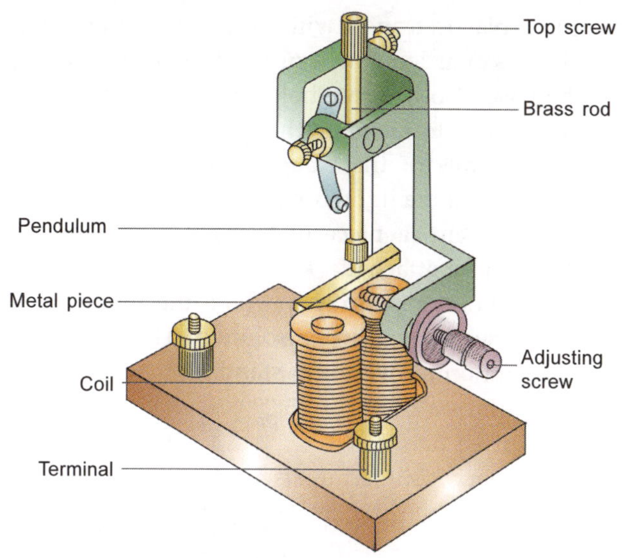

Fig. 2.1.6 Vibrating variable interrupter

(ii) It enables more accurate interruption of the primary circuit at a much lower frequency (up to 25/sec) than the Neef's hammer.

10. Electromagnetic Signal Marker (Fig. 2.1.7)

(i) Very often, it is desirable to have the *point of stimulation* also marked in the tracings when the stimulus is applied. This signal marker has a writing lever and an electro-magnet. The lever moves up or down during the make or break of the primary circuit.

(ii) When used, it is connected **in series** with the primary circuit.

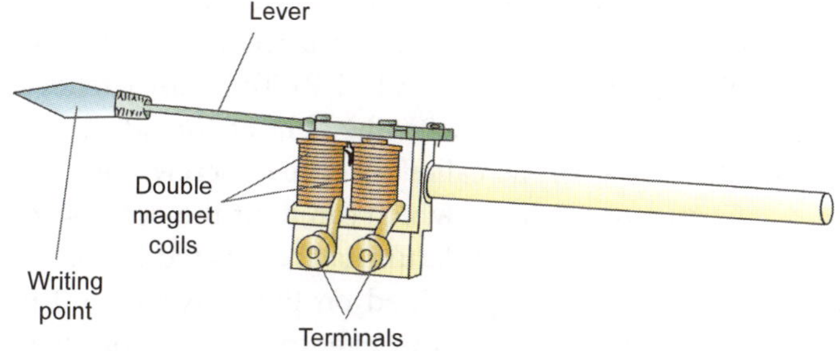

Fig. 2.1.7 Electromagnetic time marker or Signal marker

11. Kymograph

Kymograph (Greek word: Kyma means wave; graphin means write) (Fig. 2.1.8). Kymograph is thus the name given to any instrument which records movement on a moving surface. The degree of movement can be analysed from the height of the wave and its relation to time is measured by the horizontal distance. It consists of the following parts:

(i) **Electric motor**. It runs on 220 volts AC.

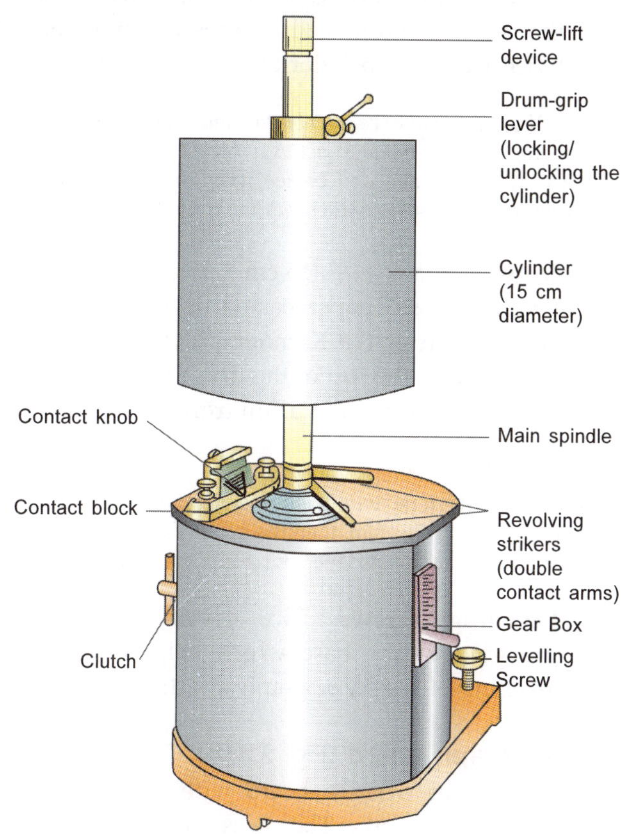

Fig. 2.1.8 Kymograph

(ii) **Shaft**

(a) It is connected to the motor vertically and can be rotated at different speeds (2.5 mm/*sec slowest*; and 640 mm/*sec fastest*).

(b) It has a *groove* on one side and a *screw-lift* at the top. A small *rectangular plug* mounted on the screw inside the shaft comes out through the groove.

(c) The rectangular plug can be raised or lowered along the groove by rotating the screw-lift at the top. It supports the weight of the drum and prevents it from sliding down during the rotation. The level of the drum can, therefore, be adjusted as desired by the top screw-lift.

(iii) **Gears**. These are employed for changing the shaft speed. A lever is provided for changing the gears.

(iv) **Clutch**. This is used to start or stop the drum and must be used every time before changing the gears. It disengages the gear from the axle of the motor.

(v) **Contact button**. It is a specially designed key mounted on the drum. It gets closed momentarily when the rotating *projecting striker* presses upon it.

(vi) **Projecting strikers** or **contact arms**. A pair of these is fixed to the base of the vertical shaft. They can be kept closed together or drawn apart by a desired distance. Accordingly, on each rotation of the drum, the contact button will be pressed either once or twice in close association at a precise interval of time.

> Note: *Thus by means of contact button and projecting strikers, the Kymograph can be made to act as a 'key' in the primary circuit; the circuit being 'made' and 'broken' when the tip of the contact arm makes and breaks contact with the contact button.*

(vii) **Drum**. It is a 6" × 6" (15 cm × 15 cm) cylinder with a white glazed paper pasted on it. It is mounted on the shaft of the Kymograph. A *drum-grip latch* provided on the top of the drum fixes the drum to axle and prevents the drum from sliding down the shaft.

> Important Note: If the writing point of the muscle lever is made up of a photographic film, then the paper pasted on the drum is first smoked with kerosene soot and then mounted.

(viii) **Levelling Screws**. Two levelling screws are provided at the base which help in the proper levelling of the kymograph in a horizontal plane.

12. Myograph Board (Fig. 2.1.9)

It is rectangular wooden board with two holes which are plugged with *corks*. The corks facilitate the pinning of tissues and electrodes. The board is layered with wax and is mounted on a *myograph stand*.

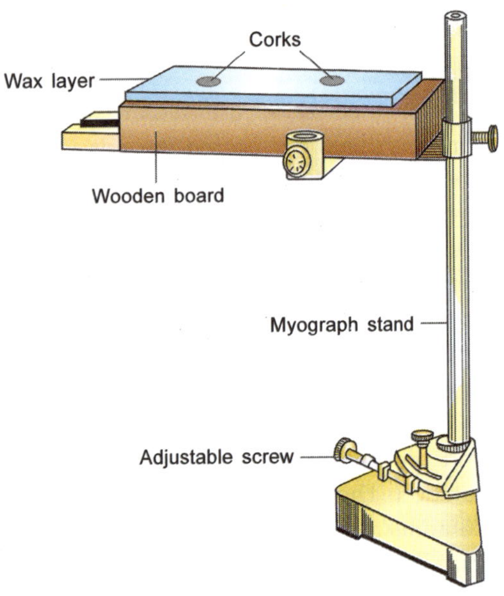

Fig. 2.1.9 Myograph board with stand

13. Myograph Stand

This is a vertical rod carrying the myograph board and can be turned on its axis so that the writing point may be applied to or removed from the drum without altering other adjustments. This is done with the help of a horizontal arm close to its base, which is heavy and a triangular metal block.

14. Lucas Chamber or Muscle Trough (Fig. 2.1.10)

(i) It is a plastic trough with an outlet at the bottom which is guarded with a rubber tubing and a clamp. The base also has two holes plugged permanently with a cork to facilitate the pinning of tissues.

(ii) To the walls of the trough, a block carrying the electrodes and a light, frictionless muscle lever with writing point (a piece of triangular photographic film) can be attached.

(iii) It is used in experiments where the tissue has to be submerged in Ringer solution. The chamber is mounted on a myograph stand.

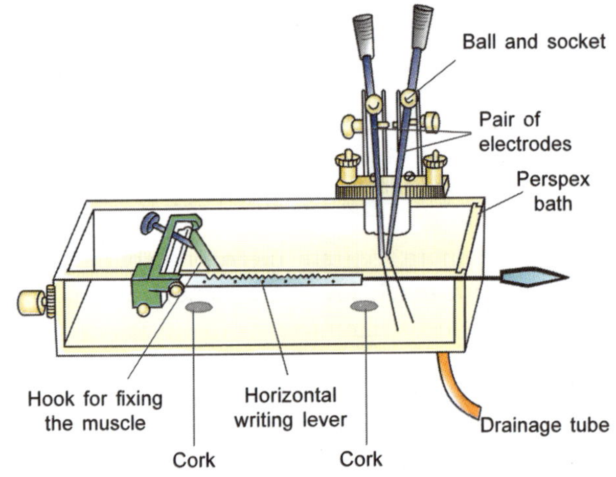

Fig. 2.1.10 Lucas chamber or muscle trough

15. Isotonic Muscle Lever

(i) It is a writing lever which can be attached to the myograph board for recording isotonic muscle contractions (Fig. 2.1.11-A). The writing point of the muscle lever is provided with a *capillary pen ink writer* or is made up of a triangular piece of photographic film (Fig. 2.1.11-B). The muscle tendon is tied to the lever with the help of thread.

(ii) There is a screw, called **after-load screw**, near the *fulcrum* of the lever which can limit the downward movement of the fulcrum to the desired level.

(iii) 3 or 4 holes are provided on the proximal end of the recording arm of the lever for suspending small weights (Fig. 2.1.11-C).

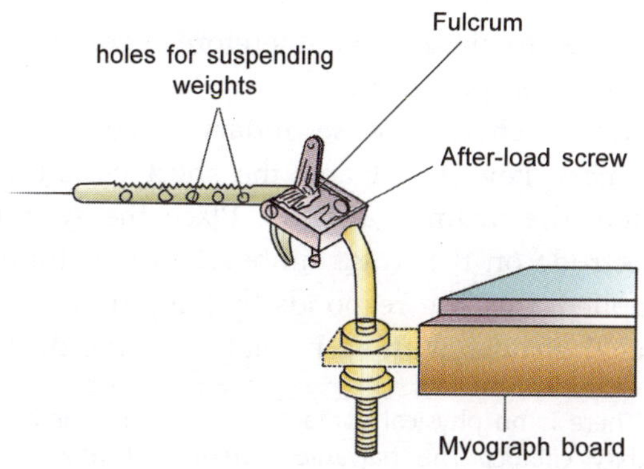

Fig. 2.1.11-A Isotonic muscle lever

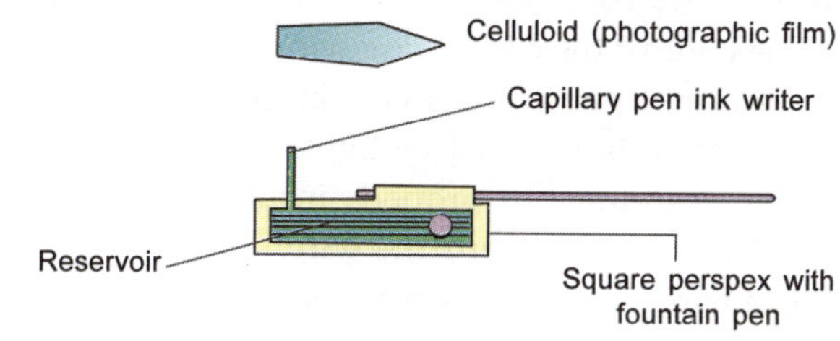

Fig. 2.1.11-B Writing points

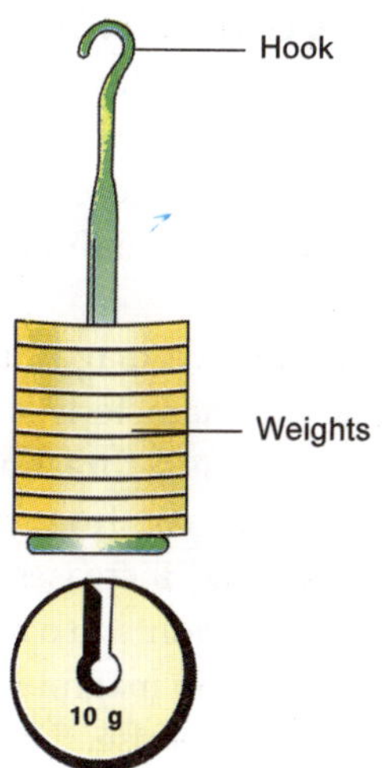

Fig. 2.1.11-C Hook and Weight

16. Starling Heart Lever

It is a sensitive writing lever for recording the isotonic contractions of the heart which are relatively weaker than skeletal muscle contractions (Fig. 2.1.12).

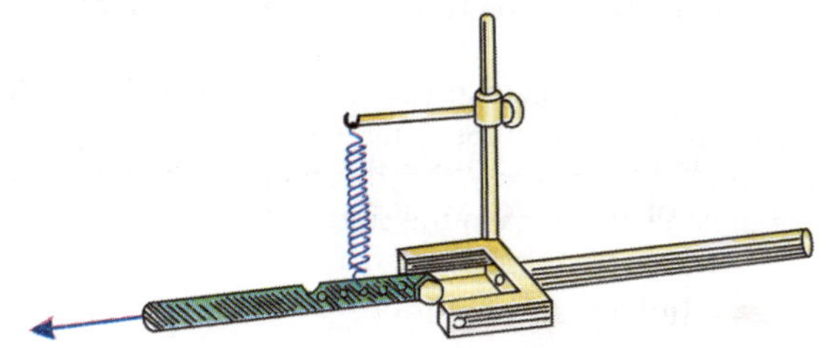

Fig. 2.1.12 Starling heart lever

17. Stimulating Electrode

(i) It is used to stimulate a tissue. It consists of two insulated copper wires held together by a piece of perspex (plastic body) with a central hole for fixing it to the myograph board (Fig. 2.1.13).

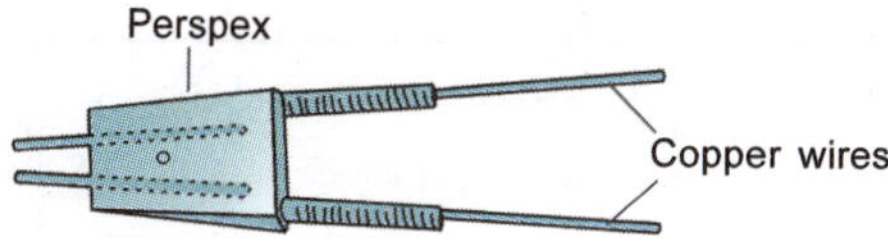

Fig. 2.1.13 Stimulating electrode

(ii) The ends of the wires are devoid of their insulation, thus the electrical circuit is completed through the tissue (muscle, nerve or heart), lying between the two wires.

18. Tuning Fork

(i) Tuning fork, vibrating frequency of 100 c.p.s (Hz) with a writing pointer attached to one of its prongs, is employed to take the time tracing (Fig. 2.1.14).

(ii) It is set vibrating and the writing point is made to write on the rotating drum. A tracing is obtained in which each wave indicates 0.01 sec (from crest to crest).

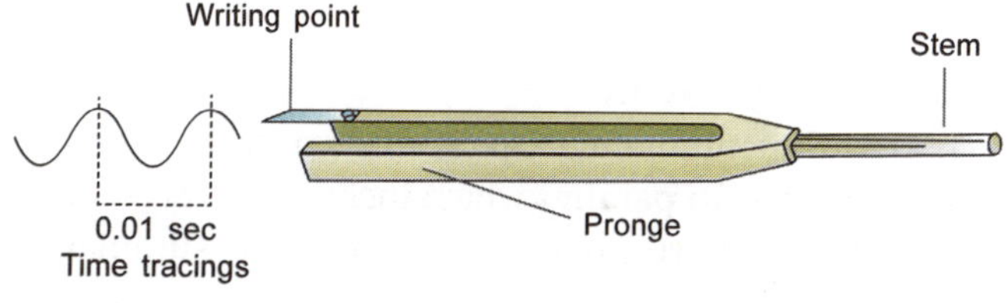

Fig. 2.1.14 Tuning Fork (100 Hz)

III. THE ELECTRICAL CIRCUITS

Two electrical circuits are employed to stimulate the live tissue: *primary* (Fig. 2.1.15) *and secondary circuits* (Fig. 2.1.16).

A. Primary circuit

1. It is the continuous current circuit and includes low voltage main (6 volts DC), primary coil, the primary key, tap key and the kymograph.
2. It is made by connecting all gadgets in **series** with the mains.
3. A constant strength of low voltage, high-ampere, direct (continuous) current flows through it. Such current must, therefore, be used with caution for stimulation to avoid tissue electrolysis and consequent damage.
4. **How to check the primary circuit** With the primary key closed keep the tap key pressed and rotate

the drum; look for an electric spark each time the projecting striker presses upon the contact button of the drum.

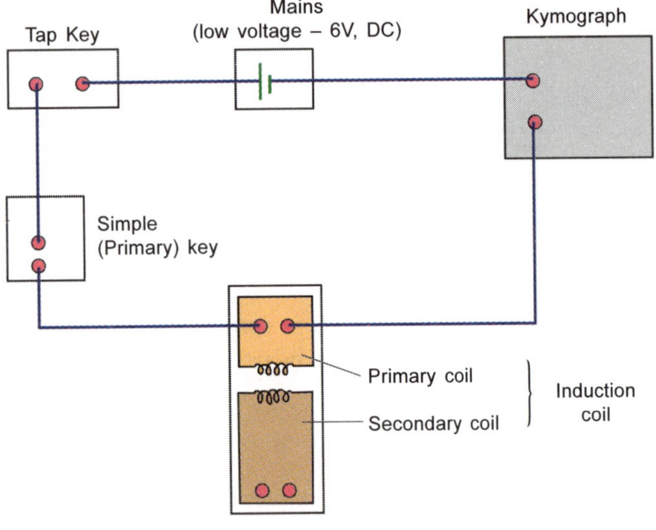

Fig. 2.1.15 The primary circuit

Important Note: All additional gadgets, such as the vibrating interrupter and the electro-magnetic signal marker, are always included in the primary circuit in **series** and never in the secondary.

B. Secondary circuit

1. It is the stimulating circuit and consists of gadget connected **in parallel** which includes the secondary coil, the short circuiting key and the stimulating electrodes (Fig. 2.1.16).
2. A constant strength of high voltage, low-ampere current flows through it which rises and falls rapidly. Their brief duration tends to minimize damage to tissue and, therefore, very useful for stimulation purposes.

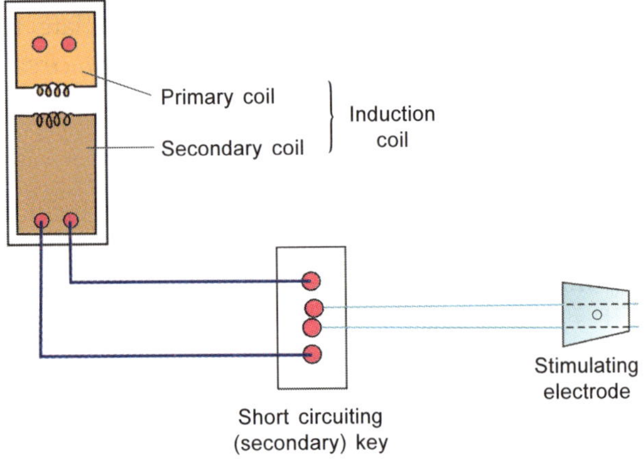

Fig. 2.1.16 The secondary circuit

3. **How to check the secondary circuit** With the primary key closed and the short circuiting key open, the drum is rotated. Place the stimulating electrode on the frog's limb; when the stimulus is applied, the frog responds by jumping away from the electrodes with each rotation of the drum.

Note: There is no physical contact between the primary and secondary circuits. The galvanic current that flows in the primary circuit induces the current in the secondary coil.

General hints for making electrical connections

1. The ends of the connecting wires should be cleaned with sand paper and made bright.
2. All connections must be tight.
3. The wires must be properly insulated. If insulation has worn off, discard the wire.
4. The wires should be kept as short as possible; long wires can be *shortened* by winding them around a glass rod or a pencil.

IV. STIMULATING CURRENT: *SOME DEFINITIONS*

Susceptibility to stimulation is the ability of the tissue to exhibit its characteristic response when suitably excited.

1. A stimulus just sufficient to elicit response is said to be of threshold magnitude and is spoken as a **threshold stimulus**.
2. A stimulus of ineffective magnitude, as judged by its failure to elicit a characteristic response from a tissue, is known as a **sub-threshold** stimulus.
3. In certain preparations e.g. frog gastrocnemius, the magnitude of response increases with increase in the strength of the stimulus to a certain point, after which further increase in magnitude of the stimulus does not augment response. The stimulus which produces maximal response is termed a **maximal stimulus**.

Important Note: Heart muscle, on the other hand, usually responds maximally to the stimuli of threshold magnitude.

4. Stimuli between threshold and maximal values are termed **sub-maximal**. Stimuli which exceed the maximal value are termed **supra-maximal**.

Important Note: Supra-maximal stimuli are to be avoided in most physiological studies, for they are prone to set up disturbance by outlasting the duration of application and induce great fluctuations in the state of the tissue.

V. THE STUDENT PHYSIOGRAPH

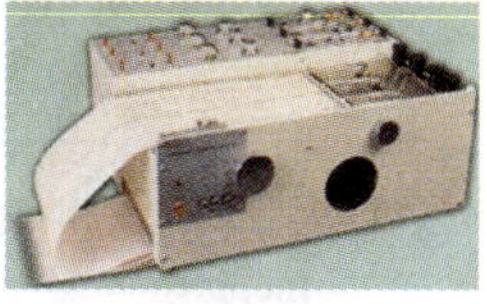

The student physiograph is a complete system design with couplers, matching transducers and pick-ups, and matching **electronic stimulator** with facility of synchronised event marker/time marker (Fig. 2.1.17). It is comprised of the following parts:

- the main console
- electronic stimulator
- couplers
- transducers, and
- accessories like electrodes, junctional boxes, etc.

The Main Console

Console Side (Fig. 2.1.17-A)

It has:

A. *Three sockets for jacks.*
   1. Top socket is for Stimulator.
   2. IN and OUT sockets for interconnecting more than one Physiograph to the same experiment. OUT of one to IN of 2nd; OUT of 2nd to IN of third... and so on.

B. *Three Screw Driver controls* as under:
   1. GAIN – to be used in calibrating the system (or increasing the amplitude of recordings beyond the limits of the Main Amplifier).
   2. DAMPING – to be used for the setting of proper damping, if over or under-damping of the record is noticed from the calibration.
   3. OFFSET, to be used for adjusting the offset, if any, at the pen.

> **Note:** Controls 2 and 3 are to be used only for a trained technician.

C. *Fuse*

D. *Mains Lead*

E. *SLOT* for paper stack.

Console Front

It has:

A. *Mains OFF/ON switch.*

B. *Speed Range Selector Knob* to select the speed range e.g. 100, 50, 25; or 10, 5, 2.5; or 1, 0.5, 0.25 mm per sec.

C. *Speed Selector Push Buttons* to select the desired speed in the range selected.

D. *Window for Paper Feeding.*

E. *Pen Lift Knob.* Turn clockwise to lift pens from the paper, and anticlockwise to put pens on the paper.

Console Top

A. *Pens and Ink Wells.* Two recording pens are provided, the upper for the main recording channel, which is 70 mm wide, and the lower for Time/Event channel.

> **Notes:**
> 1. During an experiment, while not recording, lift pens from the paper.
> 2. After finishing your work for the day, empty the ink wells (using a dropper and cotton wool) and clean the pens pressing water through a syringe.

B. *Slot* for receiving paper.

C. *Paper Guides.*

D. *Thumb Screw and Bearing.* This is used for all paper RUN or STOP during an experiment. Using the Thumb screw, the bearing can be made to lift from the paper for stopping paper movement, or press it on the paper for RUNNING it.

E. *Main Amplifier.* This has 3 controls.
   1. *50 Hz filter On/Off* for filtering 50 HZ artifacts.
   2. *Sensitivity Selector* to select sensitivity desired. With a range from 50 μV to 100 mV in 11 steps of 50, 100, 200, 500 μV and 1, 2, 5, 10, 20, 50, 100 mV.
   3. *Pen Position Control.* This is to be used for adjusting PEN baseline UP or DOWN.

> **Note:** After you have connected the experiment and selected the speed and sensitivity, turn the Console Mains ON and adjust Pen position to Centre running the paper a few cms, and mark the baseline.

F. *Coupler Housing.* To plug all couplers into this. Different, interchangeable, couplers plug-in into the housing, which is prewired to record from different couplers.

Steps for use

1. Plug in the desired Coupler, with the Physiograph Mains OFF. NEVER Plug-in Couplers when Mains are ON.
2. Lift Pens turning pen lift knob clockwise. Check ink flow.
3. Load the Paper.
4. Set up the experiment connecting the preparation/subject to the Transducer/sensor and the Transducer/sensor to the Coupler.
5. Connect Physiograph Stimulator from its "To Physiograph" jack to the corresponding jack at the side of the console. If the experiment requires Electrical Stimulation, connect OUT the terminals of the Stimulator to the Electrodes (for details *see below*).
6. Put Console Mains ON. Select desired chart speed and sensitivity.
7. Put pens on the Paper manipulating the Pen Lift Knob. Check ink flow once again.
8. Run paper a few cms, using Thumb Screw. Adjust Pen Position to Centre with Pen Position Control.

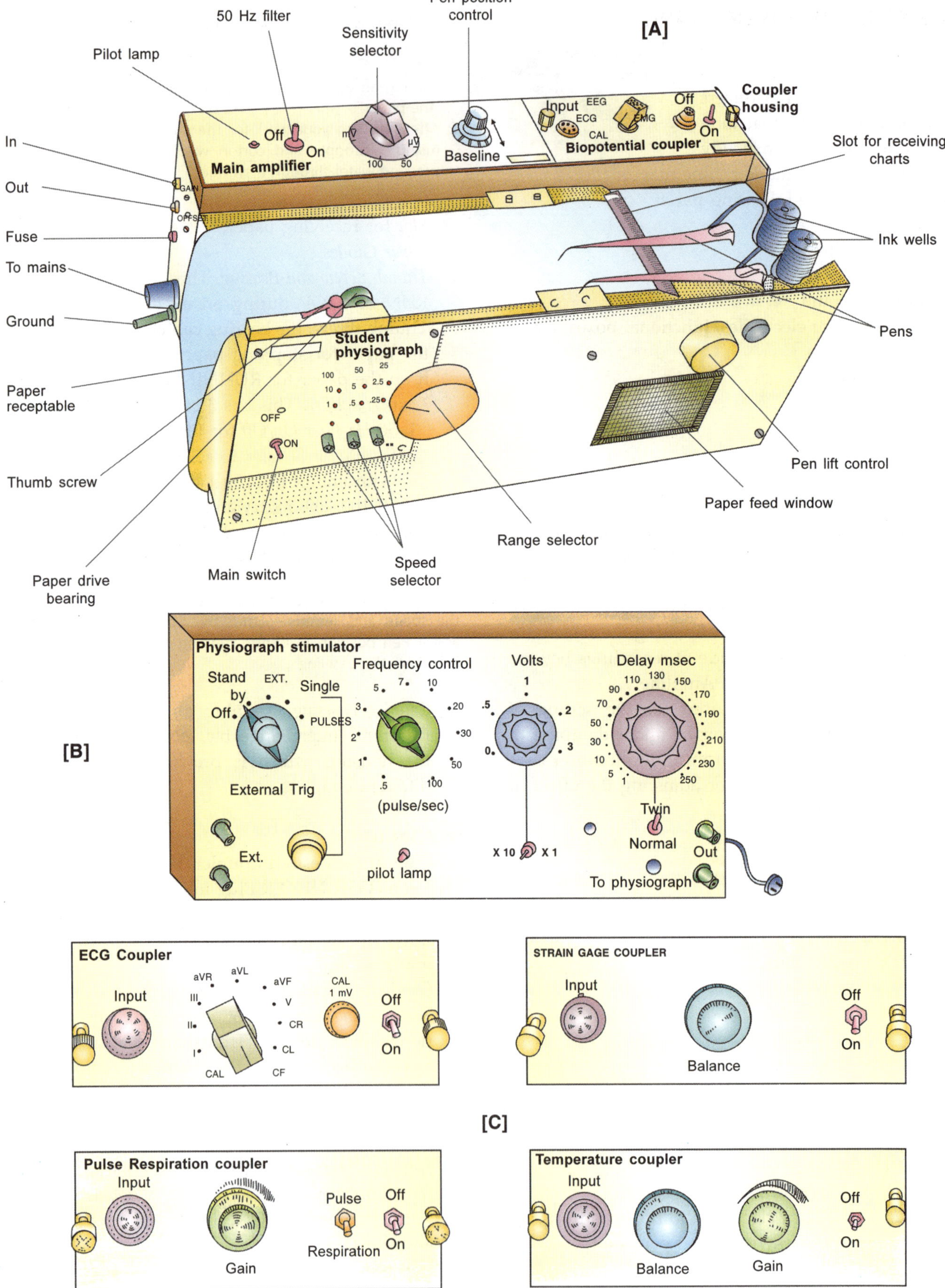

Fig. 2.1.17 The student physiograph (A), the stimulator (B) and the couplers (C)

Set Baseline while the paper is moving. Stop paper, using thumb screw.

9. Put Coupler OFF/ON to ON, and proceed with the experiment.

Note: While not recording, lift pens from the paper using Pen Lift.

Electronic stimulator

This is specially designed for use with the Physiograph (Fig. 2.1.17-B).

(1) It can be used to provide stimuli, while simultaneously energising the Time/Event marker pen, for marking of event of each stimulus.

(2) It can also give two successive Stimuli separated by predetermined delay between the two.

Controls

1. *Frequency.* 0.5 to 100 per sec in 11 steps of 0.5, 1, 2, 3, 5, 7, 10, 20, 30, 50, 100.
2. *Pulse Width.* 0.5 m/sec fixed.
3. *Output.* 0 to 30 volts continuously variable in two steps:
   (a) 0 to 3 volts with multiplier at X1
   (b) 0 to 30 volts with multiplier at X10
4. *External Trig.* Through terminals marked Ext and mode switch at EXT.
5. *Single Pulse.* Through Push Button with mode switch at Single and TWIN/NORMAL toggle switch at NORMAL.
6. ***Two Successive Stimuli.*** As for Single pulse but with TWIN/NORMAL toggle switch at TWIN.
7. *Delay.* Continuously variable between 0 to 250 m/secs. This control operates only for Twin pulses with TWIN/NORMAL switch at TWIN and represents the delay between the two pulses.
8. *Twin/Normal.* To give either a single stimulus (at NORMAL) or two successive stimuli with predetermined Delay (at TWIN).
9. *To Physiograph.* Connects the Stimulator to Physiograph. This also simultaneously connects it to Time/Event marker pen.

Use

Connect the "To Physiograph" jack of the Stimulator to its corresponding jack at the side of the Physiograph Console. This connects it to the Time/Event marker pen.

(1) **For Single Stimulation and Simultaneous Recording of event**

(i) *Mode*	Single
(ii) *Volts*	0.5 to 1.5 depending on the preparation for Minimal Shock. Increase for maximal shock.
(iii) *Twin/Normal*	Toggle switch at NORMAL.
(iv) *Out*	To electrodes.

When one presses the Push Button on the Stimulator a single pulse will go to the preparation, and simultaneously to the Time/Event pen.

(2) **For two Successive Stimuli** (separated by predetermined Delay between them)

(i) *Mode*	Single
(ii) *Volts*	2 or more depending upon preparation for maximal shock.
(iii) *Twin/Normal*	Twin
(iv) *Out*	To electrodes.
(v) *Delay*	Adjust depending upon in which part of the muscle activity the second stimulus is to be given.

When one presses the push button on the Stimulator, TWO pulses, separated by the Delay selected will go to the preparation—and simultaneously TWO pulses will go to the Time/Event pen which will record the two events.

(3) **For Number of Pulses** (increasing frequency of stimuli)

(i) *Mode*	STANDBY. Put to PULSES while giving pulses.
(ii) *PULSES/SEC*	On the number required per sec.
(iii) *Volts*	2 or more for maximal shock.
(iv) *Twin/Normal*	Normal
(v) *Out*	To electrodes.

When one brings the Mode to PULSES from STANDBY, desired pulses per sec. will go to the preparation and simultaneously to the Time/Event pen which will mark the event of each pulse. For stopping stimulation bring the mode back to STANDBY.

(4) **Use as Time Base or Event Marker**

When the Stimulator is not connected to a preparation, the OUT terminals will not be connected. The Stimulator can now be used for triggering the Time/Event pen to record either a Time Base or an Event.

As Time Base

(i) *Mode*	STANDBY; Put to PULSES while recording the desired Time base.
(ii) *Pulses/Sec*	To the number of marks per sec. Thus 0.5 will make one mark every two secs; 1 will make one mark every sec; 5 will make 5 marks every sec. and so on.
(iii) *Volts*	2
(iii) *Twin/Normal*	Normal
(iv) Out	Not connected

For stopping bring Mode to STANDBY. For recording put it to PULSES.

As Event Marker

(i) *Mode* Single
(ii) *Volts* 2
(iii) *Twin/Normal* Normal
(iv) *Out* Not connected

For making the Event, press the Push Button.

Couplers

Different couplers are designed to record different parameters. Couplers plug-in into the **coupler housing** in the main console, and all couplers are interchangeable in the same console or from console to console (Fig. 2.1.17-C). The standard range of couplers is as follows:

1. Strain Gage Coupler

Strain Gage Coupler, for recording from strain gage transducer, for the recording of the following:

(i) Arterial and venous pulse
(ii) Blood pressure
(iii) Plethysmography
(iv) Spirometry experiments
(v) BMR (basal metabolic rate)
(vi) All experiments on frog nerve-muscle preparation and heart experiments
(vii) Experiments with isolated tissue (uterus, heart, intestine, etc.)

Steps for use

(a) PLUG IN COUPLER in the Physiograph Console with the Console Mains OFF. *NEVER* plug-in with mains ON.
(b) Connect Transducer to Coupler, and preparation to Transducer.
(c) Put Console Mains ON.
(d) Select Chart Speed; Select Sensitivity on the Main Amplifier.
(e) Adjust Pen Position to centre of chart, using Pen Position control.
(f) Carefully adjust position of Transducer/preparation so that the connecting thread is 'taut', as will be indicated by a shift of Pen position. Readjust Pen position to centre.
(g) Put coupler Off/On to ON. Pen position will shift.
(h) Manipulate BALANCE control on the coupler to make Pen Position Central.

> **Note:** The Baseline (Step e) will have to be readjusted with every change of sensitivity.

Proceed with the experiment, running or stopping the paper, as required, using Thumb Screw on the console.

2. Bipotential coupler

Bipotential coupler for recording all A.C. phenomena like Electrocardiogram (ECG), Electroencephalogram (EEG), Electromyogram (EMG), Electroretinogram (ERG), etc.

CONTROLS on the Coupler are:

1. Mode for CAL; ECG; EEG (Low and high cut offs); EMG
2. CAL 100 Mv button
3. Off/On

Steps for use

(i) PLUG IN COUPLER in the Console, with the Console Mains OFF, *NEVER* plug-in with the Mains ON.
(ii) *CALIBRATE*
  (a) Console ON. Coupler ON.
  (b) Mode at CAL.
  (c) Select Sensitity of 100 µV on the Main Amplifier.
  (d) Adjust Pen to Centre with Pen Position control. Run paper using Thumb Screw.
  (e) Press for 5 secs. and Release for 5 secs, CAL button on the coupler 3 or 4 times.
(iii) *FOR RECORDING ECG*
Mode at ECG. 50 Hz filter ON. Connect Electrodes from subject to 3 pin junction box and the junction box to the Coupler. Run paper using thumb screw. Take records.
(iv) *FOR RECORDING EEG*
Mode at EEG (L or H). 50 Hz filter ON. Connect Electrodes from subject to three-pin junction box and the junction box to Coupler. Run paper using thumb screw on the console. Take records both at L and H positions of the coupler.
(v) *FOR RECORDING EMG*
Mode at EMG, 50 Hz filter ON. Connect electrodes from subject to 3-pin junction box and the junction box to coupler. Run paper using thumb screw on the console. Take records.

> **Note:** For EEG and EMG recordings, double the sensitivity by caliberating 2 cm for 100 µV instead of 1 cm.

3. ECG coupler (Fig. 2.1.17C)

CONTROLS on the Coupler are:

(i) ECG Lead Selector with CAL Position and position of leads.
(ii) CAL 1 Mv Button.
(ii) OFF/ON.

Steps for use

(i) PLUG IN COUPLER in the Console, with Console Mains OFF, *NEVER* plug-in coupler with the Mains ON.

(ii) *CALIBRATE*

(a) Console ON. Coupler ON.

(b) Mode at CAL.

(c) Select Sensitity of 1 mV on the Main Amplifier.

(d) Adjust Pen to Centre. Run paper.

(e) Press for 5 secs and release 5 sec CAL button on the coupler 3 or 4 times. If amplitude of Calibration is more, or less than 1 cm, make necessary adjustment from the screw driver contol marked GAIN at the side of the console till 1 cm amplitude is recorded both on Press and Release.

(iii) Connect from subject to 5-pin junction box, and junction box to coupler.

(iv) Run paper using thumb screw on console and take records at different positions of the Lead Selector, stopping and running paper in between each step using Thumb Screw. Briefly pause in between each Lead Selection to allow pen to come to centre.

4. Pulse/Respiration Coupler (Fig. 2.1.17C)

CONTROLS on the Coupler are:

(i) GAIN.

(ii) PULSE/RESPIRAITON selector switch.

(iii) OFF/ON.

Steps for use

(i) PLUG IN COUPLER in the Console, with the Console Mains OFF, *NEVER* plug-in with the Mains ON.

(ii) Connect sensor to subject and to coupler.

(iii) Select mode; Respiration or Pulse.

(iv) Console ON. Coupler ON. Select sensitivity and speed.

(v) Adjust Pen to Centre.

(vi) Run paper from Thumb Screw. Take records, running or stopping the paper as required using thumb screw on the console.

Vary amplitude of recording using GAIN control on the coupler.

5. Temperature Coupler (Fig. 2.1.17C)

CONTROLS on the Coupler are:

(i) BALANCE.

(ii) GAIN.

(iii) OFF/ON.

Steps for use

(i) PLUG IN COUPLER in the Console, with the Console Mains OFF, *NEVER* plug-in with Mains ON.

(ii) Connect sensor/transducer to the coupler.

(iii) Console ON. Select sensitivity and Chart speed.

(iv) Bring Pen to Centre with Pen position on the Main Amplifier. Run Paper a few cms using Thumb Screw on console.

Note: Baseline will have to be readjusted for every change in sensitivity.

(v) Coupler ON. Baseline will shift.

(vi) Return Pen to Centre using BALANCE control on the coupler.

(vii) Calibrate the Sensor/transducer within the desired temperature range using a water bath and marking Pen position at different temperatures.

(viii) Bring Pen to the desired position (centre to the edge of trace) and connect subject.

Take records running or stopping the chart using Thumb Screw on the console. You can increase or decrease the amplitude of recordings using GAIN control on the coupler.

Transducers

A wide range of *"strain gage transducers"* is in use to record different parameters. For example:

1. **Pressure volume transducer**, for the recording of pressure from –50 to +250 mmHg and small changes in volume.
2. **Volume transducer**, for recording minute changes in volume.
3. **Muscle-force transducer**, for recording all muscle activity, heart activity, force, etc.
4. **Pulse transducer**, for recording pulsation from any convenient artery.
5. **Respiration transducer**, for recording respiratory movements.
6. **Temperature transducer**, for recording surface or inside (core) temperature.

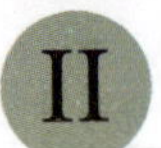

IMPORTANT VIVA-VOCE QUESTIONS

Q.1. *Why is the frog animal of choice for amphibian experiments?*

Ans. Page 75.

Q.2. *Out of the various types of the stimuli, which one is preferred and why?*

Ans. Page 75.

Q.3. *What type of current flows in the primary circuit?*

Ans. Low voltage 6 volts DC.

Note: We do not get an electric shock from this circuit.

Q.4. *Give the functions of the primary and secondary keys?*

Ans. Page 75.

Q.5. *What do you understand by short circuiting key? Why is it required in the circuit?*

Ans. Page 75.

Q.6. *Differentiate between the primary and secondary coils?*

Ans. Page 76.

Q.7. *How can the strength of the stimulating current be varied with the help of induction coil?*

Ans. Page 76.

Q.8. *What should be the criteria of an ideal stimulus?*

Ans. One of the most popular types of stimulus is the so-called ***square wave pulse***, a unidirectional current characterized by practically instantaneous onset and decay, with constant voltage from beginning to end of the pulse.

Q.9. *Give the working principle of (i) Neef's hammer; (ii) Electromagnetic signal marker and (iii) vibrating variable interrupter.*

Ans. All these instruments follow the working principle of an electric bell.

Q.10. *What is the maximum frequency of current which can be obtained by the Neef's hammer?*

Ans. Up to 40 times/sec.

Q.11. *How will you find out the time interval from the time tracings?*

Ans. Since each cycle of the tuning fork lasts 1/100 sec (10 msec), thus each wave indicates 0.01 sec from crest to crest.

Q.12. *Give the components of two electrical circuits used in amphibian experiments.*

Ans. Page 79.

Q.13. *How will you check the primary and secondary circuits?*

Ans. Page 79-80.

Q.14. *Why is primary circuit current not used for stimulating purposes?*

Ans. Page 79.

Q.15. *Explain why induced current is preferred over continuous current for stimulating purposes.*

Ans. Page 80 (Also, refer to page 92).

Q.16. *List the precautions you would like to observe for making an electrical connection.*

Ans. Page 80.

Q.17. *Define the various strengths of the stimulating currents.*

Ans. Page 80.

Q.18. *What is student physiograph? Name the different couplers used in it.*

Ans. Refer to pages 81 onwards.

STUDY NOTES

OBSERVATIONS AND DISCUSSION

....

....

....

....

....

....

....

....

Date: ....

2 Gastrocnemius Muscle and Sciatic Nerve Preparation of Frog

I. APPARATUS

Pithing needle, scissors, forceps, bone-cutter, wooden dissection board, a piece of cloth, beaker, Amphibian Ringer's solution, glass rod, cotton wool, etc.

Composition of Amphibian Ringer Solution

0.6% Nacl	:	isotonic with amphibian plasma
0.14% KCl	:	helps maintain the membrane potential
0.012% $CaCl_2$	:	helps maintain the muscle excitability and stimulates ATPase activity
0.02% $NaHCO_3$	:	provides optimal pH

II. PROCEDURE

1. Stunning of Frog

Hold the frog by its hind limbs and give a single hard blow on its head against the edge of the table. The frog becomes unconscious before it realises what has happened.

Note: A single blow is much better than the repeated blows.

2. Pithing of Frog (Fig. 2.2.1 A)

Pithing of Frog, *i.e.* destroying the brain and the spinal cord.

(i) Hold the unconscious frog in the left hand and ventroflex its head with the help of the index finger.

(ii) Feel for the depression in the mid-dorsal line joining with the posterior border of the tympanic membranes. This is the point of the junction of the skull with the vertebral column. Through this depression, insert a pithing needle into the cranial cavity. This is indicated by *sudden loss of resistance.* Destroy the brain by the rotatory movements of the needle.

(iii) Take out the needle and introduce it into the vertebral canal and, in the similar fashion, destroy the spinal cord.

3. Dissecting out the sciatic nerve (Fig. 2.2.1 B)

(i) Cut the skin of the frog all around at the middle of the trunk, and strip the skin off its hind limbs.

(ii) Lay the frog on its abdomen on the wooden dissecting board. Mobilise the tip of urostyle by cutting through the muscles along its side; lift it up and carefully cut it away, taking care not to injure, the underlying sciatic nerve. (Fig. 2.2.1 C)

(iii) Identify the sciatic plexus, isolate 1.5-2 cm long vertebral column from where sciatic plexus originates, by cutting with a bone-cutter below and above the exit of the plexus (Fig. 2.2.2).

(iv) Bisect the vertebral column by inserting pointed end of the scissor into the vertebral canal, taking care not to injure the sciatic nerve.

(v) Expose the sciatic nerve in thigh between muscle masses. Gently isolate the nerve from adjacent

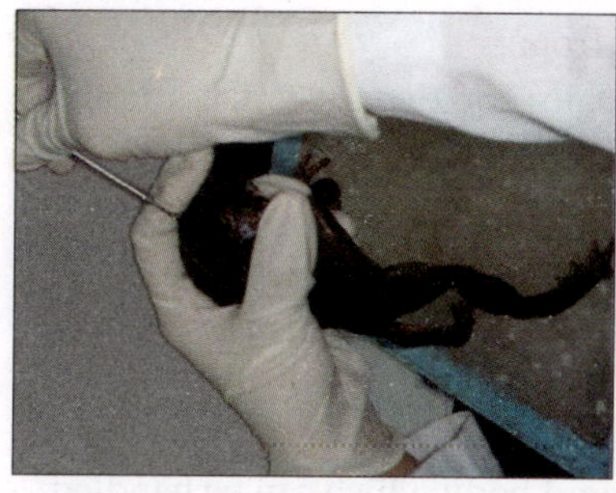
(A)

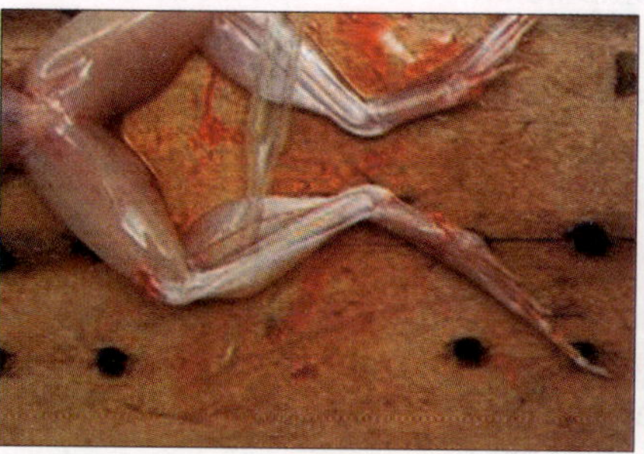
(B)

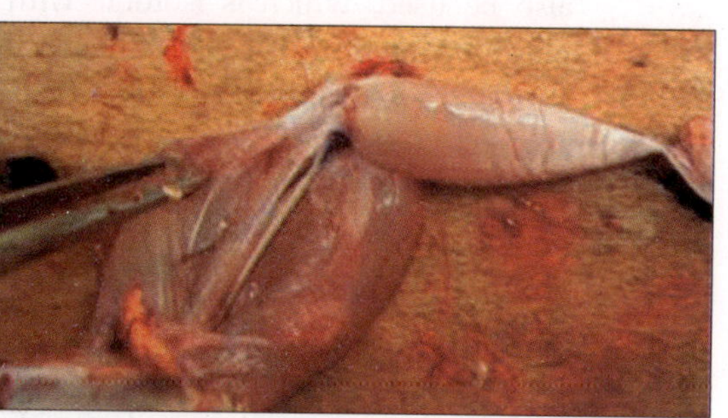
(C)

Fig. 2.2.1 (A) Pithing of frog, (B) Dissection steps, (C) Sciatic nerve-muscle preparation

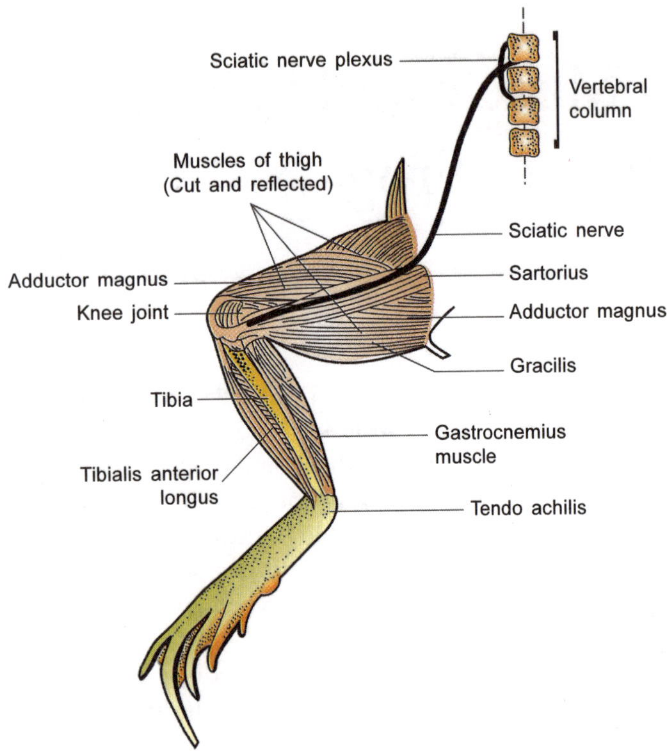

Fig. 2.2.2 Origin and course of sciatic nerve through the muscles of the thigh in a frog (hindlimb-dorsal view)

structures proximally up to the sciatic plexus and distally up to knee joint.

Important Note: Neither pull the nerve nor touch it with metal objects.

4. Dissecting out the gastrocnemius muscle

(i) Identify, disect and cut the gastrocnemius tendon from its attachment. Tie one end of the long thread around it.

(ii) Separate out the gastrocnemius muscle from the adjacent muscles by cutting through the delicate fascia in between; then free the muscle from tibia.

(iii) With the help of a bone-cutter, cut the tibia close to knee joint, and also cut femur near knee joint. Remove redundant (no longer needed) muscles other than gastro-cnemius.

Nerve muscle preparation is ready. Keep it immersed in Amphibian warm Ringer's solution, till needed for experiment.

III. PRECAUTIONS

1. Dissect out the nerve-muscle preparation by causing minimal injury to the adjacent structure.
2. Do not try to dissect out the sciatic nerve at the knee joint.
3. Waste no time after the preparation is ready as it has a limited period of useful life.
4. At no stage during the course of dissection, nerve should ever be subjected to stretching or ever allowed to come in contact with a metal object/instruments, otherwise the nerve may suffer block of conducting power.
5. Prevent drying of the preparation by moistening it with Amphibian Ringer (0.6% NaCl solution at regular interval).

IMPORTANT VIVA-VOCE QUESTIONS

Q.1. *Give the composition and functions of Amphibian Ringer solution.*

Ans. Page 87.

Q.2. *Can any other solution be used beside the Amphibian Ringer solution?*

Ans. Yes, 0.6% NaCl solution (freshly prepared) can also be used, which is isotonic with amphibian plasma. However, it has a limited value.

Q.3. *Why is the frog stunned and not anaesthesized?*

Ans. The anaesthetics used may affect the nerve, neuromuscular junction or anaesthetic like sodium pentothal may directly affect the muscle. Therefore, the frog is stunned.

Q.4. *Why is it not sufficient to destroy the brain alone?*

Ans. It is not sufficient to destroy the brain alone since spinal reflexes may interfere during dissection and the movement of the animal will make dissection impossible.

Q.5. *Why is the head ventroflexed during pithing?*

Ans. The head is ventroflexed in order to locate the triangular depression which marks the junction between the skull and vertebral column, where pithing needle has to be inserted.

Q.6. *How do you know whether the frog has been effectively pithed or not?*

Ans. A properly pithed frog:

(i) neither feels pain nor does it jerk its limbs during dissection;
(ii) exhibits complete flaccidity of the limbs;
(iii) shows loss of corneal/conjunctival reflexes.

Q.7. *What is the advantage of retaininig a small piece of vertebral column at the end of the sciatic nerve?*

Ans. The advantages are:

(i) It provides a rigid body which can be handled roughly during the dissection.
(ii) It keeps the nerve stretched over the electrodes during stimulation.

Q.8. *Why should the sciatic nerve not be allowed to come in contact with any metal object during dissection?*

Ans. Touching the nerve with metal will stimulate it and cause muscle contraction; repeated touching may lead to muscle fatigue.

Q.9. *What is the advantage of keeping the knee joint intact?*

Ans. The knee joint is kept intact:

(i) to fix it to the board along with the nerve and the muscle; and

(ii) the nerve may get cut in the process of cutting the knee joint.

STUDY NOTES

OBSERVATIONS AND DISCUSSION

....

....

....

....

....

....

....

....

....

....

....

....

....

....

....

....

Date: ....

3 Recording of a Simple Muscle Twitch

I. APPARATUS

Dissection instruments (as on page 87), Amphibian Ringer's solution, isotonic muscle lever, myograph board, weights, pins, cotton, thread, tuning fork, stimulating electrodes, kymograph with drum

II. THEORY

A single brief electrical shock of adequate stimulus applied to the nerve of a skeletal muscle gives rise to a brief contraction of the muscle followed by relaxation. This response is called a **simple muscle twitch** (SMT).

III. PROCEDURE

1. Make primary and secondary circuit connections and check them (page 80).
2. Dissect out a muscle-nerve preparation (page 87), pass a pin through the fibrous capsule of the knee joint and fix the preparation to the cork in the myograph board. Prevent drying.
3. The muscle is kept in the *after-loaded position*. How? The screw of the isotonic lever is made to touch the fulcrum, thus the whole weight of the lever is supported on the screw.
4. A 10 gm load is suspended from the lever so that the writing point may not overshoot the height of the drum during the recording of the muscle contraction.
5. Adjust the distance between the primary and secondary coils so as to obtain muscle contraction at break shock only.
6. Adjust the writing lever tangentially to the drum touching it lightly while remaining in a horizontal position. Obtain a **baseline** by setting the drum into motion at the fastest speed of 640 mm/sec.
7. With the primary key closed and the short circuiting key open, set the drum into motion (640 mm/sec) and get nerve stimulated by a single break shock. This is achieved by releasing the tap key (in the primary circuit) immediately after the first click is heard.

   A contractile response of the muscle, *i.e.* a ***simple muscle twitch***, is recorded on the paper consisting of a upstroke and a downstroke (Fig. 2.3.1). The drum is then stopped, and brought to neutral gear.

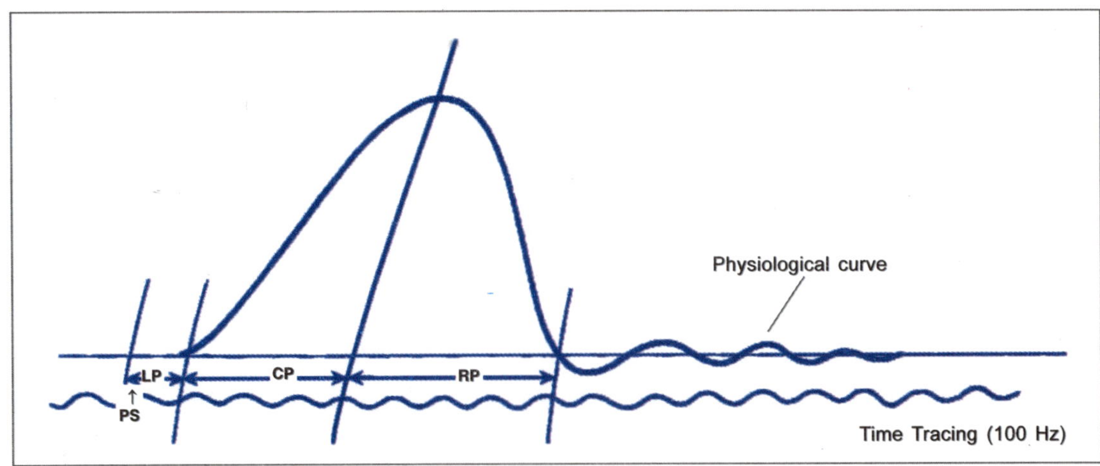

Fig. 2.3.1 A simple muscle twitch, its phases and time relationship. PS – point of stimulus, LP, CP and RP – latent, contraction and relaxation periods respectively

8. Take a time tracing below the contractile response with the help of a vibrating tuning fork (frerquency 100 c.p.s.).
9. Without moving the *pointer,* rotate the drum manually to bring the striker to the *contact button (clicking position).* The position of the pointer at this stage is recorded by gently raising the lever with the finger. This marks the **point of stimulus** (PS).
10. Rotate the drum manually and likewise mark the beginning of the contraction, the top of the contraction to baseline and end of relaxation.

Important Note: Letting the lever drop from the peak gives a more accurate division between the contraction and relaxation periods than drawing the perpendicular from the peak, because the former gives the point on the baseline where the lever would have been when it was at the peak.

11. With dividers and millimeter scale, measure the latent period (LP), contraction period (CP) and relaxation period (RP) of the simple muscle twitch from the time tracings, and determine their duration in seconds.
    [**Hint**: Each wavelength corresponds to 0.01 sec - see page 79).

(For recording on Student Physiograph, refer to page 83).

IV. PRECAUTIONS

1. Check all connections before going for dissection.
2. Level the drum.
3. Do not handle the nerve with forceps or other surgical instruments. Always use a glass seeker for this purpose.
4. Do not allow the preparation to come in contact with the frog's skin which contains poisonous secretion and, hence, toxic to the preparation.
5. Keep the preparation moist all the time with Amphibian Ringer solution.
6. When muscle is not being stimulated, the nerve should be kept off the electrodes and the tension on the muscle should be released.
7. Do not fatigue the preparation by unnecessary repeated stimulation.
8. While stimulating the nerve, make sure that the electrodes should not dip in the Ringer solution to prevent the short circuiting of the stimulating current.
9. The pointer should not be moved until different phases of the muscle-twitch have been marked out.
10. The drum should be kept in the neutral gear whenever it is to be rotated manually.

IMPORTANT VIVA-VOCE QUESTIONS

Q.1. *How does the information obtained from this experiment fit into the general scheme of body function?*

Ans. By recording SMT many phases (LP, CP, RP) as well as properties of muscle can be seen. It also shows the following properties: excitability, contractility, tonicity, elasticity, etc.

Q.2. *Give the normal durations of LP, CP and RP.*

Ans. LP: 0.01 sec; CP: 0.04 sec; RP: 0.05 sec.

Q.3. *What are the causes of the latent period?*

Ans. The duration of latent period depends on:
- (i) conduction of impulse along the nerve;
- (ii) neuro-muscular transmission;
- (iii) excitation-contraction coupling;
- (iv) stretching of series elastic elements, especially tendons, and
- (v) Inertia of the recording lever

Q.4. *What is Physiological curve? Give its normal duration.*

Ans. Physiological curve is obtained after the SMT is over and is due to the inertia of the lever. Its normal duration is 10 msec.

Q.5. *What is the difference between the isotonic and isometric muscular contraction?*

Ans. (Also, refer to page 110)

Isotonic contraction	Isometric contraction
(i) When the muscle shortens in length but the tension in the muscle remains constant.	(i) When the muscle length is not affected but the tension in the muscle changes.
(ii) External work is done.	(ii) No external work is done.
(iii) Not much of heat is produced.	(iii) Greater amount of heat is produced.
(iv) It requires much sliding over of filaments (actinmyosin).	(iv) It does not require much sliding over of filaments.
(v) LP, CP and RP all are of shorter duration.	(v) LP, CP and RP all are longer.

Q.6. *What is the role of the load suspended from the lever?*

Ans.
- (i) It lengthens the latent period but reduces the contraction and relaxation periods.
- (ii) It reduces the height of the contraction so that the graph may be obtained on the drum.

(iii) It overcomes the inertia of the lever.
(iv) It makes the lever horizontal while keeping the muscle mildly stretched.

Q.7. *Why is it important to use induced current for the experiment?*

Ans. Advantages of induced current are:
(i) There is no polarization on the electrodes.
(ii) It is of high intensity and can be changed by changing the distance between the primary and secondary coils.
(iii) It is of very short duration thus helps stimulate the tissue without causing injury to it.

Q.8. *What are the criteria of an ideal lever?*

Ans. An ideal lever has:
(i) no momentum so that it may not keep on moving;
(ii) no resistance, *i.e.* it should be weightless.

Note: Cathode ray oscilloscope comes very close to an ideal lever.

Q.9. *It is not advisable to stimulate the preparation during the first revolution of the drum. Why?*

Ans. Because at this time drum is gaining acceleration and is not running at a uniform speed.

Q.10. *Can you find out the tetanizing frequency from a simple muscle twitch?*

Ans. Yes, tetanizing frequency, *i.e.* rate of stimulation at which summation of contractions will occur will be 1/contraction period duration in msec.

Q.11. *If the time tracings are not taken, can the duration of different phases of an SMT still be determined?*

Ans. Yes, the different phases can be determined from the speed of the drum precisely known.

Q.12. *Why is the SMT recorded on a fast-moving drum?*

Ans. SMT is recorded on a fast-moving drum to find out the duration of various phases viz. LP, CP and RP.

Q.13. *Correlate the SMT and its action potential on the same time scale.*

Ans. When the muscle action potential and the twitch are plotted on the same time scale, the twitch starts about 2 msec after the start of depolarization of the membrane before repolarization is complete (Fig. 2.3.2).

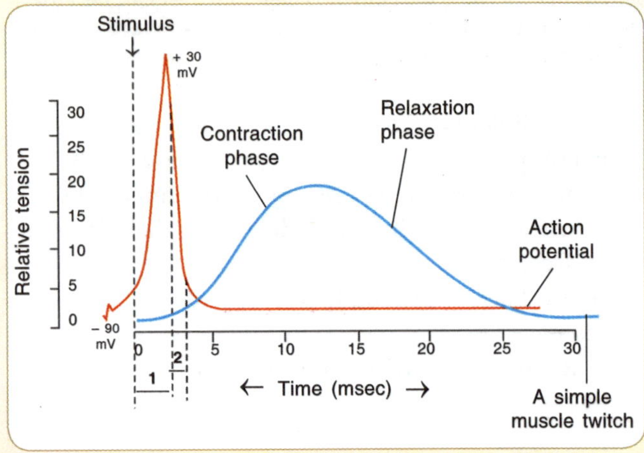

Fig. 2.3.2 A simple muscle twitch (in frog) correlated with its action potential. (1) and (2), absolute and relative refractive periods respectively.

STUDY NOTES

RESULTS

1. Express in msec the duration of:
   (i) Latent period (LP)
   (ii) Contraction period (CP)
   (iii) Relaxation period (RP)
   (iv) Total contraction-relaxation duration
   (v) Simple muscle twitch

....

2. Express the CP and RP as percentage of the total muscle twitch duration.

....

COMMENTS AND DISCUSSION

....

....

Date: ....

4 Effect of Temperature on the Simple Muscle Twitch

I. APPARATUS

The same as for recording a simple muscle twitch (page 90) except that Lucas chamber is used in place of myograph board; a centrigrade thermometer; cold and warm Amphibian Ringer solutions.

II. PROCEDURE

1. Arrange the apparatus as for recording a SMT (page 90). Use Lucas chamber in place of myograph board. Fill the chamber with Amphibian Ringer solution. Record a SMT using maximal stimulus. Note the temperature of the Ringer solution (Fig. 2.4.1).
2. Drain off the Ringer solution and replace it with fresh Ringer solution at about 38°-40°C (note the temperature precisely). Wait for at least 5 minutes; now without altering the strength of stimulus, using the same baseline and point of stimulus, record another SMT.
3. Repeat the whole procedure using cold Ringer solution at about 10-12°C (note the temperature precisely).
4. Take the time tracing in the usual manner. (For recording on Student Physiograph, refer to page 83).

III. PRECAUTIONS

1. The muscle must be immersed in the Ringer solution at different temperatures for at least 5 minutes before taking a record.
2. The temperature of warm Ringer solution should not exceed 42°C, else proteins in the preparation get denatured.
3. The effect of warm Ringer solution should be recorded before that of the cold Ringer solution.
4. The baseline, the point of stimulus and strength of stimulating current should remain unchanged for all the three tracings. This will facilitate comparison.

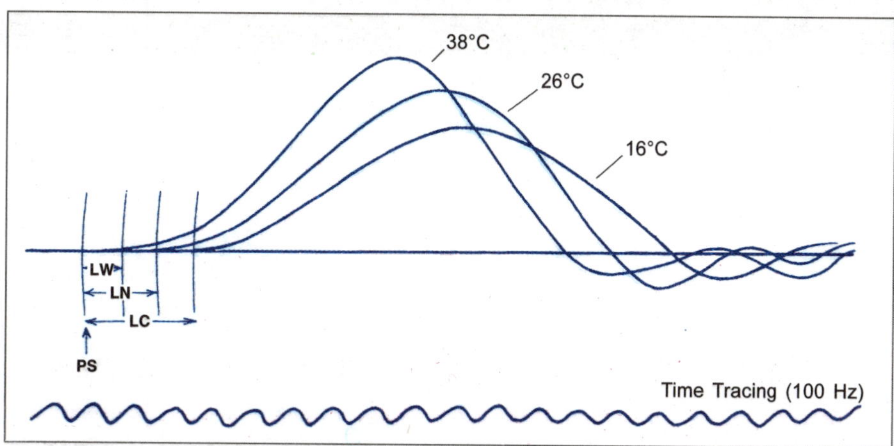

Fig. 2.4.1 Effect of temperature on the simple muscle twitch (PS: point of stimulus; LW, LN and LC: latent periods of warm, normal at room temperature and cold Ringer respectively)

IMPORTANT VIVA-VOCE QUESTIONS

Q.1. *What is the effect of cold and warm Ringer solutions on various periods and height of muscle contraction?*

Ans. *Cold Ringer* increases the duration of all phases of muscle contraction and decreases the height of contraction, whereas the *warm Ringer* solution has just the opposite effect.

Q.2. *How do the cold and warm Ringer solutions bring about their effects on muscular contraction?*

Ans. (i) Cold Ringer solution decreases the temperature of the muscle, thereby increases the viscosity and retarding some metabolic processes. Hence, depolarization is slow, thereby resulting in the decreased velocity of response.

(ii) Warm Ringer solution raises the temperature of the muscle, thereby reducing its inertia and the synaptic delays are minimized.

Q.3. *Why is it important to use maximal stimulus?*

Ans. The use of maximal stimulus will enable us to know if all the motor units have been simultaneously activated.

Q.4. *Why do the effects of Warm Ringer solution should be taken before that of cold Ringer?*

Ans. Cold Ringer inactivates the muscle. Once inactivated, it is difficult to revive it. Hence the effect of warm Ringer is observed first.

Q.5. *Why should temperature above 42°C not be used?*

Ans. See above.

Q.6. *Is the effect of temperature on muscle contraction a violation of 'All or None Law'?*

Ans. The 'All or None Law' is valid only if the environmental conditions like temperature, pH are constant. Here, as the temperature is changing, this law is not valid.

Q.7. *Why are the human muscles just as active in winter as in summer?*

Ans. This is because man being homeothermic (warm-blooded) can maintain the internal body-temperature within a narrow range in spite of wide variations in environmental temperature.

Q.8. *Give the physiological significance of this experiment.*

Ans. Efficiency of skeletal muscle contraction increases with increase in surrounding temperature within the physiological limits. This is especially useful during exercise.

Q.9. *What is heat rigor?*

Ans. When the temperature of Ringer solution exceeds 45°C, the muscle proteins get denatured. Due to this, actin and myosin filaments are unable to carry out their functions. Hence, the muscle remains in a state of permanent contraction, called heat rigor.

STUDY NOTES

RESULTS AND DISCUSSION

Tabulate your results in the Table below.

Temperature of Ringer solution	Latent period (msec)	Contraction period (msec)	Relaxation period (msec)	Height of contraction (cm)
1. At normal room temperature ....°C				
2. Warm: ....°C				
3. Cold: ....°C				

....

....

....

....

....

....

....

Date: ....

5 Effect of Two Successive Stimuli (of the same strength) on Skeletal Muscle Contraction

I. APPARATUS

The same as for recording a simple muscle twitch (page 90)

II. THEORY

1. Summation means the increase in the activity of a tissue produced by multiple stimulation as compared with the effect of a single stimulus. Summation is a property shown both by muscular and by nervous tissues, but it is most easily demonstrated in the muscle.
2. Two forms of **summation by muscle** are recognized:
   (i) ***Summation of stimuli***. It can be demonstrated by the application of multiple sub-threshold stimuli to produce muscular response.

   Note: A single stimulus of just sub-threshold magnitude produces no muscular response.

   (ii) ***Summation of contraction.*** It refers to an increase in actual magnitude of contraction as a result of multiple stimulation. It is of two types:
   (a) **Wave summation** refers to the condition produced by the passage of successive contraction waves over the same set of muscle fibres.
   (b) **Quantal summation** refers to an increase in response due to the stimulation of additional fibres by stimuli subsequent to the original.
3. If a skeletal muscle is given two successive stimuli of maximal strength, the response to the second stimulus depends upon how soon after the first stimulus it is given. The following results are obtained:
   (i) If the second stimulus falls during the latent period of the muscle, the arrival of the nerve impulse produces no additional response. The muscle is said to be *completely refractory* (non-responsive).
   (ii) If applied later, a second muscular response results, leading to further development of tension (***summation of effects***) irrespective of the phase of the muscle cycle in which the stimulus is applied, *i.e.* whether during contraction or relaxation phase. The tension resulting from the second stimulus applied successively at suitable interval may thus be considerably greater than that from the first stimulus. This phenomenon is called the ***beneficial effect*** because the second stimulus gets benefitted by the changes produced in the muscle due to the first stimulus. The important reasons underlying this phenomenon are:
   (a) release of more Ca^{2+} from sarcoplasmic reticulum;
   (b) increase in the temperature of the muscle;
   (c) decrease in internal viscosity and resistance of the muscle (series elastic element being already stretched);
   (d) decrease in the inertia of the recording system.

   Therefore, the second stimulus produces ***Beneficial Effect***.

III. PROCEDURE

1. Set a nerve-muscle preparation, fix the electrodes so as to stimulate the nerve with a maximal stimulus and record a simple muscle twitch.
2. Separate the *projecting strikers* slightly so that they may strike the *contact button* in close succession. The distance between the *strikers* is so adjusted that a second stimulus would fall in the first half of the latent period of the simple muscle twitch of the first stimulus (Fig. 2.5.1A). Record the muscle contraction using the same stimulus strength. Mark the points of stimulation.
3. Repeat the same procedure after progressively widening the distance beween the *strikers* so as the second stimulus falls:
   (i) in the second half of the latent period;
   (ii) in the contraction period;

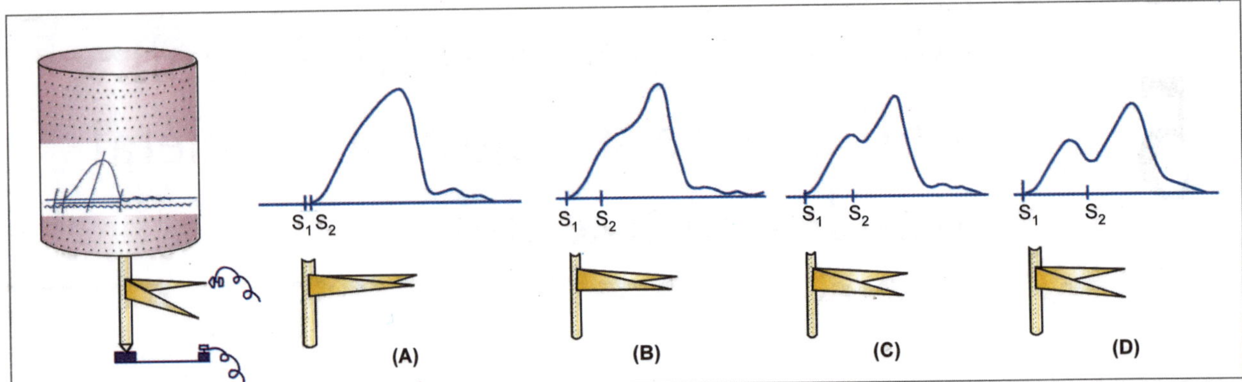

Fig. 2.5.1 Summation of contractions. Second stimulus (S_2) falls in the second half of latent period (A), contraction period (B), relaxation period - early (C) and late (D) of the first SMT

(iii) in the relaxation period; and

(iv) immediately after the relaxation period of the first SMT.

Note: Record (i) to (iv) as separate curves, marking points of stimulation every time (Fig. 2.5.1).

4. Take the time tracing in the usual manner.

Note: Describe your observations in terms of the fact whether the responses of the two stimuli are fused or discrete, and what heights of contractions are.

(For recording on Student Physiograph, refer to page 83).

IMPORTANT VIVA-VOCE QUESTIONS

Q.1. *Explain, giving reasons, the record obtained when the second stimulus falls during the different phases of the first SMT.*

Ans. (i) When the second stimulus falls on the first half of the latent period, there is no response, because the first half of the latent period is absolutely refractory and no action potential can be generated, however strong the stimulus is applied.

(ii) The height of curve is more when the second stimulus falls during the second half of the latent period or contraction period or relaxation period of the first twitch due to the phenomenon of beneficial effect.

Q.2. *What is the mechanism of the beneficial effect?*

Ans. Page 95.

Q.3. *Why is the maximal stimulus used in this experiment and not the supra-maximal?*

Ans. The maximal stimulus is used to ensure that all the motor units have been activated. The supra-maximal stimulus should not be used as already described (page 80).

Q.4. *Define summation.*

Ans. When a single response is obtained by giving two stimuli, either simultaneously or in close succession (one after the other), and the response is greater than that obtained by either stimulus alone. This phenomenon is called summation.

Q.5. *Is it the summation of stimuli or the summation of effects in this experiment? Explain.*

Ans. Here, it is the summation of effects because when the second stimulus is given all the factors underlying the phenomenon of beneficial effects are already taken care of and hence the recorded response is stronger.

Q.6. *Differentiate between summation of stimuli and summation of contractions?*

Ans. Page 95.

STUDY NOTES

RESULTS AND DISCUSSION

Describe your observations in terms of the fact whether the responses of the two stimuli are fused or discrete, and what heights of contractions are?

....

....

Date: ....

6 Effect of Increasing Strength of Stimulus on Skeletal Muscle Contraction

I. APPARATUS

As for recording a simple muscle twitch (page 90).

II. PROCEDURE

1. Arrange the nerve-muscle preparation as for recording a SMT *except* that the drum is excluded and in its place an electromagnetic signal marker is included into the primary circuit in series.
2. Put the drum in neutral gear; it need not be put on, *i.e.* it remains in stationary position. The signal marker pointer is brought in contact with the drum so that it may be in alignment with the pointer of the muscle lever.
3. Keep the *primary key closed* and *short circuiting key open,* the secondary coil is moved to the farthest away from the primary coil. The *tap-key* is briefly pressed and then released. The signal marker moves and marks the point of stimulus on the drum but the induced current will be too weak to produce a response either at *make* or *break* (Fig. 2.6.1).
4. Rotate the drum manually so that the pointer may move about a centimetre on the drum. Step by step, move the secondary coil near the primary coil by 1 cm at a time; press the *tap-key* and release it. At every point, test the response of the muscle to *make* and *break* shock separately.

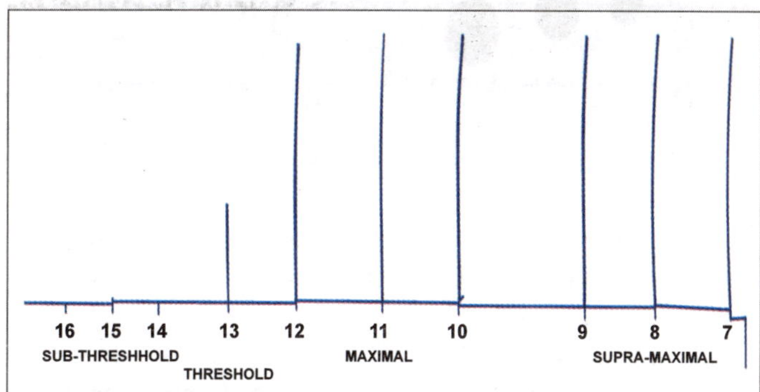

Fig. 2.6.1 Effect of increasing strength of stimulus on skeletal muscle contraction. (Note the numbers below represent distance between the primary and secondary coils in cm.)

Important Notes

1. Take care that at least 15 sec. elapse between make and break shocks to avoid beneficial effect.
2. The distance between the two coils, in cm, is not an absolute measure of the strength of the stimulus. In fact, this distance is inversely related to the strength of the stimulus.

5. Write the distance of the secondary from the primary under each make and break. The response *first* appears at the *break* shock, as the strength at break is stronger than at make (page 76). Carefully note the position of the secondary coil at this point.
6. The experiment is stopped when further increase in the intensity of stimulus is without effect on the height of the contraction.

(For recording on Student Physiograph, refer to page 83)

III. PRECAUTIONS

1. Allow sufficient time between two successive stimuli to avoid any beneficial effect.
2. Avoid unnecessary repeated stimulation of the preparation to prevent fatigue.
3. Label the graph carefully and accurately note the distance between the two coils.

IMPORTANT VIVA-VOCE QUESTIONS

Q.1. *Define: sub-threshold, threshold, maximal and supra-maximal stimulus.*

Ans. Page 80.

Q.2. *What type of Faradic shock current is being used in this experiment?*

Ans. *Break* shock is being used because it is of short duration and easy to control.

Q.3. *What is a motor unit?*

Ans. Each single motor neuron and all the muscle fibres it supplies constitutes a **motor unit.** (Fig. 2.6.2)

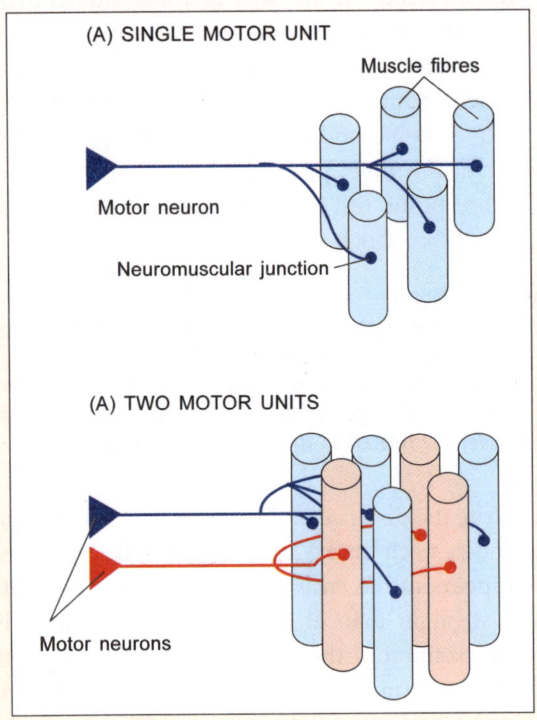

Fig. 2.6.2 Motor unit(s)

Q.4. *What is the mechanism of the graded response to increasing strength of stimulus?*

Ans. When a stimulus is sub-minimal then there is no response. As the strength of stimulus increases, a response is produced. It is maximum at the maximal stimulus. On applying supra-maximal stimulus, there is no increase in the response because by now all the motor-units have been activated.

Q.5. *Why does the strength of muscle contraction increase with the increase in the strength of the stimulus?*

Ans. The threshold of excitation of different motor neurons supplying a single skeletal muscle varies. Therefore, with the increase in strength of stimulus, more and more motor units get recruited and the height of contraction increases.

Q.6. *How is the gradation of muscular movements brought about?*

Ans. The gradation of muscle response depends on the following factors: (Fig. 2.6.3)

(i) number of motor units activated at a time, *i.e.*, recruitment of motor units.

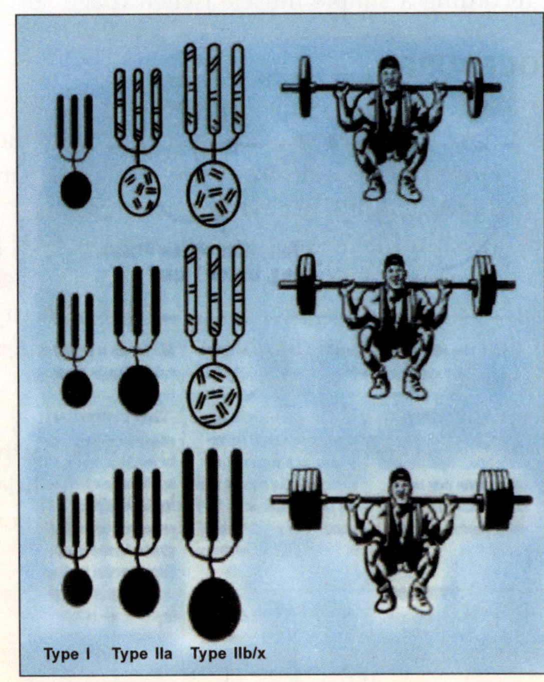

Fig. 2.6.3 Recruitment of motor units

(ii) frequency of discharge in individual nerve fiber i.e. duration for which motor units are being stimulated; and

(iii) optimal length of the muscle, the length at which they develop maximum **active** tension.

Q.7. *Define 'All or none law' in relation to this experiment.*

Ans. All or none relationship between the **stimulus** and the **response** is called all or none law. This law is applicable to an individual skeletal muscle fibre, *i.e.* each muscle fibre while contracting follows the all or none law, and always gives a maximal contraction only.

STUDY NOTES

RESULTS AND DISCUSSION

Measure the height of contractions of the tracings in cm and tabulate your findings as follows:

Sl. No.	Distance between primary and secondary coil (cm)	Height of contraction (cm)
1.		
2.		
3.		
4.		
5.		
6.		
7.		

....

....

....

....

....

....

....

....

....

....

....

....

....

....

....

....

....

....

....

....

....

Date: ....

7 Effect of Increasing Frequency of Stimuli on Skeletal Muscle Contraction (*Genesis of Tetanus*)

I. APPARATUS

As for recording a simple muscle twitch (page 90); electromagnetic signal marker; variable interrupter

II. THEORY

1. When a series of maximal stimuli are delivered to a skeletal muscle at a frequency so that successive stimuli may fall *during the relaxation phase of the previous stimulus*, there occurs an increase in the tension developed during each twitch until, after several contractions, a uniform tension per contraction is reached. This phenomenon is called as **Treppe** or **Staircase phenomenon** (German, Treppe means staircase).
2. With repeated maximal stimulation if the frequency is such that successive stimuli falls during the '*mid relaxation*' phase of the previous stimulus, the muscle relaxes but not completely. Such response is known as **Clonus**.
3. With rapidly repeated maximal stimulation during contraction phase, the activation of contractile mechanism occurs repeatedly before any relaxation has occurred and the individual responses fuse into one continuous contraction. Such response is called **Tetanus** or **Tetanic contraction**.
   (i) It is a **complete tetanus**, when there is no relaxation between stimuli; and an **incomplete tetanus** when there are periods of incomplete relaxation between the summated stimuli. These phenomena are known as **Summation of Contractions**.
   (ii) During a complete tetanus, the tension developed is approx. 4 times that developed by the individual twitch contraction.

Important Notes

1. The stimulation frequency at which the summation of contraction will occur is determined by the contraction period duration; for example, if contraction period duration is 10 msec, frequency only greater than 1/10 msec, *i.e.* 100/sec will cause summation.
2. The frequency of stimulation necessary to produce tetanus varies in different muscles. The muscle with a short latent period and contraction period will require a higher frequency of stimulation than one with a long phase of contraction.

III. PROCEDURE

1. Arrange the nerve-muscle preparation as for recording a simple muscle twitch (page 90). Do not include the drum in the circuit; connect an electromagnetic signal marker and a variable interrupter into the primary circuit in series.
2. Adjust the induction coil so as to deliver a maximal stimulus.
3. Set the variable interrupter into operation by adjusting the **vibrating rod** to provide 5 stimuli (or interruptions) per sec.
4. Start the drum at a slow speed (12.5 mm/sec), open the short circuiting key to stimulate the muscle and close it after recording 5-6 contractions on the drum.
5. The frequency of stimuli is progressively increased to 10, 15, 20, 25, 30, 35, 40 per sec. by adjusting the **screw** of the variable interrupter and take a record of muscle response (Fig. 2.7.1).
6. If even the fastest frequency possible with the variable interrupter fails to give a complete tetanus, it is disconnected and Neef's hammer is included in the primary circuit in series. This enables the delivery of higher frequency of stimuli till the muscle tetanizes.

Notes

1. Observe the type of graph recorded with the increasing frequency of stimulation.
2. Identify and label the graphs: treppe, clonus, incomplete tetanus and complete tetanus. Indicate the rate of stimulation.
3. Note the frequency of stimulation required to obtain complete tetanus.

(For recording on student physiograph, refer to page 83).

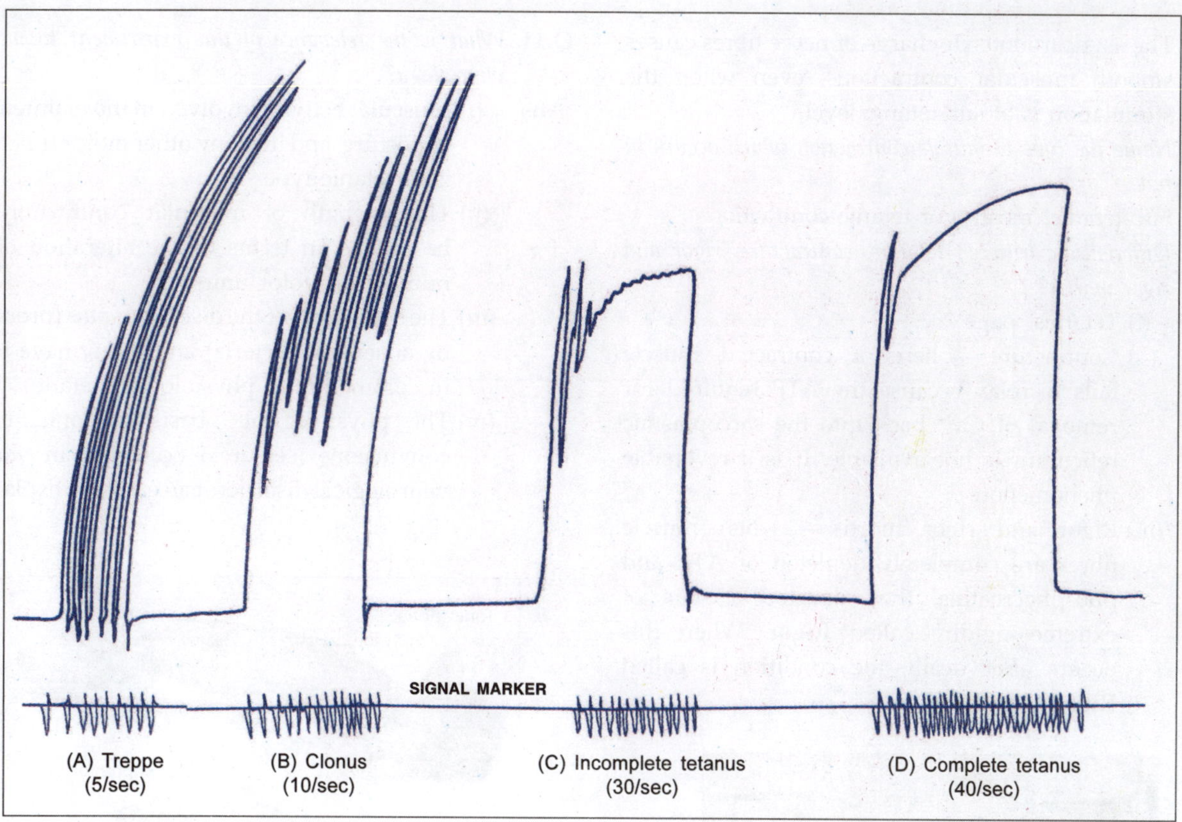

Fig. 2.7.1 Genesis of tetanus (drum speed 12.5 mm/sec)

IV. PRECAUTIONS

1. Ensure that the drum is not included in the circuit.
2. Avoid unnecessary stimulation of the preparation.
3. Do not connect the Neef's hammer and the variable interrupter simultaneously into the primary circuit.
4. Prevent the drying of the preparation.

IMPORTANT VIVA-VOCE QUESTIONS

Q.1. *Define: treppe, clonus, incomplete and complete tetanus.*

Ans. Page 100.

Q.2. *Justify that tetanus occurs due to the summation of contractions and not due to the summation of stimuli (action potentials).*

Ans. For difference between the summation of stimuli and the summation of contraction, see page 95.

Q.3. *What is the ratio of tension developed during a complete tetanus and a simple muscle twitch?*

Ans. Page 100.

Q.4. *Can you find out the minimum tetanising frequency from a given SMT record? If yes, how?*

Ans. Page 100.

Q.5. *List the factors that influence the minimum tetanizable frequency and explain their role.*

Ans. The factors that influence the minimum tetanizable frequency are:

(i) Strength of stimulation. It affects by its effect on the contraction period.

(ii) Fatigue of the muscle. If present, lesser frequency of stimulation is required for obtaining a tetanic contraction since fatigue increases the duration of the contraction period.

(iii) Temperature – the higher the temperature, the lesser the contraction period and hence the higher is the minimum required frequency.

Q.6. *What is the physiological rate of nerve stimulation during voluntary muscle contraction, and how is it maintained?*

Ans. The physiological rate of nerve stimulation during voluntary muscle contraction is 5-18/sec. These tetanic contractions are usually achieved during severe isometric exercises. But the disavantage of this is that it occludes the blood supply to the muscle. That is why Renshaw cell keeps the stimulation rate maintained at a **subtetanic level**.

The asynchronous discharge of nerve fibres causes smooth muscular contractions, even when the stimulation is at sub-tetanic level.

Q.7. *Name the type of muscle contraction which occurs in vivo.*

Ans. Sub-tetanic (mostly) or tetanic contraction.

Q.8. *Differentiate between tetanus, contracture, rigor and rigor mortis?*

Ans. (i) Tetanus, page 100.

(ii) Contracture - here, a contracted muscle fails to relax because the ATP required for removal of Ca^{2+} back into the sarcoplasmic reticulum is not available. It is a reversible phenomenon.

(iii) Rigor and rigor mortis - when muscle fibres are completely depleted of ATP and phosphocreatine, they develop a state of extreme rigidity called **Rigor**. When this occurs after death, the condition is called **Rigor Mortis**. (Fig. 2.7.2)

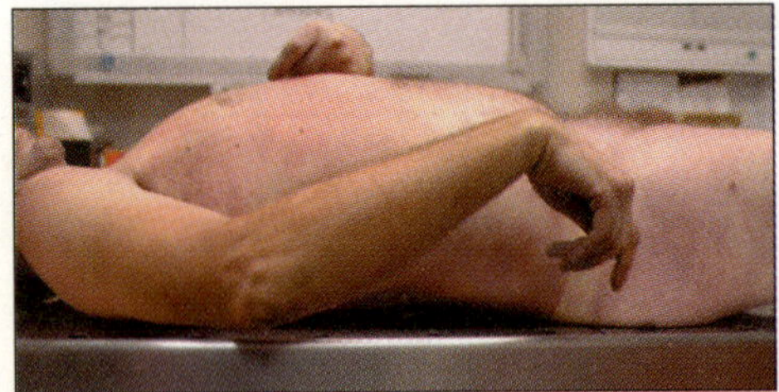

Fig. 2.7.2 Rigor mortis

Q.9. *Why can cardiac muscle not be tetanized?*

Ans. In cardiac muscles, contractile response is more than half over during the absolute refractory period (duration 180-200 msec); hence summation of contractile response is not possible, *i.e.* cardiac muscle cannot be tetanized.

Q.10. *Give examples of slow and fast muscles and their relative tetanizable frequencies.*

Ans. Extraocular muscles and some muscles of hand are fast muscles, whereas the long muscles of back and soleus are slow muscles. Fast muscles have higher tetanizing frequency.

Q.11. *What is the relevance of this experiment to medical physiology?*

Ans. (i) Muscular activity involved in the maintenance of posture, and in many other motor functions, is of tetanic type.

(ii) The strength of muscular contraction can be graded in terms of the alteration of the number of motor units.

(iii) The symptoms of the disease *tetanus* (produced by anaerobic bacteria) and *tetany* have much in common with physiological tetanus.

(iv) The physiological basis of tonic, clonic convulsions (seizures) occurring in various neurological disorders can easily be explained. (Fig. 2.7.3)

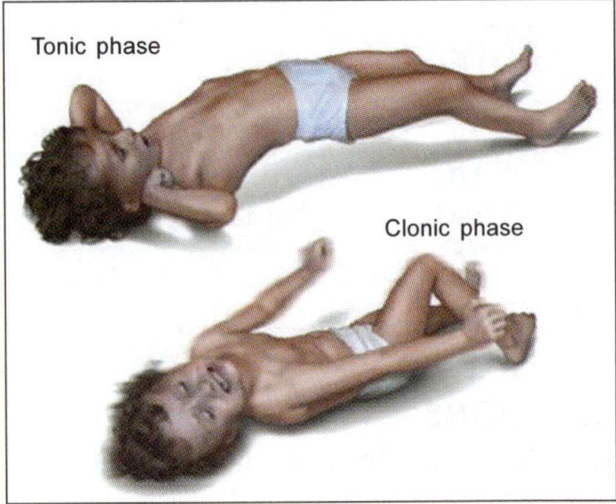

Fig. 2.7.3 Tonic and clonic convulsions

Q.12. *What type of muscular activity is involved in the maintenance of posture?*

Ans. Tetanic contraction.

Q.13. *How does tetanus differ from tetany?*

Ans. Tetanus (page 100). Tetany occurs due to decrease in ionized Ca^{2+} (<50% of normal) causing neuromuscular hyperexcitability (secondary to increase in membrane permeability to Na^{+}. This leads to cramps in extremities due to extensive spasm of skeletal muscle.

Q.14. *What is pathological tetanus?*

Ans. See Q.No. **11**.

STUDY NOTES

RESULTS AND DISCUSSION

....

....

....

Date: ....

8 Effect of Load on Skeletal Muscle Contraction (*After and Free Loaded Conditions*)

I. APPARATUS

As for recording a simple muscle twitch (page 90).

II. THEORY

The load may be applied to the muscle in two ways: *After and free loaded ways.*

1. **After-loaded** is the condition in which the load starts acting on the muscle *after* the contraction has begun, hence the muscle is not stretched by the weight during rest. However, when muscle contraction begins, it causes complete contraction of *contractile component* (actin and myosin) and no further stretching of *series elastic component* (tendon). The lifting of a weight from the ground under normal conditions is an after-loading of the muscle. (Fig. 2.8.1)

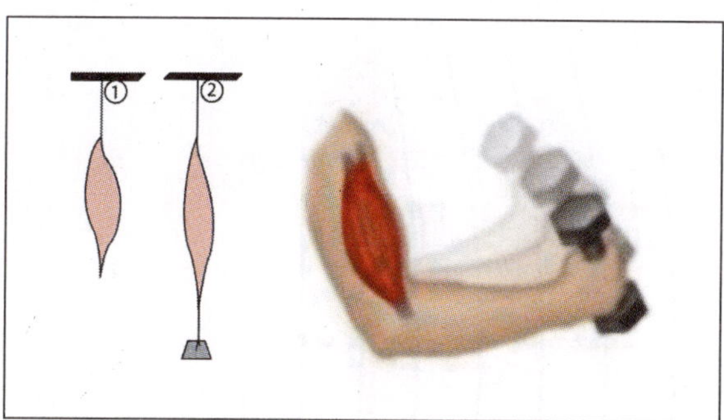

Fig. 2.8.1 After-loaded muscle preparation

2. **Free-loaded** (or *pre-loaded*) is the condition in which the load acts on the muscle *before* it begins to contract. It causes the partial contraction of *contractile component* and keeps the *series elastic component* of the muscle stretched. Therefore, muscle fibres and the muscle start the contraction not from the relaxed but from a somewhat stretched state and no time is wasted in the process after the contraction has begun. Thus the performance (measured in terms of work done) of the muscle is better than in the after-loaded condition. The continuous contraction of the antigravity muscle to maintain body posture is an example of free-loading of the muscles. (Fig. 2.8.2)

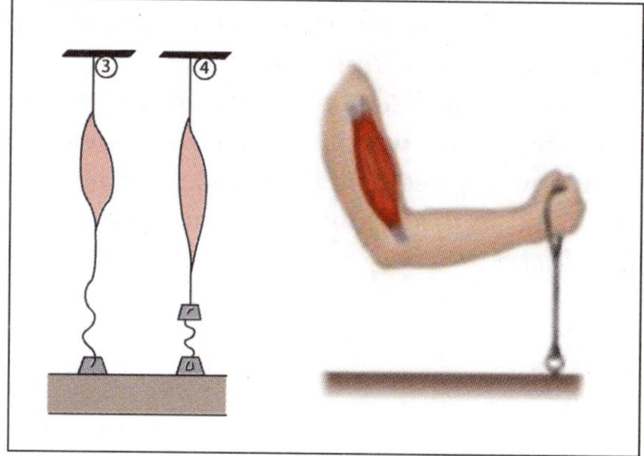

Fig. 2.8.2 Free-loaded muscle preparation

3. **Performance** of the isolated muscle. This is measured in terms of the work done during **isotonic** contraction, that is:

   Work done (W) = Force × Distance

4. The load at which maximum work is done, is called the ***optimal load***. It is about 40% of the load the muscle is just unable to lift.

> **Important Note:** Our muscles are after-loaded and free-loaded at the same time both at rest and during activities.

(Also, refer to page 110)

III. PROCEDURE

This experiment can be done in two ways: on a moving drum and on a stationary drum.

A. Recording on a moving drum

After-loaded condition

1. Arrange the nerve-muscle preparation as for recording a simple muscle twitch (page 90).
2. Hang a 10 gm weight from the lever about 1 cm

from the fulcrum. Bring the *after-load screw* just to touch the lever fulcrum. In this position of the screw, the load does not act on the muscle at rest and acts only when it contracts. In this condition, the muscle is said to be *after-loaded.*

3. Record a SMT at a drum speed of 640 mm/sec. Mark the point of stimulation.
4. Without changing the point of stimulation or strength of stimulus, add 10 gm of weight to the lever and take another SMT (Fig. 2.8.3-inset).
5. Repeat the procedure by adding 10 gm of weight each time till the muscle is unable to lift the weight any more.

Free (or pre) loaded condition

Obtain free-loaded contraction either at a different place on the drum or use a fresh drum.

1. Loosen the after-loading screw. In this position of the screw, any weight suspended from the lever will now act freely on the muscle, and stretch it at rest; and in this condition the muscle is said to be *free-loaded.*
2. Arrange the apparatus as above, hang a 10 gm weight from the lever, the writing point will descend.
3. Without changing the strength of stimulus (as used earlier) record a SMT at a drum speed of 640 mm/sec. Mark the point of stimulus.
4. Add a 10 gm weight to the lever, the writing point will descend further; lower the drum and bring the writing point to the same baseline. Without changing the point of stimulus or strength of stimulus, take another SMT (Fig. 2.8.3-inset).
5. Repeat the procedure by adding a 10 gm weight each time till the muscle is unable to lift the weight any more.

B. Recording on a Stationary Drum

After-loaded condition

1. Arrange the apparatus as for recording a SMT; do not include the drum in the circuit.
2. Hang a 10 gm weight from the lever and leave the lever in the after-loaded position (see below).
3. Record the muscle contraction produced by pressing and releasing the tap key on a stationary drum.

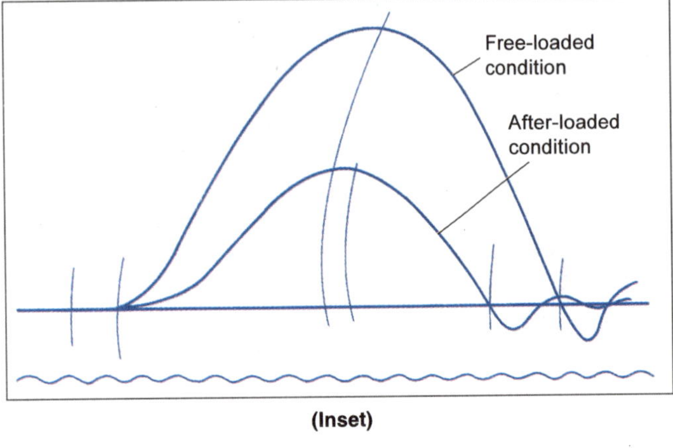

(Inset)

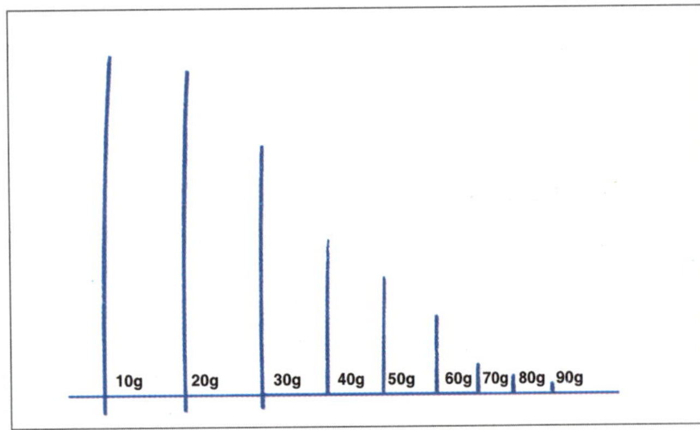

(A) After-loaded condition

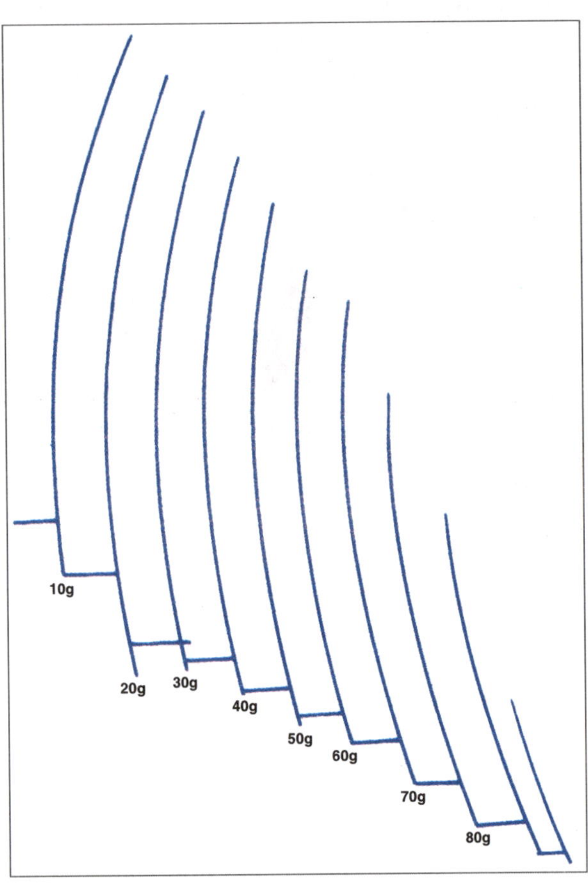

(B) Free-loaded condition

Fig. 2.8.3 Effect of load on skeletal muscle contraction (stationary drum). {Inset: free-load and after-load compared with a 10 gm weight on a moving drum}

4. After each contraction rotate the drum manually for about 1 cm; add weights by 10 gm and record the contractions till the muscle is unable to lift the weight (Fig. 2.8.3-A).

Free (or pre) loaded condition

1. Release the after-loading screw. In this free-loaded condition, the lever comes down as the muscle is stretched by the weights.
2. Stimulate the muscle and record the contraction.
3. Rotate the drum manually by 1 cm as done above. Now add weights by 10 gm and record contraction each time till the muscle is unable to lift the weight (Fig. 2.8.3-B).

(For recording on Student Physiograph, refer to page 83).

IV. CALCULATION OF WORK DONE

Calculate the work done for each weight in the after-loaded and free-loaded condition of the muscle as follows (Fig. 2.8.4):

Work done (W) = Force or load (F) × h

where 'F' is the load lifted (in gm), and
'h' is the actual height to which weight has been lifted (in cm); it can be derived from the following formula:
$h = l/L \times H$
where 'H' is the height of contraction (recorded on the drum in each case in cm); it is measured accurately by calipers;

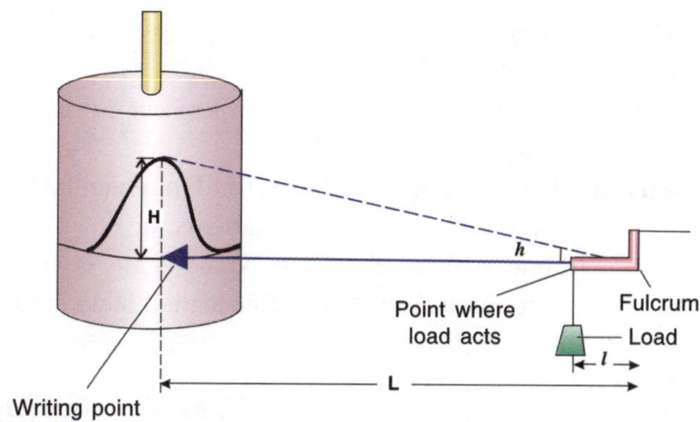

Fig. 2.8.4 Calculation of work done by the muscle

'l' is the distance between fulcrum and point where the load acts (in cm);
'L' is the distance between fulcrum and writing point of lever (in cm).

Therefore, work done (W) =

Force (or load) × l/L × H gm cm.

This should be multiplied by 981 to be expressed in **ergs**.

V. PRECAUTIONS

1. Do not alter the point of stimulus (for recording on a moving drum) and strength of stimulating current.
2. Label the whole series as after-loaded or free-loaded respectively and write the weights added under each contraction.

IMPORTANT VIVA-VOCE QUESTIONS

Q.1. *What do you understand by the term after-loaded and free-loaded conditions? Give one example for each condition.*

Ans. Page 103.

Q.2. *Why does the work output of a muscle first increase with the increase in load under free-loaded preparation and decline afterwards?*

Ans. When a muscle fibre contracts, the tension developed and, hence, the work output is proportional to the number of cross-linkages between the actin and myosin molecules. So, when the load is increased, the muscle is stretched further leading to a decrease in the number of cross-linkages, so the work output decreases.

Q.3. *What are the changes observed in response of an after-loaded muscle when the load is gradually increased?*

Ans. (i) The height of contraction gradually decreases;
(ii) The work done increases up to an optimal load, and then decreases;
(iii) A moving drum gives more details as:
(a) increase in latent period, and
(b) decrease in contraction and relaxation periods.

Q.4. *Define: resting length, initial length, equilibrium length and optimal length of a muscle.*

Ans. (i) *Resting length:* It is the muscle length at which it is present under natural conditions in the body in relaxed state.
(ii) *Initial length:* It is the muscle length before it begins to contract (either in vivo or in vitro).
(iii) *Equilibrium length:* It is the length of the relaxed muscle cut free from its bony attachment.
(iv) *Optimal length:* It is the length at which the muscle is present under natural conditions at rest in the body. At this length they develop maximum **active tension**.

Q.5. *Define optimum load.*

Ans. Page 103.

Q.6. *What is the relevance of this experiment to medical physiology?*

Ans. It is beneficial in everyday life and in rehabilitation of physically handicapped patients, if:

(i) one realises that free-loaded state is more economical than the after-loaded state; and

(ii) the concept of optimum load is understood.

Q.7. *Define free-loading and after-loading of cardiac muscle in vivo.*

Ans. In free-loaded condition, it is the degree to which the myocardium is stretched before it contracts; whereas in after-loaded condition, it is the resistance against which the ventricles pump the blood.

STUDY NOTES

CALCULATION OF WORD DONE

....

....

RESULTS AND DISCUSSION

1. Tabulate your data as follows:

	After-loaded condition	Free-loaded condition
A. Simple Muscle Twitch (with 10gm weight)		
1. Latent period (sec.)		
2. Contraction period (sec.)		
3. Relaxation period (sec.)		
4. Height of contraction (cm)		
B. Work Done (in Ergs)		
Load		
10 gm		
20 gm		
30 gm		
40 gm		
50 gm		
60 gm		
70 gm		
80 gm		

2. Plot a graph to show the relationship between the work done (in ergs) on Y-axis and the load (in gms) on X-axis. Find the *optimal load* for the given muscle in both the conditions. (Discuss your result with the table teacher.)

....

....

....

COMMENTS, RESULTS AND DISCUSSION

....

....

Date: ....

9 Genesis of Fatigue in Skeletal Muscle

I. APPARATUS

As for recording a simple muscle twitch (page 90)

II. THEORY

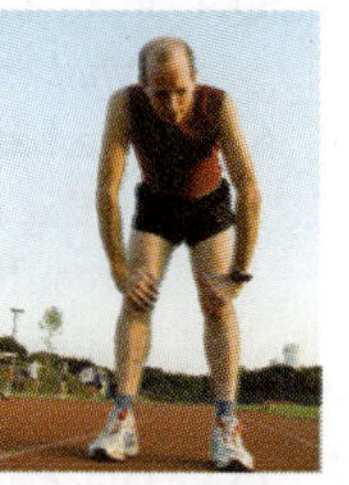

1. Fatigue is a temporary reduction of the working capacity of a cell, an organ or an organism as a whole resulting from prolonged exertion. It is a **reversible** phenomenon and passes off after a rest.
2. In an isolated nerve-muscle preparation, if rhythmic electrical stimuli are applied for some time (with a small suspended load), the amplitude of contractions will gradually fall to zero and the muscle no longer responds to stimulation. This could be due to:
   (i) lack of nutrition;
   (ii) accumulation of waste metabolites; and
   (iii) depletion of A-ch stores.

III. PROCEDURE

1. Arrange the nerve-muscle preparation as for recording a SMT (page 90).
2. Repeatedly stimulate the nerve and record the 1st, 2nd and 3rd contractions on a fast moving drum (640 mm/sec) keeping the point of stimulation same (Fig. 2.9.1).
3. Stop the drum and mark the point of stimulation.
4. Keep the point of stimulation the same and move the writing point away from the drum. Allow the drum to rotate and stimulate the nerve repeatedly by keeping the tap-key pressed so that the preparation may be stimulated once during each revolution.
5. Record every 10th contraction (to prevent overlap of responses) by applying the writing point to the drum till the muscle contractions are too feeble to be recorded.

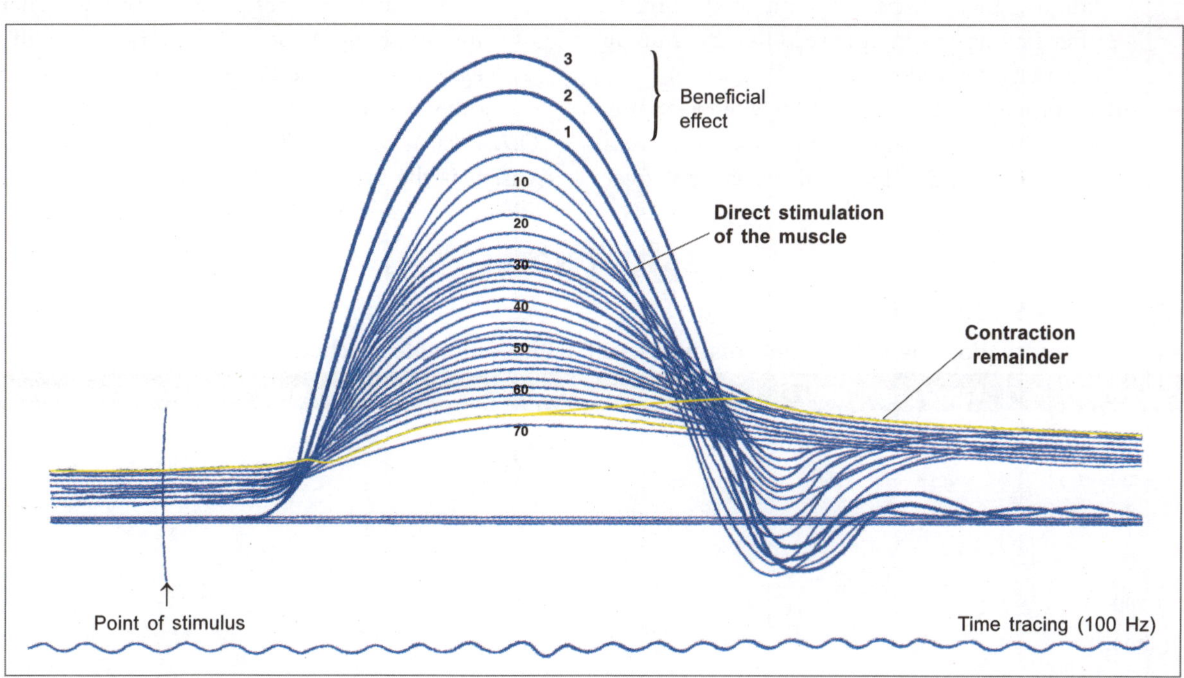

Fig. 2.9.1 Muscle curves showing fatigue as a result of repeated stimulation

6. Stimulate the muscle directly and record its response on the same baseline on a fresh portion of the paper.
7. Rest the preparation for 5 minutes. Keep pouring the fresh Ringer solution. Stimulate the nerve again and record the recovery of the muscle on the same baseline at a different point.

(For recording on Student Physiograph, refer page 83).

IMPORTANT VIVA-VOCE QUESTIONS

Q.1. *Define fatigue.*

Ans. Page 107.

Q.2. *Describe the changes that occur in a muscle as fatigue sets in.*

Ans. (i) Initially the first few contractions (3 or 4) show increase in height, because the first contraction helps the second and so on by increasing the temperature of the muscle and other related phenomena (*i.e.* beneficial effect, page 95).

(ii) With subsequent stimulation, the changes which occur are:

(a) height of contraction decreases;

(b) relaxation is inadequate and incomplete; and

(c) latent, contraction and relaxation periods increase in duration.

Q.3. *What is the first site of fatigue in an isolated nerve-muscle preparation? Justify.*

Ans. In an isolated nerve-muscle preparation, neuro-muscular junction seems to be the first site of fatigue. This can be shown indirectly as follows:

(i) To prove that the muscle is not the site of fatigue, the muscle is stimulated directly after fatigue sets in. It is seen that the muscle contracts vigorously.

(ii) To prove that nerve is not the site of fatigue. Take two nerve-muscle preparations, cross the nerves and a block of ice is kept over one of the nerve-muscle preparations. This prevents the transmission of nerve impulses. Both the preparations are stimulated till fatigue sets in one of the preparations. Now remove the block of ice and stimulate the nerve; its muscle contracts proving that nerve is not the site of fatigue.

Q.4. *Why does the baseline rise in a fatigue graph? Or What is* ***contraction remainder****?*

Ans. The baseline rises due to an incomplete relaxation of the muscle following the depletion of ATP, as a result of which the writing point does not come down to its original position. This is called as **contraction remainder.**

Q.5. *What are the causes of recovery? How can you hasten recovery process?*

Ans. Secretion of fresh A-ch; removal of waste metabolites and supply of fresh nutrition are the causes of recovery. It can be hastened by replacing the fresh Ringer solution.

Q.6. *Why does an athlete run the initial part of his race slowly and speed up only towards the finish?*

Ans. Because if he speeds up at the beginning, he draws on his anaerobic resources to provide energy for the working muscles. Then fatigue will set in earlier due to the accumulation of lactic acid and other metabolites.

Q.7. *What is the first site of fatigue in man?*

Ans. It is the synapse in the brain.

STUDY NOTES

RESULTS AND DISCUSSION

Tabulate your observations as follows and discuss result with your table teacher.

S.No. of contraction	Latent period (sec.)	Contraction period (sec.)	Relaxation period (sec.)	Amplitude of contraction (cm)
1st				
2nd				
3rd				
10th				
20th				
30th				
40th				
50th				
Direct stimulation of the muscle				

Date: ....

10 Recording of Isometric Contraction in Skeletal Muscle

I. APPARATUS

The same as for recording a SMT (page 90); isometric lever, muscle grip, calipers and weights

Isometric Lever (Fig. 2.10.1–inset)

It consists of a strong steel wire fixed at both ends, with a pointer attached to its centre. When the muscle contracts, it produces the torsion of the wire which is reflected by the movement of pointer. The muscle is prevented from shortening (*isometric contraction*) and the movement of the pointer indicates the development of tension in the muscle.

II. PROCEDURE

1. Arrange the nerve muscle preparation and electrical circuit for a single-induced stimulus.
2. *Calibration of isometric lever:* Isometric lever is fixed on the kymograph stand. Attach the weight hanger on the lever near its fulcrum. Place a weight of 10 gm on it and record a base line on the upper part of the drum. Label the line as 10 gm. Repeat the procedure by increasing the weights by 10 gm and record the baselines corresponding to increasing weights. Remove all weights and hanger after calibration (Fig. 2.10.1).

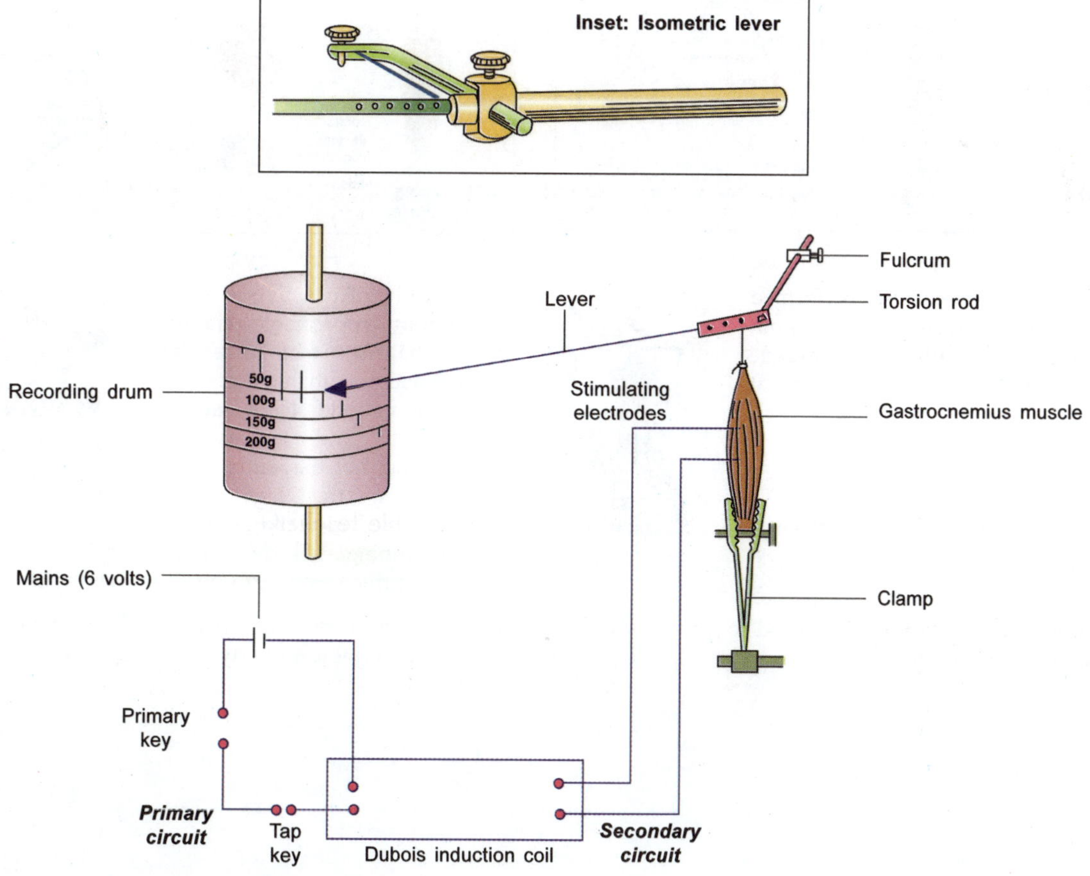

Fig. 2.10.1 Set-up for recording isometric contraction

3. Expose the gastrocnemius muscle of the pithed frog and measure its length. Remove the muscle.
4. Fix the knee joint of the preparation with the help of muscle grip (clamp) below the lever.
5. Attach the muscle tendon to the isometric lever at the same point where weight hanger was placed.
6. Measure the length of the muscle with caliper and stimulate directly the muscle by maximal stimulus. Record the tension developed (Fig. 2.10.2).
7. Repeat the procedure for different muscle lengths. Each time the record the length, corresponding passive tension and total tension developed. Increase the length of muscle by one or two mm, by lowering the muscle grip.

(For recording on Student Physiograph, refer to page 83).

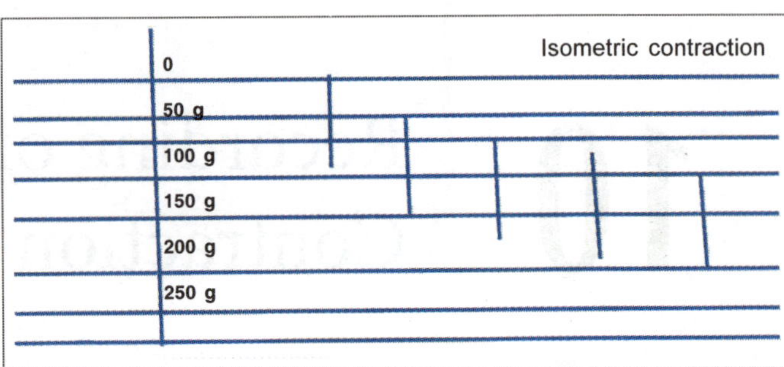

Fig. 2.10.2 Record of isometric contraction in a skeletal muscle.

IMPORTANT VIVA-VOCE QUESTIONS

Q.1. *Define resting length and equilibrium length of the skeletal muscle.*

Ans. Page 105.

Q.2. *Differentiate between isometric and isotonic skeletal muscle contraction.*

Ans.

Isometric contraction (Fig. 2.10.3)	Isotonic contraction (Fig. 2.10.4)
(i) Here muscle contracts but the length of muscle remains the same and *no external work is done.* (Also refer to page 98)	(i) Here, the length of muscle changes while tension remains constant. Therefore, *external work is done.*

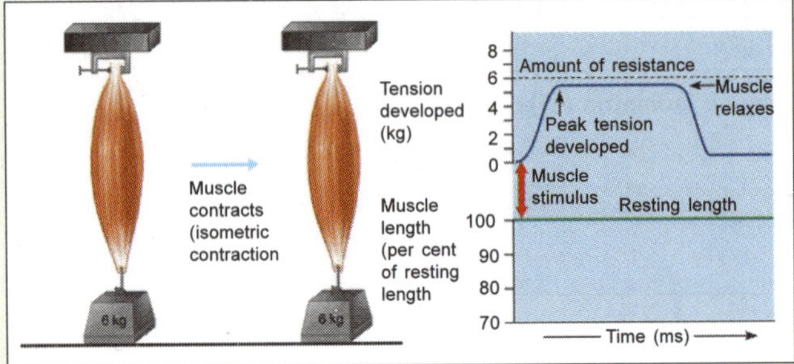

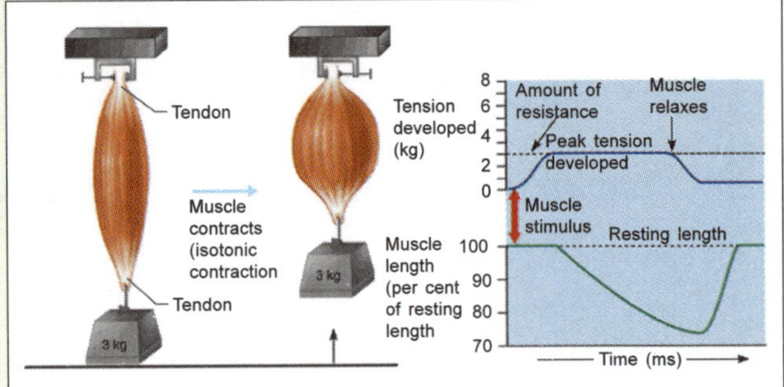

Isometric contraction (Fig. 2.10.3)	Isotonic contraction (Fig. 2.10.4)
(ii) Examples: Active exercise performed against stable resistance, without change in the length of the muscle and there is **No** visible movement at the joint. (a) muscle which helps maintain posture against gravity; (b) muscles contraction while trying to push a wall.	(ii) Examples: An active exercise without appreciable change in the force of muscular contraction, with the shortening of the muscle. Here muscle contracts and causes the movement of the joints. (a) when the legs are moved in walking and running; (b) contraction of arm muscles, while lifting a load 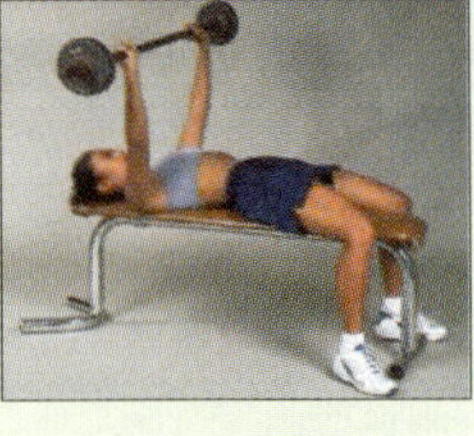
(iii) **Physiological significance:** It is used to improve tone and strength of the muscle.	(iii) It is used to strengthen muscle and its tone, and improve joint mobility.

STUDY NOTES

RESULTS AND DISCUSSION

Tabulate the results as follows and discuss with the table teacher.

Length of the muscle in cm (1)	Initial (passive) tension (gm) (2)	Total tension developed (gm) (3)	Active tension (gm) (3 – 2) (4)

Draw graphs showing the relationship of the *length* of the muscle to *passive, total* and *active tensions*.

....

....

....

....

....

....

....

....

....

....

....

....

Date: ....

11 Determination of Conduction Velocity of the Sciatic Nerve

I. APPARATUS

As for recording a SMT (page 90); reversing key (instead of short circuiting key), two pairs of electrodes

II. PROCEDURE

1. Arrange the apparatus as for recording a simple muscle twitch (page 90). Connect the reversing key in the secondary circuit instead of the short circuiting key. Connect two pairs of electrodes to the reversing key.
2. Place one pair of electrodes on the nerve at a point close to the muscle and the other pair of electrodes on the nerve close to the vertebral column.
3. Rotate the drum at the fastest speed (640 mm/sec); using the reversing key, stimulate the nerve at its *muscle end* and take a SMT (mark it as ***'M' curve***); also, mark the point of stimulus (Fig. 2.11.1).
4. Keeping the same baseline, without changing the point of stimulus or strength of stimulus, stimulate the nerve at its *vertebral end* using the reversing key and take another SMT, (mark it as ***'V' curve***) (Fig. 2.11.1).
5. Take a time tracing with the help of a tuning fork (frequency 100 Hz). Note the difference between the latent periods of the two SMTs (let it be 't' sec). This represents the time taken by the impulse to travel from one point to another.
6. Measure the distance between the central points of two pairs of electrodes (let it be 'S' cm).
7. Calculate the conduction velocity of the nerve as follows:

$$= \frac{\text{Distance travelled (S) in cm}}{\text{Time taken by nerve impulse from one point to another ('t' sec)}} \text{ cm/sec}$$

Express it in metres/sec.

(For recording on Student Physiograph, refer to page 83).

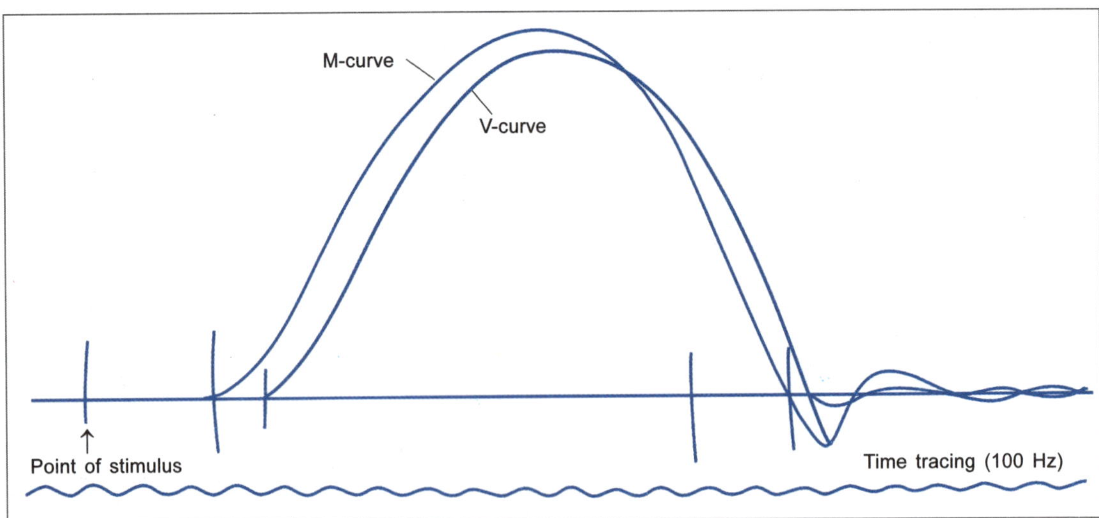

Fig. 2.11.1 Record for determining the conduction velocity of the sciatic nerve (frog)

IMPORTANT VIVA-VOCE QUESTIONS

Q.1. *What is the normal conduction velocity of the frog's sciatic nerve?*

Ans. Normally it is 40 metres/sec.

Q.2. *How are the nerve fibres classified? Give their functions.*

Ans. According to Erlanger and Gasser classification, the nerve fibres are divided into A, B and C groups. 'A' group nerve fibres are further divided into α, β, γ and δ fibres.

Fibre type Function

1. A_α Proprioception, somatic motor
2. A_β Touch, pressure
3. A_γ Motor to muscle spindles
4. A_δ Pain, temperature, touch
5. B Preganglionic autonomic fibres
6. C
   (i) *Dorsal root:* pain, touch, temperature
   (ii) *Sympathetic:* post-ganglionic sympathetic fibers.

Q.3. *Give the characteristic features of a nerve fibre based on its diameter.*

Ans. The greater the diameter of a given fiber:

(i) the greater is its speed of conduction and magnitude of spike potential;
(ii) the smaller is the duration of spike;
(iii) the lesser will be the threshold of excitation and refractory period.

Q.4. *Enumerate the factors affecting the conduction velocity in a nerve.*

Ans. Factors affecting the conduction velocity in a nerve are:

(i) Diameter of nerve fibre
(ii) Presence or absence of myelination
(iii) Temperature
(iv) Conducting media in which nerve is placed
(v) Proximity of RMP to the threshold

Q.5. *Why is the distance travelled by the nerve impulse is measured from the mid-points of the two limbs of the electrodes.*

Ans. An electrode has two limbs and since it is not known which limb is anode or cathode. Therefore, the distance is measured from the mid-points of the two limbs of the electrodes.

Q.6. *What is the relevance of this experiment to medical physiology?*

Ans. Determination of conduction velocity in a nerve helps: (Fig. 2.11.2)

(i) trace the recovery of nerve injuries;
(ii) assess the extent of damage done to a nerve due to trauma or in demyelination disorders.

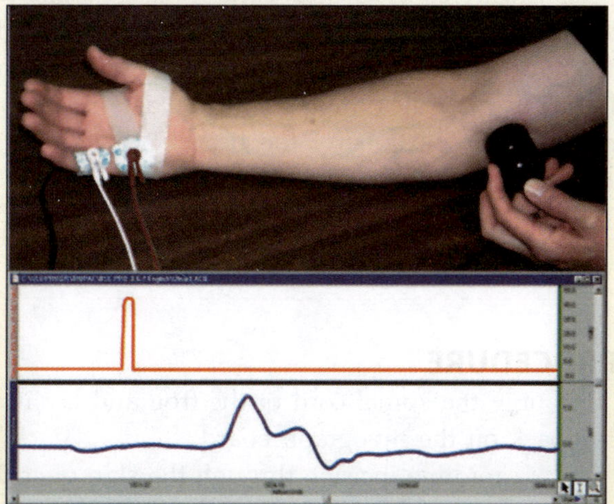

Fig. 2.11.2 Determination of nerve conduction in humans

(For further details, refer to page 297)

STUDY NOTES

CALCULATIONS

....

....

....

RESULTS AND DISCUSSION

....

....

....

Date: ....

12 Recording of a Normal Cardiogram and Effect of Temperature on It

I. APPARATUS

Myograph board, dissection apparatus, Starling heart lever, thread, cotton wool, pins, cold and warm Amphibian Ringer's solution, thermometer, kymograph, drum, dropper

II. THEORY

The frog's heart consists of 4 parts: *sinus venosus, two auricles* and *one ventricle* which beat sequentially. The heart beat originates in the sinus venosus under normal conditions. It generates impulses at the fastest rate and drives the other portions of the heart. Therefore, it is called the **cardiac pacemaker**.

> **Note:** In the mammalian heart, SA Node is the cardiac pacemaker and is located in the right atrium.

III. PROCEDURE

1. Pith only the spinal cord of the frog and lay it on its back on the myograph board.
2. Make a midline incision through the skin over the sternum, raise the cartilaginous xiphisternum and separate it from underneath by cutting through the strands of tissues.
3. Make an incision on each side of the cartilage, insert pointed end of a scissor under the pectoral girdle, keeping the blade in close contact with the bone. Divide the girdle first on one side and then on the other; raise and cut away the anterior wall of the thorax. This will expose the heart; study its parts carefully (Fig. 2.12.1).
4. Pull both forelimbs laterally and fix them in such a position so as to keep the chest wide open.
5. Slit open the pericardium and remove it. Insert a pin through the bulbus (base), fixing it to the myograph board. If this has not been done, the contracting heart will pull at both ends and the record will be greatly diminished.
6. Lift the ventricle up and pass a bent pin through its apex. Tie the pin to the Starling heart lever by means of thread. Adjust the tension on the thread (plasticine may be used) so as to keep the recording lever horizontal in contact with the drum mounted on a kymograph.
7. Rotate the drum at a slow speed of 2.5 mm/sec and take the tracing of contracting heart (**a normal cardiogram**).
8. With the help of a dropper, pour drop by drop 1-2 ml of warm Ringer solution (at about 40°C) on the heart and take the effect for 6-7 contractions (Fig. 2.12.2). Precisely note the temperature of Ringer solution.
9. Stop the drum and wait for the heart beat to return to normal. Repeat the whole procedure with cold Ringer solution (at about 10°C) on the heart and take the effect. Note the temperature precisely.

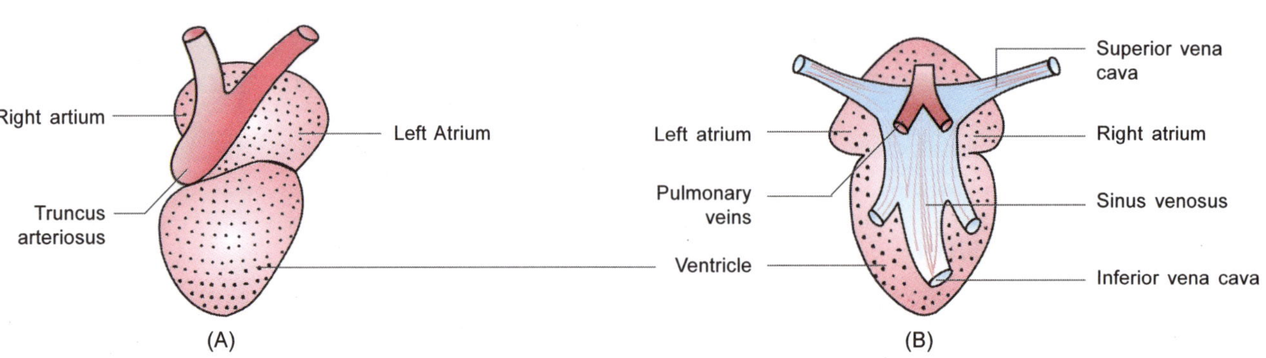

Fig. 2.12.1 Parts of a frog's heart. Anterior (A) and Posterior (Dorsal) view (B)

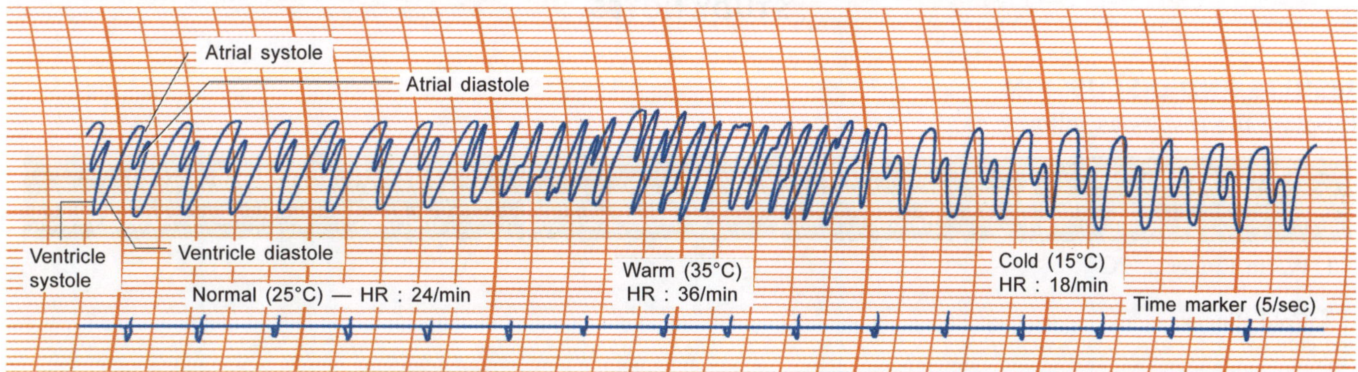

Fig. 2.12.2 A normal cardiogram and effect of temperature on it

10. Take the time record every 5 secs with the help of time signal marker.
11. In each case, note the change in rate and height of contraction of the heart.

(For recording on Student Physiograph, refer to page 84).

IV. PRECAUTIONS

1. Never use a knife while experimenting with the frog's heart, use scissors only.
2. Do not pinch the heart tissue with forceps.
3. Prevent the heart from drying by the application of Amphibian Ringer's solution at regular intervals.
4. Do not puncture the ventricle while passing a pin through its apex.
5. The temperature of warm Ringer should not exceed 42°C and take the effect of warm Ringer before the cold Ringer.

IMPORTANT VIVA-VOCE QUESTIONS

Q.1. *Label the components of a normal cardiogram.*

Ans. Refer to Fig. 2.12.2.

Q.2. *What is the effect of warm and cold Ringer solution on the rate and force of contraction of the heart?*

Ans. Warm Ringer increase both the rate and force of contraction of the heart, whereas cold Ringer has just the opposite effect.

Q.3. *Why is it necessary to fix the base of the heart?*

Ans. Page 114.

Q.4. *Is it necessary to remove the pericardium? Justify.*

Ans. The removing of the pericardium is essential as it helps:

(i) support the heart firmly from the apex;

(ii) a variable to come in direct contact with the heart muscle.

Q.5. *What is the site of action of warm Ringer on the heart? Give its mechanism of action.*

Ans. Warm Ringer increases the heart rate and height of contraction by acting on the cardiac pacemaker. Heart rate is increased due to increase in permeability of membrane to Na^+, thus increasing the frequency of discharge of pacemaker. Increase in the force of contraction is due to decrease in the viscosity. This is seen initially only.

Important: Cold Ringer has just the opposite effect.

Q.6. *What will happen if only the ventricle is warmed?*

Ans. Warming the ventricle alone increases its height of contraction, but the rhythm is unchanged.

Q.7. *How is the warming of ventricle alone brought out experimentally?*

Ans. This can be achieved by placing small bits of blotting paper soaked in warm Ringer onto the ventricle with the help of a pain of forceps, taking care of the trickling of Ringer solution onto the sinus venosus. Alternatively, ventricle can be warmed by placing platinum wire loop round the ventricle which is then connected with a battery, using a key in the circuit.

Q.8. *Where can this knowledge of the effect of temperature on cardiagram in day-to-day life in humans be correlated?*

Ans. Conditions which change the heart rate due to alteration in internal body temperature (such as fever, exercise, hypothermia) can be explained.

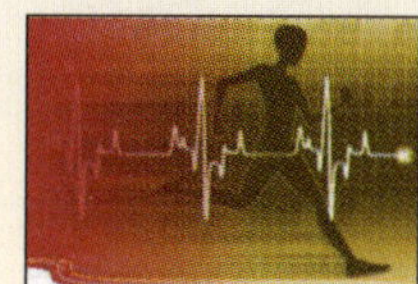

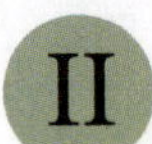

STUDY NOTES

RESULTS AND DISCUSSION

Tabulate the results as follows:

Effect of variable	Heart Rate (bmp)		Height of contraction (cm)	
	Before	After	Before	After
1. Warm Ringer .... °C				
2. Cold Ringer .... °C				

....

....

....

....

....

....

....

....

....

....

....

....

Date: ....

13 Properties of Cardiac Muscle

I. APPARATUS

The same as for recording a cardiogram (page 114); signal marker, induction coil, wire electrodes

II. THEORY

The following properties of cardiac muscle are studied:

1. Autorhythmicity
2. Phenomenon of extrasystole, compensatory pause and refractory period
3. Heart block: stannius ligature
4. All or none law
5. Staircase phenomenon
6. Summation of sub-liminal stimuli

Important note: The ***property of rhythmicity states***, that a contraction is necessarily followed by a relaxation. It is seen for quite some time even after all nerves to heart are cut, called ***autorhythmicity***. A record of normal cardiogram thus takes care of the demonstration of this property, hence, if need not to be described separately.

1. Extrasystole, compensatory pause and refractory period

(i) Normally, the ventricle contracts as a result of an impulse generated from the SA Node; however, if an artificial extra stimulus is given, it responds by contracting prematurely. This is called as ***extrasystole***, the next normal impulse coming from the SA node to the ventricle then usually falls in the **refractory period** (non-responsive period) of the extra-contraction. The ventricle, therefore, does not respond to it, and remains silent till the second normal impulse reaches it. This period of inactivity is referred as the **compensatory pause**.

(ii) The normal refractory period of heart muscle is long (ventricle 250 msec; atria 150 msec) extending up to the end of systole. Because of this, stimuli given during systole and early diastole are ineffective. This inexcitable period is called **refractory period**. By the time stimuli become effective, the muscle starts relaxing; this property thus ensures that a contraction is necessarily followed by a relaxation and some circulation is thus maintained.

Note: The duration of the normal contraction, the extra-systole and compensatory pause are together equal to **two** normal cardiac cycles.

2. Heart block: *Stannius ligatures*

The failure of conduction of impulse from one part of the heart to another is known as *heart block.*

(i) The conduction of impulse can be blocked partially or completely by mechanical pressure such as by tying a thin thread knot at various sites. These are known as **stannius ligatures** and are two in number.

(ii) The *1st stannius ligature* is tied between the sinus venosus and the atria (Fig. 2.13.1). On tying the

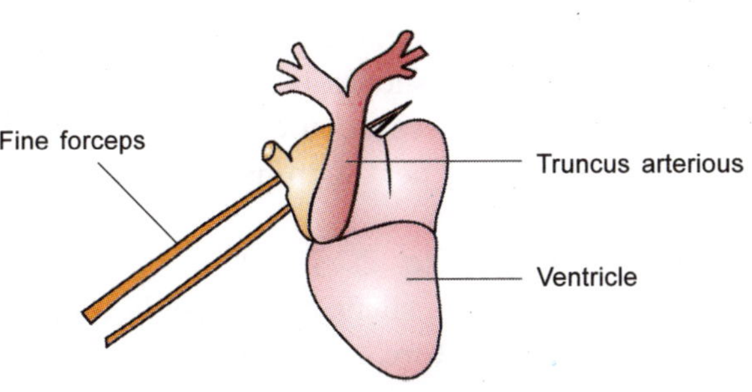

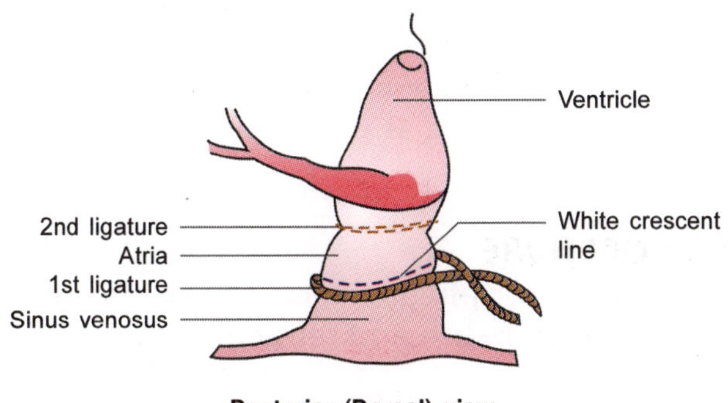

Fig. 2.13.1 The passage of the thread for the stannius ligatures

ligature the impulse from sinus venosus is prevented from reaching the atria. The sinus continues to beat but the atria and ventricle stop beating. After some time, the atria start generating their own impulse; the impulse reaches the ventricle and the atrio-ventricular segment starts beating independent of the sinus rhythm but at a slower rate than that of the sinus venosus.

(iii) The *second stannius ligature* is tied between the atria and the ventricle round the atrio-ventricular groove (Fig. 2.13.1). On tying this, the impulse from atria is prevented from reaching the ventricle. The atria continues to beat with its own rhythm while the ventricle stops beating. After a short period, the ventricle generates its own impulse and starts beating independent of atria at a much slower rate than the atrial rhythm. This is referred as the ***idio-ventricular rhythm***.

> Note: This demonstrates the property of conductivity, *i.e.* property of propagation of cardiac impulse.

3. All or none Law

The response in cardiac muscle is 'all or none' in character, *i.e.* 'all or none' relationship between the stimulus and the response. Therefore, the heart either gives no contraction at all or, if it contracts, it contracts to the maximum of its ability. This is because of the syncytial and interconnecting nature of cardiac muscle fibres.

4. Staircase phenomenon

Staircase effect/phenomenon refers to the successive increase in the first few (4 or 5) cardiac contractions after the silent heart has started beating. This is due to the mechanism of beneficial effect (page 95).

5. Summation of subliminal stimuli

If a *sub-threshold stimuli* is applied repeatedly to the heart at an interval of one half to one second, the 10th to 20th stimulus generally gives a full contraction. This shows that each stimulus even though subliminal, causes some changes in the heart muscle enabling it to respond more readily to a successive stimulus. This phenomenon is known as the **temporal summation** of subliminal stimuli.

III. PROCEDURE

A. Recording for phenomenon of extrasystole, compensatory pause and refractory period (Fig. 2.13.2-1)

1. Make primary circuit by connecting primary key, primary coil and signal marker in series to the low voltage mains. Do not include the drum in the circuit.
2. Make secondary circuit as usual using fine wire electrodes instead of muscle electrodes. Check both the circuits (page 80).
3. Arrange the preparation and record the normal cardiogram of a frog as described earlier (page 114).
4. Tie one electrode to the pin in the apex of the ventricle and another is wound round the base of the ventricle.
5. Arrange a *signal marker* in alignment with the starling heart lever to record the exact moment of stimulation.
6. Now stimulate the ventricle during the different phases of the cardiac cycle (e.g. systole, early and late diastole) and record the effects.

> **Important Notes**
> 1. Stimuli falling during systole are not responded to; and
> 2. Those falling during diastole produce a premature contraction (called **extra systole**) which is followed by a **compensatory pause.**

This experiment can also be done in a silent heart after putting the first stannius ligature.

B. Heart block: Stannius ligature (Fig. 2.13.2-2)

1. A dissected frog is mounted on the myograph board and the base of the heart is fixed to the board.
2. Pass a thread under the truncus arteriosus and brought forward at the junction of sinus venosus and atria. This marks the **white crescent line** of the heart.
3. Make a loose knot; the apex of the ventricle is then fixed to the recording lever; record the normal cardiogram.
4. Apply the first stannius ligature (page 117) so that the ventricle may stop beating. After some time, the atria generates its own rhythm and the ventricle also start beating under the influence of atrial rhythm.
5. Apply the second stannius ligature at A-V groove (see above). The ventricle stops beating and after a pause should begin beating at a much slower rate (**idio-ventricular rhythm**) while the atria continues to beat with its own atrial rhythm.

C. All or none law (Fig. 2.13.2-3)

1. The heart is made silent by the application of the first stannius ligature.
2. Arrange the connections and apparatus as described above. Adjust the writing point of the lever as to record the contraction on a stationary or slow-moving drum (2.5 mm/sec).

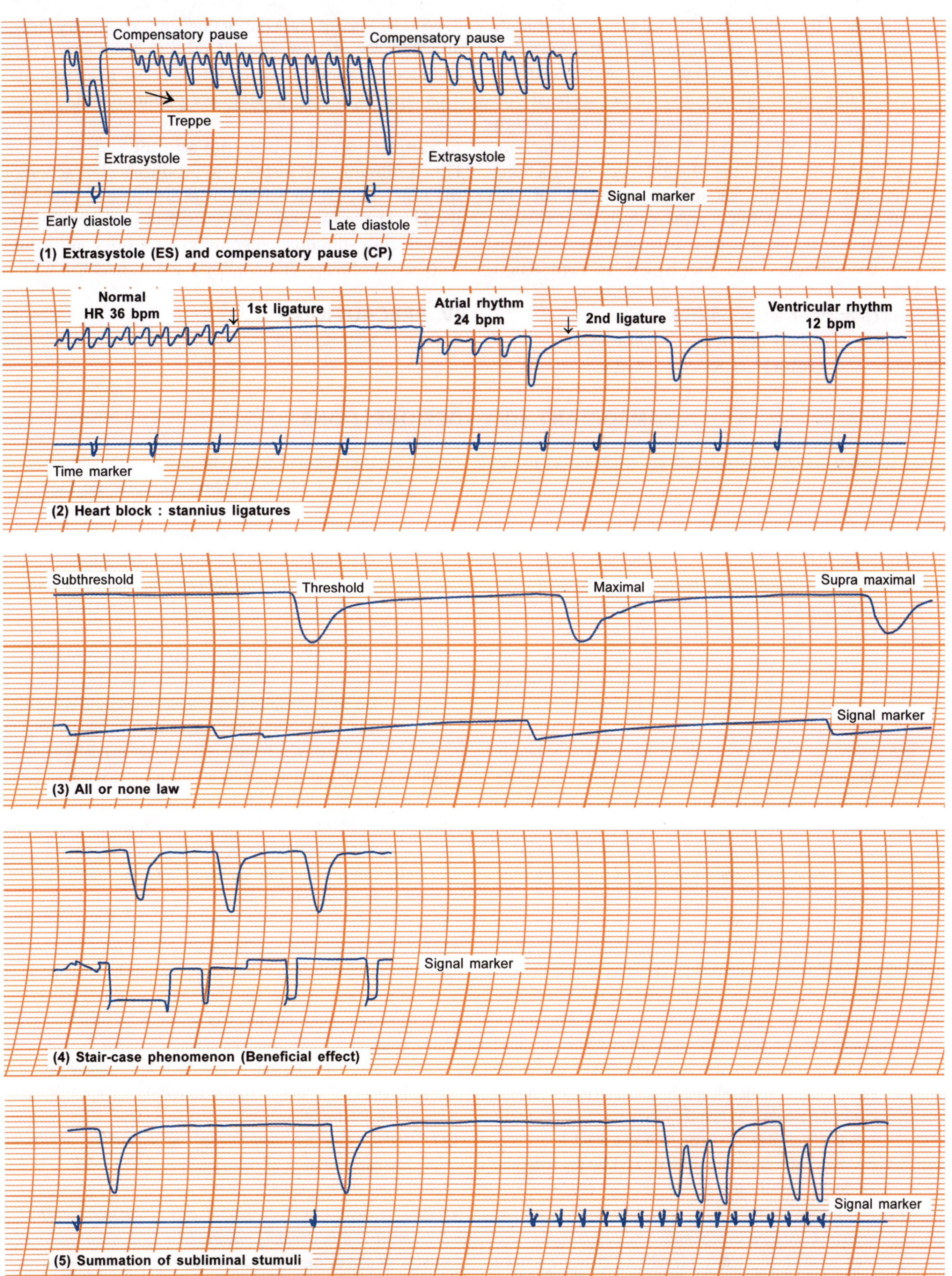

Fig. 2.13.2 Record of properties of the cardiac muscle

3. Stimulate the ventricle with subthreshold stimuli and then increase the strength of the stimulus (page 99) till there is a contraction and record it.
4. Now after every 30 seconds, further increase the strength of the stimulus, rotate the drum through 1 cm each time and record the contraction. It is seen that the height of contractions remains the same though the strength of the stimulus is being progressively increased, *i.e.* there is no relation between the strength of the stimulus and the height of contraction

D. Staircase phenomenon (Fig. 2.13.2-4)

Adjust the induction coil for a single effective shock. Stimulate the ventricle repeatedly at the intervals of 2 seconds. Record the contraction on a stationary drum at a distance of 1 cm apart. Notice that the first 4 or 5 contractions show a successive increase in amplitude. This effect is known as **staircase phenomenon**.

E. Summation of subliminal stimuli (Fig. 2.13.2-5)

Find a stimulus that just fails to produce a contraction of the heart. Repeat the stimulus several times by tapping the key at the intervals of one half to one second. The 10th to 20th stimulus generally gives a full contraction.

(For recording on Student Physiograph, refer to page 84)

IV. PRECAUTIONS

The same as described earlier on page 115.

IMPORTANT VIVA-VOCE QUESTIONS

Q.1. *Define the terms: Extra-systole and compensatory pause.*

Ans. Page 117.

Q.2. *Why is the extra-systole followed by a compensatory pause?*

Ans. Page 117.

Q.3. *How will you differentiate between atrial and ventricular extra-systole?*

Ans. Differentiation between atrial and ventricular extra-systole can be made from E.C.G. only.

Q.4. *Give the physiological significance of compensatory pause.*

Ans. Page 117.

Q.5. *What are the factors predisposing to extra systole in humans?*

Ans. Predisposing factors for extra-systole in humans are:

(i) excess intake of coffee or alcohol or tobacco; this leads to the formation of micro-thrombi.
(ii) anxiety;
(iii) hyperthyroidism;
(iv) hypoxia, and
(v) electrolyte imbalance, etc.

Q.6. *How many extra-systoles per minute are regarded as normal? When do they become clinically significant?*

Ans. 2-4 extra systoles/minute are regarded as normal in humans. This may result from excessive smoking, lack of sleep, ingestion of too much coffee or alcohol. When they become very frequent (>6 per minute) or occur in a diseased heart e.g. myocardial infarction, they should be regarded as clinically significant.

Q.7. *Define absolute and relative refractory period in cardiac muscle. Give their significance.*

Ans. (i) *Absolute refractory period (ARP)* begins from the time the firing level is reached until the repolarization is about 1/3 complete. During this period, no stimulus, no matter how strong, can initiate the fresh impulse. Since contractile response is more than half over during ARP, therefore, the summation of contractile response is not possible, *i.e.* **cardiac muscle cannot be tetanized**.

(ii) Relative refractory period (RRP) begins at the end of ARP until the repolarization is complete. During this period, stimulus stronger than normal stimulus can cause excitation and the cardiac muscle responds by contracting prematurely. This is called *extra systole.*

Q.8. *What purpose is served by a long refractory period for the cardiac muscle?*

Ans. Long refractive period in cardiac muscle prevents it from tetanization (see above), thereby ensuring the continuous flow of blood into the circulation.

Q.9. *Define all or none law.*

Ans. Page 118.

Q.10. *What unit of a tissue obeys all or none law?*

Ans. In a skeletal muscle and nerve, an individual fibre obeys 'all or none' law, whereas, in the *heart*, the unit being the entire atria or entire ventricle.

Q.11. *Why should the interval between stimuli be half a minute to demonstrate the all or none phenomenon?*

Ans. This is to prevent the summation of stimuli or beneficial effect.

Q.12. *Define: staircase phenomenon and summation of subliminal stimuli.*

Ans. Page 118.

Q.13. *How will you demonstrate experimentally that the heart is a functional syncytium?*

Ans. This can be demonstrated by studying the property of all or none law in a cardiac muscle.

STUDY NOTES

RESULTS AND DISCUSSION

Date: ....

14 Effect of the Stimulation of the Vagus Nerve and White Crescentic Line on the Cardiogram

I. APPARATUS

The same as for recording properties of cardiac muscle, page 117; nerve stimulating electrodes, signal marker

II. THEORY

1. A large number of sympathetic and parasympathetic (vagal) fibres end on SA node and conducting tissues. Sympathetic fibres also supply the ventricular muscles.
2. The stimulation of vagus decreases heart rate and conduction but has no effect on ventricular contraction.
3. The stimulation of sympathetic fibres increases heart rate, conduction and force of contraction.
4. The ***white crescentic line (WCL)*** is located at the junction between the sinus venosus and the atria. It is the region where vagus nerve (pre-ganglionic fibers) ends over a group of nerve cells (ganglia) thus forming a synapse. The nerve cells of the ganglion give rise to post-ganglionic fibres. Therefore, the stimulation of the WCL will have the same effect as the stimulation of the vagus.

III. PROCEDURE

A. Dissection to expose vago-sympathetic trunk

1. Pith a frog and open its chest to expose the heart. Prolong the incision upwards to the lower jaw.
2. Cut the platysma muscle and remove the tissue running from the angle of the jaw to expose the thin petrohyoid muscle running from the base of the skull to the posterior cornua of the hyoid bone. The glossopharyngeal and hypoglossal nerves are seen superficially crossing the petrohyoids (Fig. 2.14.1).
3. Along the lower border of the petrohyoid muscle running from above downwards are:
   (i) the laryngeal nerve;
   (ii) the carotid artery and
   (iii) the vagus nerve.
   Isolate the vagus nerve carefully by means of a thin glass rod and pass a thread beneath the nerve. The nerve must be kept moist with Amphibian Ringer solution and handled with the great care.

> **Note:** The vagus nerve, in fact, is seen accompanied by the sympathetic trunk, together called as ***vago-sympathetic trunk***. This bundle can be identified easily as it runs across and superficial to the shining tendon of the levator scapulae.

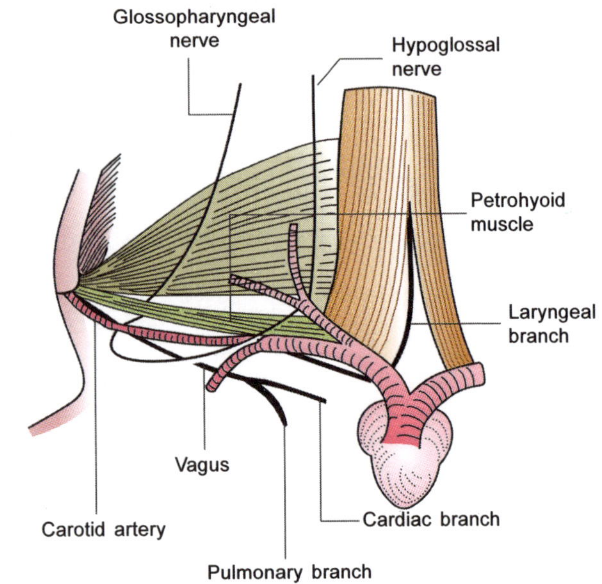

Fig. 2.14.1 The course and relations of the vago-sympathetic trunk in the frog

B. Stimulation of vago-sympathetic trunk

1. Arrange the apparatus for recording normal cardiogram (page 114).
2. Place the vago-sympathetic trunk on the electrode which are connected to the secondary coil.
3. Record normal cardiogram.
4. Now, stimulate the vago-sympathetic trunk through Neef's hammer (*i.e.* at high frequency) at different strengths and record the effect. The heart beat becomes slower and weaker (Fig. 2.14.2).
5. Stimulate with a strong current. The heart stops in diastole (**Vagal Inhibition**).

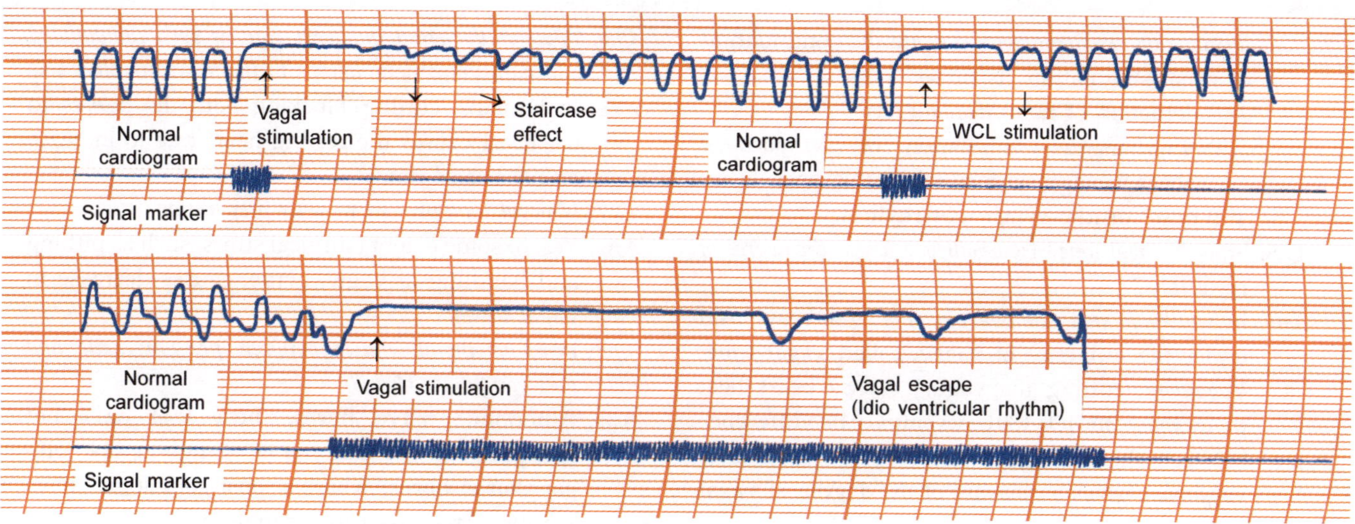

Fig. 2.14.2 Stimulation of vagus nerve and white crescentic line in the frog.

6. Continue the stimulation. After some seconds the ventricle begins to beat but at a very slow rate. This phenomenon is called **Vagal Escape**. Record 4 or 5 ventricular contractions. Mark on the graph the beginning and end of vagal stimulation, label the *vagal escape* (Fig. 2.14.2).
7. Stop the stimulation; the heart begins to beat at the normal rhythm. Record the normal cardiogram.

Important Notes

1. Stimulation of vago-sympathetic trunk may cause *a double effect,* the vagal effect being always the first. The sympathetic effect generally appears only after the stoppage of the stimulus.
2. In many cases, it is found that only one vagus has an action, the other producing either a sympathetic effect or none at all. It is advisable, therefore, to find both the vagi.
3. In the frog the vagus fibres to the heart are **never** equally distributed between the nerves on both sides.

C. Stimulation of white cresentic line

Identify the white crescentic line (page 122) and stimulate it. Record the effect. It will have the same effect as the stimulation of the vagus.

(For recording on Student Physiograph, refer to page 84).

IV. PRECAUTIONS

The same as described earlier on page 115.

IMPORTANT VIVA-VOCE QUESTIONS

Q.1. *Mention the parts of the mammalian heart supplied by the autonomic nerves. Is there any difference between supply of right and left vagus?*

Ans. (i) *Sympathetic supply* to the heart comes from the nerve cells located in the T_1 to T_5 spinal segments. Cardiac sympathetic fibres supply the nodal tissues (SA node and AV node) and muscles of atria and ventricles.

(ii) *Parasympathetic supply* to the heart is via two vagus nerves (right and left) with their cell bodies located in the medulla in the nucleus ambiguus. Its fibres are distributed to the SA node, AV node and muscles of atria. **No vagal motor fibres are distributed to the ventricles.** There is no difference in the supply of right and left vagus to the heart. However, in some individuals, it is the right vagus which is dominant whereas in others, the left vagus.

Q.2. *What are the effects of the stimulation of sympathetic and parasympathetic nerves on the heart?*

Ans. (i) Sympathetic stimulation produces:

(a) increase in the heart rate (positive chronotropic effect)

(b) increase in the force of contraction of the myocardium (positive inotropic effect)

(c) increase in conductivity in conduction tissue (positive dromotropic effect)

(d) increase in the excitability of the heart (positive bathmotropic effect)

(ii) Stimulation of para-sympathetic produces just the opposite (negative) effects.

Q.3. *What type of cells constitute the white crescentic line?*

Ans. It is the cells of the post-ganglionic parasympathetic neurons.

Q.4. *What is* **vagal escape**? *What are its causes?*

Ans. Vagal escape is the resuming of heart beat from

a phase of cardiac arrest, despite the continuation of vagal stimulation. Its causes are:

(i) depletion of neurotransmitter;
(ii) simultaneous stimulation of sympathetic fibers in vago-sympathetic trunk, and
(iii) onset of idio-ventricular rhythm.

Q.5. *What is vagal tone? How will you assess the degree of vagal tone?*

Ans. In adults, at rest, the heart beat @ 70-80 beats/min under the influence of vagus, called **vagal tone.** *Vagotomy* (cutting the vagus) causes heart beat to increase to 160-180 beats/min. The difference between the resting heart rate before and after vagotomy gives a measure of the **degree of vagal tone**.

Q.6. *What is the effect on heart rate, if both sympathetic and parasympathetic nerves to the heart are blocked?*

Ans. In humans, cutting/blocking both the nerves to the heart causes the resting heart rate to increase to 100 beats/min.

Q.7. *Is vagal tone present in your preparation?*

Ans. Yes, to some extent (surgical stress, such as pithing and handling of vagus nerve, causes decrease in vagal tone).

Q.8. *What is the difference between pre-ganglionic and post-ganglionic fibres?*

Ans. Autonomic nerve fibres, those that have not synapsed in the autonomic ganglion are pre-ganglionic fibres, whereas post-ganglionic fibres are the fibres distal to a ganglion.

STUDY NOTES

RESULTS AND DISCUSSION

....
....
....
....
....
....
....
....
....
....
....
....
....
....
....
....

Date: ....

15 Effects of Variables on the Intact Frog's Heart

I. APPARATUS

The same as in the previous experiment (page 122), and

(i) Adrenaline solution : 1 in 10,000
(ii) Nicotine solution : 0.5% and 7%
(iii) Atropine solution : 0.5%

II. THEORY

1. *Adrenaline* acts equally on both α and β-adrenergic receptors located on the target cells. The cardiac tissue has only β_1-receptors on them, stimulation of which brings about a positive chronotropic and positive inotropic effect (page 123).
2. *Nicotine* acts on the nicotinic cholinergic receptors which are present at the neuromuscular end plates and peripheral autonomic ganglia. Nicotine, when applied to the frog's heart, acts on parasympathetic ganglia located on the white crescentic line.
   (i) In low concentrations (0.5%), it stimulates the post-ganglionic parasympathetic fibres producing bradycardia; and
   (ii) In high concentration (7%), it blocks the ganglion by producing *persistant depolarization.* Thus, after application of nicotine:
      (a) vagal stimulation will be less effective or ineffective depending upon the extent of paralyzation of the ganglia caused by nicotine; and
      (b) white crescent line stimulation, however, will still remain effective as the stimulus will be able to excite the post-ganglionic fibres beyond the blocked regions.
3. Post-ganglionic parasympathetic neurons on the cardiac muscles secrete A-ch at their nerve endings. The A-ch receptors on the cardiac muscle are *muscarinic receptors* which are blocked by *atropine.* Thus after the application of 0.5% atropine solution, the peripheral nerve endings of the post-ganglionic fibres are blocked, and the stimulation of either vagus or WCL will now be ineffective.

III. PROCEDURE

1. Arrange the preparation as in the previous experiment (page 122) and take a normal cardiogram on slow moving drum (2.5 mm/sec).
2. First stimulate the vagus nerve and check for the inhibition of the heart. Then stimulate the white crescentic line (WCL), a similar response is obtained. Wait till normal contractions reappear.
3. Pour a few (3 or 4) drops of adrenaline solution on the heart and record its effect. Before its effect wears off, record again the effects of the vagal and the WCL stimulation. Wash the heart with Ringer's solution till the normal cardiogram is obtained (Fig. 2.15.1).
4. Pour 1-2 drops of 0.5% nicotine solution on the heart, and record the effect. Stimulate the vagus again and compare the effect with those obtained before adding nicotine. Next stimulate the WCL and similarly compare. Wash the heart with Ringer solution till normal cardiogram is obtained.
5. Pour a drop of 0.5% solution of atropine. Now, stimulate the vagus first and then the WCL and record the effects.

Compare the results with (3) and (4).

Important: Label the record properly at each step.

(For recording on Student Physiograph, refer to page 84)

IV. PRECAUTIONS

The same as described earlier on page 115.

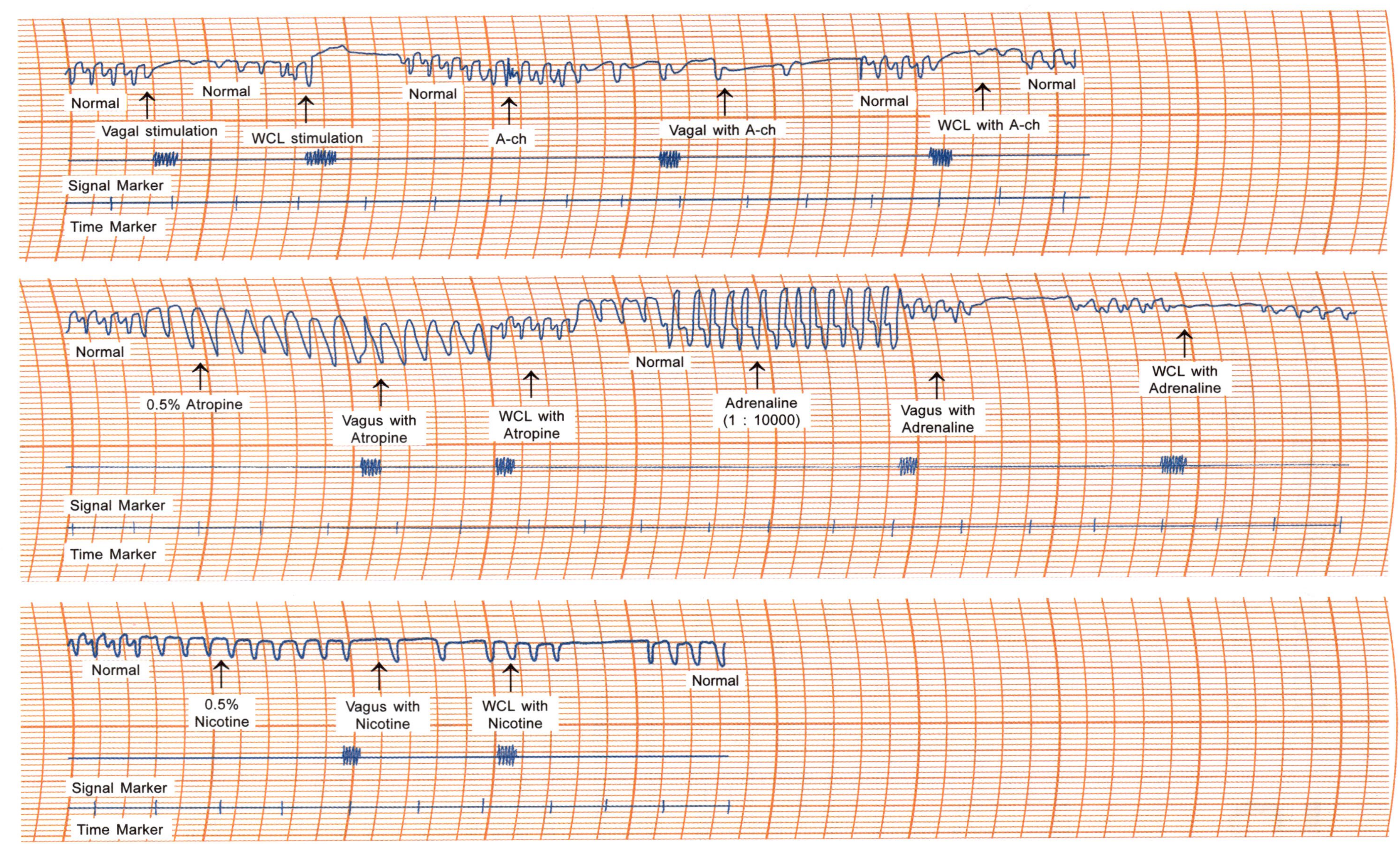

Fig. 2.15.1 Effect of variables on the intact frog's heart

IMPORTANT VIVA-VOCE QUESTIONS

Q.1. *Explain the effect of the local application of adrenaline, nicotine and atropine on the heart.*

Ans. Page 125.

> **Note:** The local application of atropine blocks the A-ch receptors producing chemical vagotomy and hence resting heart rate and force of contraction increases.

Q.2. *What is the importance of checking the effects of vagal and WCL stimulation on each time after adding a new drug?*

Ans. If the blockage by a drug is at the receptors of the target organ, then neither vagal nor WCL stimulation is effective. If, however, the blockage is at the ganglia, only vagal stimulation will be ineffective.

Q.3. *Why does transient depolarization of a neuron excite the activity of the heart, whereas persistent depolarization inactivates it?*

Ans. The persistent depolarization of a neuron inactivates the sodium channels and thereby prevents the generation of action potential, whereas transient depolarization brings the resting membrane potential towards its firing level.

Q.4. *Does nicotine affect the sympathetic or para-sympathetic system?*

Ans. Nicotine affects both sympathetic and parasympathetic systems, since it blocks the receptor on the post-ganglionic neurons, irrespective of the system it belongs to.

Q.5. *Name the blockers of non-adrenergic receptors or name the agents that block cholinergic receptors.*

Ans.
(i) A-ch receptors on all autonomic (sympathetic and parasympathetic) post-ganglionic neurons and neuromuscular end plate respond to *low* doses of the drug nicotine and are, therefore, called *nicotinic receptors*. They are antagonized by *hexamethonium at autonomic ganglia* and by *tubocurarine* at *skeletal muscle.*

(ii) The A-ch receptors on the smooth muscle, cardiac muscle and gland cells are not stimulated by nicotine but are stimulated by muscarine (a mushroom poison); they are called *muscarinic receptors* and are blocked by *atropine.*

STUDY NOTES

RESULTS AND DISCUSSION

....

....

....

....

....

....

....

....

....

....

....

....

....

Date: ....

16 Effects of Variables on the Isolated Frog's Heart

I. APPARATUS

The same as for recording a cardiogram (page 114); Amphibian Ringer's solution; perfusion bottle (Mariotte); Syme's cannula; solution: 1% $CaCl_2$, 1% KCl, 1% NaCl, 1 : 100000 adrenaline, 1 : 1000000 A-ch

II. THEORY

1. The heart when cut out of the body, continues to beat for some time and then gradually dies. The mammalian heart dies more quickly (1-2 minutes) under these conditions than the frog's heart. Death results because of the lack of oxygen and appropriate nutrients.
2. If the heart is perfused with a fluid which is iso-osmotic with the blood, has similar composition of electrolytes as blood, and adequate oxygen supply is maintained, the heart will continue to beat for much longer time.

Important Note: There is no need for any special administration of oxygen for the frog's heart; the oxygen dissolved in the perfusion fluid is sufficient to keep the heart alive.

III. PROCEDURE

1. Expose the heart of a pithed frog, lift the ventricle up and identify sinus venosus.
2. Pass a fine thread around the sinus venosus (page 114).
3. With the help of sharp scissors, make a small slit in the sinus and introduce Syme's cannula and tie the thread around the neck of the cannula. Do not tie the ligature on the WCL.
4. Cut the heart out of the frog.
5. Connect the cannula with the perfusion bottle containing Amphibian Ringer's solution. The perfusion pressure is adjusted by adjusting the height of the reservoir above the level of the frog's heart, and with the help of the pinch-cork (which helps to maintain a constant rate of flow of Ringer's solution to the heart). (Fig. 2.16.1)

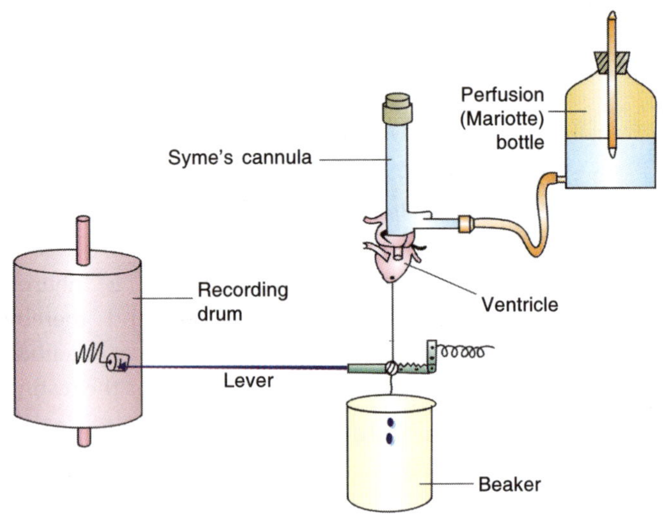

Fig. 2.16.1: Perfusion of the frog's heart

6. Perfuse the heart with Ringer solution and record normal cardiogram.
7. ***Effect of change of perfusion pressure:*** Raise the level of the Syme's cannula and this raises the pressure of the flow. Take the record of the heart beat. Bring the pressure to the previous level and again record the heart beat.
8. ***Effect of ions and drugs:*** The effect of the following agents should be recorded by adding solutions directly through the Syme's cannula. One agent should be added at a time; record the effect and wait until normal contraction returns (Fig. 2.16.2).
   (i) 1 ml of 1% $CaCl_2$
   (ii) 1 ml of 1% KCl
   (iii) 1-2 ml of 1% NaCl
   (iv) 0.5 ml of 1 in 1,00,000 solution of adrenaline
   (v) 0.5 ml of 1 in 1,00,00,00 A-ch solution.

Important Note: Perfusion pressure should be maintained constant throughout the experiment while recording the effect of variables.

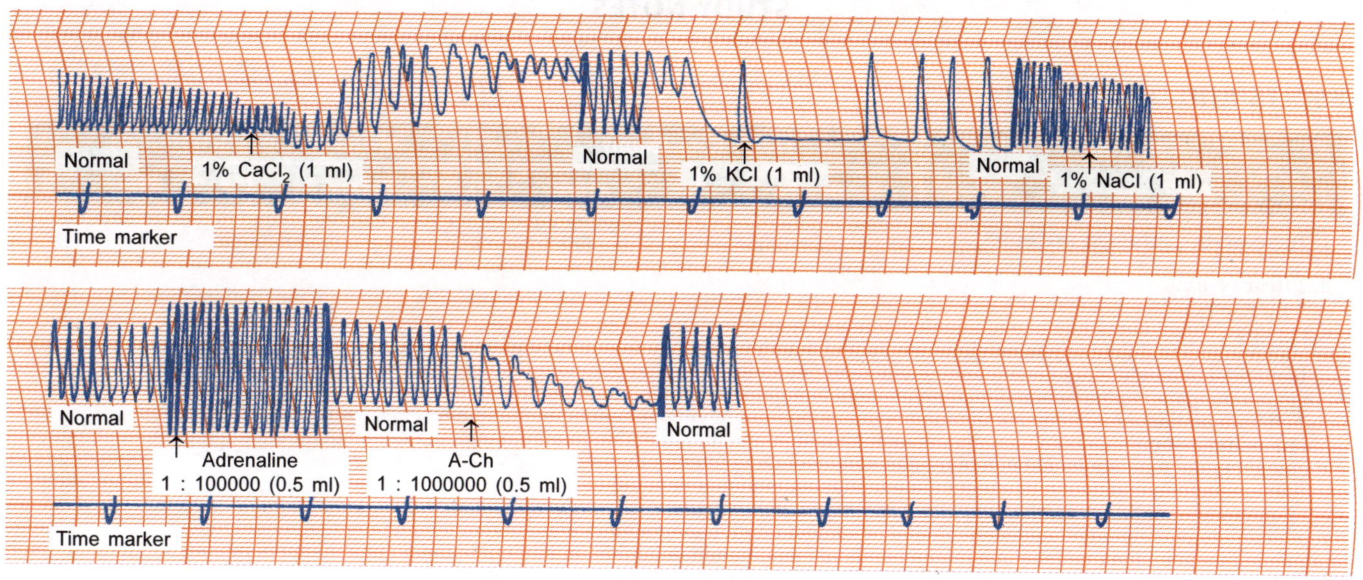

Fig. 2.16.2 Effect of ions and drugs on the frog's heart (isolated preparation)

IMPORTANT VIVA-VOCE QUESTIONS

Q.1. *How does the intact heart preparation differ from that of an isolated one?*

Ans. In an isolated heart preparation, the effect of variables produces direct action on the heart whereas in an intact preparation, the effect of variables on the heart is due to the balanced action: immediate effects produced are due to direct action on the heart and late effect due to reflex action.

Q.2. *What will be the effect of changing in the reaction (acid/alkaline) of perfusing fluid on the heart?*

Ans. (i) Addition of an acid (e.g. NaH_2PO_4) to Ringer solution causes heart contractions to decrease. Therefore, its beats become smaller and the heart finally stops in diastole.

(ii) Addition of an alkali (e.g. NaOH) to Ringer solution causes an incomplete relaxation of heart and finally it stops in a contracted condition.

Q.3. *What is the effect of increasing the perfusion pressure?*

Ans. Increase in perfusion pressure increases the initial length of cardiac muscle fibre. Hence, the force of contraction increases (Frank Starling Law of the heart).

Q.4. *Explain the effects and mechanism of the action of various ions and drugs on the heart.*

Ans. See Table 2.16.1.

Table 2.16.1 Effect and mechanism of action of various ions and drugs on the isolated frog's heart

Agent	On Heart Rate	On Force of Contraction
(i) $CaCl_2$	*No effect*	Increases in $[Ca^{2+}]$ in ECF, *increases* myocardial contractility as$[Ca^{2+}]$ in ICF also increases; with marked increase in $[Ca^{2+}]$ in ECF, calcium rigor may occur
(ii) KCl	*Decreases* (because RMP of nodal tissues decreases)	*Decreases* due to decrease in RMP of atrial and ventricular muscles; finally heart stops in diastole
(iii) NaCl	*No effect*	Na^+ competes with Ca^{2+} in contractile process and may *decrease* the contractility
(iv) Adrenaline	*Increases* (increases Na^+ influx of nodal tissues)	Increases as Ca^{2+} influx of myocardial fibre increases
(v) A-ch	*Decreases* (hyperpolarizes the nodal membrane by causing K^+ influx)	*Decreases* secondary to decrease in Ca^{2+} influx of myocardial fibres

STUDY NOTES

RESULTS AND DISCUSSION

Effect of	Heart Rate (bpm)		Force of Contraction (cm)	
	Before	After	Before	After
1. Increase in perfusion pressure				
2. Effect of ions (i) $CaCl_2$ (ii) KCl (iii) NaCl				
3. Effect of drugs (i) Adrenaline (ii) A-ch				

....

....

....

....

....

....

....

....

....

....

....

....

....

Date: ....

17 Perfusion of Blood Vessels in the Frog

I. APPARATUS

The same as for recording a cardiogram (page 114); perfusion (Mariotte's) bottle; drop counter, signal marker, stimulating circuit, mercury key.

Drop Counter: It consists of an arrangement by which each drop of the perfusate that falls on the diaphragm (of drop counter) depresses the lever so as to complete the *mercury key* contact and thereby to mark a stroke on the signal marker.

Stimulating Circuit: It consists of two pin electrodes from the secondary coil of the DuBois Raymond induction coil. One pin electrode is connected to the spinal cord and the other to any part on the body of the frog as an **indifferent electrode**. The primary coil is connected to the signal marker, Neef's hammer, primary key and drop counter with the low voltage mains in series.

II. THEORY

In this experiment, the influence of some of the reactions on the circulation of the intact organism is demonstrated.

1. The effect of adrenaline as a vasoconstrictor and of A-ch as a vasodilator is seen;
2. The spinal cord is stimulated to check for the vasoconstrictor fibres; and
3. Also, to check whether these reactions are operating locally or centrally.

III. PROCEDURE

1. Use a perfusion (Mariotte's) bottle connected by rubber tubing to a cannula. Fill this bottle with Amphibian Ringer's solution after clamping the rubber tubing.
2. Stun the frog, then **without pithing** it, decapitate it (remove both hemispheres) by cutting off the upper jaw between the tympanic membranes.
3. Open the chest, pass a fine ligature round the aorta and introduce a small glass cannula into the vessel. Fix the cannula in the aorta by tying the ligature round its neck (Fig. 2.17.1-inset).
4. Make a wide incision through the sinus venosus and suspend the frog by its lower jaw.
5. Fill the cannula with Ringer's solution to drive out all the air and then connect it to the perfusion bottle by the rubber tubing. Fix the perfusion bottle at about 40-60 cm above the cannula to give enough perfusion pressure. The perfusion fluid will begin to leak out from the sinus venosus and falls off the frog's toes (Fig. 2.17.1).
6. The rate of flow may be recorded either by counting the number of drops falling per 30 seconds on drop counter or by collecting them in a measuring cylinder and noting the level at one minute interval throughout the experiment.
7. *Effect of drugs: adrenaline and acetyl-choline (A-ch)*
   (i) When the outflow becomes constant, inject 1 ml of 1 in 100000 **adrenaline** solution by means of a syringe into the rubber tubing and note the *decrease* of the outflow due to vasoconstriction.
   (ii) Perfuse with Ringer solution for some time to get back the original rate of flow. Now inject 1 ml of 1 in 100000 **A-ch** solution and note the *increase* in the outflow due to vasodilation.
8. *Effect of spinal cord stimulation:* Stick one pin electrode into the spinal cord of the frog and the other into the tissue close to the opening of the spinal canal or any other part on the body of the frog. Stimulate the spinal cord and note the vasoconstriction; as a result, the capacity of the vascular system decreases and so does the rate of the flow of drops.

> **Note:** There might be at first an initial increase in the outflow due to the emptying of the blood vessels by the contracting muscles (**squeezing effect**).

9. *Effect of destruction of the spinal cord:*
   (i) Destroy the spinal cord by passing a needle down the spinal canal. Compare the outflow before and after the destruction. If the frog is

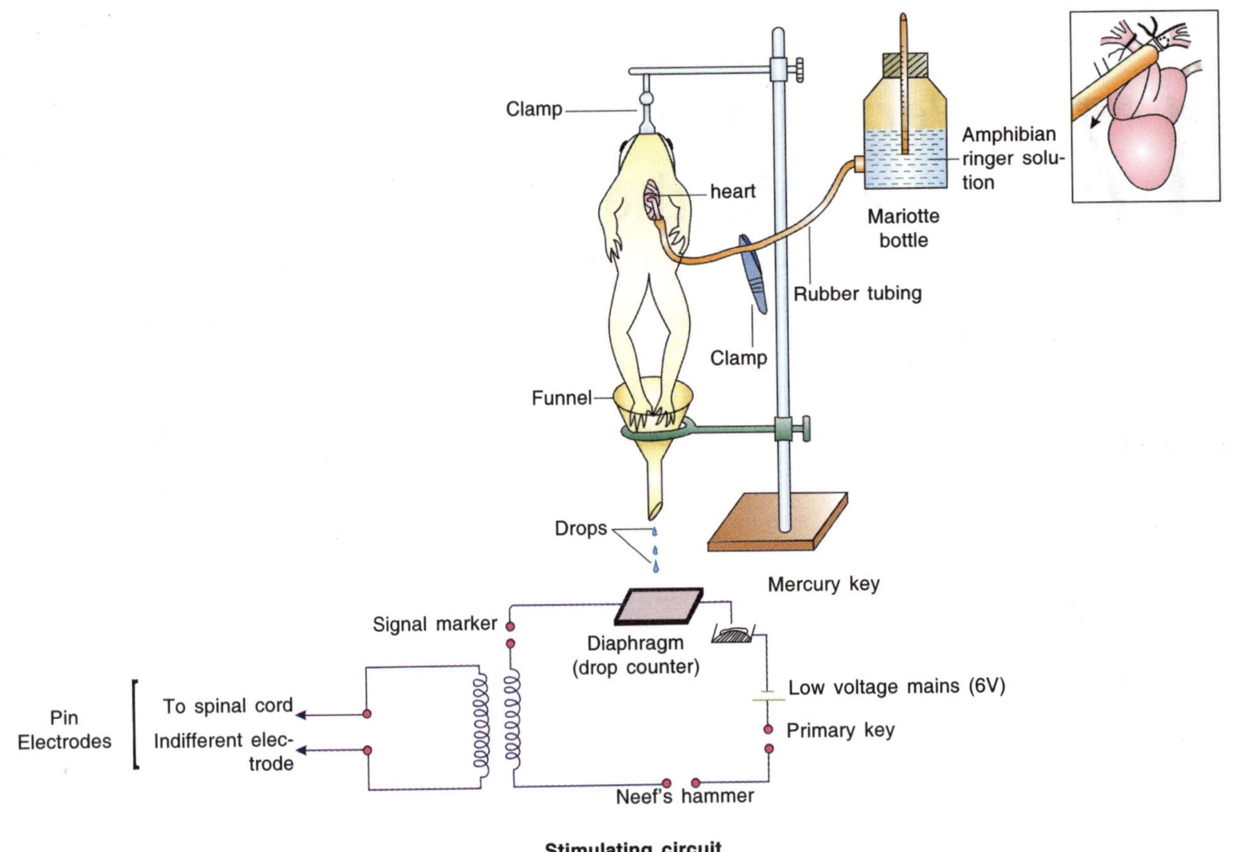

Fig. 2.17.1 Arrangement for the perfusion of blood vessels in the frog. Inset: Introduction of cannula into the aorta

in a good condition, there is an increase in the outflow due to vasodilation, the tonic effect of the CNS being abolished.

(ii) Repeat the injection of adrenaline; it produces the same effect, which proves that its action is independent of the CNS.

Important Note: As the experiment proceeds, fluid will escape from the blood vessels into the tissues which will become swollen and tense, *i.e.* oedematous. The perfusion rate will become less and less and the preparation will become useless.

(For recording on Student Physiograph, refer to page 84).

IMPORTANT VIVA-VOCE QUESTIONS

Q.1. *Describe the action of the various drugs and explain whether their action is local or central.*

Ans. On injecting a vasodilator substance such as A-ch, there is an initial vasodilatation of the blood vessel of the body with the result that the number of flow of drops decreases. But later, the capacity of the blood vascular system increases as a result of vasodilatation and, hence, the rate of flow of drops increases. Similarly, a vasoconstrictor agent (e.g. Adrenaline), initially there is squeezing effect due to which the rate of drops increases. Later on, the capacity of the vascular system decreases and so does the rate of drops.

Note: The action is local; see above.

Q.2. *What is the cause of oedema and why does it slow up the flow?*

Ans. See above.

Q.3. *What is the difference between perfusion and transfusion?*

Ans. In perfusion, the perfusate does not remain in the body of the animal but is drained out; in transfusion, the fluid remains in the system.

Q.4. *Decribe the path of perfusate.*

Ans. Aorta → blood vessels → sinus venosus → outside

Note: The heart is totally bypassed and only the blood vessels are perfused.

STUDY NOTES

RESULTS AND DISCUSSION

Date: ....

18 Capillary Circulation (Frog Web)

I. APPARATUS

Frog, myograph board with stand, pithing apparatus, thread, chemicals: histamine, adrenaline (1 in 100000); acetic acid (1%), warm and cold Ringer solutions; compound microscope

II. THEORY

Many important aspects of circulation may be learnt by the observation of a living tissue under the microscope. The web of the frog's foot is an ideal tissue for such study since it is thin enough to transmit light and can be examined without injury to the intact animal.

III. PROCEDURE

1. Anaesthetise a frog by injecting 0.5 ml of 1% urethane solution intraperitoneally.
2. Wrap the frog in a moist cloth, and place it on a wooden board, with a web of one foot spread out over a hole made in a waxed board.
3. With pins fasten the toes of the frog to the board, but do not stretch the web.
4. Using myograph stand, support the myograph board just above the stage of a microscope, with the hole in the myograph board just over the centre of the stage. Adjust the mirror so that light may be directed through the web.
5. The web is placed under low power objective (X10) of a microscope, and the circulation observed through the eye piece. Care is taken to avoid the drying up of the web by applying 0.6% saline solution to its surface.

IV. OBSERVATIONS

(1) Find an artery, a vein and the capillaries. These can be identified by noting the branching of blood vessels and direction of the flow of blood.

(2) Compare the rate of flow. Note the pulsations in the arteries.

(3) Compare the diameter of different types of blood vessels.

(4) Find a capillary and follow a RBC along it. Note the change in the shape of the corpuscle.

(5) Find a WBC and observe its movements and process of its emigration (*diapedesis*) from the vessel into the surrounding lymph spaces.

(6) Pour a few drops of warm saline (about 40°C) and then cold (about 20°C). Note the vasodilatation and vasoconstriction produced respectively.

(7) Apply a drop of histamine to the web and observe the vasodilatation produced. Wait for 15-20 minutes, to get back to the original rate of flow.

(8) Now, apply a drop of adrenaline (1 in 100000) to the web and observe the vasoconstriction.

(9) Dissect out the sciatic nerve on the same side, pass a ligature round the nerve, tie it and nerve is cut central to the ligature. Note the vasodilatation, called ***paralytic vasodilatation***. Stimulate the peripheral end of the sciatic nerve and note vasoconstriction.

(10) Apply a drop of 1% acetic acid to the web and study its effect. Note the ***inflammatory*** changes in the blood vessel. The stream of blood at first increases, but later on, after 10-15 minutes, decreases, the capillaries become packed with blood cells due to the exudation of the plasma. The WBCs form a layer between the walls of the veins and the RBCs.

IMPORTANT VIVA-VOCE QUESTIONS

Q.1. *Enumerate various factors regulating blood flow through capillaries.*

Ans. (i) *Local vasodilators include:* hypoxia, fall in blood pH, hypercapnea, increase in blood osmolality, increase in body temperature, K^+, lactic acid.

(ii) *Local vasoconstrictors include:* 5HT (serotonin), decrease in body temperature. Adrenaline is the systemic vasoconstrictor whereas histamine is a systemic vasodilator.

Q.2. *Describe the changes produced during inflammation.*

Ans. See above.

STUDY NOTES

RESULTS AND DISCUSSION

Date: ....

19 Postural and Protective Reflexes in the Frog

I. APPARATUS

Frog, dissecting instruments, stimulating apparatus, 0.5% H_2SO_4; 1% dilute acetic acid

II. THEORY

Various types of motor activities - voluntary or automatic (reflex), postural or protective are controlled by the CNS. By appropriately placed section we can isolate a portion of the CNS from the other parts and study the movements of the animal controlled by this isolated portion of the CNS.

1. ***Normal Reflexes – Characteristic features:***
   - (i) Weak stimuli produce localized homolateral reflexes; moderate stimuli produce homolateral and contralateral reflexes; strong stimuli produce a maximal escape reaction which is a jump. This is called **spreading of reflexes**.
   - (ii) Weak stimuli may be produced by touching or stroking a sensory surface, while a pin is a suitable device for producing moderate or strong stimuli.

> **Important Note:** The frog should not be held in the hand for testing reflexes since it will make every effort to escape, and certain localized reflexes cannot be produced.

   - (iii) *Summation of stimuli:* Stimuli which are too weak to produce a response may become effective upon repeated application. It occurs over many neurons converging on the **final common path**.
   - (iv) *Facilitation:* Once a reaction has been obtained, it may immediately be repeated more readily than after a period of rest. The initial tests raise the central excitatory state to threshold level. This is called facilitation.
2. ***Postural Reflexes***
   - (i) *Posture:* Observe the normal resting posture of a frog, the head is held in a lower position. Compare the posture of excitement or alertness, in which the head is held high. These positions are controlled by the degree of the extension of the forelimbs.
   - (ii) *Proprioceptive reflexes:* Place a frog board in the normal position. Incline the board in various planes and note how the legs resist gravity to maintain posture.
   - (iii) *Righting:* Place a frog on its back and observe how it rights itself. Take two pieces of cardboard, and apply one on the dorsal and one on the ventral surface of the body. Hold these in position by means of a rubber band. Now place the frog on its back. Although righting is attempted yet it cannot be completed successfully because of a confusion of sensory impulses. Usually, the reflex is accompanied by a succession of asymmetric stimuli from the skin surface. Equal pressure on both sides of the body prevents this progressive asymmetric stimulation.
3. ***Decerebration,*** *i.e.* removal of cerebral cortex.

   The frog has no cortical motor area, such as is found in mammals. There are, however, connections with a primitive motor system whereby voluntary movement is produced. Decerebration is, accordingly, well tolerated. Such frogs may swim, jump, right and can respond to many reflexes. Voluntary movement, however, is entirely absent. The posture is normal or slightly exaggerated by the development of the increased extensor tone of the muscles of the forelegs, which are antigravity muscles. Both resting and alert posture are still possible. The posture of the hind legs is essentially normal.

III. PROCEDURE

A. Intact frog

Study the behaviour of the intact frog:

1. Its posture;
2. Its response to stimulation of various kinds such as response to:
   - (i) nocuous stimuli,

(ii) how it swims when placed in a bowl of water,
(iii) how it moves up on an inclined board etc.;
3. Note how it rights itself when placed on its back; and
4. Observe its respiration.

B. Decerebrate frog

1. Remove the cerebral hemisphere by cutting with sharp scissors, along a line passing through the caudal border of the eyeball (the upper blade of the scissors is placed on this line whereas the lower blade remains inside the mouth). Apply a small piece of cotton soaked in Ringer solution to the cut surface.
2. Observe the frog's behaviour again. At first there is some *shock*. After a few minutes, the headless frog assumes a posture either normal or slightly exaggerated. After the frog has made some recovery, apply the following tests:
   (i) put the frog on its back; it rights itself;
   (ii) put on a tilted board; it will not fall;
   (iii) put it into a basin of water; it will swim like a normal frog;
   (iv) apply a small piece of paper soaked in dilute acetic acid on its back; it may be removed with considerable skill;
   (v) suspend the frog vertically on a stand by its jaw;
      (a) immerse a leg in a beaker filled with 0.5% H_2SO_4, the leg will be withdrawn (***flexor reflex***); wash the leg by dipping it in a beaker of water;
      (b) repeat and count the seconds until withdrawal occurs; there is an appreciable latency of response. On further repetition, latency is decreased. However, upon resting for 5 minutes, the latency becomes longer again. This illustrates *facilitation* (page 136).

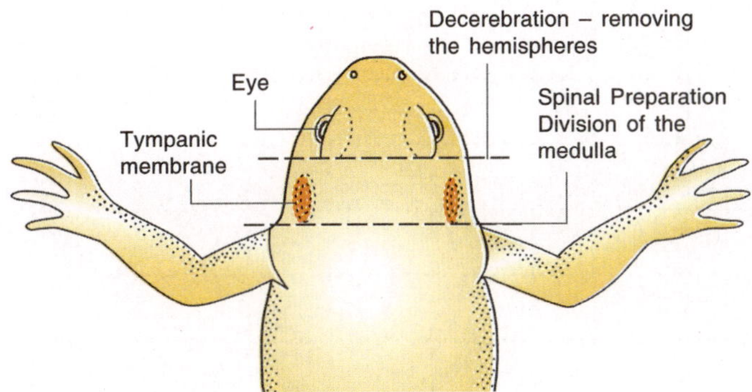

Fig. 2.19.1 Decerebration and spinal preparation in the frog

Important Note: All these observations illustrate that a frog without his hemispheres behaves in every respect like a normal frog, except for the absence of the so-called spontaneous movements.

C. Spinal frog

Cut off the head in front of a line passing behind the tympanic membrane. This leaves the animal with only the spinal cord portion of the CNS intact, called **spinal preparation**.

1. Immediately after the section is made the frog lies as if dead (*stage of spinal shock*).
2. The muscles are completely relaxed (flaccid/loss of muscle tone).
3. Stroking or pinching the skin will not elicit any response. Observe all the above parameters after the spinal shock passes off (usually in 3-5 minutes). Note the difference in attitude e.g. head end of the body is no more raised; observe the righting, etc.

Spinal reflex

Suspend the frog on a stand by its lower jaw. Study the different properties of *withdrawal reflex* by applying nocuous stimulus:
(i) mechanical stimulus (pinching with foreceps); and
(ii) chemical stimulus (acetic acid of different concentration).

Important Note: Spinal frog responds to nociceptive stimuli by the flexion of the leg, indicating that ***flexor reflex is of spinal origin***.

1. **Irradiation**: Pinch one toe gently. The same limb is gradually withdrawn with only a slight reflex movement of the corresponding limb. Increase the stimulus more and more; the movement increases also. At first, the same limb responds; with stronger movements, opposite limb begins to take part in the reflex, and finally, the whole frog.
2. **After discharge**: Note that in every case, the reflex movements outlast the duration of the application of the stimulus.
3. **Summation**: Stimulate a toe with a weak single induction shock, repeated at regular intervals. One single shock does not produce a reflex, but the repeated shocks, although weak, cause the summation of stimuli and produce reflex movements.
4. ***Measurement of the reflex time (Turk's method):*** Take a beaker full of 0.5% H_2SO_4 and immerse the hind limb of the suspended frog. Note, the length of time from the beginning of the stimulus to the reflex withdrawal of the limb. Wash off the acid with water.
5. **Inhibition**: Having determined the reflex time of your preparation, place a small artery clip/bull

dog on the forelimb of the frog; wait until the frog stops moving and then determine the reflex time again. It will now be much longer on account of the inhibitory action of the second stimulus. Wash off the acid and take the clip away. Measure the reflex time again to show that it is the same as in (4).

D. Destruction of the spinal cord

Make an estimate of the tone of the limb muscles of the frog by moving the joints. Now destroy the spinal cord by pushing the pithing needle down the vertebral column. They should now be completely flaccid. *Test for reflexes* – these also should have disappeared.

IMPORTANT VIVA-VOCE QUESTIONS

Q.1. *How does the body react to different strengths of stimuli?*
Ans. Page 136.

Q.2. *How are weak or strong stimuli applied to elicit a response?*
Ans. Page 136.

Q.3. *Define the terms: summation of stimuli, facilitation, righting reflex, decerebration.*
Ans. Page 136.

Q.4. *What do you understand by the term spinal shock? Give its normal duration.*
Ans. Definition, page 137.
The duration of spinal shock is a direct function of the degree of encephalization of motor functions, *i.e.* level of development of cerebral functions. Therefore, it lasts for a few minutes in frogs, a few hours in dogs and cats, a few days in monkeys and for about 3 weeks in men.

Q.5. *Define nociceptive stimulus.*
Ans. Stimulus which is damaging or injurious to the body tissues e.g. pain, is called nociceptive (noxious) stimulus.

STUDY NOTES

RESULTS AND DISCUSSION

Procedure	Spontaneous behaviour (normal attitude, swimming)	Withdrawal reflex	Righting reflex	Reflex time
1. Intact frog				
2. Decerebrate frog				
3. Spinal frog				
4. After destruction of the spinal cord				

....

....

....

....

....

....

....

Unit III
Human Experiments

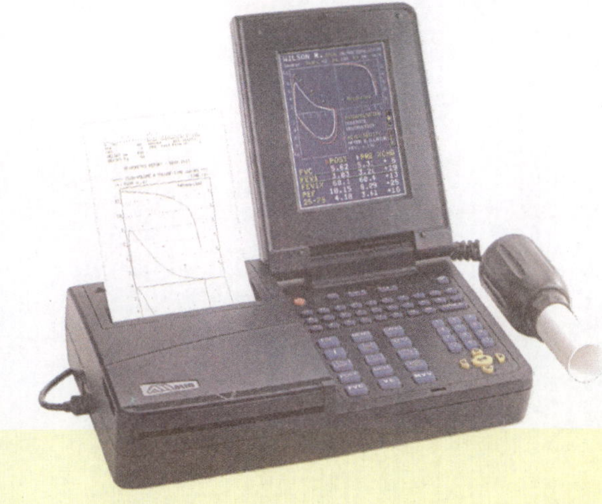

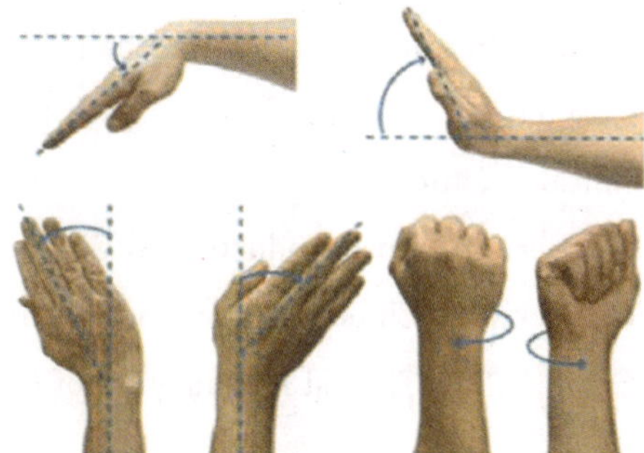

1 Phenomenon of Human Fatigue by Mosso's Ergograph and HandGrip Spring Dynamometer

I. APPARATUS

Mosso's ergograph, hand grip spring dynamometer, metronome, kymograph, sphygmomanometer and weights

Mosso's Ergograph

Ergograph for isotonic exercise. It consists of:

1. A **wooden board** fitted with two pairs of **clamps** (curved plates) for fixing the forearm of the subject and a pair of **finger holders** (metal tubes) for fixing the index and ring fingers in position (Fig. 3.1.1).

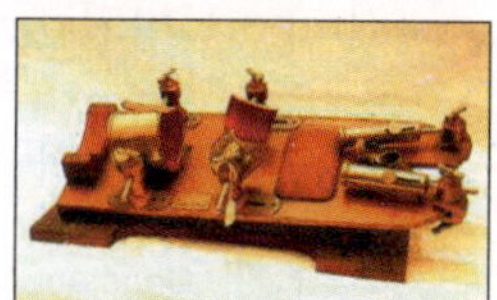

2. A **hook** (for suspending weights) attached to a cord, is made to hang over the **pulley**. The other end of the cord is attached to a **sliding plate** which moves to and fro.
3. The sliding plate carries a **lever system** to record the movements on a kymograph. The other end of the plate is connected through a sling to the middle finger of the hand.
4. Alternatively, the sliding plate is fitted with a **chart holder**. A pencil or a ballpoint pen can be fitted

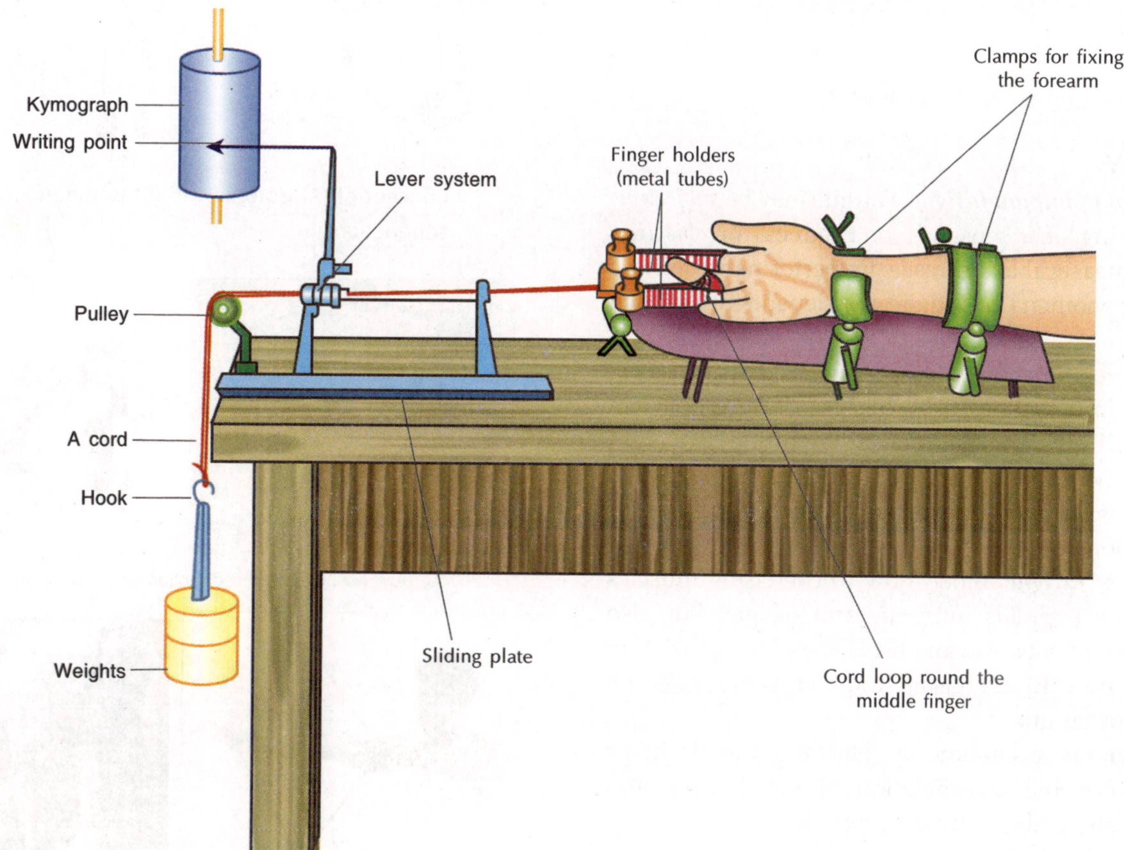

Fig. 3.1.1 Mosso's ergograph

vertically over the chart paper so as to record the movements of the chart holder when it moves.

Hand Grip spring Dynamometer

Ergograph for isometric exercise

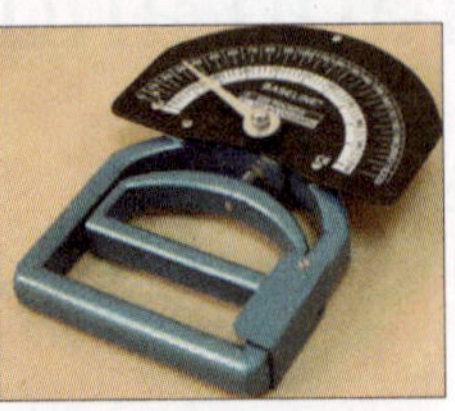

It consists of two parallel metallic hollow bars, called the **handles**. These are connected together through a flexible elliptical **metallic strip**. The whole apparatus can conveniently be held within the palm and when compressed, metallic strip offers a great deal of resistance to compression. A **graduated pressure scale** is also provided between the bars for direct estimation of compression force (Fig. 3.1.2).

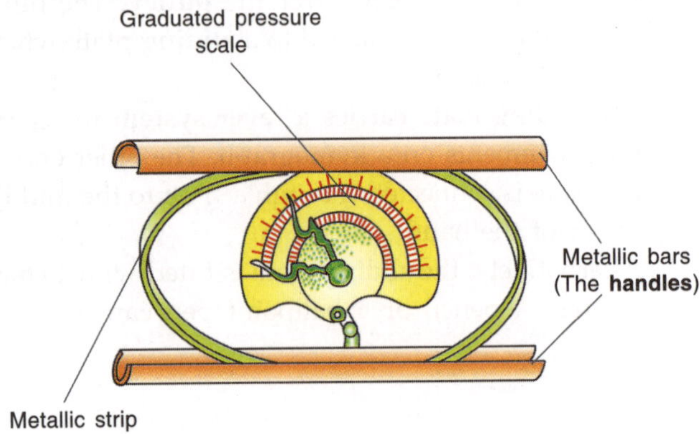

Fig. 3.1.2 Hand grip spring dynamometer

II. THEORY

1. ***Concept of human fatigue.*** Fatigue may be *subjective, i.e.* feeling of a sensation of tiredness or *objective, i.e.* a measurable decrease in performance. These two phenomena of fatigue are dependent on each other.
2. The development of fatigue in voluntary contracting muscle can be shown by the use of an ergograph in which work is performed in lifting a weight (as in Mosso's ergograph) or in compressing a high tension coil spring (as in hand grip spring dynamometer).
3. ***Cause of fatigue.*** Blood flow to exercising muscles not only supplies nutrients and oxygen but also removes metabolites and heat. Therefore, restricting blood flow to exercising muscles accelerates the onset of fatigue.
   (i) **Venous occlusion** by blocking the drainage causes the accumulation of metabolities and waste in the exercising muscles.
   (ii) **Arterial occlusion** affects both supply of oxygen and nutrients, and removal of metabolites and wastes. Therefore, it causes the onset of fatigue early and more effectively.

   Thus, the occlusion of blood supply to the forearm results in fatigue due to the accumulation of metabolites (lactic acid) or hypoxia. The associated pain is due to the accumulation of ***Lewis P factor*** in the ischaemic muscle, stimulating nerve endings. The *P-factor* may consist of more than one factor e.g. K^+, adenine and lactic acid.
4. During muscular contraction, the blood vessels supplying the muscles are squeezed by the high extramural pressure. **During isotonic contraction,** the muscle gets a chance for liberal blood flow during relaxation, but in **isometric contraction** blood flow to muscle remains restricted throughout its activity. Therefore, there is not much scope for further impairment of circulation if blood flow is occluded by some other means. That is why circulatory occlusion hastens the onset of fatigue to a much greater extent in case of isotonic exercise than in case of isometric exercise. (Fig. 3.1.3 and 3.1.4) (Important: For details, refer to page 110)

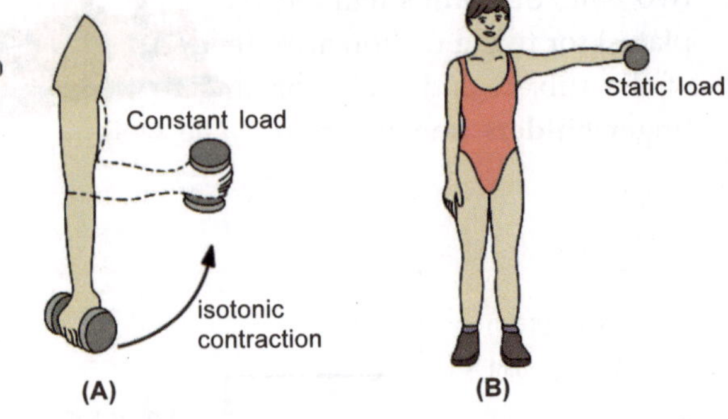

Fig. 3.1.3 Concept of (A) Isotonic and (B) Isometric muscle contraction

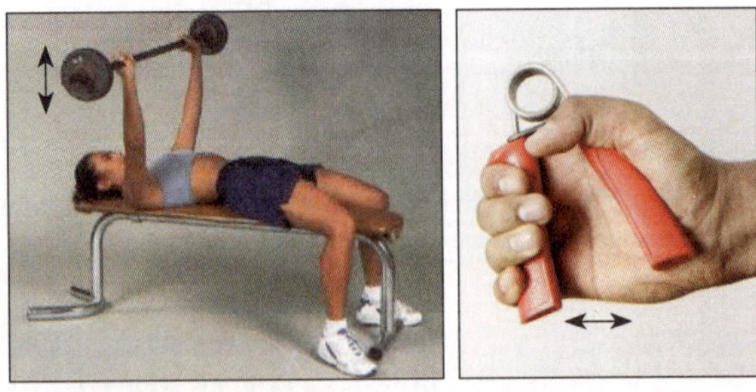

(A) (Arrows indicate the direction of movement)

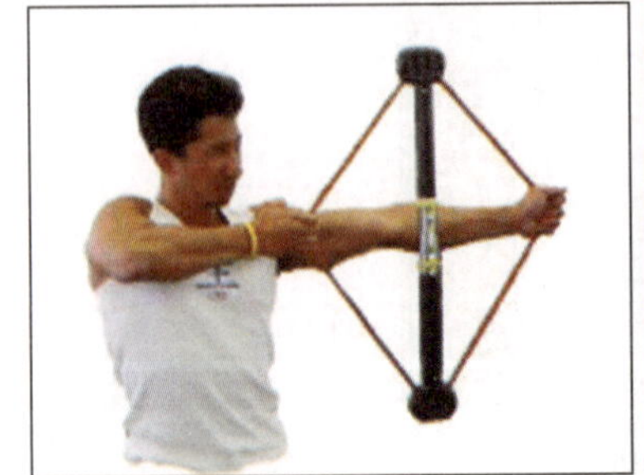

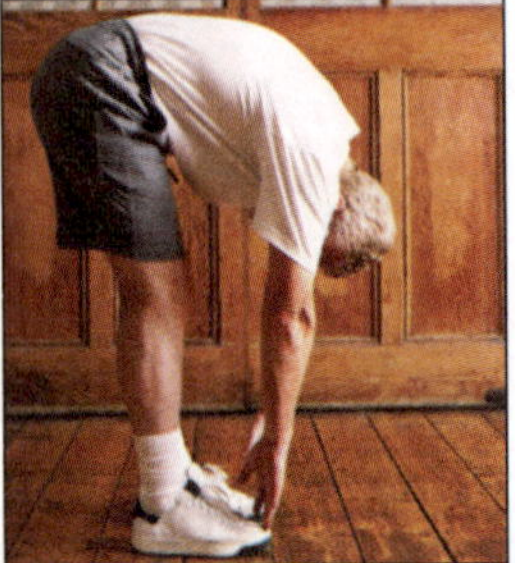

(B)

Fig. 3.1.4 Examples : (A) Isotonic and (B) Isometric muscle contraction

5. ***Site of fatigue.*** The fatigue developing in maximal voluntary muscular effort, first occurs in the central nervous system, followed by neuro-muscular junction and lastly in the muscle proper.

III. PROCEDURE

A. Mosso's Ergograph

Ergograph for isotonic exercise

1. Lay kymograph on its side and arrange the writing lever to write on a very slow moving drum. Alternatively, arrange a spring loaded writing device or ballpoint pen in the Mosso's ergograph and a paper on the platform underneath.
2. Fix the forearm on the ergograph by means of clamps. Put the middle finger in the loop to be pulled, and insert the index and ring fingers into the fixed metal tubes provided in the ergograph.
3. Adjust the subject position and various adjustable points in the ergograph in such a way that the forearm is properly fixed, and at the same time the subject is comfortable.
4. With the middle finger extended, suspend a weight (say 2 or 3 kg) according to the subject's requirement on the ergograph. The weight should be such that the subject must exert a real effort to lift it up. 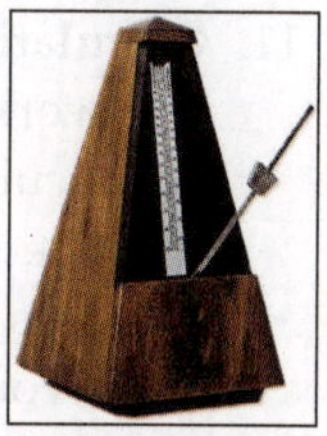
5. Set the *metronome* at one beat per two seconds, *i.e.* to a frequency of 30/min.

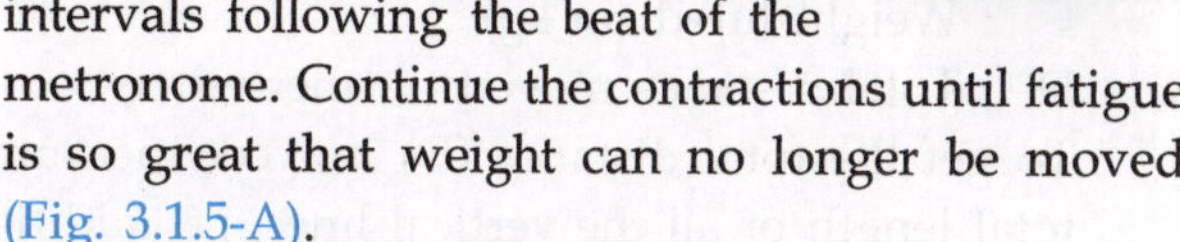

6. Ask the subject to make a series of **maximal contractions** without moving the shoulder at regular intervals following the beat of the metronome. Continue the contractions until fatigue is so great that weight can no longer be moved (Fig. 3.1.5-A).
7. Study the effect of rest pause for 10-15 minutes on the graph.
8. Next, study the effect of encouragement (motivation) on the graph.
9. Wrap the sphygmomanometer cuff round the upper arm of the subject and inflate the cuff to 40 mmHg to *occlude venous flow only*. Repeat the whole procedure and note the effect of venous occlusion (Fig. 3.1.5-B).
10. After a period of rest pause, now raise the pressure of the cuff well above the expected systolic blood pressure (150 mmHg) to produce *arterial as well as*

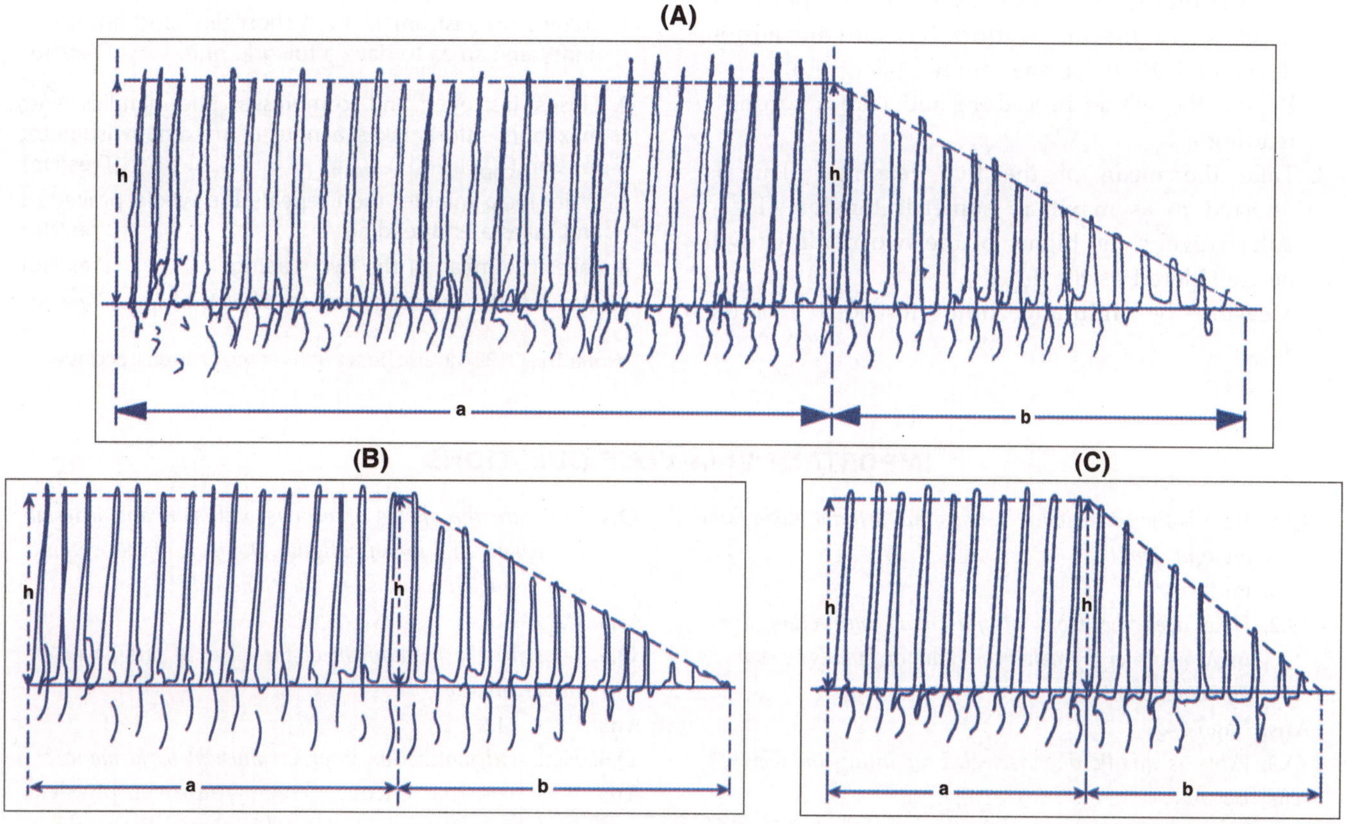

(A) h h a b

(B) h h a b

(C) h h a b

$$\text{TOTAL DISTANCE MOVED (D)} = \frac{\text{AREA OF TRIANGLE } (1/2 \text{ b X h}) + \text{AREA OF RECTANGLE } (\text{a X h})}{\text{TOTAL LENGTH OF THE BASE } (\text{a + b})} \times \text{NUMBER OF CONTRACTIONS}$$

Fig. 3.1.5 Mosso's ergographic tracings (A) with circulation intact; (B) venous occlusion and (C) arterial occlusion

venous occlusion. Repeat the whole procedure and note its effect (Fig. 3.1.5-C).

11. **Calculation of work done**

The work done (W) in each of the above cases may be calculated from the force, *i.e.* weight lifted (F) and the total distance (D) moved as revealed by the lines on the paper, *i.e.* W = F × D, where

W : Work done (in kg metres)

F : Weight lifted (in kg)

D : Total distance moved (in metres)

To get the total distance (D) moved, measure the total length of all the vertical lines, *i.e.* addition of all vertical amplitudes. Alternatively, it can also be determined as shown in the diagram.

D (cm) = No. of contractions × average height of contraction (A in cm), where

$$A = \frac{\text{Area of triangle (1/2 base × altitude) + Area of rectangle (length × breadth)}}{\text{Total length of the base}}$$

(B) HandGrip spring Dynamometer

Ergograph for isometric exercise.

1. Allow the subject to study the instrument for a short time; ask him to hold the dynamometer in right hand so as to have a full grip of it; then instruct him to close his eyes and to compress the handles with maximum effort. Measure the tension developed. Wait for one minute. (Fig. 3.1.6)
2. Repeat the whole procedure and take a second's reading.
3. Take the mean of the two readings. This is referred to as **maximal isometric tension** (T_{max}). Alternatively, the higher of the two readings will be considered as the T_{max}.
4. Measure the **endurance time*** for 60-80% of the T_{max}.

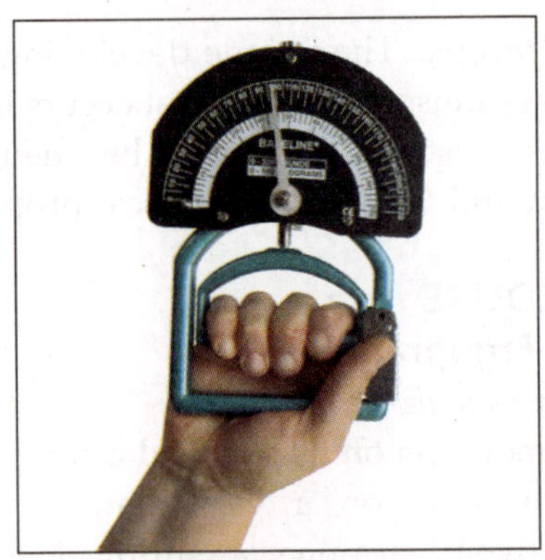

Fig. 3.1.6 Handgrip spring dynamometer in use

(*This is the time of the onset of fatigue while performing isometric exercise on handgrip dynamometer.*)

5. Measure the **endurance time** for 60-80% of T_{max}, first with venous occlusion and then with the arteries occluded.

OSPE

Aim: To measure your own **Endurance Time** for 60-80% of the T_{max} with the help of hand grip spring dynamometer

Procedure steps: Refer above

Checklist

1. Studies the instrument for a short time and holds it in right hand so as to have a full grip of it. **(Yes/No)**
2. Closes his eyes and compresses the handles with maximum effort; takes a note of maximum isometric tension (T_{max}). **(Yes/No)**
3. Waits for a minute, then repeats the whole procedure and takes a 2nd reading. **(Yes/No)**
4. Takes the mean of the two readings. **(Yes/No)**
5. Measures the endurance time for 60-80% of T_{max}. **(Yes/No)**

Note: This OSPE can also be set with venous or arterial occlusion.

IMPORTANT VIVA-VOCE QUESTIONS

Q.1. *How is the occlusion of venous and arterial blood flow brought about?*

Ans. Page 143.

Q.2. *How does the mode of muscular contraction differ in Mosso's ergograph from that of Handgrip spring dynamometer?*

Ans. Page 142.

Q.3. *Why is middle finger selected for lifting the weight?*

Ans. Because

(i) it is the longest and strongest of all the other fingers.

(ii) it can easily be fixed in proper position so as to exert optimal effort to lift the weight.

Q.4. *Compare the effects of venous occlusion and arterial occlusion on human fatigue. Do they affect isotonic and isometric exercise in the same way?*

Ans. Page 142.

Q.5. *Describe the mechanism of the onset of fatigue in an intact muscle.*

Ans. Page 142.

Q.6. *How will motivation improve physical performance?*

Ans. It is seen that encouragement improves physical performance temporarily. This shows that fatigue has a cortical component.

Q.7. *Describe how you will demonstrate the site of fatigue in an intact muscle.*

Ans. Fatigue the finger, the muscle, even when fatigued by voluntary effort, will still respond to peripheral nerve stimulation, indicating that the fatigue must have developed centrally first of all.

Q.8. *What will be the effect of the following factors on the work done by the muscle during Mosso's ergography?*

(i) Increasing the weights to be lifted
(ii) Changing the frequency of contractions
(iii) Increasing the rest pauses

Ans. Either increasing weights be lifted or increasing the frequency of contractions, onset of fatigue will be early due to hypoxia and accumulation of metabolites. Increasing the rest pause, delays the onset of fatigue since the working muscles get enough time to recover.

Q.9. *How does fatigue of the isolated nerve-muscle preparation differ from that of the intact organism?*

Ans. In isolated nerve-muscle preparation blood supply to the contracting muscle is sacrificed, hence fatigue sets in quite early.

Q.10. *Name one condition each in which muscle performance gets impaired due to venous occlusion and arterial occlusion.*

Ans. Venous blood supply to a muscle gets impaired due to thrombosis secondary to *thrombophlebitis* (Fig. 3.1.7 A), and due to arterial occlusion in *Buerger's disease* (Fig. 3.1.7 B), a disease characterized by the inflammation of the coats of arteries. (Heavy smoking is a precipitating factor.)

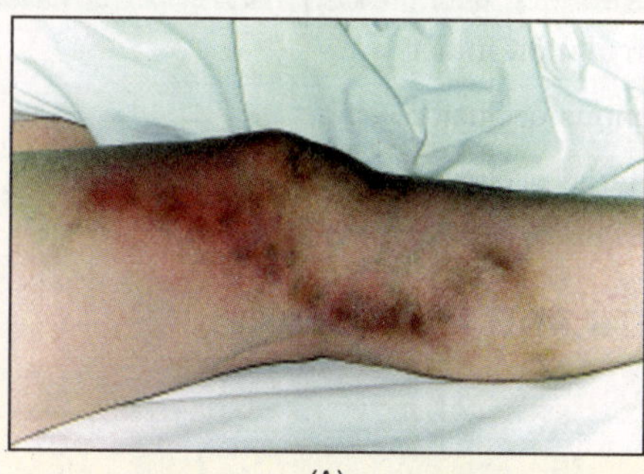

(A)

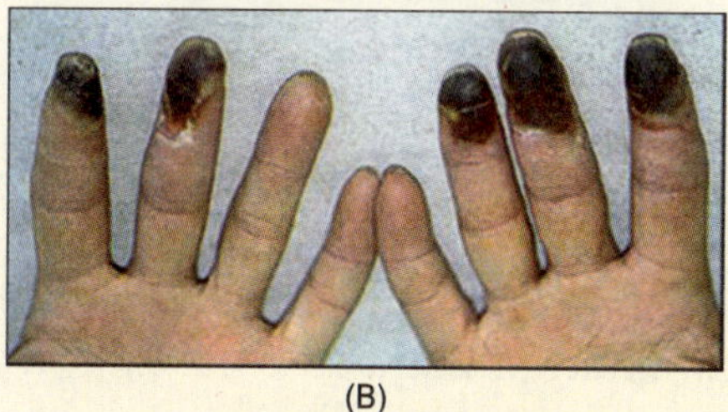

(B)

Fig. 3.1.7 (A) Thrombophlebitis and (B) Buerger's disease

Q.11. *Differentiate between isotonic and isometric exercise.*

Ans. Refer to pages 110 and 142.

STUDY NOTES

RESULTS

A. MOSSO'S ERGOGRAPH

Sl. No.	Weight	Metronome frequency	Circulation	Onset of fatigue		Percentage Change compared with (1)	
				Duration	Work done	In duration	In work done
1.	.... kg	30/min	Intact			–	–
2.	.... kg	30/min	Venous occlusion				
3.	.... kg	30/min	Arterial occlusion				

Give reasons for the stopping (like unbearable fatigue or pain) and effect of motivation/encouragement (if any):

....

....

....

....

....

....

B. HANDGRIP SPRING DYNAMOMETER

Procedure	Endurance time for 60-80% T_{max}	Percentage decrease compared to (1)
1. With circulation intact		–
2. With venous occlusion		
3. With arterial occlusion		

COMMENTS AND DISCUSSION

....

....

....

....

....

....

....

....

....

....

....

....

....

....

Date: ....

2 Electromyography (E.M.G.)

I. APPARATUS

Subject, cathode ray oscilloscope, pre-amplifier, ether or spirit, recording electrodes (needle or surface silver chloride electrodes) and electrode paste (to minimise resistance)

II. THEORY

1. An electromyogram is a recording of electrical activity from a muscle during its activity. The procedure of recording the electromyogram is called ***electromyography*** *(E.M.G.)*. The electrical potentials developed in the muscle are so small that they must be amplified before they are recorded.
2. In normal human skeletal muscle, the fibres do not contract individually, and the functional unit of neuromuscular activity is the ***motor unit.*** Thus at rest, there is a slow asynchronous discharge by the motor units. This results in little (if any) spontaneous activity in the skeletal muscle. Therefore, muscle in relaxed state does not show any electrical activity (*i.e. potentials*). Potentials are produced when the muscle contracts.
3. With the minimal voluntary activity a few motor units discharge and with increasing voluntary efforts more motor units are brought into play. This process is called ***recruitment of motor units.*** Therefore, with increase in the force of contraction the amplitude of potentials is also increased.
4. In **needle E.M.G.**, three types of activities are observed:
   (i) *insertional activity;*
   (ii) *spontaneous activity;* and
   (iii) *voluntary activity.*

   (i) ***Insertional activity***
   (a) Introduction of needle into the muscle produces a brief burst of electrical activity (duration 0.5–1.0 sec.) due to mechanical damage by needle movement.
   (b) It appears as *positive* or *negative* high frequency spike in a cluster.
   (c) *Increased in:* denervated muscle and myotonia
   (d) *Decreased in:* muscular individuals and myopathies

   (ii) ***Spontaneous activity***
   (a) In normal individuals, it is absent *except* in the end plate zone where '*miniature end plate potentials*' are spontaneously recorded.
   (b) *End plate potentials* appear as monophasic negative waves up to 100μV and of 1–3 msec duration, called *end plate noise.*
   (c) The abnormal spontaneous activities include: fibrillations, fasciculations and cramps (Fig. 3.2.1).
   (d) *Fibrillations:* These are spontaneously occurring action potentials from a *single* muscle fibre that fire regularly at a rate of 0.5–15Hz with an amplitude of 20–200μV and duration of 1–5 msec (Fig. 3.2.1). These are biphasic and triphasic waves with initial positivity and are seen in:
   - lower motor neuron diseases
   - diseases of neuromuscular junction (myasthenia gravis), and
   - denervation hypersensitivity

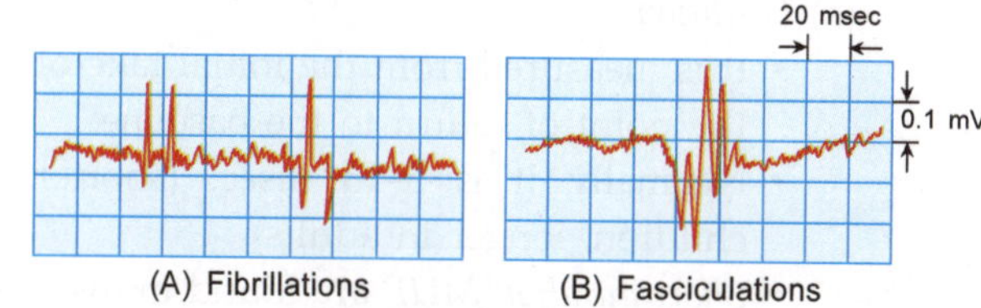

(A) Fibrillations (B) Fasciculations

Fig. 3.2.1 Abnormal spontaneous activity

   (e) *Fasciculations:* These are spontaneous contraction of a number of muscle fibres either from a whole or a part of motor unit. They occur randomly and irregularly at variable rates (between 1 and 500 per minute) (Fig. 3.2.1). Benign fasciculations can occur in normal individuals due to

muscle cramps, otherwise these are seen in:
- syringomyelia
- thyrotoxicosis, and
- uremia

(f) In *cramps*, spontaneous discharges of potential occur at 40–60Hz with an abrupt onset and cessation. The cramps occur in:
- some normal individuals
- salt depletion
- myxoedema
- pregnancy, and
- uremia

5. Potential produced by the excitation of an individual motor unit is called **Motor Unit Potential (M.U.P.).**

(i) It represents the sum of the muscle action potentials supplied by a motor neuron. Therefore, it has a higher amplitude and longer duration than action potential produced by a single muscle fibre.

Note: The number of muscle fibres in a motor unit varies from 3–6 in extraocular muscles to 120–165 in leg and back muscles.

(ii) It is characterised by their firing pattern and appearance.

(a) *On mild contraction*, the *MUP* fires at 5–15 Hz.

(b) *Recruitment of M.U.P.* leads to additional firing of M.U.Ps during muscle contraction which depend on ***size principle***, *i.e.* on initiation of voluntary contraction of muscle, the motor units are recruited in an orderly fashion; the smallest appearing first, larger later and the largest still later.

(iii) *M.U.Ps* is also characterised by its *duration*, *amplitude*, *phases* and *rate of rise of fast component*. (Fig. 3.2.2).

(a) *Duration*
- It is measured from the initial take-off to the point of return to the baseline.
- Normally it is 5–15 msec. (shorter in children, longer in adults)
- *Short duration MUP* are found in disorder associated with loss of muscle fibres *e.g.*:
  - myopathies,
  - myasthenia gravis;
  - early stage of reinnervation after nerve damage.
- *Long duration MUPs* are seen in
  - motor neuron diseases (lower motor neuron lesion), and
  - neuropathies.

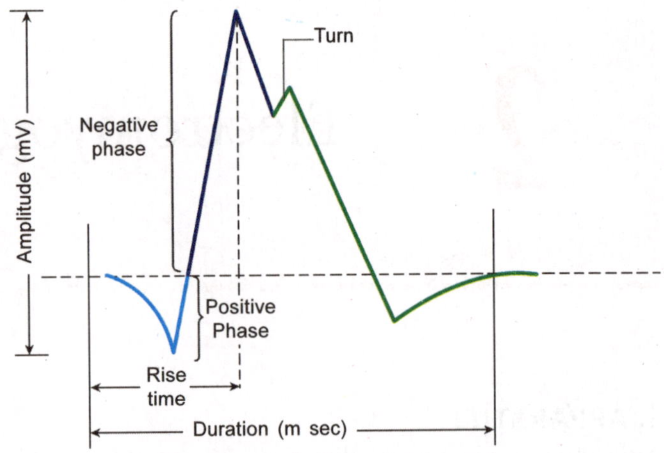

Fig. 3.2.2 Normal motor unit potential – MUP (as recorded by needle E.M.G.)

(b) *Amplitude*
- It is measured peak to peak (Fig. 3.2.2). Normal: 0.5mV to 2mV.
- It depends upon:
  - size, density and type of muscle fibres;
  - age of the subject, and
  - muscle temperature (decreasing muscle temperature results in higher amplitude and longer duration of M.U.Ps.).

(c) *Phase*
- M.U.P. recorded by needle shows an inverted *triphasic* potential (positive-negative-positive: Fig. 3.2.2)
- M.U.P. with more than 4 phases is called *polyphasic potential*. Some potentials show directional changes without crossing the baseline and these are known as *turns*.
- Polyphasic potential and turns are most frequently seen in myopathies where there is the regeneration of fibres and increased fibre density.

(d) *Rise time*
- It is the duration from initial *positive* to subsequent *negative* peak. Normal: up to 500 µsec.
- It is an indicator of the distance of needle electrode from the muscle fibre. A greater rise time signifies the resistance of the intervening tissue.

(iv) ***Factors affeting M.U.P.***

(a) *Age:* Duration and amplitude increases while firing rate decreases in linearity with age.

(b) *Sex:* The M.U.P. amplitude and rise time are more in men compared to women due to a larger diameter of muscle fibre in men.

(c) *Type of the muscle, **i.e.**,* muscle fibres in a motor unit.

(d) *Location of needle in the muscle:* Superficial, deep or near end plate. The amplitude is smaller when needle electrode is superficial and higher when the needle is deep into the muscle.

(e) Degree of muscle contraction, and

(f) Temperature

6. ***Factors affecting E.M.G.:*** See above.

III. PROCEDURE

(A) Equipment set up for E.M.G. recording

1. *Sweep speed:* 5–10 msec/division
2. *Amplification*
   (i) 50 μV/division for studying spontaneous activity; and
   (ii) 200 μV/division for motor unit potentials (M.U.P.)
3. *Filter setting:* 20–10,000Hz., *i.e.* low cut: 20Hz; high cut: 10,000Hz. Before performing E.M.G., a proper knowledge about anatomy, nerve and root supply and function of the muscle is necessary. Here procedure for recording E.M.G. for biceps brachii ($C_{5,6}$ roots, musculocutaneous nerve) is briefly described.

(B) Procedure for Surface E.M.G.

1. Ask the subject to lie supine with the arm extended and forearm pronated.

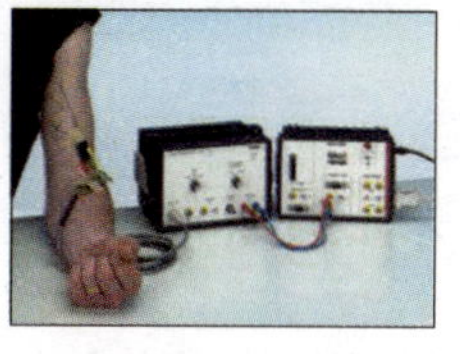

2. The skin overlying biceps muscle is cleaned with ether or spirit.
3. Using electrode paste, a set of three electrodes are fixed on a small area of the skin over the biceps muscle (one for grounding, and the other two act as exploring electrodes for recording E.M.G.).
4. The electrodes are connected through the preamplifier to the cathode ray oscilloscope (CRO); record for resting potentials.
5. The subject is asked to flex the *biceps* muscle by the supination of forearm or flexion of the elbow. Observe the potentials.
6. The subject is asked to flex the test arm against resistance. Again observe the potentials.

(C) Procedure for Needle E.M.G.

1 and 2. The same as steps 1, 2 above.

3. Fix the ground electrode as described above, step 3.
4. The needle electrode is inserted into the bulk of the biceps muscle in the mid arm.

5, 6 and 7. The same as steps 4, 5 and 6 above.

8. Move the needle electrode in different directions in the biceps muscle and record any change in the potentials.

IV. OBSERVATIONS

Observe (Fig. 3.2.3) and draw the pattern of E.M.G. under:

(i) Resting condition

(ii) On minimal voluntary effort

(iii) On maximal voluntary effort

Note: Observations need to be evaluated in view of important points described under the theory (page 147).

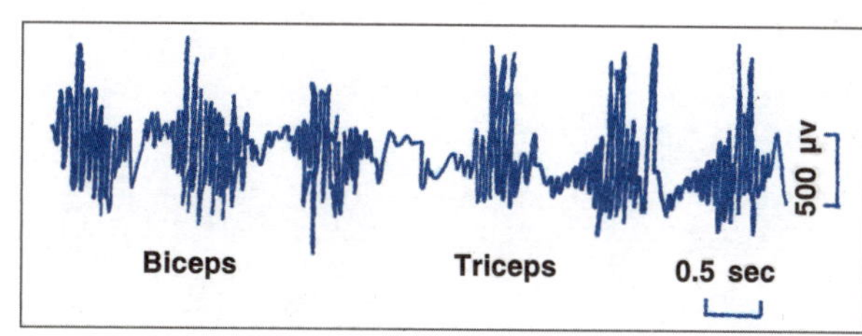

Fig. 3.2.3 Electromyogram from biceps and triceps muscle during alternate flexion and extension at the elbow

V. PRECAUTIONS

Refer to page 296.

IMPORTANT VIVA-VOCE QUESTIONS

Q.1. *Define the term: electromyogram and electromyography.*

Ans. Page 147.

Q.2. *Why is there no potentials in muscle under resting condition? Why does it increase with an increase in the force of muscular contraction?*

Ans. There are no potentials during resting conditions since there is no discharge of motor neurons. As a result, acetyl choline is not released, and no potential change occurs. As muscular contraction force is increased, larger potentials are obtained due to more number of fibres being recruited.

Q.3. *Mention the factors which determine the gradation of muscle response.*

Ans. The gradation of muscle response depends on:

(i) Number of motor units activated at a time during any reflex activity

(ii) Frequency of discharge in an individual nerve fibre, *i.e.* duration for which motor units are being stimulated.

(iii) Optimal length of the muscle, *i.e.* the length at which they develop maximum active tension.

Q.4. *Experimentally how will you demonstrate the phenomenon of the recruitment of motor units?*

Ans. With recording electrodes placed on thenar eminence, instruct the subject to move his thumb slowly. By adjusting the grades of the movement of the thumbs we will be able to record motor unit potentials of different amplitudes and slopes. This demostrates the phenomenon of the recruitment of motor units in higher grades of action.

Q.5. *Differentiate between insertional and spontaneous activity.*

Ans. Page 147.

Q.6. *Name the types of activities observed in needle E.M.G.*

Ans. Page 147.

Q.7. *Name the abnormalities associated with spontaneous activities during needle E.M.G.*

Ans. Page 147.

Q.8. *What type of electrical activity is observed due to muscle cramps? List the major causes of cramps.*

Ans. Page 148.

Q.9. *What is motor unit potential? What does it represent?*

Ans. Page 148.

Q.10. *What do you understand by the term size principle?*

Ans. Page 148.

Q.11. *Enumerate the characteristics of motor unit potential (M.U.P.).*

Ans. Page 148.

Q.12. *Give the causes of variations in M.U.P.*

Ans. Page 148.

Q.13. *What happens to M.U.P. in hypothermia?*

Ans. Page 148.

Q.14. *What is polyphasic potential? Give its clinical significance.*

Ans. Page 148.

Q.15. *Name the factor that can influence E.M.G.*

Ans. Hint: Factors affecting E.M.G. (Page 147 and 148).

Q.16. *Give the clinical uses of E.M.G.*

Ans. Hint: Factors affecting EMG (Q. 15).

STUDY NOTES

RESULTS, COMMENTS AND DISCUSSION

....

....

....

....

....

....

....

....

....

....

....

....

....

....

....

Date: ....

3 Recording of Systemic Arterial Blood Pressure

I. APPARATUS

An examination couch, sphygmomanometer, stethoscope

II. THEORY

1. The arterial blood pressure (B.P.) is the pressure exerted by a column of blood on the vessel-wall while flowing through it.
2. **Components**
   - (i) *Systolic BP.* It is the maximum pressure exerted during systole; Normal: 100-130 mmHg (*average* 120 mmHg).
   - (ii) *Diastolic BP.* It is the minimum pressure exerted during diastole; Normal: 70-85 mmHg (*average* 80 mmHg).
   - (iii) *Pulse pressure.* It is the difference of systolic and diastolic BP; Normal: 40 mmHg (average).
   - (iv) *Mean BP.* It is the average pressure throughout the cardiac cycle and computed as:
     Diastolic BP + 1/3 pulse pressure;
     Normal: 95-100 mmHg (*average* 96 mmHg).
3. Clinically B.P. is expressed as SBP/DBP; *Normal:* 120/80 mmHg.

> **Note:** Current recommendations from WHO refer to <120/<80 mmHg as optimal BP.

4. Systolic B.P. undergoes considerable fluctuation, e.g. increased by excitement, anxiety, nervousness, after meals, etc. and decreased by rest and during sleep. Therefore, for resting measurements the subject should be quiet for at least five minutes before the measurements are made.

III. PROCEDURE

Systemic arterial B.P. can be measured by two methods: *direct and indirect method.*

A. Direct Method

In this method a cannula is introduced into an artery and secured in position with the help of a ligature; the other end of the cannula is connected to a mercury manometer, consequently the mercury column will rise. The measurement of B.P. is made by noting the pulsations in the mercury column. This measures the ***End Pressure,*** *i.e.* lateral wall pressure (**lateral pressure**) plus the increment of pressure caused by the conversion of kinetic energy of flow into pressure energy from the point at which cannula is tied with the artery.

Disadvantage: This method is unsafe, inconvenient and involves high risk of infection. It is appropriate only for research purposes such as measurement of B.P. in animals.

B. Indirect Method

PRINCIPLE: It involves the balancing of pressure in a bag, *i.e. Air Pressure* against the pressure of the blood in an artery. The air pressure is estimated by means of mercury or air (aneroid) manometer.

APPARATUS: Sphygmomanometer, Fig. 3.3.1 (devised by Riva-Rocci). It consists of:

1. An **inflatable flat rubber bag** covered by a non-distensible cloth envelope called **Riva-Rocci Cuff**. The cavity of the bag is connected by a long rubber tube to a manometer and by a short tube to a **rubber pump**; by this means the bag can be inflated to any desired pressure (Fig. 3.3.1-C).
2. A **small valve** is provided between the pump and the bag which permits the escape of air and reduction of the pressure as required to compensate tissue resistance.
3. The **manometer** is a U-shaped tube, one limb being broader than the other. The broader limb is the reservoir for mercury and the narrow limb is graduated from 0 to 300 mm, with the smallest division corresponding to a reading of 2 mmHg.
4. The inflatable bag dimensions **for adults** are: 23 × 12.5 cm; width of this bag varies with the age of the individual:
   - (i) below 1 year: 2.5 cm
   - (ii) below 4 years: 5 cm
   - (iii) below 8 years: 8 cm
   - (iv) adult: 12.5 cm.

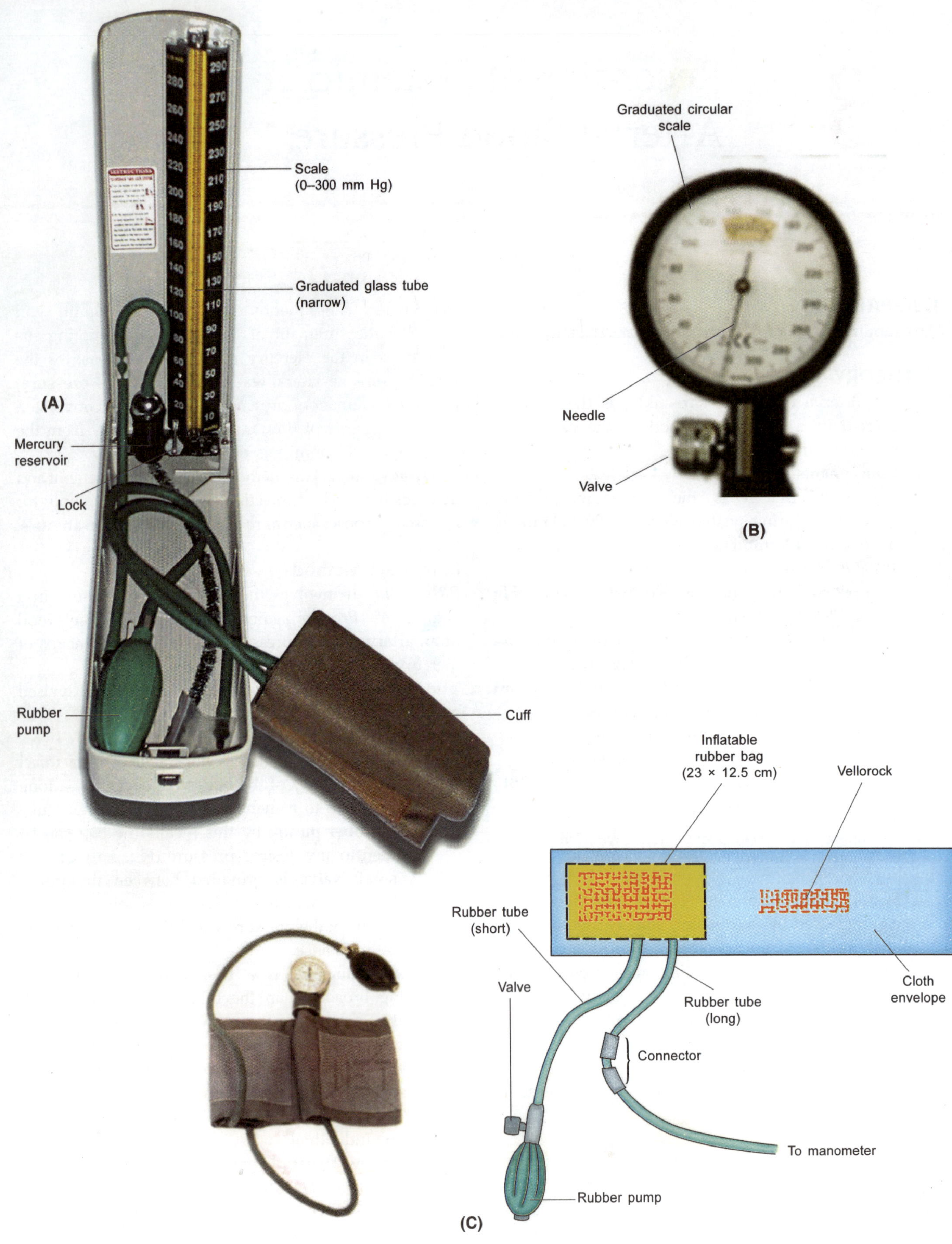

Fig. 3.3.1 (A) Mercury Sphygmomanometer; (B) Air (Aneroid) Manometer and (C) Riva-Roci Cuff

To overcome tissue resistance, ***Rule of Thumb*** involves that the inflatable arm bag should be 20% wider than the arm diameter and length should cover 2/3rd of the arm circumference (a length-to-width ratio of 2:1). Therefore, wider cuff should be used for recording the B.P. in *obese* individuals and in lower limbs to overcome tissue resistance.

PROCEDURE: Two methods are commonly in use for the measurement of systemic arterial B.P.: **palpatory** and **auscultatory** method. (Fig. 3.3.2)

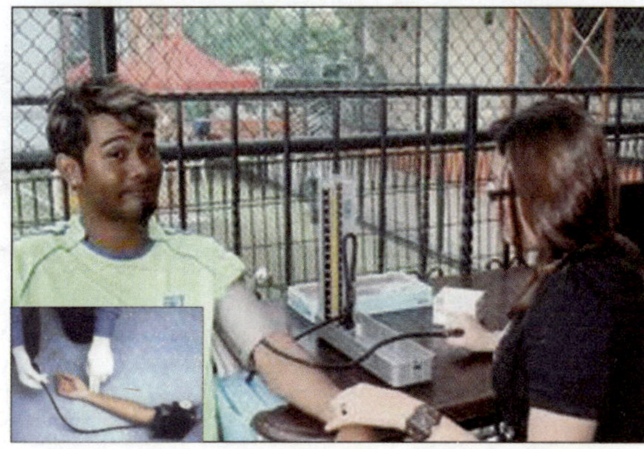

Fig. 3.3.2 Palpatory method to record Blood Pressure (Inset : note the position of the fingers to palpate radial artery)

1. **Palpatory Method**. Steps:
   (i) Allow the subject to sit comfortably in a chair or to lie supine on the examination couch for 5 minutes.
   (ii) The uninflated cuff of sphygmomanometer is wrapped firmly around the bare upper arm 2.5-3 cm above the elbow joint (ante- cubital fossa) at the heart level (Fig. 3.3.2).

   Note: The sleave should not be rolled up such that it has a tourniquet effect above the blood pressure cuff.

   (iii) Feel for the radial pulse and inflate the rubber bag to increase the pressure 20-30 mmHg above the point at which the radial pulse will disappear at the wrist.
   (iv) Now deflate the cuff slowly, releasing the pressure @ 2-3 mmHg/sec; while lowering the pressure, keep palpating the radial artery and reading is taken just when pulse starts reappearing. This gives the systolic B.P.
   (v) *Disadvantages*
      (a) Diastolic B.P. cannot be estimated.
      (b) Systolic B.P. estimated is lower than the actual by 6-10 mmHg because:
         • When the pressure in the 'cuff' just balances the brachial artery pressure, only a small amount of blood flows through the artery which may not be sufficient enough to produce a pulse wave.
         • Some time is taken by the blood to flow from the brachial artery to radial artery. During this mercury column falls further.

2. **Auscultatory Method**. This method was introduced by Russian physician, **Korotkoff**, in 1905. Take the following steps:

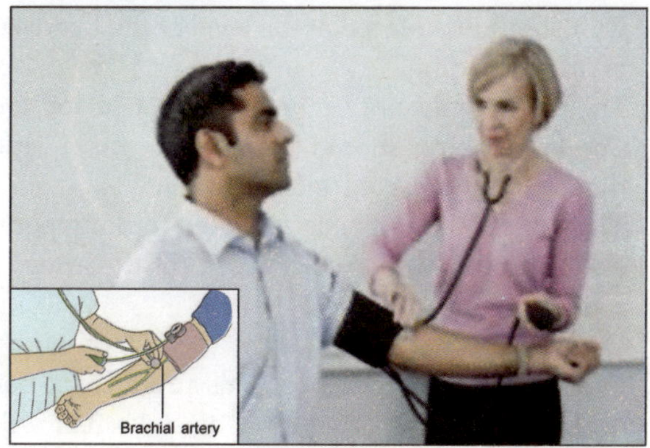

Fig. 3.3.3 Auscultatory Method to record Blood Pressure (**Inset** : note the position of the stethoscope to auscultate brachial artery)

   (i) Allow the subject to sit comfortably in a chair or to lie supine on the examination couch for 5 minutes.
   (ii) The uninflated cuff of sphygmomanometer is wrapped firmly around the upper arm 2.5-3 cm above the elbow joint at the heart level (Fig. 3.3.3).
   (iii) Place the chest piece of stethoscope over the arm medial to the tendon of biceps where the pulsations of brachial artery are felt (Inset Fig. 3.3.3). Under ordinary circumstances, if a stethoscope is placed over an artery, no sound can be heard, as the *streamline flow* of blood through the unconstricted blood vessel produces no sound.
   (iv) Inflate the cuff rapidly until the pressure in it is well above the systolic B.P. as measured by the palpatory method. The brachial artery gets occluded by the cuff and no sound can be heard with the stethoscope.
   (v) Now gradually lower the cuff pressure by opening the valve till a clear sharp tapping sound is heard. The cuff pressure at which the sound is heard first, gives a measure of *systolic B.P.*
   (vi) The pressure in the cuff is further progressively lowered (@ 2-3 mmHg/sec), while listening for the appearance of the ***sound of Korotkoff's***

(Fig. 3.3.5). The sound undergoes a series of changes in quality and becomes dull and muffled (in most individuals), to disappear finally. The cuff pressure at which the sound becomes muffled or disappears is the *diastolic B.P.*

(vii) Express the B.P. as SBP/DBP (mmHg); take two or three readings.

IV. PRECAUTIONS

1. The subject should be quiet for at least five minutes before the measurements are taken.
2. Cuff should be placed at the level of the heart while taking a reading.
3. The cuff should not be tied too tight or too loose.
4. The cuff tubing should lie over the inner side of the arm and directed inferiorly (Fig. 3.3.3).
5. The cuff should not be left inflated for long periods, else it produces the reflex spasm of the artery and a high reading will be obtained.
6. Do not apply pressure over the artery with the chest piece of stethoscope. This produces a partial obstruction of the artery and diastolic B.P. will be underestimated.
7. The cuff should not be left inflated for long periods, especially in persons suffering from purpura or tetany.
8. In suspected hypertensive individuals, cuff pressure should be raised well above 200 mmHg (or estimated systolic BP by palpatory method) to detect ***auscultatory gap*** (page 155).
9. The mercury column should not be deflated more than 2-3 mm/sec, otherwise it can lead to a significant underestimation of SBP and overestimation of DBP. The column should be read to the nearest 2 mmHg.
10. Check for the 'zero' error on mercury manometer, *i.e.* neither the column of the mercury should be above or below the zero reading with the cuff completely deflated. Otherwise, false lower or higher recording of BP will be made. (Fig. 3.3.4)

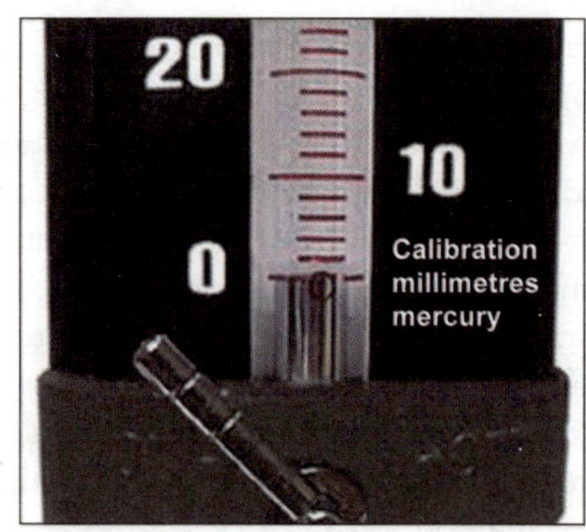

Fig. 3.3.4 "Zero error"–mercury manometer

OSPE

Aim: To record the blood pressure of the subject provided.

Procedure steps: Refer to page 151

Checklist

1. Checks for the 'zero' reading on the mercury manometer. **(Yes/No)**
2. Wraps uninflated cuff of sphygnomanometer firmly around the bare upper arm 2.5-5 cm above the elbow joint at the heart level. **(Yes/No)**
3. Inflates the cuff rapidly until the pressure in it is well above the systolic BP. **(Yes/No)**
4. Deflates the cuff slowly, releasing the pressure @ 2-3 mmHg/sec.
5. Records the BP first by palpatory method. **(Yes/No)**
6. Checks for the normal functioning of the diaphragm of the stethoscope by lightly tapping its diaphragm with a finger. **(Yes/No)**
7. Places the ear piece of the stethoscope properly into the ears directed forwards and medially along the direction of ear canals. **(Yes/No)**
8. Feels for the pulsations of the brachial artery and then places the chest piece of the stethocope over the arm medial to the tendon of biceps. **(Yes/No)**

IMPORTANT VIVA-VOCE QUESTIONS

Q.1. *Define B.P. and give the significance of its components.*

Ans. Definition, page 151.

(i) *Systolic B.P.* indicates the force with which the heart is working.

(ii) *Diastolic B.P.* is a measure of total peripheral resistance.

(iii) *Pulse pressure* determines the volume of the pulse.

(iv) *Mean B.P.* determines the pressure head for an organ on which its blood flow depends. All cardiovascular reflexes are sensitive to changes in mean B.P.

Q.2. *Enumerate the precautions while recording the B.P.*

Ans. See above.

Q.3. *Recording B.P. in an obese person with standard size cuff, would give it the same reading?*

Ans. Using a standard size cuff in obese individuals will fail to overcome tissue resistance (see rule of thumb, page 153) resulting in a falsely high measurement of B.P.

Q.4. *Give the merits and demerits of palpatory method.*

Ans. Disadvantage of palpatory method, page 153.

Merits: This method provides a rough estimation of

systolic B.P. which is of help to detect auscultatory gap in hypertensive individuals.

Q.5. *What are sounds of Korotkoff's? How are they produced?*

Ans. These sounds are produced by **turbulent flow** in the artery which can be heard during auscultation distal to obstruction when compression is slowly released. Four phases of sounds are recognized (Fig. 3.3.5).

Q.6. *What is **auscultatory (silent) gap**? How can it be avoided?*

Ans. It is seen in hypertensive persons while recording B.P. by auscultatory method. In such individuals, occasionally sound may disappear temporarily during phase I and II, covering a range of 40-50 mmHg pressure and reappear again. The cause of this **silent gap** is not known. This causes the marked under-estimation of systolic B.P. if cuff pressure is only raised to a level at which sounds are absent. This can be avoided by estimating the systolic B.P. first by palpatory method.

Q.7. *Why should the cuff be placed at the level of the heart while reading is being taken?*

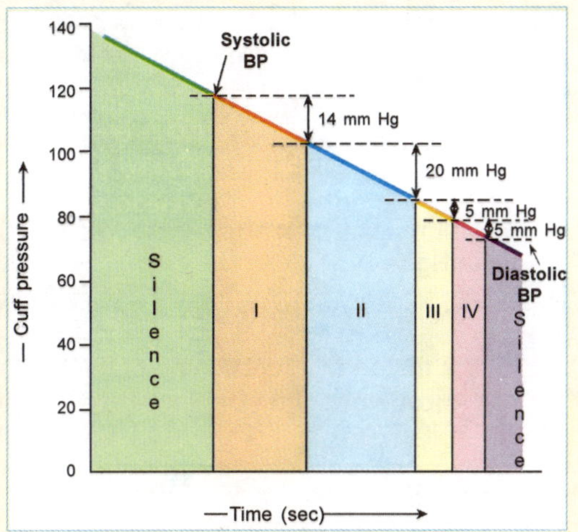

Fig. 3.3.5 Sounds of Korotkoff's

Phase I : Clear faint, tapping sound for first 10-14 mmHg fall of pressure
Phase II : Murmuring or musical quality of sound during next 15-20 mmHg fall in pressure
Phase III : Clear loud sound during the next 5-7 mmHg fall of pressure
Phase IV : Dull and muffled sound for the last 5-6 mmHg fall of pressure and finally the sound disappears.

Ans. The pressure in any vessel below heart level is increased and that in any vessel above the heart level is decreased by the effect of gravity. The magnitude of the gravitational effect being 0.77 mmHg for each cm vertical distance is above or below the heart. For example, mean B.P. in a large artery 50 cm below the heart will be: 100 + (0.77 × 50) = 138 mmHg.

Q.8. *Name some factors affecting B.P.*

Ans.
(i) *Age:* Both systolic and diastolic B.P. increase with age, systolic B.P. increases more than the diastolic B.P. Roughly, systolic B.P. in adults is (100 + age in years).
(ii) *Sex:* In females, before menopause systolic B.P. is 4-5 mmHg less than that in males of the same age. This may be due to oestrogen.
(iii) *Body built:* obesity (page 153).
(iv) *Exercise* (page 157).
(v) *Posture* (page 157).
(vi) *Gravity:* Refer to Q. 7.
(vii) *Sleep:* Systolic B.P. falls in early hours of sleep by 15-30 mmHg due to the generalised relaxation of blood vessels.

Q.9. *How will the B.P. reading be affected if an over-or under-sized cuff is used?*

Ans. In either situation, reading is higher than the normal since more air needs to be pumped into the bag to overcome the tissue resistance.

Q.10. *Is there any difference in BP readings between the two arms?*

Ans. In healthy individuals, there is *no* difference in the B.P. readings between the two arms.

Q.11. *Why does the graduated manometer scale show the highest mark of 300 mmHg?*

Or

Is it possible that the systolic B.P. in an individual can go beyond 300 mmHg?

Ans. The maximum limit of intramyocardial tension which can normally be generated in a healthy individual corresponds to 300 mmHg.

Q.12. *What is 'zero error'? How does it affect the recording?*

Ans. Page 154.

STUDY NOTES

OBSERVATIONS AND RESULTS

Tabulate your results as follows:

A. Palpatory Method

1. 1st reading ....

2. 2nd reading ....

B. *Auscultatory Method*

	Systolic B.P. (mmHg)	Diastolic B.P. (mmHg)	Pulse pressure (mmHg)	Mean B.P. (mmHg)
1. 1st reading				
2. 2nd reading				
3. 3rd reading				

Important note: A minimum of two readings should be taken at intervals of at least 1 minute, and the average of those readings should be used to represent subject's BP. If there is >5 mmHg difference between the first and second reading, additional 3rd reading should be obtained, and then the average of these three readings is used.

COMMENTS

Explain if there is any difference in the systolic B.P. readings measured by two methods.

....

....

....

....

....

....

....

....

....

....

....

....

....

....

....

Date: ....

4 Effect of Posture and Exercise on Blood Pressure

I. APPARATUS

The same as in the previous experiment, page 151.

A. Effect of Posture on Blood Pressure

Theory

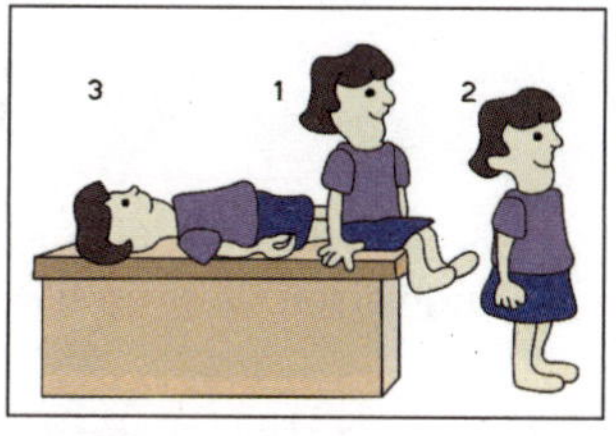

1. Changes in both systolic and diastolic B.P. are common with change in body posture; alteration in the diastolic B.P. is for much longer duration compared to systolic component.
2. In standing posture diastolic B.P. increases; in sitting remains normal and decreases in lying posture. *Mechanism*: on sudden standing:
   (i) Peripheral pooling of blood in dependent parts decreases venous return, thereby cardiac output decreases, so systolic B.P. falls by 6-23 mmHg. This reflexly via baroreceptor discharge, increases the diastolic B.P.
   (ii) Increase in peripheral resistance increases the diastolic B.P.

   Thus, upon sudden standing from lying or sitting position, increases the diastolic B.P. However, it will return back to normal level after 1-2 minutes of change in posture due to the operation of baroreceptor reflexes.

Procedure

1. Ask the subject to lie supine quietly on a couch for 5-10 minutes, record the pulse rate and B.P. with sphygmomanometer by both methods. Do not untie the cuff.
2. Ask the subject to sit up and immediately note the pulse rate and B.P. (by auscultatory method only) every minute for 3-4 minutes.
3. Similarly, make the subject stand from lying position and repeat the whole procedure.
4. Compare the B.P. recorded during the two positions with the lying position.

Precautions

1. B.P. should be recorded by keeping brachial artery at the heart level in all positions.
2. Since changes in the B.P. are sudden and of short duration, therefore B.P. should be recorded within 30-60 seconds of change in posture.
3. To avoid loss of time, do not untie the cuff.

B. Effect of Exercise on Blood Pressure

Theory

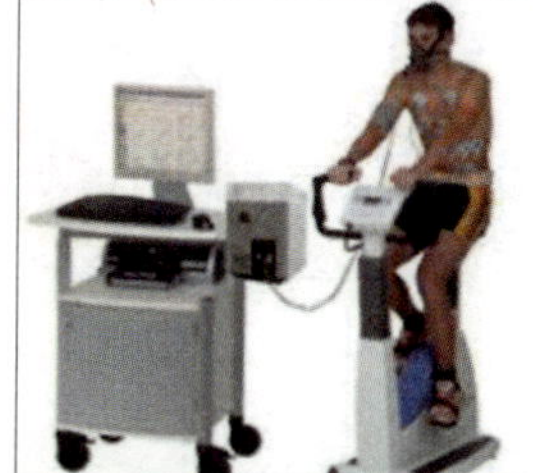

1. Effect of exercise on systemic arterial B.P. varies with the intensity (severity) of exercise and with the type of individual (trained or untrained).

Type of individual	Intensity of exercise					
	Mild		Moderate		Severe	
	SBP	DBP	SBP	DBP	SBP	DBP
Trained	-	-	-	-	+↑	-
Untrained	+↑	-/+↓	++↑	+↑	+++↑	+ to ++↑

(–): no change; +, ++, +++: mild, moderate, severe; ↑: increase; ↓: decrease

2. Systolic B.P. increases in linearity with the severity of exercise at all ages and may increase up to 200 mmHg. Increase is mainly due to increased sympathetic activity in response to exercise.
3. In mild to moderate exercise, diastolic B.P. shows either no change or slightly increases. (or may even fall due to drastic vasodilatation in working muscles). In severe exercise, it increases slightly due to vasoconstriction in non-working muscles and the skin.
4. B.P. comes back to normal within 5-7 minutes after stopping exercise due to the relaxation of muscles which produces vasodilatation.

Procedure

1. Allow the subject to sit quietly for 5-10 minutes, take the heart rate (radial pulse) and B.P. (auscultatory method) and make a note of them.
2. *The exercise.* Various forms of physical activities can be performed as a mode of exercise like climbing upstairs, jumping, hopping, bending, etc.; the common ones which are used in the laboratory are:
   (i) Hop twenty times on each foot, raising the body, 15-20 cm for 4-5 minutes.
   (ii) Let the subject perform the **two-step exercise test** for 4 to 5 minutes. Here, the subject ascends to the top of **two steps** and walks down the other side. This is counted as one trip. He should then turn and start the second trip. The rate of ascent and descent should be controlled by a metronome (Fig. 3.4.1).

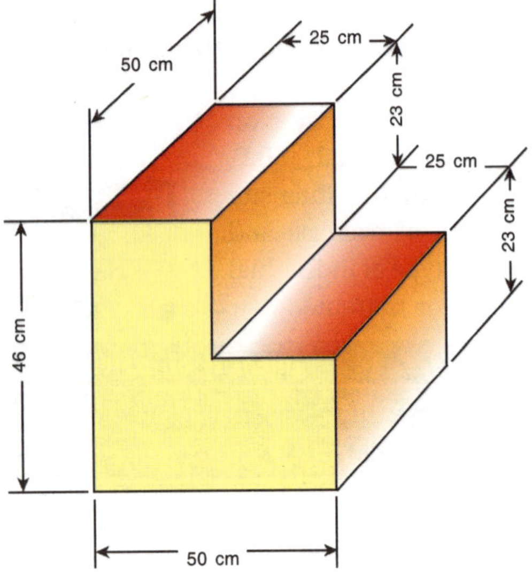

Fig. 3.4.1 Two-step exercise testing

Important Note: In case the subject feels intolerably breathless, fatigued in legs, giddy or pain, constriction or suffocation in chest during the exercise, ask him to discontinue the exercise immediately.

Note: Alternatively, a bicycle or treadmill ergometer (Page 191) can also be used as a mode of exercise.

3. Immediately after the stoppage of exercise, record the heart rate and B.P.

Note: To avoid loss of time, have the sphygmomanometer prepared before the exercise with the disconnected **cuff** in position.

4. The heart rate and B.P. recording should be continued every minute till the resting values are obtained. Note the time of recovery.

OSPE

Aim: To record the effect of sudden change in posture from sitting to standing on B.P. of the subject provided.

Procedure steps: Refer to page 157.

Checklist

1. Checks for the proper functioning of B.P. apparatus and stethoscpe. **(Yes/No)**
2. Records the resting B.P. of the subject first by palpatory method and then by auscultatory method. **(Yes/No)**
3. Instructs the subject to stand up immediately without untying the cuff. **(Yes/No)**
4. Records the BP of the subject by auscultatory method only within 30-60 secs of change in posture. **(Yes/No)**
5. Records the BP, keeping the cuff at the heart level. **(Yes/No)**
6. Also, makes a note of the pulse rate. **(Yes/No)**

IMPORTANT VIVA-VOCE QUESTIONS

Q.1. *What is postural hypotension?*

Ans. In this condition, there occurs a fall in the B.P. with a sudden change in posture. This is due to the autonomic insufficiency. This condition is associated with dizziness, dimness of vision and fainting attacks.

Q.2. *Why is it necessary to make a note of pulse rate while observing the effect of exercise on B.P.?*

Ans. The effect of exercise on B.P. varies with the intensity of exercise. Heart rate is a measure of level of exercise (page 193).

Q.3. *Why should B.P. be recorded within 30-60 secs of change of body posture?*

Ans. Page 157.

Q.4. *What is the effect of exercise on B.P.?*

Ans. Page 157.

Q.5. *What is steady state exercise (or) what should be the minimum duration of exercise for most variables to reach constant values?*

Ans. Page 190.

STUDY NOTES

OBSERVATIONS

(A) EFFECT OF POSTURE ON B.P.

Posture	Pulse rate (per minute)	Systolic/Diastolic B.P. (mmHg)	Pulse pressure (mmHg)
1. Lying (after 5-10 minutes of rest)			
2. On sitting (i) immediate (ii) after 1 minute (iii) after 2 minutes (iv) after 3 minutes			
3. On standing (i) immediate (ii) after 1 minute (iii) after 2 minutes (iv) after 3 minutes			

(B) EFFECT OF EXERCISE ON B.P.

	Heart rate (b.p.m.)	Systolic/Diastolic B.P. (mmHg)	Mean B.P. (mmHg)
1. Resting (after 5-10 minutes of rest)			
2. Immediately after 4-5 minutes of exercise			
3. Recovery: (i) 1 min. after exercise (ii) 2 min. after exercise (iii) 3 min. after exercse (iv) 4 min. after exercise (v) 5 min. after exercise			

RESULTS, COMMENTS AND DISCUSSION

....

....

....

....

....

....

Date: ....

5 Measurement of Blood Flow by Venous Occlusion Plethysmography

I. APPARATUS

Plethysmograph (airtight chamber), float recorder, sphygmomanometer, recording drum, time marker, hot and cold water (± 10°C of ambient temperature)

Plethysmograph (Fig. 3.5.1)

1. It consists of a **rigid walled container**, so arranged that the forearm or hand can be placed into it.
2. An airtight seal being obtained by means of a **rubber collar**
3. The plethysmograph proper is connected to a recording tambour by means of a stiff-walled (pressure) rubber tubing. A safety valve is placed in the system to protect the tambour. This should be kept open except at the time of taking actual records.

Float recorder or Volume recorder

It consists of a chamber (capacity 225 ml) made of copper foil open at the bottom, and floating in a **tank** over a central tube. The chamber is so shaped that the movement is directly proportional to the volume. It is pivoted at one end, and has an **adjustable balance weight** with a **screw**. A **writing lever** attached at one

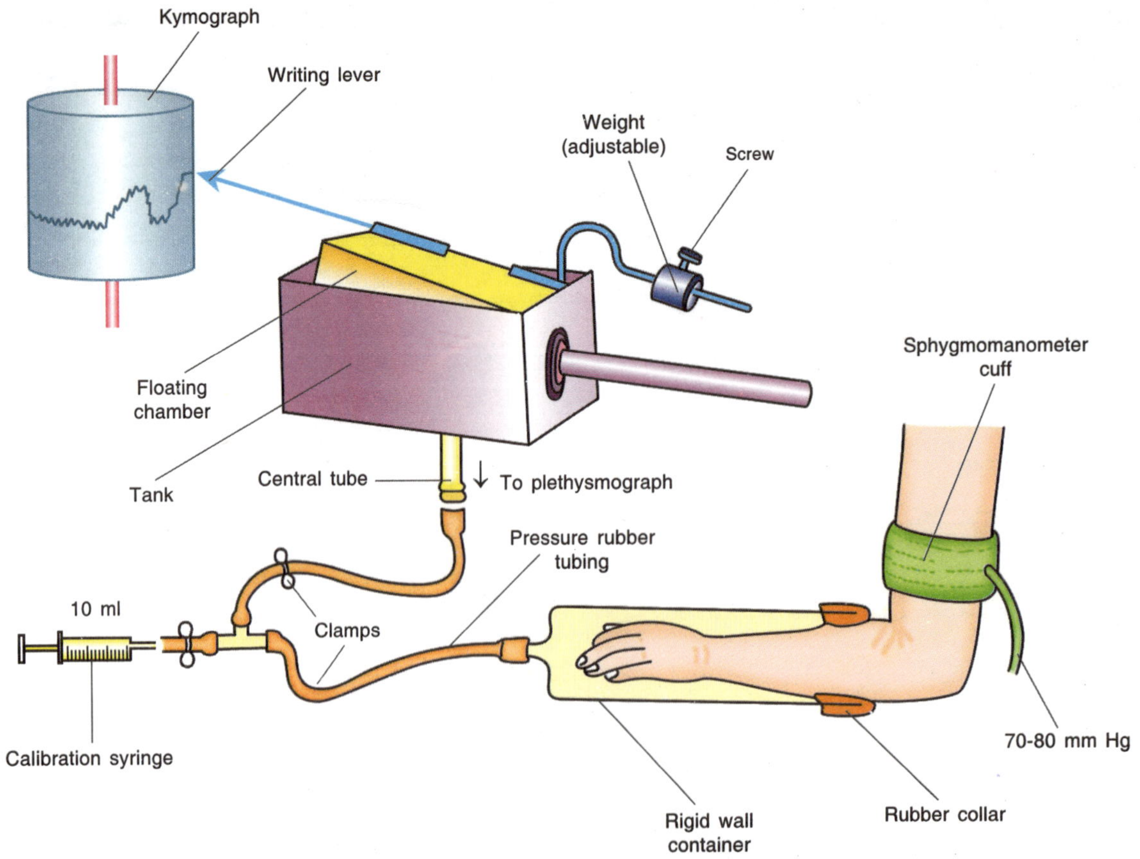

Fig. 3.5.1 Plethysmograph and float recorder: an arrangement for recording blood flow of the forearm is shown.

end of the chamber records its movements directly on the kymograph.

II. THEORY

1. If only the venous return from an organ is stopped, the volume of the organ increases because arterial blood continues to flow into the organ. A rough idea of the flow of blood through the organ at rest can be obtained by measuring the rate of arterial inflow immediately following venous occlusion. The rate of change of volume thus is equal to the rate of inflow of blood.
2. ***Measurement of blood flow in the forearm by venous occlusion plethysmography***
   (i) The forearm is composed mainly of muscle and bone with relatively little skin. Therefore, its blood-flow can be measured by enclosing the forearm in a plethysmograph and recording changes in its volume. When a cuff is applied above the elbow at a pressure just below the diastolic pressure (*i.e.* 70-80 mmHg) of the subject for 30 seconds, not only the entry of arterial blood into the forearm is impaired, but also for some time venous blood cannot return to the heart. The blood collected in the forearm causes it to swell and its volume increases. The increase in the volume displaces the air from the plethysmograph into a volume recorder whose movements can be recorded on a kymograph.
   (ii) At 25°C, full venoconstriction occurs. Therefore, if ambient temperature is 25°C, as in winters, then with a further fall of temperature no appreciable decrease in the blood-flow is observed.

Note: Hand blood flow is principally through skin whereas the forearm blood flow is principally through the muscles.

III. PROCEDURE

1. Calibrate the volume recorder by injecting known volume of air each time. How? First fill the volume recorder with water and balance it by adjusting the screw on the weight, so that the pointer may write horizontally on the kymograph. Now using a syringe inject 10 ml of air each time taking care that tube to plethysmograph is clamped. After calibration is over clamp the calibration tube as well (Fig. 3.5.2).
2. Adjust the speed of the kymograph to about 2.5 mm per second and arrange the time-marker.
3. Determine the blood pressure of the subject using sphygmomanometer.
4. ***To determine the blood-flow through forearm,*** insert the forearm into the plethysmograph so that the upper end of the plethysmograph may be close to the elbow. This ensures that the maximum possible musculature of the forearm is included.
5. Tie the sphygmomanometer **cuff** round the upper arm on the same side. Suddenly inflate the cuff and raise the pressure between 70-80 mmHg (or 10-15 mmHg below the estimated diastolic B.P. of the subject) for 30 seconds and record the volume change. Release the pressure to zero (Fig. 3.5.2).
6. Calculate the rate of blood flow through the forearm from the volume change and time (30 seconds here).
7. ***To study the blood-flow through the hand,*** the same procedure is used but instead of the forearm insert the hand into the plethysmograph so that the plethysmograph diaphragm may lie against the wrist. The study of blood flow through the hand gives mainly an index of blood flow through the skin.
8. ***Effect of temperature***
   Principle: Insert the forearm or hand into a precalibrated plethysmograph filled with water and

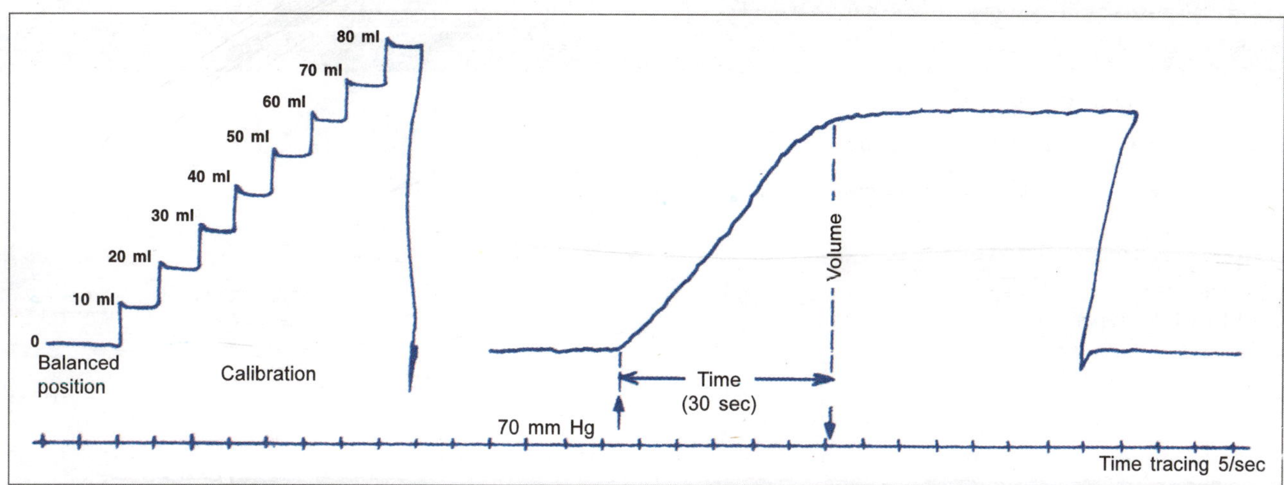

Fig. 3.5.2 Plethysmographic tracing for measurement of blood flow through the forearm by venous occlusion plethysmography

find out the volume change by water displacement technique.

(i) For the direct effect of temperature fill the plethysmograph with the warm water (usually 10°C above the ambient temperature) and maintain the water temperature. After 5 to 7 minutes record the volume change as already described above.

(ii) To study the effect of cold, take out the water and empty the plethysmograph, and fill it with the cold water (usually 10°C below the ambient temperature) and repeat the whole procedure.

9. *To demonstrate autonomic reflex due to temperature,* dip the opposite forearm or hand in warm or cold water and then record the blood-flow.

10. *Effect of exercise.* Ask the subject to close and open the fist inside the plethysmograph at the rate of 20 per minute for 3 minutes. Now suddenly raise the cuff pressure between 70-80 mmHg to cut off the venous outflow; record the volume change and measure the blood flow.

11. ***Reactive hyperaemia.*** To demonstrate reactive hyperaemia, first inflate the sphygmomanometer cuff pressure to 70-80 mmHg for 30 seconds and measure the blood flow. Then suddenly increase the cuff pressure to 200 mmHg and maintain it for the stoppage of circulation for 5 minutes. Suddenly, release the pressure to 70-80 mmHg and record the enhanced filling of the relaxed vessels. This increased blood-flow is then substracted from the resting blood-flow to determine the reactive hyperaemia.

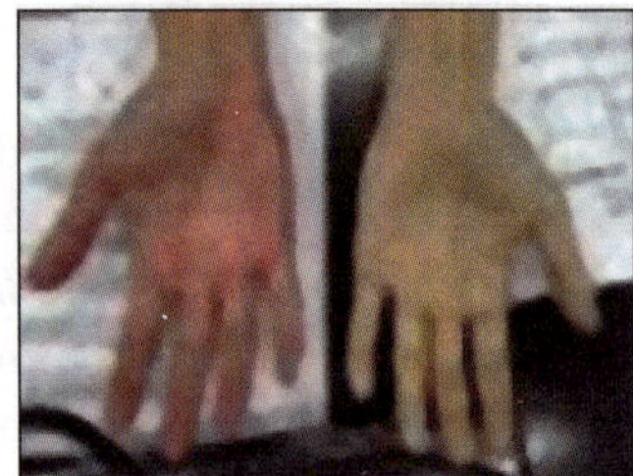

Note: The recording can also be made using a volume transducer on a student physiograph, page 85.

IMPORTANT VIVA-VOCE QUESTIONS

Q.1. *Give the principle underlying the working of venous occlusion plethysmograph.*

Ans. Page 160.

Q.2. *How does the blood-flow through the skin differ from that of the muscle?*

Ans. Page 161.

A.3. *Why does the pressure of the cuff need to be raised above the diastolic BP of the subject?*

Ans. Page 161.

Q.4. *What is the effect of temperature on the blood-flow through the forearm?*

Ans. Blood flow through the forearm increases in linearity with the rise of the ambient temperature within the physiological limits. However, at 25°C, full venoconstriction occurs. Therefore, if ambient temperature falls below 25°C, no appreciable decrease in the blood-flow will be observed.

Q.5. *Define the term reactive hyperaemia.*

Ans. Increased flow of blood after temporary ischaemia is called reactive hyperaemia.

STUDY NOTES

RESULTS AND DISCUSSION

	Blood flow through		Remarks (if any)
	forearm	hand	
1. At ambient temperature ... °C			
2. At 10°C above the ambient temperature			
3. At 10°C below the ambient temperature			
4. Effect due to: (i) Autonomic reflex (ii) Exercise (iii) Reactive hyperaemia			

....

....

....

Date: ....

6 Recording of a 12-Lead Electrocardiogram *(E.C.G.)*

I. APPARATUS

Electrocardiograph, or student physiograph with ECG coupler; patient cable with leads, subject, electrodes, cardiac jelly, examination couch, etc.

Electrocardiograph: ECG machine

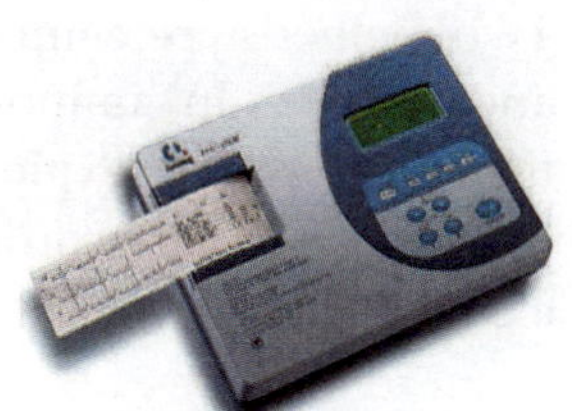

Electrocardiograph is an instrument for making permanent record of small potential variations which occur in different parts of the body due to the electrical activity of the heart. It consists of:

1. **Cathode ray oscilloscope**. It is a voltage amplifier recorder system with an arrangement to record the deflection of galvanometer.
2. An arrangement to run the recording paper at a desired speed
3. The other parts of an electrocardiograph are shown in Fig. 3.6.1.

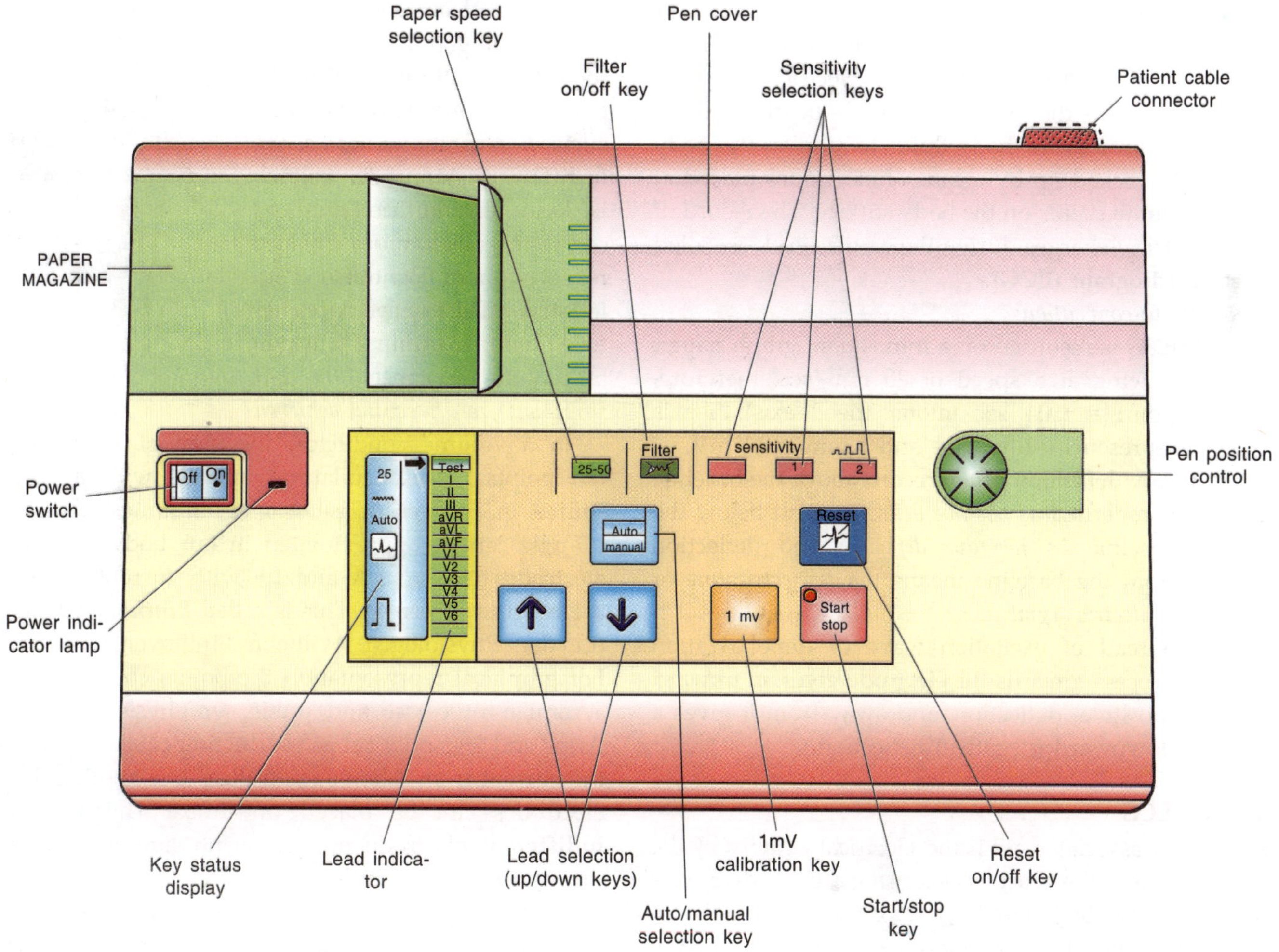

Fig. 3.6.1 An electrocardiograph – controls and connectors

Cardiac jelly

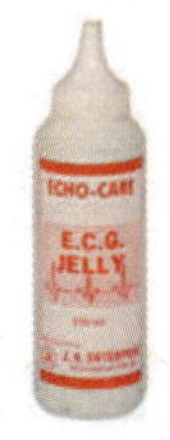

It is a conducting paste which contains very fine particles of sand or glass; when rubbed on the skin it produces erythema locally; therefore, electrical activities can be picked up nicely.

Electrodes

These are rectangular flat discs (dimension 7.5 cm × 5 cm) made up of non-corrosive metal. These can be applied and fixed on suitable body surface by means of rubber straps. They conduct electrical current.

Student physiograph with ECG coupler

Refer to page 84.

ECG coupler consists of:

1. One **off/on** control
2. The **lead selector** with the following positions: CAL, I, II, III, aV_R, aV_L, aV_F, V, CR, CL, CF
3. A **push button** marked CAL 1 mV, for checking calibration
4. An input socket

II. THEORY

Body is a volume conductor, *i.e.* body fluids are good conductor of electricity. Therefore electrical changes generated inside the heart with each heart beat are conducted through the body fluids to all over the body and can be picked up by means of electrodes placed at certain definite points on the body surface. The record of these electrical charges during the cardiac cycle is called **Electrocardiogram (ECG).**

Recording conventions

1. ECG is recorded on a mm square graph paper, moving at a speed of 25 mm/sec; therefore, 1 mm = 0.04 sec (along the X-axis). Y-axis represents the voltage and 1 mm = 0.1 mV.
2. Any deflection of the record above the baseline is regarded as *positive deflection,* and below the baseline as *negative deflection;* no deflection from the baseline means the *isoelectric line* or *isoelectric segment.*
3. Spread of excitation wave or depolarization process towards the electrode gives an upward (positive) deflection, and away from it gives a downward (negative) deflection.

Normal ECG

The waves associated with the electrical activity of the various parts of the heart tissue during each cardiac cycle are represented by letters P, Q, R, S, T and U (Fig. 3.6.2). The characteristic features of each wave are described in Table 3.6.1.

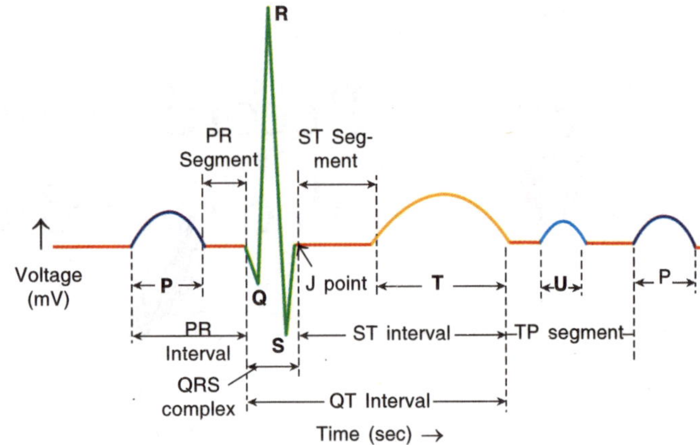

Fig. 3.6.2 Normal Electrocardiogram (ECG)

Electrocardiography: *Basis of recording of ECG*

Two methods are employed for recording ECG: *unipolar* and *bipolar.* In unipolar method, ECG is recorded using one **active (exploring) electrode** while in bipolar method, ECG is recorded using two active (exploring) electrodes.

(A) Unipolar recording

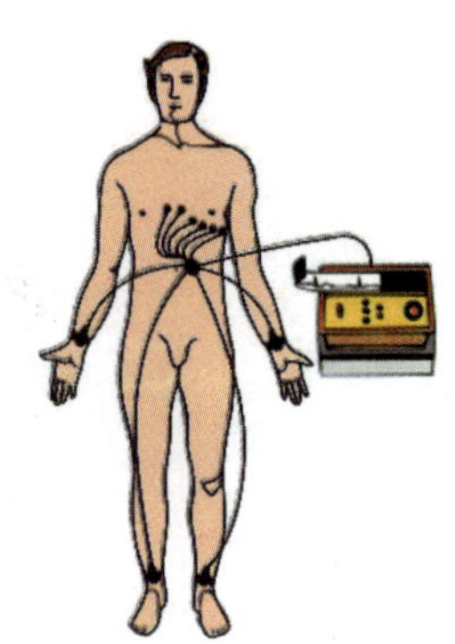

Here two electrodes are used for recording purposes: one is the **active** (exploring) electrode, placed on the area of the body surface; and the other is the **indifferent** electrode, which is kept at **zero** potential by connecting electrodes placed respectively on right arm (RA), left arm (LA) and left foot (LF) to a central terminal through 5000 ohms resistance.

How is zero potential achieved?

In a volume conductor, the sum of potentials at the points of an equilateral triangle with a current source in the centre is **zero** at all times. A similar triangle can be approximated in our body by placing electrodes on RA, LA and LF with current source as the heart at its centre. This is called ***Einthoven Triangle*** (Leyden Physiologist, Wilhelm Einthoven, 1860-1927). For graphical representation the points chosen are two acromian processes and pubic symphysis (Fig. 3.6.3). Arms and legs only act as conducting cables. Therefore, the current from 3 limbs neutralizes one another, hence electrodes can be placed on limbs. Therefore, this **indifferent** electrode undergoes no significant change during the cardiac cycle.

Thus in unipolar record, ECG records potential changes which affect the active electrode only. A record obtained in this method is labelled by letter 'V' which means a 'vector'.

Table 3.6.1 Characteristic features of normal ECG waves

ECG component (Fig. 3.6.2)	Cause	Duration and magnitude		Remarks
1. P-wave	Atrial depolarization	0.08-0.1 sec;	0.5 mV	Always inverted in aV_R
2. Isoelectric period	–	0.04 sec;	–	–
3. QRS complex (ventricular complex)	Ventricular depolarization	0.08-0.12 sec;	1.5-2 mV	(i) Q-wave due to septal activation (ii) R-wave due to activation of major part of both the ventricles (iii) S-wave due to activation of basal parts of ventricles
4. Isoelectric period or *ST segment*	–	0.04-0.08 sec	–	Measured from end of S-wave to the beginning of T-wave
5. T-wave	Ventricular repolarization	0.27 sec;	0.5 mV	–
6. Isoelectric period	–	0.04 sec;	–	–
7. U-wave	Slow repolarization of papillary muscles	0.08 sec;	0.2 mV	–
8. P-R interval	Atrial depolarization and conduction in bundle of HIS	0.13-0.16 sec;	–	Measured from the beginning of P-wave to the beginning of R-wave (if Q-wave is absent)
9. Q-T interval	Ventricular depolarization and repolarization	0.40-0.43 sec;	–	Measured from the beginning of Q-wave (or R-wave) to the end of T-wave
10. S-T interval	Ventricular repolarization	0.32 sec;	–	Measured from end of S-wave to the end of T-wave
11. T-P segment	Polarized (resting) state of whole heart	0.2 sec at HR 75 bpm		Duration inversely related to HR
12. J point	Point between S-wave and S-T segment	–	–	Point of no electrical activity

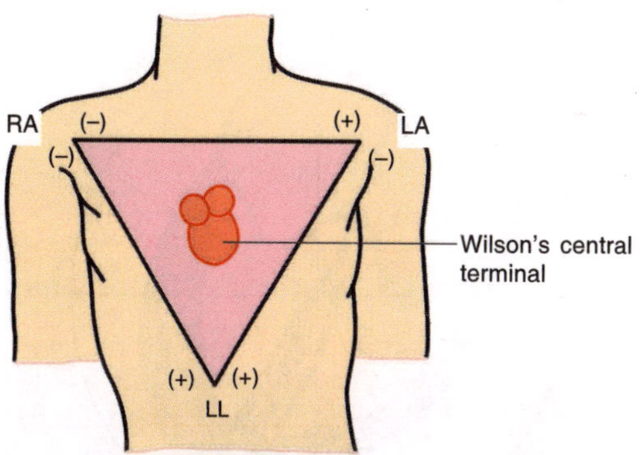

Fig. 3.6.3 Einthoven's Triangle Superimposed on Chest (LA: left arm; RA: right arm; LL: left leg)

In unipolar recording, the following unipolar leads are used:

Name of unipolar lead	Position of exploring electrode
A. Limb Leads	
1. V_L	Left arm
2. V_F	Left foot
3. V_R	Right arm
B. Precordial Leads of Wilson	
1. V_1	4th intercostal space to the right of sternum
2. V_2	4th intercostal space to the left of sternum
3. V_3	mid-way between V_2 and V_4
4. V_4	5th left intercostal space in mid-clavicular line
5. V_5	5th left intercostal space in anterior axillary line
6. V_6	5th left intercostal space in mid-axillary line

Augmented limb leads of Goldberger

These are unipolar limb leads with slight modification in the recording technique. The augmented limb leads are the recording between one limb connected to the positive terminal of ECG machine and the other two limbs are connected through electrical resistance to the negative terminal of the ECG machine. This arrangement increases the size of potentials by 50% without any change in configuration (pattern) from the non-augmented record; therefore,

Vector of augmented limb lead = 3/2 vector of unaugmented limb lead

Augmented limb leads are designated by letter 'a' prefixed to the name of the limb lead. Therefore, these are aV_R, aV_L and aV_F. Thus,

$$aV_R = V_R - \left(\frac{V_L + V_F}{2}\right)$$

$$2aV_R = 2V_R - (V_L + V_F) \quad \text{.. (i)}$$

Since $V_R + V_L + V_F$= Zero (Einthoven triangle)

$$V_R = -(V_L + V_F) \quad \text{.. (ii)}$$

From (i) and (ii)

$$2aV_R = 2V_R + V_R$$

$$aV_R = 3/2\ V_R$$

(B) Bipolar Recording

Here ECG is recorded using two active electrodes. Therefore, the deflection recorded here at any moment represents the algebraic sum of the potentials of two constituent leads.

Bipolar leads or classical (standard) limb leads of Einthoven are:

1. Lead I : records the difference in potential between RA and LA ('LA' positive)
2. Lead II : records the difference in potential between RA and LF ('LF' positive)
3. Lead III : records the difference in potential between LA and LF ('LF' positive)

Thus,

Lead I, records $(V_L - V_R)$, therefore, main QRS deflection is the same as in aV_L

Lead II, records $(V_F - V_R)$, therefore,main QRS deflection is the same as in aV_F

Lead III, records $(V_F - V_L)$, therefore, main QRS deflection is the same as in aV_F

Important Note: Standard (or classical) limb lead II is often used for cardiac monitoring as the positioning of the electrodes most commonly resembles the pathway of current flow, a normal atrial and ventricular depolarization. Moreover, on analysis it can be shown that at any given instant (moment) the sum of potentials in Lead I and Lead III equals the potentials in Lead II,

i.e. Lead II = Lead I + Lead III

$$V_F - V_R = (V_L - V_R) + (V_F - V_L)$$
$$= V_F - V_R$$

Why is it necessary to have 12 leads ECG?

The ECG leads are the pair of electrodes across which the electrical potential is measured. There are 12 conventional E.G.G. leads which can be divided into *Frontal plane leads* and *Horizontal plane leads.*

A. **Frontal plane leads**: *The six limb leads* (I, II, III, aV_R, aV_L and aV_F)

1. These limb leads view the heart in a *vertical (frontal) plane*: These leads record the electrical activity (*i.e.* wave of depolarization and repolarization) moving up and down, and left and right across the heart.
2. *Orientation of frontal plane leads* or the view of the heart.
   (i) An imaginary line joining the positive and negative electrode of a lead is called *axis of the lead*. It measures the *angle of orientation of the lead* and is expressed in degrees (Fig. 3.6.4).
   (ii)

	Lead					
	I	II	III	aV_R	aV_L	aV_F
Angle of orientation	+0°	+60°	+120°	-150°	-30°	+90°

   (iii) (a) Leads I and aV_L are called the *left lateral leads* and they view the left lateral wall of the heart predominantly formed by the left ventricle.
   (b) Leads II, III and aV_F are called the *inferior leads* as they view the inferior surface of the heart whch rests on the diaphragm. This may be formed by both right and left ventricles.

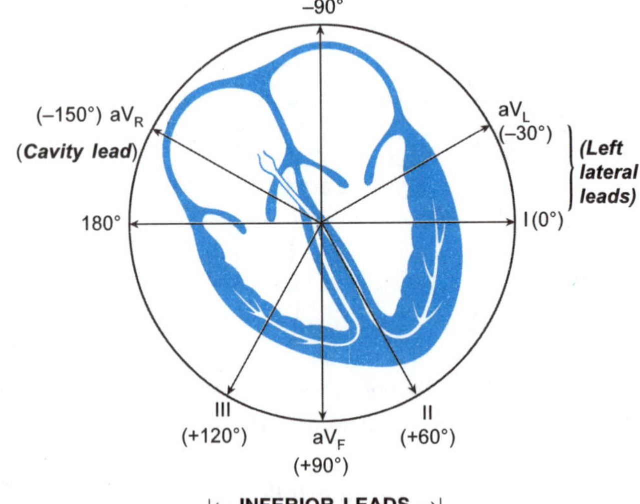

Fig. 3.6.4 Angle of orientation of frontal plane leads

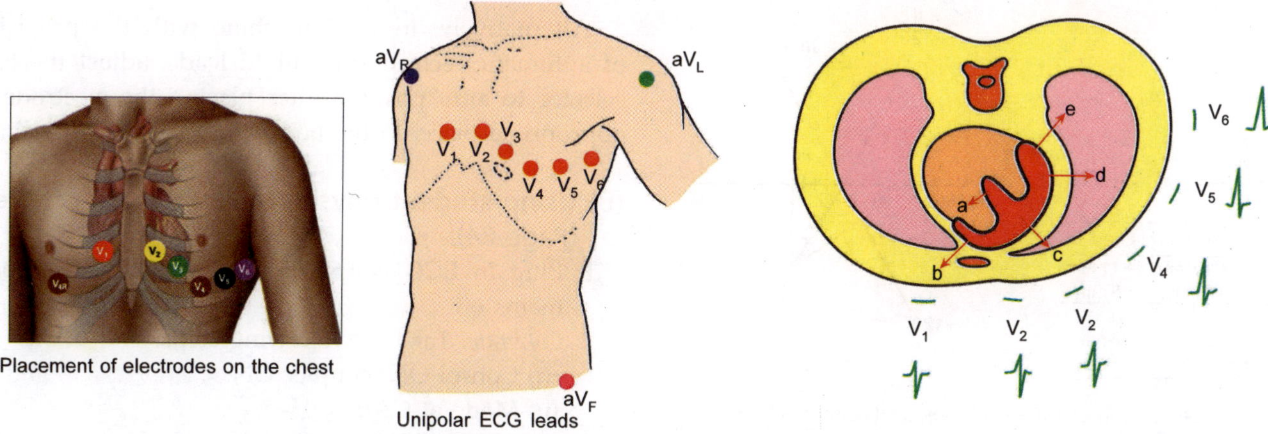

Fig. 3.6.5 "Cross-section through chest showing precordial leads and their relation to heart' (a, b, c, d and e show the order in which the electrical impulse spreads through the ventricles)

(c) Lead aV_R is oriented to the cavities of the heart, whatever may be the position of the heart.

B. **Horizontal plane leads**: *The Precordial leads* (V_1 to V_6)

1. These leads are arranged across the chest in a *horizontal plane* (Fig. 3.6.5) and view electrical forces moving anteriorly and posteriorly. To make the six precordial leads, each chest electrode is made positive in turn using the active electrode.
2. In most of the individuals, heart is placed obliquely in the chest. Thus leads V_1 and V_2 lie directly over the right ventricle, V_3 and V_4 over the interventricular septum and V_5 and V_6 over the left ventricle (Fig. 3.6.5).
3. (i) Leads V_1 through V_4 are referred as the *anterior leads*. This may be formed by both right and left ventricles; and

   (ii) Leads V_5 and V_6 are referred as *left lateral leads* (see above).

Summary

1. Left lateral leads : Leads I,aV_L; V_5 and V_6
2. Anterior leads : Leads V_1 to V_4
3. Inferior leads : Leads II, III and aV_F
4. Cavity lead : aV_R

Cardiac vector or cardiac axis

Since the classical (standard) limb leads I, II and III are the records of the potential difference between two points, therefore, deflection in each lead at any moment indicates the magnitude and direction in the axis of the electromotive force (EMF) generated in the heart. This is called as **cardiac vector** or **cardiac axis**.

Calculation of cardiac axis

Cardiac axis at any given moment can be calculated from any two classical limb leads. How?

In an Einthoven triangle, if perpendiculars are dropped from the mid-points of the sides of the equilateral triangle, the lines will intersect at the centre of the electrical activity (Fig. 3.6.6-A). Thus, the Einthoven triangle can be modified in such a way that the leads intersect each other at a common central point without altering the mathematical relationship of the leads. The lead potentials are seen to be placed as in the diagram (Fig. 3.6.6-B).

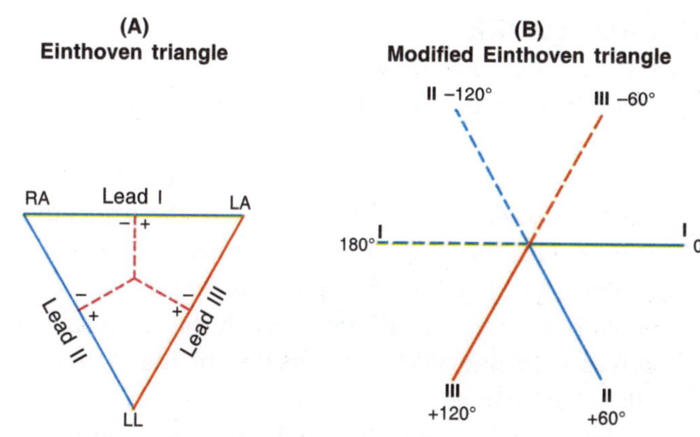

Fig. 3.6.6 Calculation of cardiac axis

The electrical axis of the heart is plotted using the average QRS deflection in any two classical limb leads. This is called as *mean QRS vector*. The average QRS deflection is the distance equal to the height of 'R' wave minus the height of the largest negative deflection in the QRS complex (Fig. 3.6.7).

The distance equal to the average QRS deflection is measured off from the mid-point of the sides of the triangle representing that lead; perpendiculars are extended from the distance measured off. An arrow is drawn from the centre of the electrical activity to the point of intersection of perpendiculars. This represents the magnitude and direction of the mean QRS vector.

The *normal direction* of the ***"mean QRS vector"*** is -30° to +110°.

(i) -30° to +30° is normal *left axis deviation* (LAD). It represents the horizontal position of the heart.

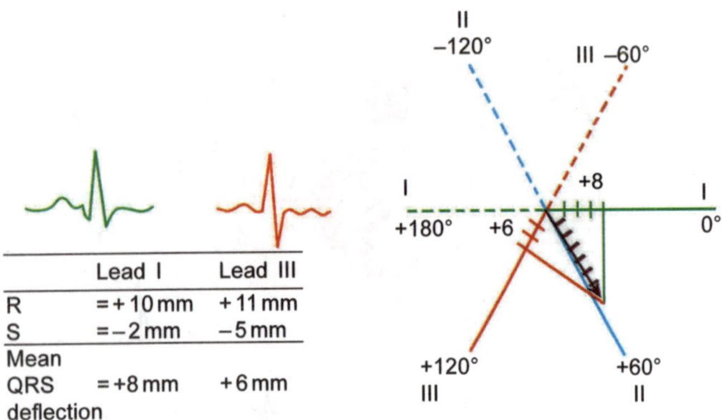

Fig. 3.6.7 Calculation of mean QRS vector (12 mm; +55°)

(ii) +75° to +110° is normal *right axis deviation* (RAD). It represents the vertical position of the heart.

(iii) +30° to +75° represents the oblique position of the heart; position in which heart is placed in the chest in most of the individual.

If the calculated axis falls to the left of –30 or to the right of +110°, then 'abnormal' left or right axis deviation is said to be present.

III. PROCEDURE

(A) Using electrocardiograph

1. Ask the person to lie supine on the bed comfortably.
2. Check that the instrument is satisfactorily earthed.
3. Rub cardiac jelly and then apply firmly the limb leads marked RA, LA, RL and LL to the respective limbs with the help of rubber straps.
4. Adjust the speed of chart paper at 25 mm/sec, and obtain a record of calibration such that 1 mV input gives a 10 mm vertical deflection of the stylus on the chart paper.
5. Adjust the lead selector knob so as to record the activity in lead I, II, III, aV_R, aV_L and aV_F in that order.
6. Apply chest electrodes at the appropriate position on the chest after applying the cardiac jelly; adjust the lead selector knob to chest position and record the activity in chest leads V_1 to V_6 in that order.
7. Label the appropriate strip of the chart paper according to the leads recorded.

Alternatively, in ECG machine with the provision of automatic recording of all 12 leads, adjust the lead selector to **auto** position after placing the electrode at appropriate place on the body and take the recording.

(B) Using student physiograph and ECG coupler (Page 84)

1. Plug in **ECG coupler** in the consol with consol mains off.
2. *Calibrate.* Take the following steps:
   (i) Consol ON, coupler ON.
   (ii) Mode at CAL.
   (iii) Select sensitivity of 1 mV on the main amplifier.
   (iv) Adjust pen to centre and run paper.
   (v) Press 5 secs and release 5 secs CAL button on the coupler three or four times. If the amplitude of calibration is more or less than one cm, make necessary adjustment from the control marked GAIN.
3. Connect from subject to 5-pin junction box through the patient cable and then connect the junction box to the coupler.
4. Run the paper and take the record at different positions of the lead selector (as already described above).

IV. PRECAUTIONS

1. Ensure that the required voltage is available at the mains and the instrument is satisfactorily earthed.
2. The subject should be comfortable and should not wear any magnetic/metallic article which might interfere with the electric signals of low voltage.
3. Ensure all leads are in good/firm contact with the body surface.
4. Must obtain a record of **calibration** before the actual ECG record is taken.
5. Record the activity in 12 leads in a proper sequence: I, II, III, aV_R, aV_L, aV_F and V_1 to V_6 and label the record accordingly.
6. Use right leg for grounding the subject for eliminating 50 Hz interference.

IMPORTANT VIVA-VOCE QUESTIONS

Q.1. *Define: Electrocardiogram (ECG), Electrocardiography and Electrocardiograph.*

Ans. Electrocardiogram (ECG) is the record of electrical activity of the heart tissue; **Electrocardiography** is the procedure of reading ECG with the help of **Electrocardiograph** (ECG machine).

Q.2. *Give the uses of ECG.*

Ans. ECG provides useful information about the following:
(i) Position of heart in the chest, whether horizontal, oblique or vertical
(ii) The relative size of cardiac chambers and cardiac muscle
(iii) Heart rate, rhythm and conduction of cardiac impulse

(iv) Type of conduction block
(v) Origin of new rhythm centres (extra-systole and arrhythmias)
(vi) Site, duration and extent of ischaemic damage to the myocardium
(vii) Effect of electrolyte disturbances and of drugs

Q.3. *Why is it necessary to have a record of 12 leads ECG?*
Ans. Refer to page 166.

Q.4. *What is 50 Hz filter?*
Ans. The 50 Hz filter permits recording even under the conditions of severe main electricity line frequency interference. However, it also reduces the high frequency response of the amplifier. Therefore, it should not be used unless absolutely necessary.

Q.5. *How can ECG free from main line frequency interference be obtained?*
Ans. This can be obtained as follows:
(i) use only a single grounding electrode from the subject
(ii) keep electrodes resistance below 10,000 ohms
(iii) unplug all unnecessary equipment from the main power in the room where the recordings are being made
(iv) keep all AC cords as far away as possible from the subject.

Q.6. *How is indifferent electrode constituted?*
Ans. Page 164.

Q.7. *Why is right leg also connected for recording the ECG?*
Ans. Page 168.

Q.8. *How is heart rate and rhythm determined from the ECG?*
Ans. See below.

Q.9. *How is mean QRS vector determined?*
Ans. Page 167.

Q.10. *Classify the main abnormalities in ECG.*
Ans. Abnormalities in ECG are broadly of three types:
(i) Heart block,
(ii) Origin of new rhythm centres: extra-systoles and arrhythmias,
(iii) ischaemic myocardium disorders: angina pectoris and myocardial infarcts.

Q.11. *Give the clinical significance of P-R interval.*
Ans. Definition (page 165), duration of more than 0.2 sec, indicates delayed conduction in bundle of HIS; duration of less than 0.13 sec, indicates impulse has probably arisen in the AV node.

Q.12. *What is the third degree heart block? What complications may it cause?*
Ans. In this condition, there is complete interruption of the conduction of cardiac impulse between atria and ventricles (**complete heart block**). If it sets in suddenly, then there occurs a delay before ventricles start beating at their own rate. This might lead to **Stoke's Adams Syndrome.**

Q.13. *What is Stoke's Adams Syndrome?*
Ans. In the third degree heart block, ventricle standstill lasts for a few seconds. The systemic blood pressure falls to a very low level and blood supply to brain becomes inadequate, resulting in dizziness and fainting. This is called Stoke's Adams syndrome.

Q.14. *Give the clinical significance of J-point.*
Ans. J-point is a point of no electrical activity. Its elevation, as small as 1 mm from its original position, is suggestive of ischaemia to the myocardium.

Q.15. *Name the conditions in which cardiac axis becomes abnormal.*
Ans. (i) Abnormal right axis deviation is seen in: right bundle branch block, right ventricular hypertrophy and posterior (or inferior) myocardial infarction (MI).
(ii) Abnormal left axis deviation is associated with: left bundle branch block, left ventricular hypertrophy and antero-lateral MI.

STUDY NOTES

ANALYSIS AND INTERPRETATION OF ECG

1. Determine the ventricular rate and rhythm. How?
   (i) *Ventricular rate or heart rate per minute* = 1500/distance between two consecutive R-R waves in mm.
   (ii) *Ventricular rhythm:* count the number of mm squares between two consecutive R-R waves in different leads; see whether it is similar or not.
2. Similarly, determine the *atrial rate and rhythm* by finding the distance between two consecutive P-P waves.

3. Analyse for the following:

		Form	Duration	Amplitude	Remarks
	(i) P-wave				
	(ii) QRS complex				
	(iii) T-wave				
	(iv) PR interval				
	(v) QT interval				
	(vi) ST interval				
	(vii) ST segment				
	(viii) TP segment				

4. Calculate the mean electrical axis of QRS complex and give ***comments*** for your findings.

....

....

....

....

....

....

....

....

....

....

....

Date: ....

7 *Stethography:* Study of Respiratory Movements

I. APPARATUS

Stethograph, Marey's tambour, stop watch, stand, kymograph, drum and time marker

Stethograph

It is an instrument for recording the chest wall movements occurring during respiration. The process of recording the respiratory movements is known as ***Stethography.*** It consists of: (Fig. 3.7.1)

1. **A corrugated rubber tube** (60 cm long, 2 cm diameter), one end of which is blind and the other end is connected through a **pressure rubber tubing** to *Marey's tambour.* A hook and metallic chain arrangement enables the stethograph to be tied around the chest wall.
2. **Marey's tambour**. It is provided with a metallic cup or a flat saucer shaped connection with its top covered with a *latex* or *rubber diaphragm.* To the bottom is fixed a metal tube which is connected with the stethograph through a pressure rubber tubing. The pressure variations occurring within the corrugated rubber tube are thus transmitted faithfully onto the rubber diaphragm. A **pointer** sits on the rubber diaphragm to record its movements on the kymograph.
3. ***Working of a stethograph.*** Because of the corrugation of the rubber tube, there is little or no change in the mean radius of the tube during stretching. So with expansion of chest wall during inspiration, the tube stretches and its length increases; since mean radius remaining constant, any increase in volume of air inside the tube is associated with a fall of pressure. The diaphragm of the Marey's tambour thus gets depressed and its lever records a down stroke with each inspiration. The opposite sequence occurs during the expiratory phase, which is then recorded as an upstroke.

II. PROCEDURE

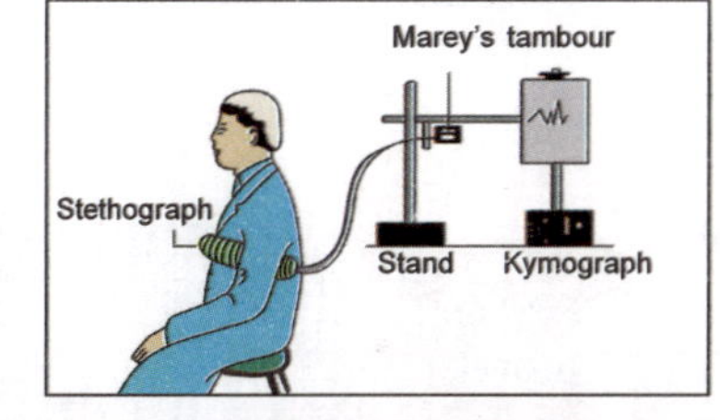

1. The subject sits quietly and comfortably on a stool with his back towards the recording apparatus and the stethograph tied across the chest at the level of nipples (*i.e.* 4th intercostal space).
2. The corrugated tube is left partially stretched so that the respiratory movements may produce pressure changes in it.

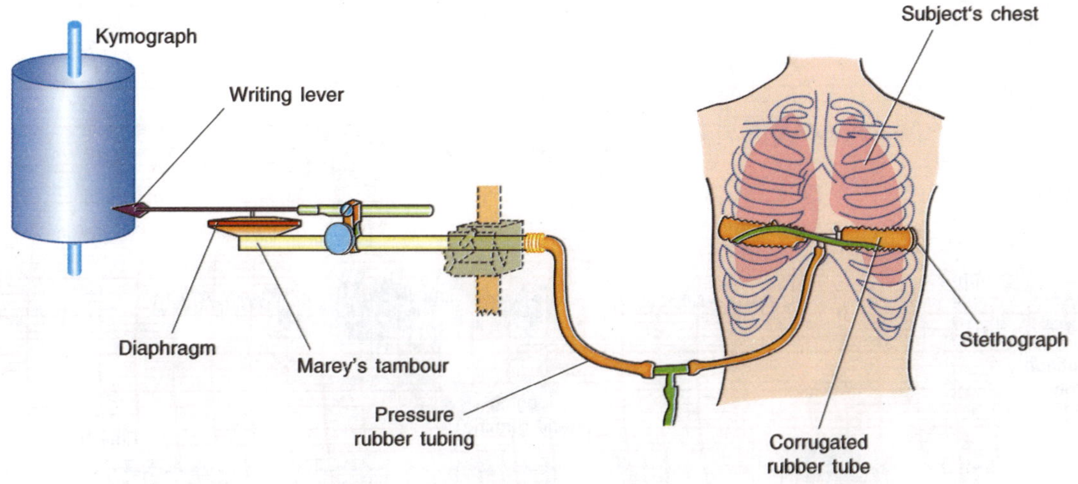

Fig. 3.7.1 A stethograph

3. The connecting pressure tube is joined to the Marey's tambour, which is then mounted along with a time marker on the same stand. The two levers are brought in the same vertical line and made to touch the kymograph drum.
4. ***Normal respiration***. The drum is set to move at a slow speed (2.5 mm/sec); record the normal respiratory movements and note:
   (i) the rate of respiration,
   (ii) the relative duration of inspiration and expiration, and
   (iii) presence or absence of pause between inspiration and expiration, or between expiration and inspiration.
5. ***Effect of swallowing*** (Fig. 3.7.2)
   (i) Ask the subject to take a mouthful of water and hold it in his mouth without swallowing. Make a record of the normal respiration and then direct him to **swallow** the water once during expiration and a second time during inspiration; mark on the drum simultaneously. Note the inhibitory effect of deglutition on respiration.
   (ii) Ask the subject to drink water (about 250 ml) from a glass in a continuous swallowing movement, and note its effect on the respiratory movements.
6. ***Effect of voluntary hyperventilation***. Record normal respiration. Stop the drum, instruct the subject to breathe in and out as deeply and as rapidly as possible for 1-2 minutes. Switch on the drum and stop hyperventilation, and pay no further attention to breathing. Record the respiratory movements till it comes back to normal (Fig. 3.7.2).
7. ***Effect of Exercise***. Record normal respiration. Stop the drum and ask the subject to exercise (jogging on the same spot) for 2 minutes. Connect the stethograph to the kymograph and record respiratory movements.
8. ***Study of breath holding time*** (Fig. 3.7.2)

   A. Effect after inspiration and expiration

   The subject sits quietly for a few minutes breathing normally. Instruct him to hold his breath as long as possible in the following positions:
   (i) at the end of quiet expiration
   (ii) at the end of maximum expiration
   (iii) at the end of quiet inspiration
   (iv) at the end of maximum inspiration

Note: Between each breath holding, the subject should wait for 3-5 minutes.

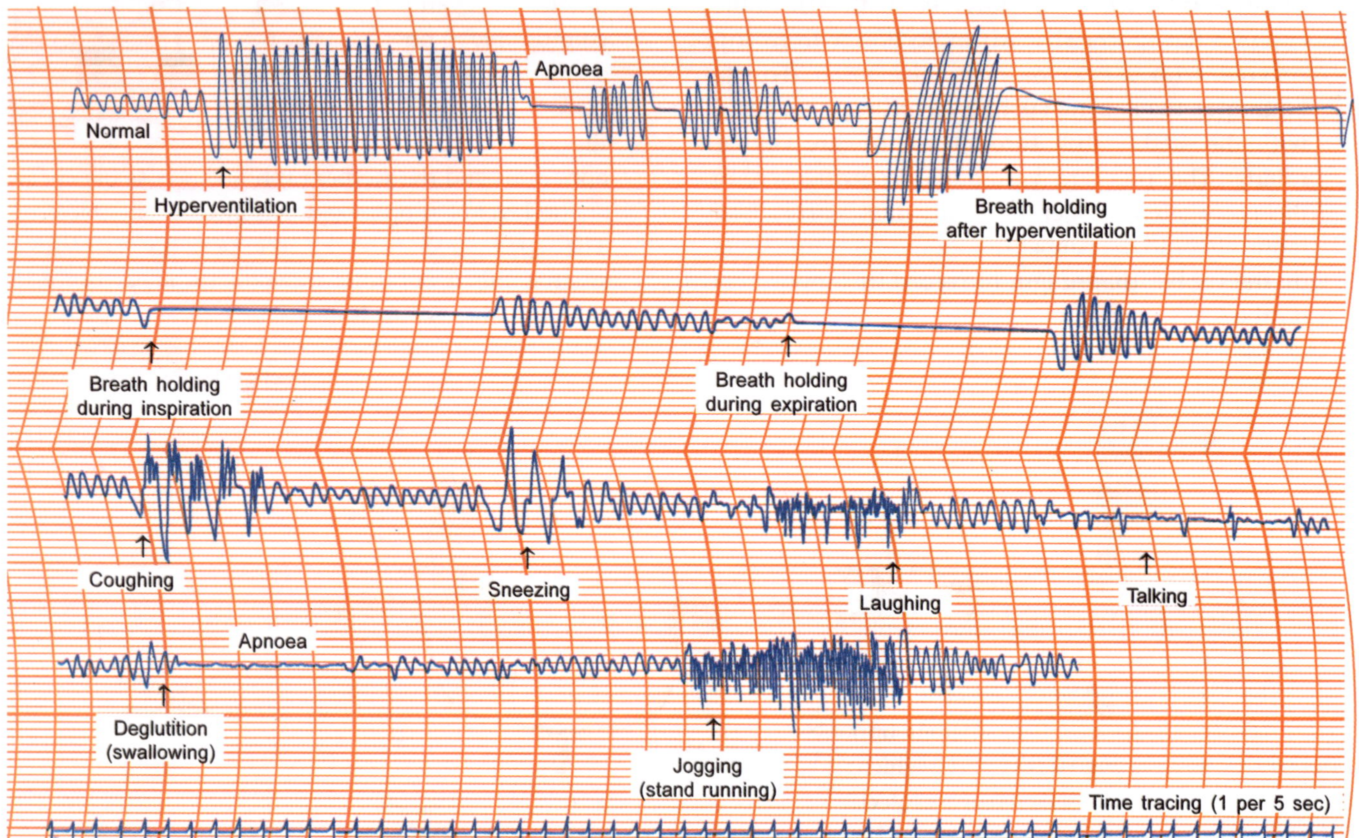

Fig. 3.7.2 Stethographic recording during various manoeuvres

B. Effect after voluntary hyperventilation

Record normal respiration, stop the drum; ask the subject to hyperventilate for 30-45 seconds, start the drum and record the last 2-3 of the deep breaths, and then ask the subject to hold his breath. Compare this breath holding time with 8A above.

C. Effect after exercise

Record normal respiratory movements; stop the drum and with stethograph on his chest the subject exercises by jogging on the same spot for 2 minutes. Start the drum and then ask the subject to hold his breath. Note the effect.

9. ***Effect of sneezing, coughing, laughing, talking*** (Fig. 3.7.2)

The subject sits quietly for a few minutes breathing normally, and then the effect of the following manoeuvres is recorded on the respiratory movements:

(i) sneezing
(ii) coughing
(iii) laughing, and
(iv) talking.

Important Note: To observe the effect of various factors on the respiratory movements, the stethographic recording is started about 5-6 breaths before and stopped only when the rate and depth have returned to the resting level.

III. PRECAUTIONS

1. Do not let the subject see the recording.
2. Do not allow the subject to hyperventilate voluntarily beyond 2 minutes.
3. The stethograph tied across the chest should neither be too tight nor too loose.
4. Do not forget to record 4-5 normal breaths before the effect of any parameter is observed; stop only when the recordings have come back to resting level.

OSPE

Aim: To record the respiratory movements of the subject provided.

Procedure steps: Refer to page 171.

Checklist

1. Checks for the appartus. **(Yes/No)**
2. Makes the subject sit quietly and comfortably on a stool with his back towards the recording apparatus. **(Yes/No)**
3. Ties the stethograph firmly (neither too loose nor too tight) across the chest at the level of nipples. **(Yes/No)**
4. Explains the procedure to the subject and gives proper instructions. **(Yes/No)**
5. Sets the kymograph to move at a slow speed (2.5 mm/sec) and records the normal respiratory movements. **(Yes/No)**
6. Takes the time tracing using the signal marker. **(Yes/No)**

Important note: Stethographic recording during various manoeuvres such as hyperventilation, breath holding, coughing, sneezing, talking, swallowing or jogging may be asked as a separate OSPE. Do not forget to record 4-5 normal breaths before the effect of any parameter is observed after giving proper instructions to the subject.

IMPORTANT VIVA-VOCE QUESTIONS

Q.1. *What is the working principle of a stethograph?*

Ans. Page 171.

Q.2. *Why should a stethograph be tried at the level of nipples?*

Ans. At this level respiratory movements are maximum.

Q.3. *Why is corrugated tube partially stretched and tied across the chest?*

Ans. Page 171.

Q.4. *What is deglutition apnoea? Give its physiological significance.*

Ans. During a swallowing movement, respiration gets inhibited in whatever stage of the cycle the swallowing was initiated. This is called deglutition apnoea. The afferent impulses travel in glossopharyngeal (IX) nerve which inhibits the respiratory centre. The reflex is protective in nature and prevents the aspiration of food particles into the respiratory passage.

Q.5. *Why is the subject not allowed to see the recordings?*

Ans. If the subject sees the recording, he will become self-conscious and respiratory movements get altered; the actual effect thus fails to occur.

Q.6. *Give the normal duration of breath holding time in a healthy person.*

Ans. 45-55 secs.

Q.7. *Define* **breaking point** *and give its causes.*

Ans. The point at which breathing can no longer be voluntarily inhibited is called the breaking point. It is due to:

(i) increased arterial pCO_2; and
(ii) decreased arterial pO_2.

Q.8. *How can breath holding time be prolonged?*

Ans. Breath holding time can be increased:

(i) If 100% oxygen is breathed prior to breath holding; this increases the alveolar pO_2. In this way, the time can be increased by 15-20 secs.

(ii) If prior to breath holding, the person hyperventilates the room air for approx. 1 minute, therefore CO_2 is washed off and arterial pCO_2 falls. The breath holding can be increased by 1 minute.

(iii) After removal of carotid bodies

(iv) Psychological factors. For example, subjects can hold their breath longer when they are told their performance is very good although it may not be so.

Q.9. *Describe the effect of voluntary hyperventilation on the respiration.*

Ans. Hyperventilation increases the alveolar pO_2 and decreases the pCO_2; any fall in alveolar pCO_2 inhibit the respiration to a point till normal CO_2 levels are built up again. Therefore, voluntary hyperventilation for about 2 minute produces **apnoea** followed by the restoration of respiration, this cycle keeps on repeating but with a decreasing duration of apnoea until the normal respiration is restored.

Q.10. *How can high alveolar pO_2 be achieved with maximum voluntary efforts? Explain.*

Ans. Alveolar pO_2 can increase to a maximum of 140 mmHg only (normal 100 mmHg). As total atmospheric pressure of 760 mmHg, 620 mmHg (573 by pN_2 and 47 by pH_2O) remains constant, now by hyperventilation, even if whole CO_2 gets removed, O_2 will contribute only 140 mmHg pressure.

Q.11. *What are the consequences of prolonged hyperventilation?*

Ans. Refer to Q.9.

Q.12. *Define: periodic breathing, Cheyne-Stokes breathing and Biot's breathing.*

Ans. Repeated sequence of apnoea followed by respiration is called **periodic breathing**. If the onset of this breathing is gradual, it is called Cheyne-Stokes breathing (see **Ans.** 9); if onset is abrupt (sudden), it is referred to as Biot's breathing.

Q.13. *Describe the effect of following manoeuvres on the respiration: coughing, sneezing and talking.*

Ans. (i) Both coughing and sneezing begin with a deep inspiration followed by forceful expiration; however, in sneezing expiration is a continuous process.

(ii) Effect of talking. In the expiratory phase, there is a staircase pattern because all syllables are formed in this phase.

Q.14. *Differentiate between maximum voluntary ventilation and hyperventilation due to exercise.*

Ans. Effect of maximum voluntary ventilation, (MVV), refer to Q.No.9. During exercise, pulmonary ventilation increases in parallel with increase in oxygen consumption but during maximum exercise it is always of a lesser extent than MVV. This shows that respiration is not the main limiting factor in muscular exercise.

STUDY NOTES

RESULTS AND DISCUSSION

Express your results as follows:

1. Normal respiration:

   (i) rate of respiration ....

   (ii) duration of inspiration ....

   (iii) duration of expiration ....

2. Effect of swallowing

   ....

   ....

3. Effect of voluntary hyperventilation. (Analyse the record and explain the effects obtained.)

   ....

   ....

4. Effect of exercise

....

....

5. Effect of breath holding time (calculate for different manoeuvres and explain the differences).

....

....

....

....

6. Effect of:
   (i) sneezing

   ....

   ....

   (ii) coughing

   ....

   ....

   (iii) laughing

   ....

   ....

   (iv) talking

   ....

   ....

COMMENTS

....

....

....

....

....

....

....

....

Date: ....

8 *Vitalography:* Effect of Posture on the Vital Capacity

I. APPARATUS

Subject, vitalograph, nose clip, mouth piece

Vitalograph

It is the instrument used to measure the vital capacity (VC). The procedure of recording the VC is called **Vitalography**.

1. Vitalograph is a double-walled metallic cylindrical chamber containing water between the two cylinders. The cavity of the inner cylinder at its lower end is connected with the help of one-way breathing valve to a corrugated rubber tubing to which a mouth piece is attached (Fig. 3.8.1).
2. An inverted cylinder, called of **Bell** of light weight material (aluminium), floats on the water and surrounds the inner cylinder completely. The tip of the Bell carries a **hook** to which is attached a **chain** which passes over a frictionless pulley. The other end of the chain carries a **weight** which counter-balances the bell.
3. As the volume of air in the **bell** increases, it moves up and its displacement movement can be recorded with the help of a **pointer** pivoted to the overhead pulley.
4. The **pointer** is held in place with a guard so that when the pulley rotates, the pointer sweeps over the circular scale on the pulley through an arc proportional to the rise of the bell. The graduation on the pulley directly gives the volume of air collected under the bell.

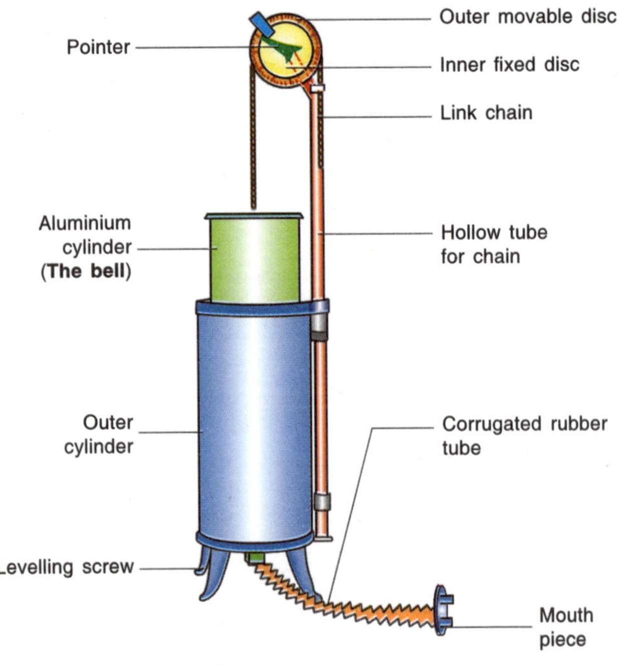

Fig. 3.8.1 A vitalograph

II. THEORY

1. ***Vital Capacity (VC)***. It is the maximal volume of air which can be expelled from lungs by forceful effort following a maximal inspiration *(one stage VC)*.
   Two stage VC. VC measured in two stages:
   Stage 1: The subject is asked to breathe in maximally after a normal expiration; then he takes a few normal breaths.
   Stage 2: The subject is asked to breathe out maximally after a normal expiration.
   The sum of stage 1 and 2 volumes gives the **two-stage VC**. It is slightly larger than **one-stage VC**.
   Normal: 4.8 litres in males and 3.2 litres in females
   It can be computed as: TV + IRV + ERV (page 180).
2. *Advantages of VC*
   (i) It provides useful information about the strength of the respiratory muscles; therefore, maximum inspiratory and expiratory effort can be assessed.
   (ii) It gives the useful information about other aspects of pulmonary function through FEV_1 (page 181).
3. *Factors Affecting VC*
   Physiological
   (i) Physical dimension, *i.e.* size and development of the subject
   VC in males is 2.6 L/m^2 BSA; and in females, 2.1 L/m^2 BSA

VC is more in males because of (a) large chest size, (b) more muscle power and (c) more BSA (body surface area).

(ii) Age: VC decreases in old age due to the loss of the elasticity of lungs. (With aging, elastic fibres get replaced by fibrous tissue).

(iii) Strength of respiratory muscles: VC increases in swimmers and divers.

(iv) **Posture**: in standing position VC is more as compared to sitting or lying positions, because in standing position, (a) decrease in venous return, decreases the pulmonary blood flow and (b) diaphragm descends down, thus increasing inspiration.

(v) Pregnancy: VC decreases.

Pathological

(i) VC decreases in the diseases of the respiratory system. For example: poliomyelitis, pulmonary fibrosis, respiratory obstruction, emphysema, pleural effusion, pulmonary oedema, pneumothorax, etc.

(ii) Ascites, *i.e.* accumulation of fluid in the abdominal cavity; it causes VC to decrease.

III. PROCEDURE

1. The space between the outer and inner cylinder is filled 3/4th with water.
2. Set the pointer over the circular scale to zero. How?
   Let the inverted **bell** dip completely into the water; apply pressure from above so that the top of the bell may come to lie at the top of the double walled cylinder. Now the pointer is set to 'zero' manually.
3. The subject is made to stand facing the vitalograph; insert a mouth piece between the teeth and the lips.
4. Ask the subject to take a deep (maximal) inspiration through the nostrils and hold the breath.
5. Clip his nostrils either with a nose clip or with fingers (to prevent leakage of air) and instruct him to exhale completely and forcefully into the mouth piece.
6. Note that the vitalograph bell is raised and the pointer moves; take the reading on the scale attached to the pulley.
7. After a pause of 1-2 minutes, set the apparatus and take second reading.
8. Repeat the whole procedure for the third time also; make a note of maximum value of the three readings to get the best result.
9. After a rest period of 2-3 minutes, repeat the whole procedure; take the three readings, each in sitting and lying (supine) posture respectively.

OSPE

Aim: To record the vital capacity of the subject with the help of vitalograph.

Procedure steps: Refer to page 176.

Checklist

1. Checks for the leak in the apparatus. **(Yes/No)**
2. Sets the pointer over the circular scale to zero. **(Yes/No)**
3. Asks the subject to stand facing the vitalograph with mouthpiece inserted between the teeth. **(Yes/No)**
4. Asks the subject to take a deep inspiration through the nostrils and holds the breath. **(Yes/No)**
5. Clips the subject's nose and instructs him to exhale completely and forcefully into the mouthpiece. **(Yes/No)**
6. Takes reading on the scale attached to the pulley. **(Yes/No)**

Note: The effect of posture on the vital capacity may be asked as a separate OSPE.

IMPORTANT VIVA-VOCE QUESTIONS

Q.1. *What is the principle of the working of a vitalograph?*

Ans. Page 176.

Q.2. *How will you check for the leak in the system?*

Ans. Let the vitalograph bell float on the water; apply pressure from above while the corrugated rubber tubing is obstructed to prevent escape of any air. If there is a leak in the system, the bell will begin to move down.

Q.3. *Why is it necessary in order to obtain the best results, maximum of three readings should be considered?*

Ans. The vitalography procedure is effort-dependent. Moreover, the subject will breathe with his nostrils clipped for the first time through a closed system.

Q.4. *Give the normal values of vital capacity in an adult male and a female.*

Ans. Page 176.

Q.5. *What is the effect of the change in posture on vital capacity? Explain.*

Ans. See above.

Q.6. *Enumerate the factors influencing the vital capacity.*

Ans. Page 176.

Q.7. *What is two-stage vital capacity?*

Ans. Page 176.

Q.8. *Enumerate the precautions that must be taken for this experiment.*

Ans. (i) Ensure there should be no leak in the system.

(ii) Set the 'zero' of circular scale accurately before starting the procedure.

(iii) Spirometer should be filled properly with water.

(iv) Follow the instructions properly.

(v) To obtain the best results, maximum of three readings should be considered.

STUDY NOTES

RESULTS

Tabulate your results for vital capacity (in mL) as follows:

Position	First reading	Second reading	Third reading	Maximum of three readings
1. In standing position				
2. In sitting position				
3. In lying position				

COMMENTS AND DISCUSSION

....

....

....

....

....

....

....

....

....

....

....

....

....

....

Date: ....

9 *Spirometry:* Determination of Lung Volumes and Capacities

I. APPARATUS

Spirometer, mouthpiece, nose clip, Wright's peak flow meter

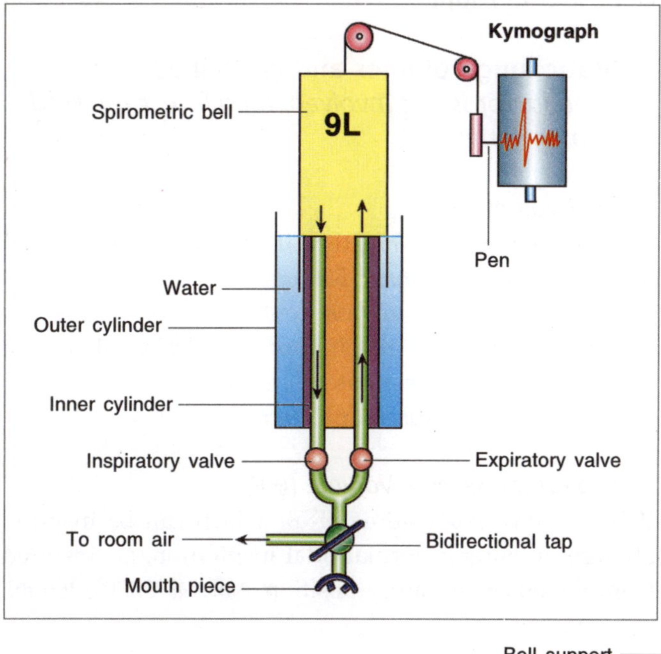

Spirometer

It is an instrument used routinely in physiological and clinical studies for the determination of lung volumes and capacities. It consists of: (Fig. 3.9.1)

1. A **double-walled cylindrical chamber** containing water between the two cylinders, water to maintain an airtight seal.
2. **A Bell**. It is cylinder of 9 litres capacity made of light weight metal which dips into this water from above. The top of the **bell** carries a **hook** to which a chain is attached. The chain passes over a frictionless pulley and carries a counter weight and a pen. This pen moves up and down as the volume of air in the bell decreases or increases, thus the

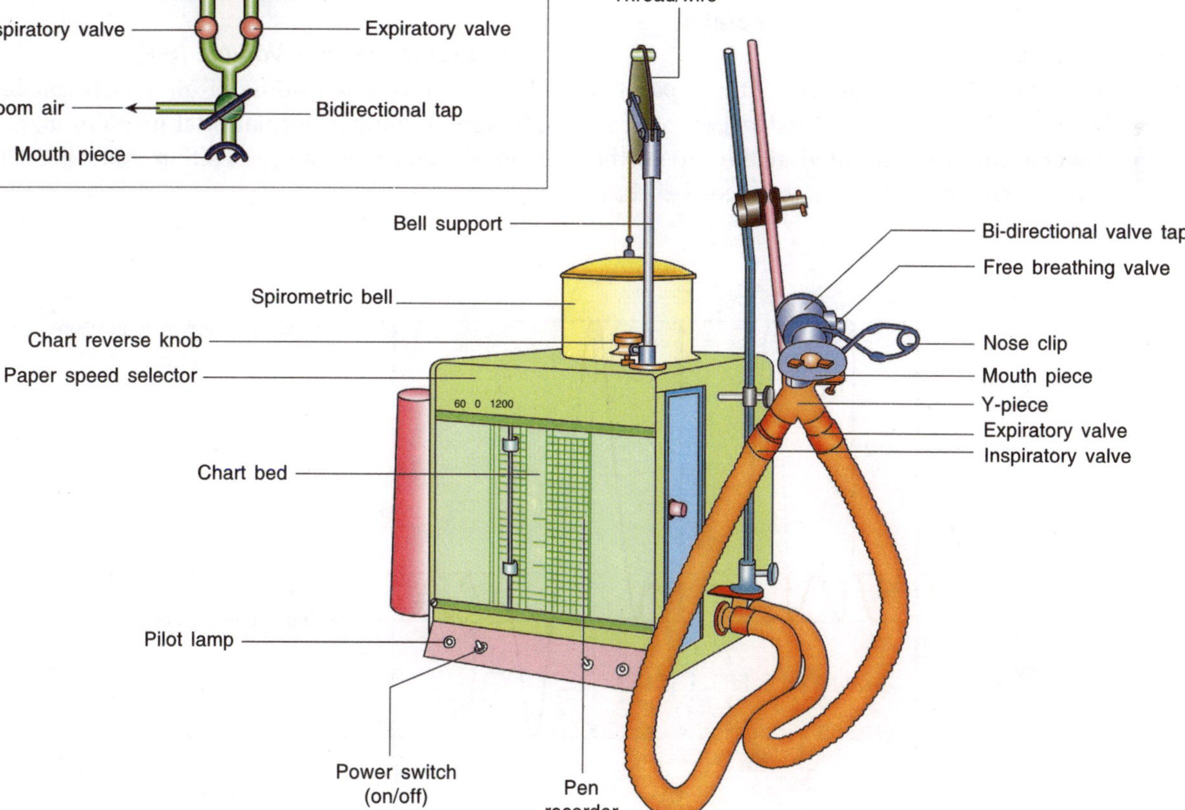

Fig. 3.9.1 A spirometer: components and controls; **Inset** shows its working

bell displacements are recorded on the kymograph. (Fig. 3.9.1-inset)

3. **The kymograph**. It carries a mm square graph paper which is calibrated for time as well as for volume. The speed of the kymograph drum can be selected with the help of **selector lever** that has marking of 60-0-1200.
   (i) 60 mm/min for normal spirometric recordings,
   (ii) 1200 mm/min for recording of timed vital capacity, and
   (iii) 'zero' mark is neutral position, in which kymograph does not move.
4. **Pilot lamp with power switch**. It glows when the power switch is put in the 'On' position.
5. **Breathing assembly,** *i.e.* breathing valves with mouth piece:
   (i) There are two **unidirectional breathing valves,** one for inspiration and the other for expiration. These are connected with the help of Y-shaped piece to a free-breathing valve.
   (ii) **Free breathing valve** is 25 mm bore metallic tube having **bidirectional tap** which can be turned to allow the subject either to breathe room air or spirometric air
6. **Soda lime absorber** to remove CO_2 from the expired air
7. **Inlet** for filling O_2 or any other gas into the bell
8. **Tap** to drain the water from the apparatus
9. **Levelling screws**
10. **Slot** - present on the right side door of the apparatus provides an outlet for the recorded paper.
11. **Chart reverse knob** is provided at the top of the cabinet; by turning it clock-wise, the recorded chart is wound up again.
12. **Chart paper**: Calibration
    (i) Y-axis represents volume:
    1 mm = 30 ml.
    (ii) X-axis represents time
    (a) at drum speed: 60 mm/min;
    1 mm = 1 sec.
    (b) at drum speed: 1200 mm/min; 20 mm = 1 sec.

II. THEORY

A convenient way of measuring the lung volumes and capacities is by using a **spirometer**, and the procedure of recording these is called ***spirometry***. The various lung volumes and capacities are shown on a spirogram (Fig. 3.9.2) and can be divided into two broad headings: **static** and **dynamic**.

A. Static lung volumes and capacities

Time factor is not involved, therefore, expressed in ml or litres

Volumes

1. Tidal Volume (TV)

It is the volume of air breathed in or out of lungs, during quiet respiration. *Normal: 500 ml.*

(i) Decreases due to less contraction of respiratory muscles; *causes:* respiratory muscles weakness or depression of respiratory centre.
(ii) Increases in muscular exercise.

2. Inspiratory Reserve Volume (IRV)

It is the maximal volume of air which can be inspired after completing a normal tidal inspiration, *i.e.* inspired from the end-inspiratory position. *Normal: 2000-3200 ml.*

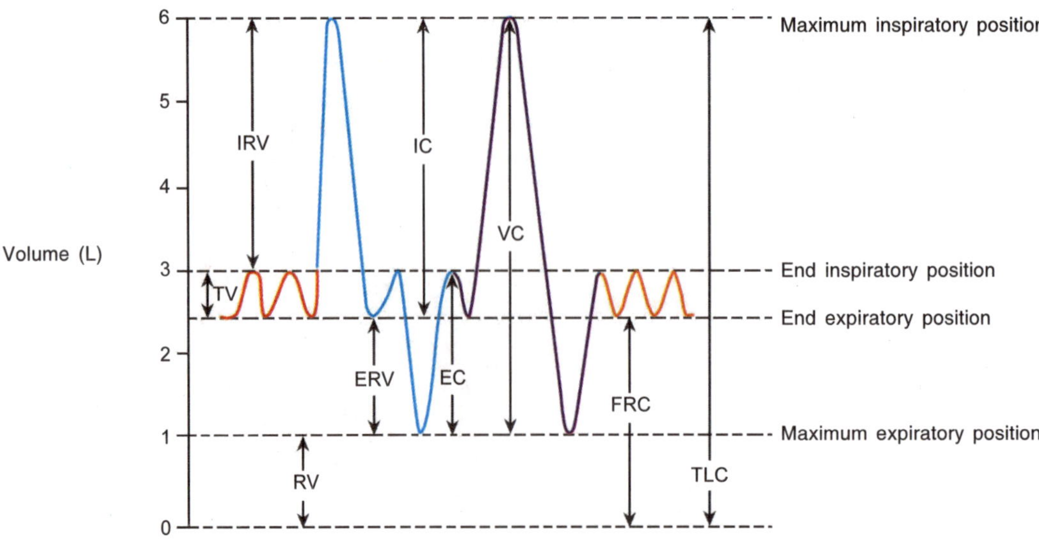

Fig. 3.9.2 A spirogram showing various lung volumes and capacities (Abbreviations as given in text)

3. Expiratory Reserve Volume (ERV)

It is the maximal volume of air which can be expired after a normal tidal expiration, *i.e.* expired from the end-expiratory position. *Normal: 750-1000 ml.*

4. Residual Volume (RV)

It is the volume of air which remains in lungs after a maximal expiration. *Normal: 1200 ml.*

5. Closing Volume (CV)

It is the lung volume above residual volume at which airways in the lower, dependent parts of the lungs begin to close off because of the lesser transmural pressure in these areas.

Capacities

1. Inspiratory Capacity (IC)

It is the maximal volume of air which can be inspired after completing tidal expiration, *i.e.* from the end-expiratory position. It can be computed as: TV + IRV.

Normal: 2500-3700 ml.

2. Vital Capacity (VC)

Refer to page 176.

3. Functional Residual Capacity (FRC)

It is the volume of air which is contained in the lungs at end-expiratory position, *i.e.* after the completion of tidal expiration. It can be computed as: RV + ERV.

Normal: 2.5 litres.

4. Total Lung Capacity (TLC)

It is the volume of air contained in the lungs after a maximal inspiration. It can be computed as: VC + RV. *Normal: 6 litres.*

> **Important Note:** With the exception of functional residual capacity, total lung capacity and residual volume, all other lung volumes and capacities can be measured with the help of a simple spirometer.

B. Dynamic Lung Volumes and Capacities

Time dependent, therefore, expressed in ml/min or L/min

1. Timed Vital Capacity (TVC) or Forced Vital Capacity (FVC)

If VC is recorded on a kymograph (spirograph) at the known speed, the volume of air expelled can be timed. Thus, FVC is the maximum volume of air which can be breathed out as 'forcefully' and 'rapidly' as possible following a maximum inspiration. Thus TVC is exactly similar to VC except that there is a special stress on *rapid, forcible and complete exhalation.*

Components of TVC (FVC):

(i) FEV_1 (Forced Expiratory Volume in 1 sec), *i.e.* volume of FVC expired in the first sec of exhalation. *Normal: 80% of FVC.*

(ii) FEV_2 (Forced Expiratory Volume in 2 sec), *i.e.* volume of FVC expired in the first two secs of exhalation. *Normal: 95% of FVC.*

(iii) FEV_3 (Forced Expiratory Volume in 3 sec), *i.e.* volume of FVC expired in the first three secs of exhalation. *Normal: 98-100% of FVC.*

Clinical Significance of TVC (FVC): To distinguish between 'restrictive' and 'obstructive' lung disorders (page 185).

2. Forced Expiratory Flow during 25-75% of Expiration ($FEF_{25-75\%}$)

This is the mean expiratory flow rate during middle 50% of FVC. Some workers call it erroneously as 'Maximum Mid Expiratory Flow Rate' (MMEFR). *Normal: 300 L/min.* It is a sensitive indicator of small airway disease where most of chronic obstructive pulmonary diseases (like bronchial asthma, emphysema) start.

The time taken for $FEF_{25-75\%}$ is called *'Mid Expiratory Time' (MET). Normal: MET 0.5 sec*; increases in obstructive lung disorders.

3. Minute Ventilation (MV) or Pulmonary Ventilation (PV)

This is the volume of air expired or inspired out of the lungs in one minute. Therefore,

$$PV = TV \times RR \text{ per min}$$
$$= 500 \times 12$$
$$= 6\text{L/min, normally.}$$

4. Maximum Breathing Capacity (MBC) or Maximum Voluntary Ventilation or Maximum Ventilation Volume (MVV)

It is the largest volume of air that can be moved into and out of the lungs in one minute by maximum voluntary effort. *Normal: 90-170 L/min* (average 100 L/min).

5. Pulmonary Reserve (PR) or Breathing Reserve (BR)

That is, maximum amount of the air above the pulmonary ventilation, which can be breathed in and out of lungs in one minute.

It can be computed as: MVV − PV.

It is usually expressed as percentage of MVV, *i.e.* (MVV − PV) × 100/MVV; and called as percentage pulmonary reserve or ***Dyspnoeic Index (DI)***.

Normal % PR (DI) ≥ 60-70% (usually 90%).

If <60%, Dyspnoea is usually present.

III. PROCEDURE

1. Fill the space between the two cylindrical chambers 3/4th with water; put the inverted **bell** from above so as to dip into this water.
2. With the free breathing valve open move the bell manually 3 to 4 times up and down to wash it with the fresh room air; finally fill it with room air.
3. The subject is made to sit comfortably in a stool facing the spirometer, nose is clipped and the mouthpiece is inserted between the teeth and the lips. Allow him to breathe in the room air; this is done to make him familiar to breathe through the mouthpiece with the nose clipped.

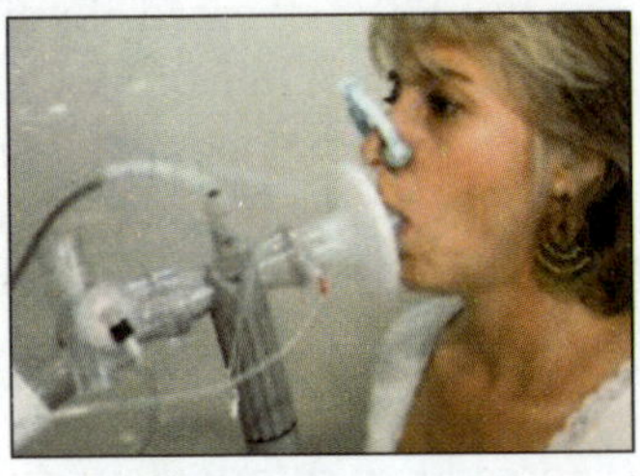

4. After a gap of one minute, the free breathing valve is turned to connect the subject to spirometer; immediately start the kymograph at a speed of 60 mm/min and record normal breathing for about one minute. This is used for computing the tidal volume, respiratory rate and the resting pulmonary ventilation.
5. The subject is then instructed to breathe in with maximum effort from the end of resting expiration and subsequently to breathe out completely with maximum effort. He is beforehand instructed not to breathe in while he is breathing out. At least three such forced vital capacity (FVC) curves are obtained and the maximum (best performance) of the three values is taken for calculation purposes.
6. Change the speed of kymograph to 1200mm/min and repeat the whole procedure (step 5) but with the specific instructions to the subject to breathe out completely as rapidly and forcibly as he can. Repeat this thrice and evaluate the best record for calculating out the timed vital capacity and its component.
7. Bring the speed of kymograph to 60 mm/min, the subject is now instructed to breathe in and out as rapidly and deeply as he can for a period of 15 seconds. The pulmonary ventilation (tidal volume × respiratory rate) thus calculated from the record, is called the maximum breathing capacity (MBC) or maximum voluntary ventilation (MVV).
8. ***Peak expiratory flow rate (PEFR).*** It is the maximum velocity (litres/minute) with which air is forced out of the lungs in a single forced expiratory effort. *Normal: 350-400 L/min.*

Note: It is used to assess large central airway obstruction.

Procedure

(i) The subject stands or sits upright on a chair or in bed.

(ii) The subject takes as deep a breath as he can and then places the mouthpiece in his mouth, gripping it lightly with his teeth and sealing it with his lips. He then blows out as hard as possible in a short sharp blast.

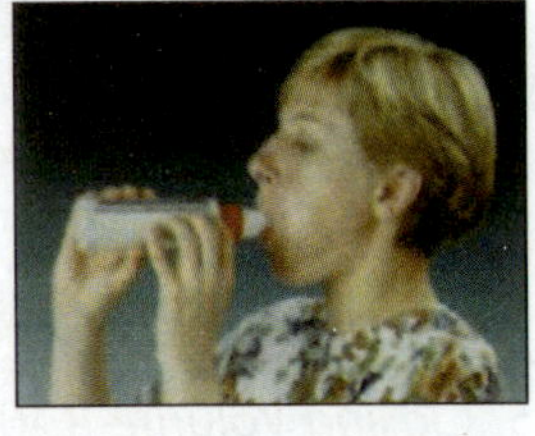

(iii) During the test, the subject should be carefully watched to ensure that no leaks occur between the mouthpiece and his lips.

(iv) PEFR can be read directly from the dial of the **Wright's peak flow meter** (Fig. 3.9.3).

(v) Take three readings after an adequate period of rest between each attempt. Note the maximal value.

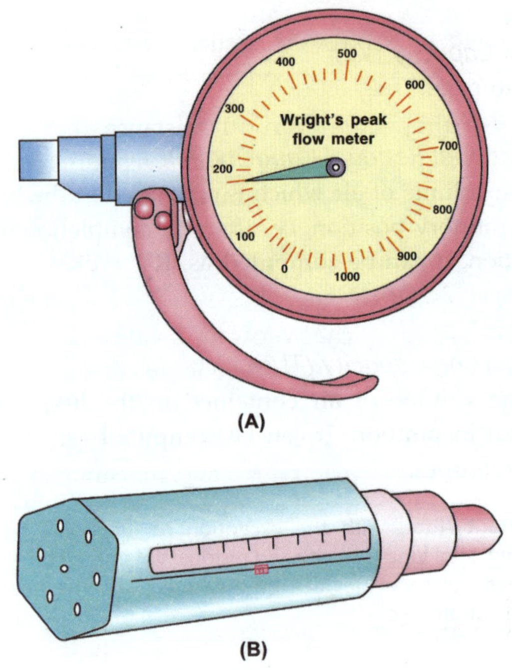

Fig. 3.9.3 (A) Wright's peak flow meter and (B) Mini Wright peak flow meter

IV. CALCULATIONS

(A) Static lung volume and capacities

These are computed from the forced vital capacity (FVC) spirogram recorded at 60 mm/min speed.

1. **TV.** Place a ruler across the record to cut maximum number of expiratory tops (expiration being more stable); draw another line parallel to the first to cut the maximum number of inspiratory tops (Fig. 3.9.4).

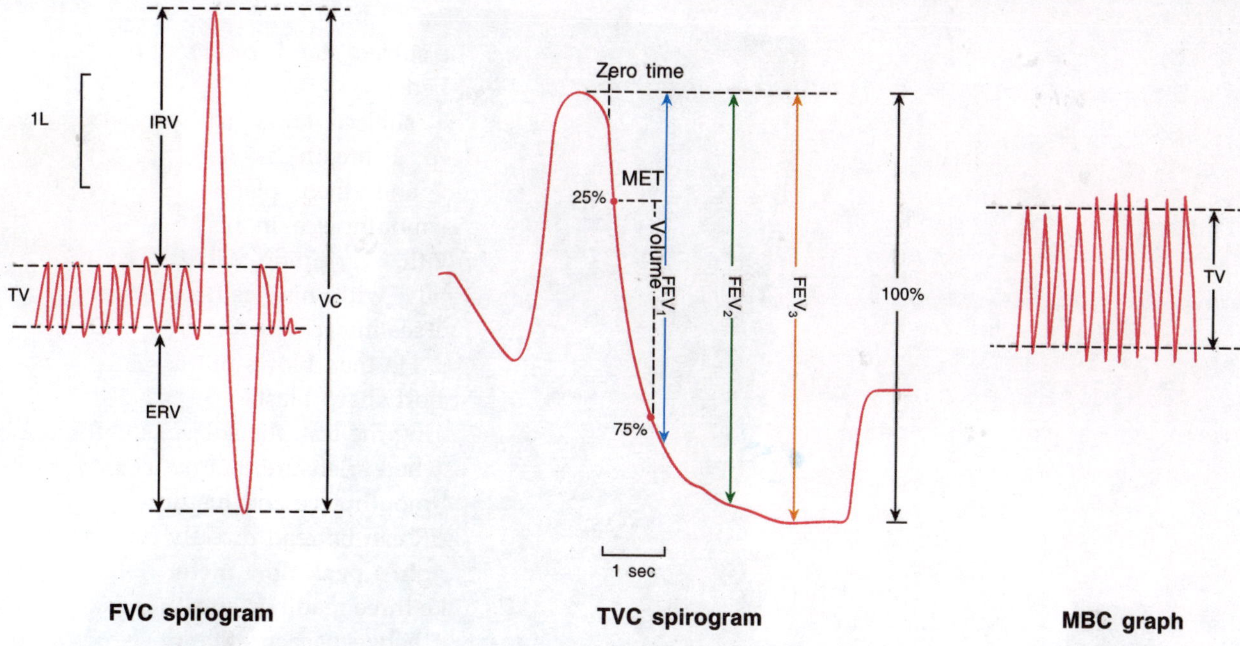

Fig. 3.9.4 Calculation of lung volume and capacities (Abbreviations as given in text)

The TV (ml) = the vertical distance between two lines (mm) × 30

2. **IRV** (ml) = the vertical distance between End inspiratory and maximum inspiratory positions (mm) × 30.

Note: 1 mm along the y-axis = 30 ml, page 180.

3. **ERV** (ml) = The vertical distance between End expiratory and maximum expiratory positions (mm) × 30
4. **VC** (ml) = the vertical distance between maximum inspiratory and maximum expiratory positions (mm) × 30 = TV + IRV + ERV.
5. **IC** (ml) = TV + IRV

(B) Dynamic lung volume and capacities

1. **TVC** (FEV_1, FEV_2, FEV_3). These are computed from TVC spirogram recorded at 1200 mm/min speed. Mark 'zero' point (or time) (*i.e.* point where inspiration ends and expiration begins), move 20 mm (= 1 sec) right to the point marked; drop a perpendicular line from the second point onto the expiratory tracing. This will give the volume of air expired in the first second of exhalation (FEV_1) (Fig. 3.9.4). Express it either as absolute volume in ml or as the percentage of FVC. Similarly, determine FEV_2 and FEV_3 by moving 40 mm and 60 mm respectively to the right of 'zero' time.
2. **$FEF_{25-75\%}$**. Divide expiratory tracing on TVC spirogram into 4 equal parts; draw two perpendicular lines, one vertical from 75% mark and the other horizontal from 25% mark. The vertical and horizontal distances from the point of intersection denote the volume of air expired and time (MET) respectively. The flow rate thus can be computed.
3. **Minute Ventilation (MV)**. Count either the number of inspiratory or expiratory tops over a period of 15 seconds from FVC spirogram (let it be N), then MV (ml/min) = N × 4 × TV.
4. **MBC**. Calculate it from MBC graph like the MV; express in L/min (Fig. 3.9.4).
5. **Pulmonary reserve (PR)**. Calculate from the MV and MBC (refer to page 181).

Important Note: These days ***computerized multifunctional spirometers*** (Fig. 3.9.5) are available which allow high-quality measurements for all static and dynamic lung volumes, to be made virtually breath by breath. These spirometers display to high-resolution graphic display as well as the *predicted curves*. The generated reports may be seen on the display or can be printed. All *pulmonary function test* parameters with actual, predicted and percentage predicted values, as well as normal range with the option of interpretation and lung age can also be obtained. Moreover, all tests performed are presented with both the selected test highlighted and the percentage variation from best.

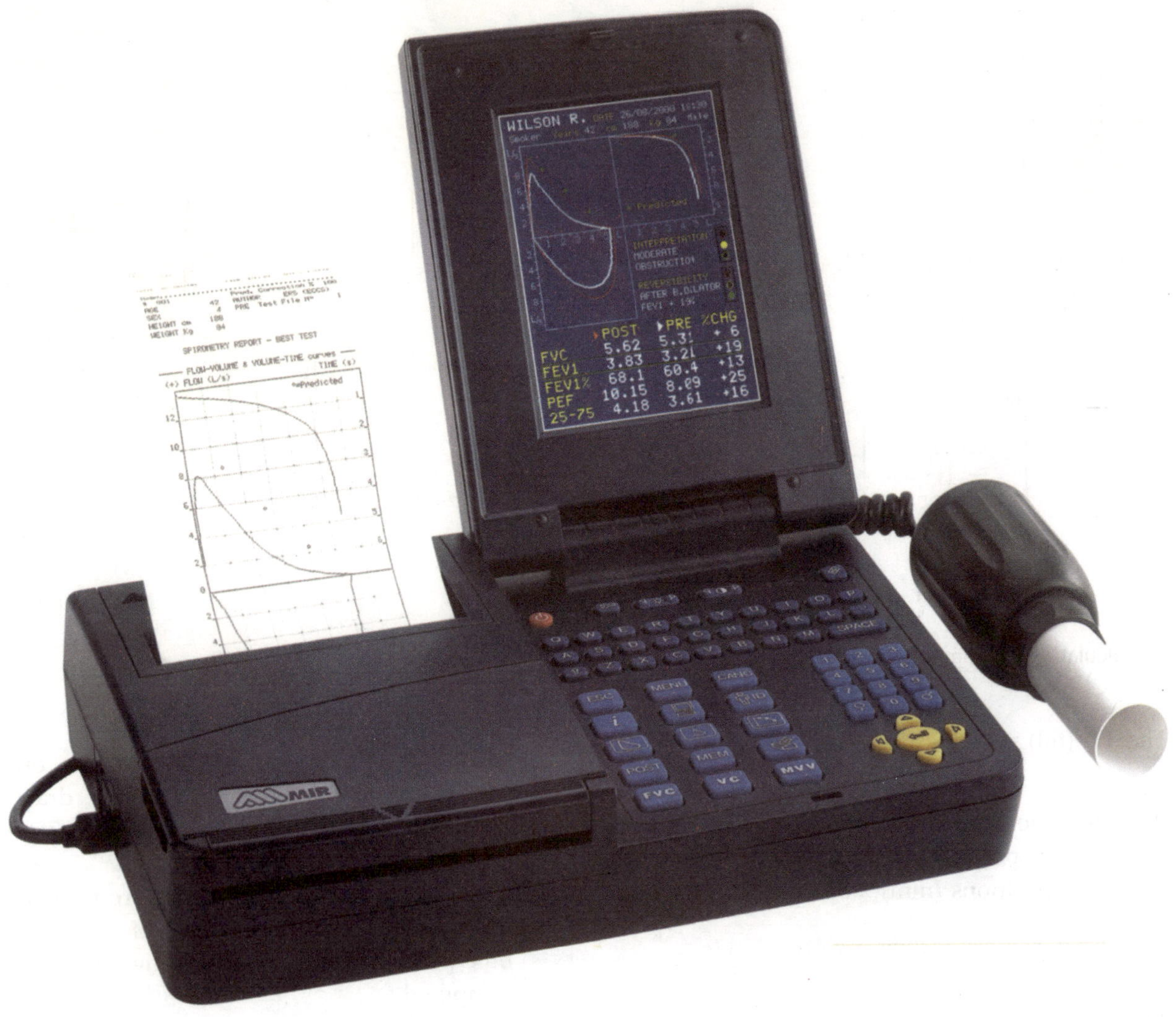

Fig. 3.9.5 Computerized multifunctional spirometer with graphic display

OSPE

Aim: To assess the Peak Expiratory flow rate (PEFR) of the subject provided.

Procedure steps: Refer to page 182.

Check list

1. Asks the subject to stand up holding the peak flow meter facing him. (Yes/No)
2. Explains the procedure to the subject. (Yes/No)
3. Instructs him to take a deep breath. (Yes/No)
4. Asks the subject to place the mouthpiece in his mouth, gripping it lightly with his teeth and sealing it with his lips. (Yes/No)
5. Instructs him to blow out rapidly, completely and forcefully into the mouthpiece. (Yes/No)
6. Checks for leak at the mouth. (Yes/No)
7. Takes the reading directly from the dial of peak flow meter. (Yes/No)

IMPORTANT VIVA-VOCE QUESTIONS

Q.1. *Name the lung volumes and capacities which cannot be measured by simple spirometry.*

Ans. Functional residual capacity (FRC), total lung capacity (TLC) and residual volume (RV) cannot be measured by simple spirometry.

Q.2. *Name the factors that influence the vital capacity.*

Ans. Page 176.

Q.3. *Give the physiological significance of FRC.*

Ans. FRC by maintaining the residual volume constant, acts as a buffer and allows the continuous exchange of gases to occur even during expiration. Thus it prevents sudden change in the partial pressure of gases in the blood.

Q.4. *Name the conditions in which FRC increases.*

Ans. FRC is increased in the conditions of hyper-inflation of the lungs; this may result from: old age, emphysema, bronchial asthma, etc.

Q.5. *What is the importance of FEV_1?*

Ans. FEV_1 helps to distinguish between restrictive and obstructive lung disorders:

(i) in restrictive disorders (kyphosis, scoliosis), VC decreases while FEV_1 is normal; TLC, flow rates and MVV also fall as VC decreases.

(ii) in obstructive disorders (bronchial asthma, emphysema), VC is normal while FEV_1 decreases.

Note: FEV_1 is a much more sensitive index (*i.e.* most reproducible) of the severity of obstructive lung disorders but it does not allow for the differentiation of the various causes of obstruction.

Q.6. *Give the physiological significance of pulmonary reserve.*

Ans. Page 181.

Q.7. *Why are all lung volumes and capacities usually measured from end-expiratory position?*

Ans. This position is more stable, because at this position the tendency of lungs to recoil from the chest wall is just balanced by the tendency of the chest wall to recoil in the opposite direction.

Q.8. *Name the methods of determining FRC.*

Ans. FRC can be determined by two methods:

(i) open circuit method - nitrogen wash out method, and

(ii) close circuit method – helium dilution method.

Q.9. *What is close-circuit spirometry. When is it done?*

Ans. When a person inspires from and expires into the same spirometer, it is called close-circuit spirometry. It is usually done to measure the basal metabolic rate (page 186).

Q.10. *What is computerized spirometry? How does it differ from conventional spirometry?*

Ans. Page 183.

Q.11. *How does spirometry help, the differentiation of small and large airway obstruction?*

Ans. Refer to Q.5.

STUDY NOTES

RESULTS AND DISCUSSION

Tabulate your results in the following table:

S. No.	Parameters	Value		Remarks
		Observed	Predicted	
1.	TV (ml)			
2.	IRV (ml)			
3.	ERV (ml)			
4.	IC (ml)			
5.	VC (ml)			
6.	FEV_1 (ml)			
7.	$FEF_{25\text{-}75\%}$ (L/min)			
8.	MV (L/min)			
9.	MBC (L/min)			
10.	% PR (DI)			

....

....

....

....

....

....

....

Date: ....

10 Measurement of Basal Metabolic Rate : (*BMR*)

I. APPARATUS

Spirometer with a recording kymograph or Benedict Roth apparatus for determining oxygen consumption, O_2 cylinder, nose clip, mouth piece, dettol, cotton, barometer, height and weight measuring equipment, charts for the correction of gas volumes, Dubois nomograms for normal BMR values and for finding body surface area

II. THEORY

1. The heat production or energy expenditure of the body for minimal level of activity is referred as **basal metabolism**. The measurement of the rate of heat production (metabolism) under resting (**basal**) conditions is called the **basal metabolic rate** (BMR).
2. *Basal conditions necessary for the measurement of BMR.* The subject should be:
   (i) at complete physical and mental rest (half an hour rest is given preceding the test after overnight sleep and rest),
   (ii) in a post-absorptive state (should have had nothing by mouth for the past 12-18 hours), thus avoiding the effect of digestion and absorption,
   (iii) in a comfortable environmental temperature (usually 20-25°C) during the test.

   Under such circumstances, a portion of energy liberated is used to maintain the activity of vital organs (brain, heart, lungs, kidney, liver, etc.) but greater part is converted into 'heat' to maintain the body temperature and thus prevent it from falling below normal.
3. Test is carried out in the awake subject in recumbent position. Clinically, it is convenient to determine BMR by estimating the oxygen consumption of the subject under basal conditions. It is expressed as : kcal/hour/m^2 body surface area (BSA).
4. *Normal values for adults*
   (i) In males: 40 kcal/hour/m^2 BSA,
   (ii) In females: 37 kcal/hour/m^2 BSA

   Clinically, BMR is considered within normal limits if the values are within ±10% of the normal values. It is expressed with a prefixed '+' or '–' sign indicating the per cent by which subject's O_2 consumption is above or below the normal value.
5. *Clinical significance.* BMR is of value:
   (i) for prescribing a diet of adequate calorific value;
   (ii) for diagnosing various pathological conditions, especially in hypo- and hyper-thyroidism;
   (iii) to note the effect of different types of foods and drugs on the BMR

III. PROCEDURE

By Indirect calorimetry (Fig. 3.10.1)

All commonly used clinical forms of basal metabolism apparatus employ the indirect principle, wherein oxygen consumption is measured and translated into terms of heat production by the application of appropriate factors. Therefore, there should be no one in the room excepting the subject, the operator and an assistant. In calculating the metabolism from the O_2 consumption, one assumes a respiratory quotient (RQ) of 0.80.

Steps

1. Note the temperature of the spirometer and the barometric pressure. Record the height (cm) and weight (kg) and note the age and sex of the subject.
2. Allow the subject to rest on a couch for half an hour before the test.
3. Fill the **bell** of the apparatus with 100% O_2.
4. Connect the subject to the apparatus through the mouthpiece and clip the nose. By adjusting the two-way tap, allow the subject to breathe from the atmosphere for a few minutes.
5. Turn the two-way tap and connect the subject to the spirometer so that he may inspire O_2 from the **bell** and expire into the same apparatus (**this is called closed-circuit spirometry**). Record the oxygen consumption for six minutes.

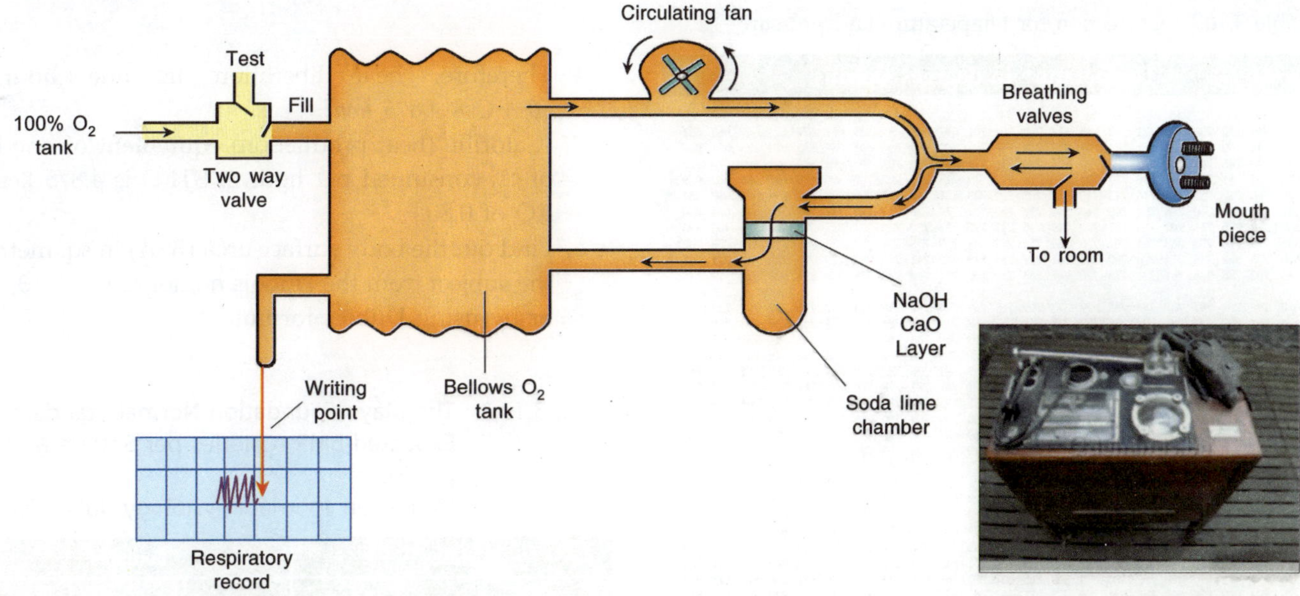

Fig. 3.10.1 Diagram of the connections of closed-circuit spirometry. **(Inset:** Sanborn metabulator or Benedict Roth apparatus)

Note: The CO_2 breathed out is removed by soda lime contained within the inner chamber of the spirometer.

6. As the oxygen is consumed, the bell is lowered and simultaneously tracing of respiratory movements is recorded on the moving drum. This gives the record of O_2 consumption on the calibrated graph paper for required time interval (see below).
7. If necessary, repeat the whole procedure after rest for 10 minutes and take mean of the two readings.

IV. CALCULATIONS

A. Calculations of oxygen consumption per minute

$$= \frac{\text{Initial level of } O_2 - \text{Final level of } O_2 \text{ (after 6 minutes)}}{6}$$

Note the initial level of oxygen under the **bell** from the record chart paper, and again the final level at the end of the experiment.

B. Calculation of BMR

1. Volume of O_2 consumed per minute at BTPS = ***'A' litres.***
2. Hence O_2 consumed in 1 hour = ***60·A litres;*** convert this O_2 volume at BTPS to STPD by using correction factor "C" (factor for the temperature of gas and barometric pressure, STPD; refer to standard temperature of O°C or 32°F and barometric pressure of 1 atmosphere, *i.e.* 760 mmHg) (Refer to Fig. 3.10.2 or Table 3.10.1).
3. Corrected volume of O_2 consumed at STPD in 1 hour = ***60·A·C litres.***

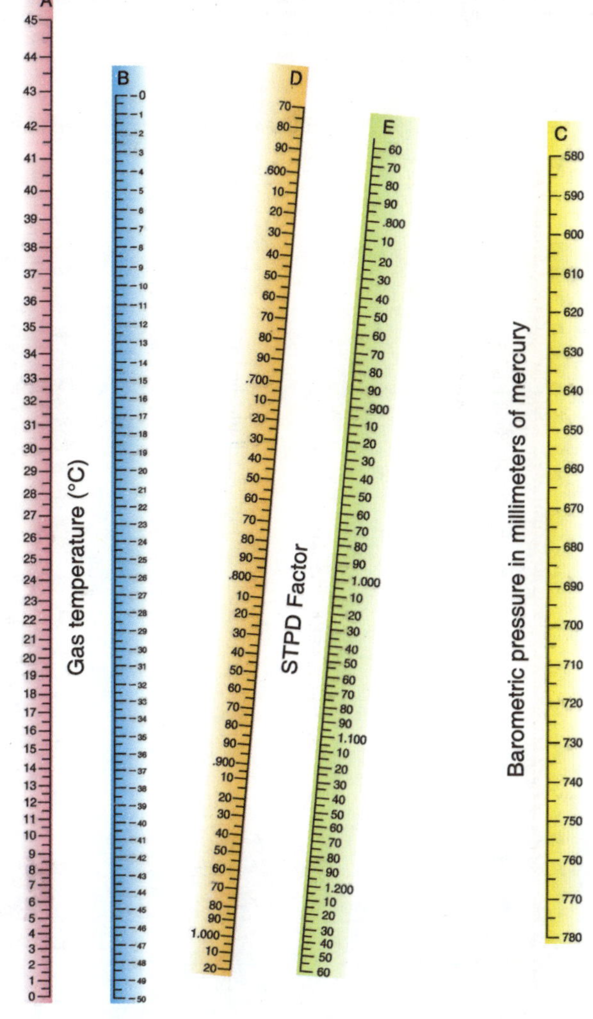

Fig. 3.10.2: Nomogram for determining STPD factors for the reduction of saturated gas volumes to dry volumes at 0°C and 760 mm Hg

Table 3.10.1 Correction for temperature and pressure

	Temperature in degrees Celsius																				
	15	16	17	18	19	20	21	22	23	24	25	26	27	28	29	30	31	32	33	34	35
600	.735	.732	.728	.725	.721	.718	.715	.712	.708	.704	.701	.697	.693	.689	.685	.681	.677	.673	.669	.665	.661
605	.742	.739	.735	.731	.727	.724	.721	.718	.714	.710	.707	.703	.699	.695	.691	.687	.683	.679	.675	.671	.667
610	.748	.745	.741	.737	.733	.730	.727	.724	.720	.716	.713	.709	.705	.701	.697	.693	.689	.685	.680	.676	.672
615	.754	.751	.747	.744	.740	.737	.734	.730	.726	.722	.719	.715	.711	.707	.703	.699	.695	.691	.686	.682	.678
620	.760	.757	.753	.750	.746	.743	.740	.737	.733	.729	.725	.721	.717	.713	.709	.705	.701	.696	.692	.688	.684
625	.767	.764	.760	.756	.752	.749	.746	.742	.739	.735	.731	.727	.723	.719	.715	.711	.707	.702	.698	.694	.690
630	.773	.770	.766	.762	.758	.755	.752	.749	.745	.741	.737	.733	.729	.725	.721	.717	.713	.708	.704	.700	.696
635	.779	.776	.772	.768	.764	.761	.758	.755	.751	.747	.743	.739	.735	.731	.727	.723	.719	.714	.710	.706	.702
640	.785	.782	.778	.774	.770	.767	.764	.761	.757	.753	.749	.745	.741	.737	.733	.729	.725	.720	.716	.711	.707
645	.792	.788	.784	.781	.777	.773	.770	.767	.763	.759	.755	.751	.747	.743	.739	.735	.731	.726	.722	.717	.713
650	.798	.794	.791	.787	.784	.780	.777	.773	.769	.765	.761	.57	.752	.748	.744	.740	.736	.732	.727	.723	.719
655	.804	.800	.797	.793	.790	.786	.783	.779	.775	.771	.767	.763	.758	.754	.750	.746	.742	.738	.733	.729	.724
660	.810	.806	.803	.799	.796	.792	.789	.785	.781	.777	.773	.769	.764	.760	.756	.752	.748	.744	.739	.735	.730
665	.816	.812	.809	.805	.802	.798	.795	.791	.787	.783	.779	.775	.770	.766	.762	.758	.754	.749	.745	.741	.736
670	.822	.819	.816	.812	.809	.805	.801	.797	.793	.789	.785	.781	.776	.772	.768	.764	.760	.755	.751	.746	.742
675	.828	.825	.821	.818	.815	.811	.807	.803	.799	.795	.791	.787	.782	.778	.774	.770	.766	.761	.757	.752	.748
680	.834	.831	.827	.824	.821	.817	.813	.809	.805	.801	.797	.793	.789	.784	.780	.776	.771	.767	.763	.758	.754
685	.841	.837	.833	.830	.827	.823	.819	.815	.811	.807	.803	.799	.794	.790	.785	.782	.777	.773	.769	.764	.760
690	.848	.844	.841	.837	.833	.829	.825	.821	.817	.813	.809	.805	.800	.796	.792	.788	.783	.779	.775	.770	.765
695	.854	.850	.847	.843	.839	.835	.831	.827	.823	.819	.815	.811	.806	.802	.798	.794	.789	.785	.780	.776	.772
700	.860	.856	.853	.849	.845	.841	.837	.833	.829	.825	.821	.817	.812	.808	.804	.800	.795	.791	.786	.781	.777
705	.866	.862	.859	.855	.851	.847	.843	.839	.835	.831	.827	.823	.818	.814	.810	.806	.801	.796	.792	.787	.783
710	.872	.868	.865	.861	.857	.853	.849	.845	.841	.837	.833	.829	.824	.820	.816	.812	.807	.802	.798	.793	.788
715	.878	.874	.871	.867	.863	.859	.855	.851	.847	.843	.839	.835	.830	.826	.822	.818	.813	.808	.804	.799	.794
720	.885	.881	.877	.873	.869	.865	.861	.857	.853	.849	.845	.841	.836	.832	.828	.824	.819	.814	.810	.805	.800
725	.891	.887	.883	.879	.876	.872	.867	.863	.859	.855	.851	.847	.842	.838	.834	.830	.825	.820	.816	.811	.806
730	.897	.894	.890	.886	.882	.878	.874	.869	.865	.861	.857	.853	.848	.844	.840	.836	.831	.826	.822	.817	.812
735	.904	.900	.896	.892	.888	.884	.880	.875	.871	.867	.863	.859	.854	.850	.846	.842	.837	.832	.827	.822	.817
740	.910	.905	.902	.898	.894	.890	.886	.881	.877	.873	.869	.865	.860	.856	.852	.848	.843	.838	.833	.828	.823
745	.916	.912	.908	.904	.900	.896	.892	.887	.883	.879	.875	.871	.866	.862	.857	.853	.848	.844	.839	.834	.829
750	.922	.918	.914	.910	.906	.902	.898	.893	.889	.885	.881	.877	.872	.868	.863	.859	.854	.849	.845	.840	.835
755	.928	.924	.920	.916	.912	.908	.904	.899	.895	.891	.887	.883	.878	.874	.869	.865	.860	.855	.851	.846	.841
760	.934	.950	.926	.922	.918	.914	.910	.905	.901	.897	.893	.889	.884	.880	.875	.871	.866	.861	.857	.852	.847
765	.941	.936	.932	.928	.924	.920	.916	.911	.907	.903	.899	.895	.890	.886	.881	.877	.872	.867	.863	.857	.852
770	.947	.943	.939	.935	.930	.926	.922	.917	.913	.909	.905	.901	.896	.892	.887	.883	.878	.873	.869	.863	.858
775	.954	.949	.945	.941	.936	.932	.928	.923	.919	.915	.911	.907	.902	.898	.893	.889	.884	.879	.875	.869	.864
780	.960	.956	.952	.948	.943	.939	.935	.930	.926	.921	.917	.913	.908	.904	.899	.895	.890	.885	.880	.875	.870

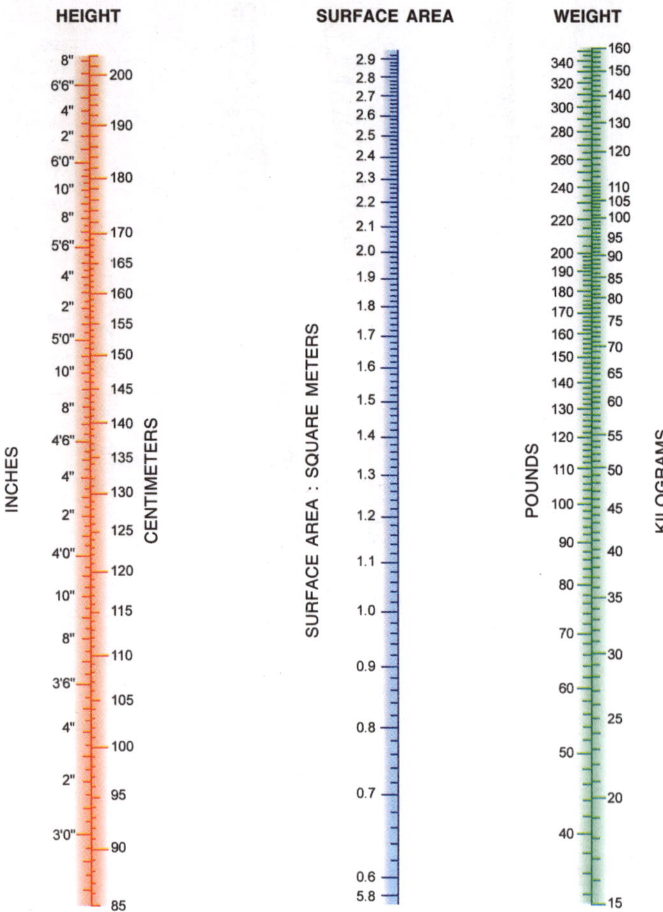

Fig. 3.10.3 Dubois nomogram for the calculation of body surface area

4. Therefore, heat liberation in one hour = ***60·A·C × 4.875 kcal.***
   {Calorific (heat production) equivalent of one litre of O_2 consumed per hour at STPD is 4.875 kcal at RQ of 0.80.}
5. Find out the body surface area (BSA) in sq. metre of the subject from the Dubois nomogram (Fig. 3.10.3) or by using Dubois formula

Table 3.10.2 The Mayo Foundation Normal Standards for Expected BMR (Calories per Square Meter per Hour) (American Journal Physiology, July, 1936)

Males		Females	
Age at last birthday	Mean	Age at last birthday	Mean
6	53.00	6	50.62
7	52.45	$6^1/_2$	50.23
8	51.78	7	49.12
$8^1/_2$	51.20	$7^1/_2$	47.84
9	50.54	8	47.00
$9^1/_2$	49.42	$8^1/_2$	46.50
10	48.50	9-10	45.90
$10^1/_2$	47.71	11	45.26
11	47.18	$11^1/_2$	44.80
12	46.75	12	44.28
13-15	46.35	$12^1/_2$	43.58
16	45.72	13	42.90
$16^1/_2$	45.30	$13^1/_2$	42.10
17	44.80	14	41.45
$17^1/_2$	44.03	$14^1/_2$	40.74
18	43.25	$15^1/_2$	40.10
$18^1/_2$	42.70	$15^1/_2$	39.40
19	42.32	16	38.85
$19^1/_2$	42.00	$16^1/_2$	38.30
20-21	41.43	17	37.82
22-23	40.82	$17^1/_2$	37.40
24-27	40.24	18-19	36.74
28-29	39.81	20-24	36.18
30-34	39.34	25-44	35.70
35-39	38.68	45-49	34.94
40-44	38.00	50-54	33.96
45-49	37.37	55-59	33.18
50-54	36.73	60-64	32.61
55-59	36.10	65-69	32.30
60-64	35.49		
65-69	34.80		

(BSA in m^2 = $W^{0.425} \cdot H^{0.725} \cdot 71.84$
= 0.425 log W + 0.725 log H + log 7184 – log 100
where, W = Body weight in kg
H = Height in cm)

Normal body surface area = 1.7-1.8 sq. metres.

6. Hence the BMR of the subject =

$$\frac{60 \cdot A \cdot C \times 4 \cdot 875}{\text{Body surface area}} \text{ kcal/m}^2\text{/hour}$$

7. Find out the **expected BMR** for the subject from the Table 3.10.2 according to the age and sex of the subject.
8. Determine the percentage deviation (above '+' or below '–') of the estimated BMR from accepted **normal** standard

i.e. percentage BMR =

$$\frac{\text{Calculated BMR - Expected BMR}}{\text{Expected BMR}} \times 100$$

IMPORTANT VIVA-VOCE QUESTIONS

Q.1. *Define BMR*

Ans. Page 186.

Q.2. *List the conditions necessary for the measurement of BMR.*

Ans. Page 186.

Q.3. *Give the normal value of BMR.*

Ans. Page 186.

Q.4. *What is the clinical significance of BMR?*

Ans. Page 186.

Q.5. *Explain how various factors influence basal metabolic rate.*

Ans. (i) *Age.* In children, BMR is higher compared to adults, because children possess greater BSA in proportion to their weights. As age advances, BMR decreases.

(ii) *Sex.* Metabolic rate is slightly higher in males compared to females due to larger BSA.

(iii) *Body surface area (BSA).* BMR is directly proportional to BSA.

(iv) *Body temperature.* For every rise of 0.5°C of internal body temperature, BMR increases by 7%, as the chemical reactions in the body are speeded up.

(v) *Climate.* Exposure to *cold* increases the BMR as there is subsequently more heat production by the body to maintain the normal body temperature. Exposure to *heat* has an opposite effect.

(vi) *Diet.* BMR increases after meals—maximum rise seen after a protein meal and minimum with carbohydrate or fat diet. Proteins cause increase in cellular metabolism to maximum (***specific dynamic action of food***).

For example, 125 gm of protein increases BMR by 25-35%; carbohydrates or fats of same calorific value increase BMR by 5-10% only.

(vii) *Exercise.* This results in an increase in O_2 consumption, so BMR increases.

(viii) *Endocrine.* Hormones which increase the tissues metabolic activities, increase the BMR e.g. hormones of adrenal cortex adrenal medulla, thyroid gland and anterior pituitary gland.

(a) In thyrotoxicosis, BMR increases and BMR decreases in the myxoedema.

(b) Anterior pituitary hormones increase BMR through the release of thyroid stimulating hormones and growth hormones.

(ix) *BMR* increases in fever and pregnancy.

(x) *Pressure.* Moderate decrease in atmospheric pressure does not affect the BMR, but a fall of pressure to 1/2 the atmospheric pressure at sea level, increases the BMR due to fall in arterial pO_2. That is why at a high altitude BMR rises.

STUDY NOTES

OBSERVATIONS, CALCULATIONS, RESULTS AND DISCUSSION

....

....

....

....

Date: ....

11 Energy Cost of Work: Cardio-Respiratory Responses to Steady State Exercise

I. APPARATUS

The same as in the previous experiment (page 186); bicycle ergometer, stethoscope, clinical thermometer, metronome, B.P. apparatus, measuring tape, stop watch

II. THEORY

1. Energy is constantly used by the body and the rate of utilization is determined by (i) BMR; (ii) physical activity and (iii) specific dynamic action of food. The extra amount of O_2 consumed during performance of a work of moderate severity is a ***measure of the energy cost of work***.
2. To assess the energy utilized during a specific activity, it is necessary to know the energy utilized for basal metabolism. Substract this from the total energy utilized calculated from the spirometric record of O_2 consumption obtained after the steady-state has been reached during exercise.
3. The metabolic requirements of the body at rest or during exercise are met with by supplying O_2 to tissues and by removing CO_2 from them. The series of linked mechanisms which operate to establish this, are primarily *governed by cardiovascular and respiratory system.*
4. In order to load these mechanisms maximally, large muscle groups must be engaged during exercise. For this reason, *treadmill* and *bicycle ergometers* are most commonly used, which enable a known power output to be used.
5. ***Steady-state*** *or constant power output.* In this test, a power output is maintained constant for long enough for most variables to reach relatively constant steady-state values. Rapid increase in O_2 consumption and CO_2 output occurs in the first 2 to 4 minutes at a given workload, but changes thereafter are small. Thus, after 4 to 5 minutes of exercise at a constant work rate, a steady state is assumed to have been reached for the measurement of cardio-respiratory responses.

III. PROCEDURE

1. Note the temperature of the spirometer and the barometric pressure. Record the height (cm) and weight (kg) and note the age and sex of the subject.
2. Note the heart rate of the subject by auscultation over the precordium and the BP with sphygmomanometer again by auscultation method.
3. Arrange the spirometer and measure the resting oxygen consumption (as described earlier, page 186); also make a note of resting parameters like TV, frequency of breathing, minute ventilation (page 181).
4. After a short rest period, the subject is asked to sit on a bicycle ergometer; adjust the metronome and he is instructed to pedal the bicycle at a rate of 50 times per minute, which is equivalent to about 130 revolutions per minute (r.p.m.) at the wheel (Fig. 3.11.1).
5. Adjust the **tension load** (**breaking resistance**: T_1-T_2) at the belt at 2 kg; he is then asked to respire from the mouthpiece while it is connected to the atmosphere. For first 5-6 minutes, the pedalling rate is kept constant and the heart rate, respiratory rate and B.P. are noted (take 3 readings of each).
6. When three readings are consistent, the subject presumably has reached a *steady state* and is then connected to the spirometer (filled with oxygen and fitted with soda lime for the absorption of CO_2). A one-minute record should be taken and O_2 consumption during this period determined. Also note the exact r.p.m. of the wheel from the revolution counter attached to the bicycle wheel.
7. Calculate the O_2 consumption per minute during the period of exercise (page 187). Also, calculate the respiratory parameters from the same record.
8. Allow the subject to recover and note his heart rate, respiratory rate and BP during recovery each minute.

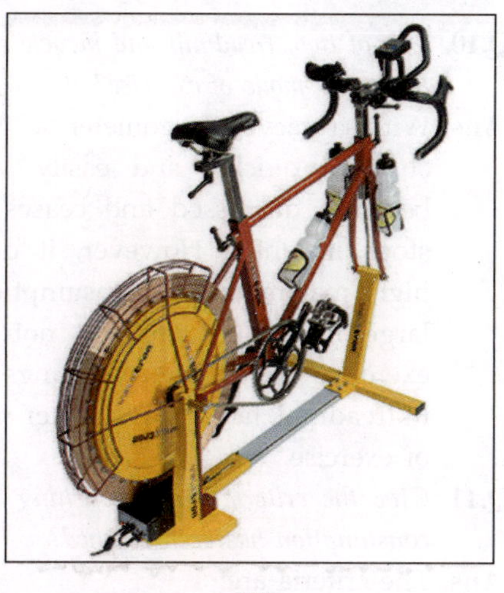

(A)

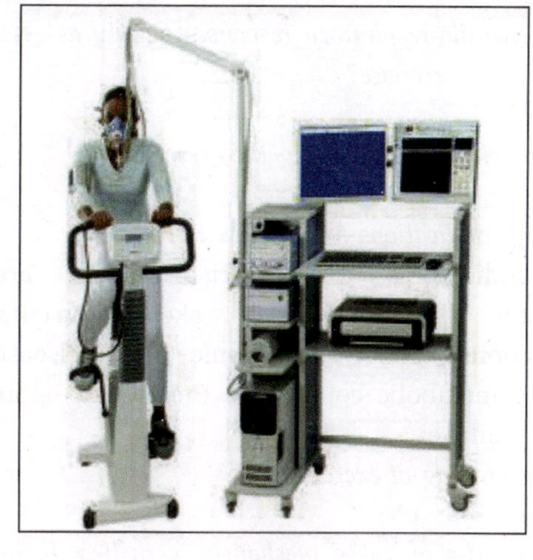

(B)

Fig. 3.11.1 (A) Bicycle ergometer and (B) Exercise set-up

Important Note: Before starting the exercise test every subject is instructed to signal with his hand in case he feels intolerably breathless, fatigued in legs, giddy, pain, constriction or suffocation in the chest.

IV. CALCULATIONS

(A) Calculation of energy cost of work

The oxygen consumption measured before and during the performance of a moderately severe work would give the energy cost of work. Energy cost is expressed either as:

(i) litres of O_2 consumed per minute (page 187), or

(ii) calories per minute (see below).

(B) Calculation of work done (W)

Work done (W) in kpm/min:

= [Distance] × [force]

= [Wheel circumference (m) × r.p.m.] × [tension (kg)]

(distance) *(breaking resistance: $T_1 - T_2$)*

kpm (kilo pond meter) is the unit of work, whereas **power** is the rate at which work is done. Therefore, kpm may be converted to power output (watts) by multiplying with a factor of 0.1635

(since kpm/min × 0.1635 = watt).

Note: Power output is the correct dimension for the rate of continuous expenditure of biological energy.

(C) Calculation of mechanical efficiency

$$\text{Mechanical efficiency} = \frac{\text{Output}}{\text{Input}} \times 100$$

Output = Work done in kpm/min

(426.7 kpm/min = 1 kcal).

Input = O_2 consumption in L/min

(1 litre of O_2 consumed at STPD gives out 5 kcal).

Thus, mechanical efficiency:

$$\frac{W(\text{kpm/min})/426.7}{O_2 \text{ consumption (L/min)} \times 5} \times 100$$

IMPORTANT VIVA-VOCE QUESTIONS

Q.1. *What is the relevance of this practical to medical physiology?*

Ans. The physiologist's interest is:

(i) to assess the work capacity of healthy individuals;

(ii) to determine the physical fitness of population groups; and

(iii) to improve the performance of athletes, sportsmen and military personnel.

The physician's interest is to use these tests as:

(i) in aiding the diagnosis of the heart and lung disease;

(ii) pre- and post-operative measurement of cardio-thoracic patients;

(iii) rehabilitation of cardiac invalids; and

(iv) screening workers for disability compensation.

Q.2. *Why is there a need for classifying exercise?*

Ans. What is mild exercise for one individual may be moderate for the second, and severe for the third; classification thus helps to understand the adaptation of body responses to exercise at a given load.

Q.3. *Define steady state exercise.*

Ans. Page 190.

Q.4. *Why are cardio-respiratory responses mainly assessed in response to exercise?*

Ans. Page 190.

Q.5. *Give the criteria for stopping the exercise.*

Ans. Page 191.

Q.6. *Give contraindications for exercise testing.*

Ans. Contra-indications for exercise testing are: locomotor disturbances, skeleto-muscular dysfunctions, anxiety, ischaemic heart disease, unstable metabolic conditions, threatening signs of heart failure

Q.7. *Give the grading of exercise.*

Ans. Refer to Table 3.11.1

Q.8. *Give the series of linked mechanism activated during exercise to meet the metabolic demand of the body tissue.*

Ans. The series of linked mechanisms are: capacity to breathe, to transport O_2 by the blood, to perfuse the active muscles and remove CO_2 from tissues.

Q.9. *Describe a treadmill ergometer.*

Ans. Treadmill is a motor driven belt over which a subject stands (Fig. 3.11.2). As the belt slips under his feet, he is obliged to simulate walking in order to prevent himself from falling. The spread of walking will depend upon the speed at which the belt moves; the latter can be adjusted at a desired level. The intensity of workload can also be increased by giving a slope to the belt.

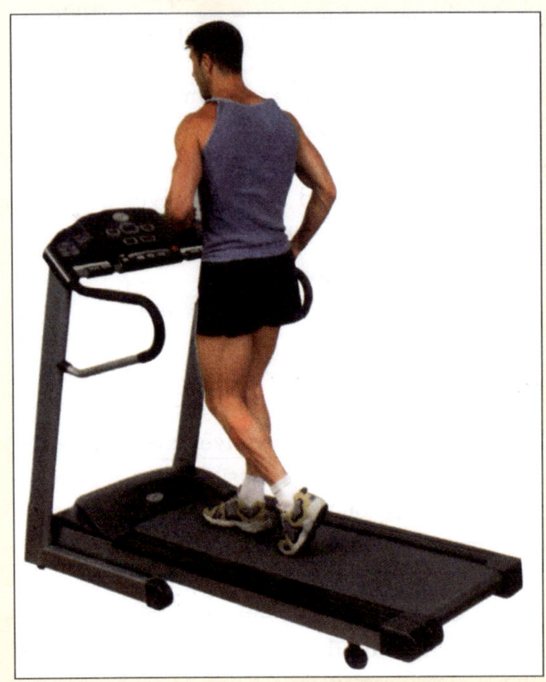

Fig. 3.11.2 A treadmill ergometer

Q.10. *Out of two, treadmill and bicycle ergometer, which is the better mode of exercise?*

Ans. With a bicycle ergometer a workload can be changed quickly and easily, and if a person becomes distressed and ceases pedalling, work stops instantly. However, it does not produce high maximum O_2 consumption since all the large muscle groups are not engaged during exercise. All these shortcomings can be overcome in treadmill, hence it is a better and natural source of exercise.

Q.11. *Give the criteria for establishing that maximum O_2 consumption has been reached?*

Ans. The criteria are:

(i) O_2 consumption reaches a plateau.

(ii) Achievement of maximum heart rate: 220 - Age (in years).

(iii) RQ increases more than 1.15.

(iv) Blood lactic acid increases more than 70-80 mg/dL (normal: 20-40 mg/dL).

Q.12. *Define: O_2 deficit and O_2 debt.*

Ans. It takes a few seconds for the circulation to deliver extra O_2 required by the working muscles. Therefore, regardless of the severity of exercise, there occurs a *O_2-deficit* at the beginning of the exercise, which remains throughout the whole exercise period. This O_2 deficit is repaid after the stoppage of exercise, in the form of O_2-debt. Therefore, the extra amount of O_2 consumed during recovery above the resting level is called *O_2 debt.* (Fig. 3.11.3)

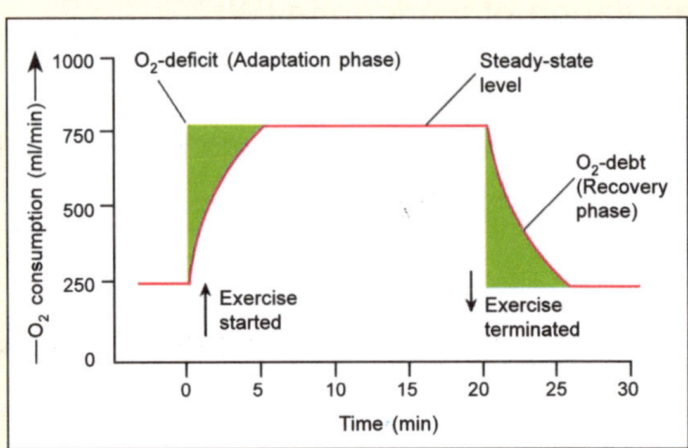

Fig. 3.11.3 Oxygen deficit and oxygen debt

Q.13. *What is warm-up effect?*

Ans. A light training done prior to actual exercise is called warm-up. It helps to decrease the O_2 deficit by increasing the blood-flow and nutrients to the working muscles.

Table 3.11.1 WHO classification of grading of exercise

Grade	Level	Relative load index	Metabolic (energy) expenditure test (METS)	Heart rate
I	Light (mild)	<25% of V_{O_2} max	<3 METS	up to 100 bpm
II	Moderate	25-50% of V_{O_2} max	3-4.5 METS	101-125 bpm
III	Heavy	51-75% of V_{O_2} max	4.6-7 METS	126-150 bpm
IV	Very heavy(severe)	>75% of V_{O_2} max	>7 METS	>150 bpm
V_{O_2} max: maximum O_2 consumption; METS: multiples of resting O_2 consumption				

STUDY NOTES

OBSERVATIONS AND CALCULATIONS

Table 3.11.2 Observations made during energy cost of work

Parameter	At rest	During steady state exercise	Remarks (if any)
(A) Cardiac			
1. Heart rate per minute			
2. BP (mmHg)			
(i) Systolic			
(ii) Diastolic			
(iii) Mean			
(iv) Pulse pressure			
(B) Respiratory			
1. Tidal volume (ml)			
2. Respiratory rate/min			
3. Pulmonary ventilation (L/min)			
(C) Energy Cost			
1. O_2 consumption (L/min)			
2. Calories/min			
(D) Mechanical Efficiency			

....

....

RESULTS

....

....

COMMENTS AND DISCUSSION

....

....

Date: ....

12 Cardio-Pulmonary Cerebral Resuscitation (*C.P.C.R.*)

I. GENERAL

Cardio-pulmonary-cerebral resuscitation (C.P.C.R.) is an emergency life-saving procedure. It is given as quickly as possible to a person presented with cardio-respiratory arrest.

Cardio-respiratory arrest is defined as the abrupt failure of the heart or respiration or both to maintain an adequate cerebral circulation.

Causes of cardio-respiratory arrest

A. *Acute conditions*
   1. Drowning
   2. Anaphylactic shock
   3. Coronary thrombosis
   4. Cardiac surgery
   5. Electrocution
   6. Poisoning with drugs (especially barbiturates): Accidental/suicidal.
   7. Inhalation of poisonous gases like carbon monoxide.
   8. Head injury
   9. Overdose or hypersensitivity to general anaesthetic agents or muscle relaxants (e.g. curare).

B. *Chronic conditions*
   1. Chronic lung disease
   2. Congestive heart failure
   3. Progressive obstruction to the air flow e.g. foreign body inhalation

Signs and symptoms of cardio-respiratory arrest

1. The person becomes unconscious with cold, moist and pale skin
2. Presence of weak or no pulse
3. Blood pressure not recordable
4. Dilatation of pupil due to increased sympathetic discharge

First-aid measures

1. Ensure that the airway is clean. To remove mucus or other secretions from the air passage, a stick with cotton wrapped at one end can be used.
2. Extend the neck so that the tongue may not fall back and block the airway.
3. All tight clothing such as tight collar should be loosened.
4. In case of drowning, turn the patient upside down by holding his ankles so as to remove water; also, apply strong pressure on the abdomen.

II. PROCEDURE

(A) Pulmonary resuscitation: Artificial respiration

This is an important factor in resuscitation and so it should be started as quickly as possible. Administer pure oxygen, if available; **CO_2 must not** be given with it since these subjects with respiratory failure are already suffering from an accumulation of CO_2.

For pulmonary resuscitation, several methods are used to provide **artificial respiration**; these are broadly divided into *manual* and *mechanical* methods.

Manual methods

They are less effective than the mechanical methods but are more useful because they are:

1. easy to perform,
2. do not need any apparatus, and
3. can be employed by a learner as a first-aid measure till medical services become available.

1. Mouth-to-mouth breathing (Fig. 3.12.1)

Steps:

(i) The subject is made to lie flat (supine).
(ii) Clear the airway; this can be achieved by administering a slap on the middle of the back to jerk the tongue forward.
(iii) Extend the neck, close the nostril and open the mouth of the subject.
(iv) Take a deep inspiration yourself; apply your mouth to the subject's mouth and exhale forcefully into the subject's mouth.

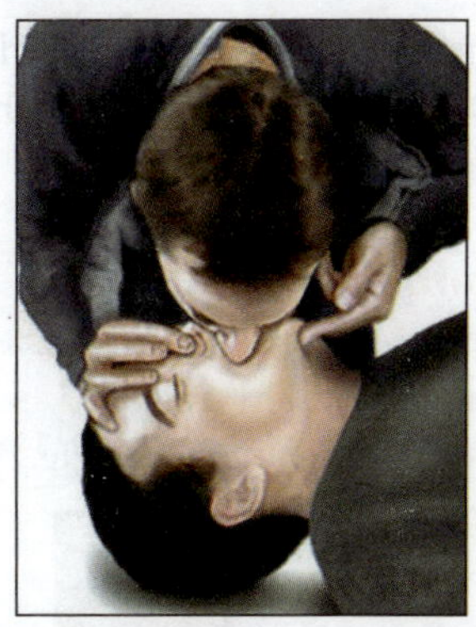

Fig. 3.12.1 Mouth-to-mouth breathing

(v) Look at the chest for expansion; watch for gastric distension.
(vi) Maintain a rate of 10-12 breaths per minute.

Important Notes

(1) Mouth-to-mouth breathing is ideally suited for infants and children, and the steps are the same as mentioned above.
(2) Always give one deep breath rather than 2 or 3 short breaths at the same time.
(3) It is the easiest to perform and is often the best but the single disadvantage lies in the fact that the tongue of the subject keeps falling back thus obstructing air flow.

2. Holger-Nielsen Method

Back pressure-arm lift (BPAL) method. Steps:

(i) The subject is made to lie prone (better for saliva drainage). The arms are abducted at the shoulders and elbows flexed; the head is turned to one side resting on the hands (Fig. 3.12.2).
(ii) The operator kneels down with one knee near the subject's head. The subject's arms are held just above the elbow; the operator gently straightens himself, while raising the subject's arms until resistance is felt. During this manoeuvre the thorax expands and intrathoracic pressure drops and inspiration takes place.
(iii) The subject's arms are then gently dropped.
(iv) The operator's hand and fingers spread apart are placed on the back of the subject immediately below the scapulae; the operator sways forward till his elbows are extended vertically above the subject. This procedure produces active expiration.
(v) The whole cycle is repeated 12 times per minute.

Important Note: This is most valuable method of resuscitation on victim with respiratory failure, such as rescue from drowning. It is used by the International Red Cross.

3. Sylvester Brosche Method.

Steps:

(i) The subject is made to lie in prone position.

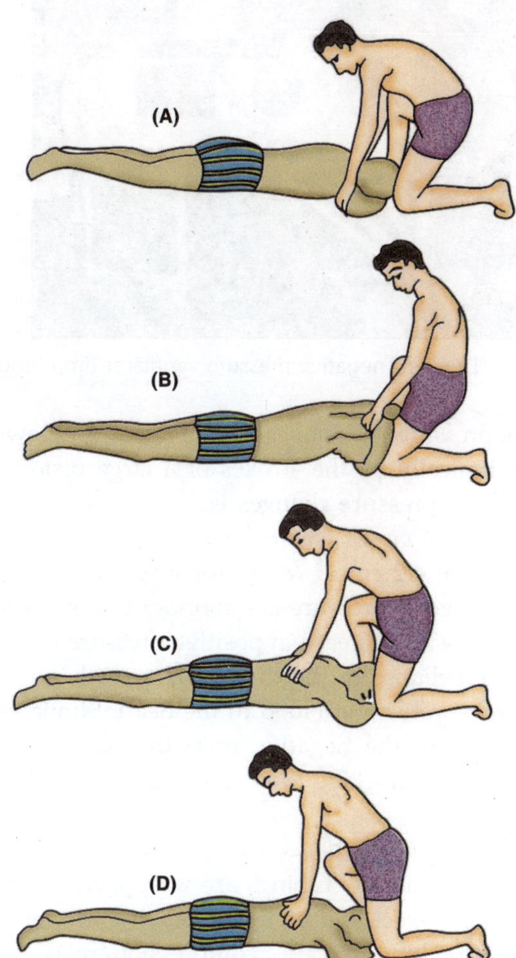

Fig. 3.12.2 Holger Nielsen Method. (A) Placing hands for arm lift; (B) arm lift; (C) backing hands for back pressure; (D) Back pressure

(ii) The operator kneels behind the subject and supports his head behind his own (operator's) knees.
(iii) The subject's forearm is held at the wrist and placed across the lower part of the chest.
(iv) The operator slowly rocks forward on straight elbows until his arms are nearly vertical; keeping the arms straight presses down on the lower part of the subject's chest wall for 2 seconds. This procedure produces active expiration.
(v) The operator then draws the subject's arms upwards, outwards and backwards in a sweeping movement as far as they can go. This produces inspiration.
(vi) The whole cycle is repeated 12 times per minute.

Mechanical Methods

1. Drinker's Method

(i) It was developed by Drinkers at Harward. In this, an iron respirator cabinet is used, the head of the subject remaining out of the cabinet and the rest of his body inside it (Fig. 3.12.3).

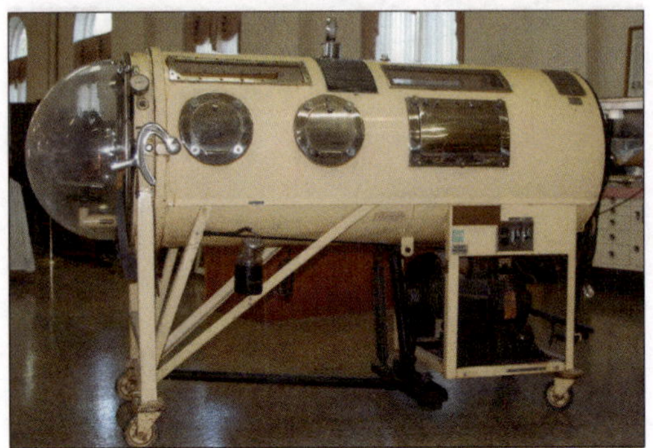

Fig. 3.12.3 Drinker's negative pressure ventilator (iron lung)

(ii) The pressure in metal cabinet is raised and lowered rhythmically by the strokes of a large piston. The range of pressure changes is:
(a) 0 to +4 cm of water, for expiration.
(b) -10 to -12 cm of water, for inspiration.
The range of pressure is important to note because on excessive increase in positive pressure may lead to the collapse of the thorax along with occlusion of veins returning blood to the heart. Similarly, an increase in the negative pressure may cause the thorax to burst due to expansion.

2. Paul-Bunnell Method

In this method hollow tubings are wrapped around the chest of the subject and air is forced rhythmically into the pressure tubings to cause compression/relaxation of the thorax.

3. See-Saw or Rocking Method (Fig. 3.12.4)

Here, the victim is laid on his back on a stretcher. Tie the ankles together, place the strap over the shoulders and the stretcher is rocked up and down 8 to 9 times per minute through an angle of ±45°. This causes the movement of diaphragm secondary to abdominal visceral movements and thus stimulates respiration.

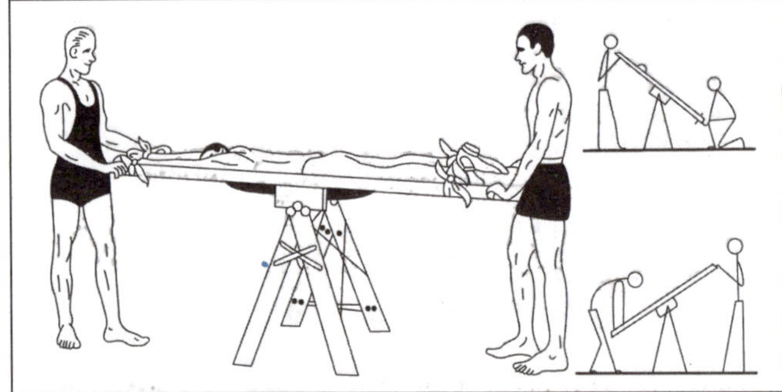

Fig. 3.12.4 See-saw method for artificial respiration

(B) Cardiac resuscitation

In cardiac arrest the heart stops either in *systole* or *ventricular fibrillation*. Asystole is revived by *external (or closed) cardiac massage* and ventricular fibrillation either by *internal (or open) cardiac massage* or by the use of an *electric shock defibrillator*.

1. External (or closed) cardiac massage

Principle. The heart is compressed between the sternum and the vertebral column and then released so that circulation may be established and maintained. (Fig. 3.12.5)

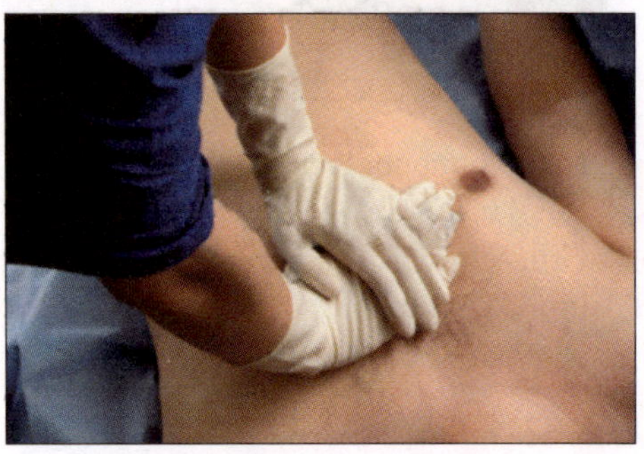

Fig. 3.12.5 External (closed) cardiac massage

Methods of compression

Steps:

(i) Place the heel of the hand over the site of compression (at the junction of upper 2/3rd and lower 1/3rd of sternum).
(ii) Place the heel of the second hand over the first, parallel to it.
(iii) The fingers should not touch the body.
(iv) The elbow should be straight.
(v) The force should be vertically downwards.
(vi) The movement should be at the shoulders so that the body weight of the operator may be transmitted through the hand to the sternum; compress by 4-5 cms.
(vii) Maintain a rate of 70-80/minute.

In Infants:

(i) Place the thumb over the middle of the sternum and fingers supporting the back.
(ii) Two fingers of the hand pressing over the sternum can also be used.
(iii) Maintain a rate of 100-120/minute.
(iv) Compress by 2-3 cm.

Important Notes

1. Avoid vigorous compression, which can lead to the fracture of ribs. Compression should, however, be sufficient to produce a palpable pulse at the wrist.
2. (i) In resuscitation by one person, maintain a ratio of 15 compressions to two breaths. Compression rate should be maintained at 70-80/minute so that with frequent interruptions for respiration, rate of 65-70/minute may be attained.
   (ii) If resuscitation is carried out by two persons, a ratio of 5:1 should be maintained with an effective compression rate of 70/minute and respiration 14/minute.

2. Internal (or open) cardiac massage (Fig. 3.12.6)

This method should be used only in a hospital in operation theatre. It is done either during operation or in the post-operative stages of cardiac arrest.

Procedure: A 5 cm long incision is given in the left 4th intercostal space in the midclavicular region (without anaesthesia). The hand of the doctor is placed below the heart after inserting it into the thorax and the heart is pressed upwards towards the thoracic cage.

In terminal cases, it is advisable to open the pericardium and squeeze the heart between the fingers and thumb.

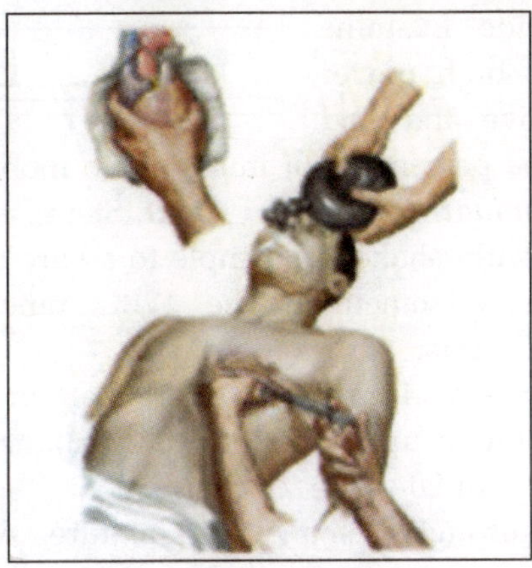

Fig. 3.12.6 Internal (open) cardiac massage

3. Electric shock defibrillator (Fig. 3.12.7)

This is a method of choice in abolishing ventricular fibrillation. The electric shock may be delivered via electrodes placed across the chest cavity or directly to the heart in open cardiac preparation.

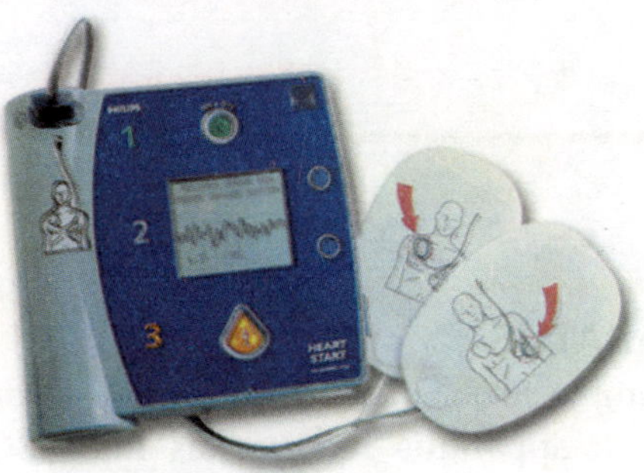

Fig. 3.12.7 Electric shock defibrillator

Important Note: Ventricular fibrillation can also be abolished by the following procedure:

1. Intravenous (I/V) administration of 100 ml soda bicarb 8.4% solution (to wash out the accumulated metabolites).
2. I/V calcium chloride 5 to 10 ml of 1% solution (to maintain cardiac contractions).
3. Convert fine fibrillations into coarse fibrillations by giving I/V or intracardiac injection of 0.5 ml adrenaline (1:1000).

IMPORTANT VIVA-VOCE QUESTIONS

Q.1. *Give the advantages and disadvantages of mouth-to mouth breathing.*

Ans. Page 195.

Q.2. *What is the method of choice for resuscitation in a victim of drowning?*

Ans. Page 195.

Q.3. *What is the physiological basis in the use of a defibrillator?*

Ans. Since the fibrillating ventricles cannot pump the blood effectively and the circulation of blood stops causing immediate death, electric shock application converts the fibrillation into flutter so that the ventricular contractions may become effective enough to pump the blood into the circulation.

Q.4. *Give the indications for CPCR.*

Ans. Page 194.

Q.5. *What are the signs and symptoms of cardio-respiratory arrest?*

Ans. Page 194.

Q.6. *How is resuscitation carried out simultaneously when there is one rescuer or there are two rescuers?*

Ans. Page 196.

Q.7. *What special measures should be taken while giving cardiac massage to infants and children?*

Ans. Page 196.

STUDY NOTES

COMMENTS AND DISCUSSION

....

....

....

Date: ....

13 Semen Analysis: Sperm Count and Motility

I. APPARATUS

Fresh sample of semen; 4% sodium bicarbonate in 1% phenol; apparatus required as for WBC counting (page 27).

II. THEORY

1. Semen (or seminal fluid) analysis reflects the events and function of testes and accessory sex organs of the male. The examination of semen is one of the tests for male fertility.
2. A fresh specimen of semen is liquid when ejaculated but clots immediately in vitro, therefore it should be examined 15-20 minutes after ejaculation during which the fluid undergoes secondary liquefaction.
3. A sample of semen collected after **3 to 4 days of sexual abstinence** shows the following characteristic features:
   - (i) Colour: white, opalescent.
   - (ii) Specific gravity: 1.028.
   - (iii) pH: 7.35 to 7.50.
   - (iv) Average volume: 2.5 to 3.5 ml per ejaculate.
   - (v) Count: 80-120 million/ml (average 100 million/ml).
   - (vi) Motility: 100% with more than 80% sperms having normal morphology.
   - (vii) Reaction: Alkaline (sperms get rapidly immobilized in an acidic medium).

Important Note: The volume of semen and sperm count decreases rapidly with repeated ejaculation. 50% of men with count of 20-40 million/ml and essentially all of these with count less than 20 million/ml are **sterile**.

III. PROCEDURE

1. Obtain a fresh sample of semen after masturbation collected in a penicillin (small) bottle; wait for 15-20 minutes so that it may undergo secondary liquefaction.
2. *To assess the sperm motility*, place a drop of semen on the cover slip and invert it on a rim of plasticine on the slide. Examine under high power objective and find out the percentage of immobile to mobile sperms.

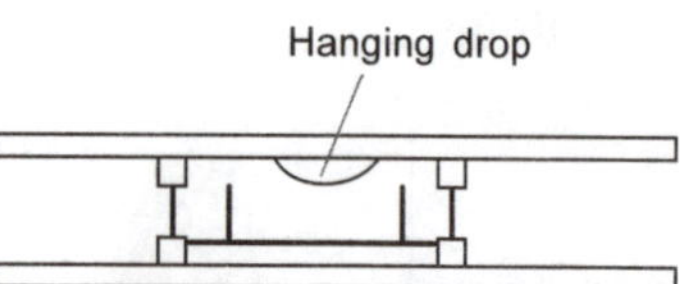

3. *Determination of sperm count*. Steps:
   - (i) Gently shake the sample to assure uniformity.
   - (ii) Draw semen in the WBC pipette up to 0.5 mark.
   - (iii) Draw in 4% sodium bicarbonate in 1% phenol solution up to the mark 11, making a dilution of 1 in 20 (page 27).
   - (iv) Thoroughly shake the mixture, discard the first few drops and then charge the counting chamber. Ensure uniform distribution.
   - (v) Count the sperm under high power in the four WBC squares (Fig. 3.13.1) (follow rules for counting, page 20).

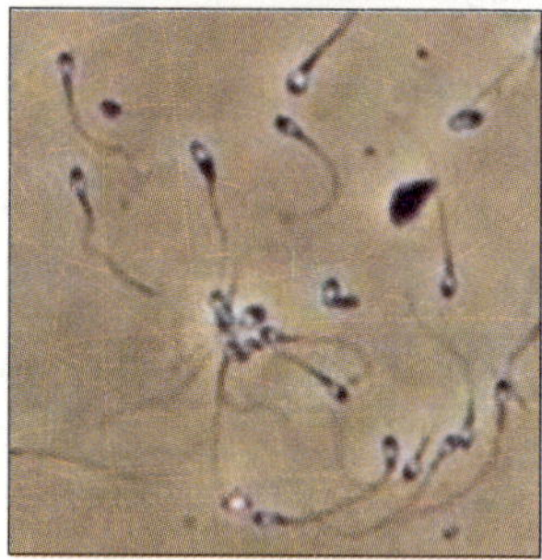
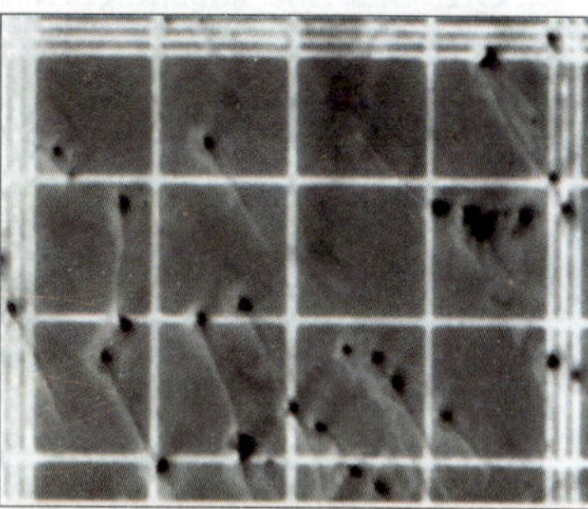

Fig. 3.13.1 Sperm as seen under high power

4. *Calculation*

   Number of sperms in 1 μL of sample
   = N × 10/4 × 20 (for details, refer to page 27)
   Number of sperms in 1 ml (*i.e.* 1 cu.cm) of sample
   = N × 50 × 1000 (as 1 cc = 1000 μL)
   N × 50,000

Note: Follow the same precautions as already described under procedure for RBC count, page 19.

IMPORTANT VIVA-VOCE QUESTIONS

Q.1. *Give the normal composition of semen.*

Ans. See above.

Q.2. *Explain the significance of semen analysis.*

Ans. (i) to find whether the male is fertile or not;
(ii) to detect the percentage of abnormal sperm;
(iii) to detect pathological and genetic disorders like cryptorchidism and klinefelter's syndrome.

Q.3. *Give the mechanism of coagulation and secondary liquefaction.*

Ans. (i) Mechanism of coagulation. Semen contains fibrinogen and thromboplastin but no prothrombin or thrombin. Its coagulation involves the conversion of its fibrinogen into fibrin (exact mechanism is not known).
(ii) **Mechanism of liquefaction**. The secondary liquefaction of the fibrin is due to specific enzyme, fibrinolysin (plasmin) present in the prostatic fluid. 2 ml of prostatic fluid at body temperature can liquefy 100-1000 ml of clotted plasma in 18 hours.

Q.4. *What is the maximum duration of fertilizing capacity of sperms within the female genital tract?*

Ans. The maximum duration of fertilizing capacity is 24-48 hours.

Note: Motility may persist for 48-60 hours.

Q.5. *What should be the minimum sperm count to label a male fertile?*

Ans. 40 million/ml.

Q.6. *At what sperm count is an individual essentially sterile?*

Ans. Less than 20 million/ml.

Q.7. *Define: Azoospermia, oligospermia, necro-spermia.*

Ans. *Azoospermia:* Total absence of sperms in a sample of semen
Oligospermia: sperm count less than 20 million/ml
Necrospermia: A condition in which seminal sperms are not alive (*dead sperms*)

Q.8. *How long may the sperm appear in the semen of an individual after bilateral vasectomy?*

Ans. For first two months after vasectomy viable sperms may be released from the ampulla.

STUDY NOTES

OBSERVATIONS AND CALCULATIONS

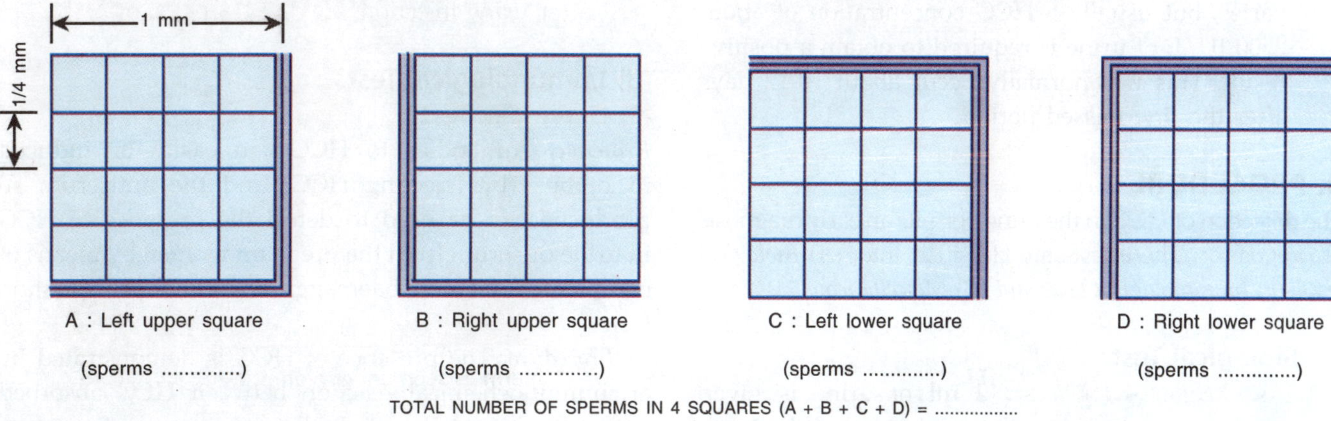

Fig. 3.13.2 Enter the observations after counting the sperms in the corresponding squares

RESULTS AND COMMENTS

....

....

Date: ....

14 Pregnancy Diagnostic Tests

I. THEORY

1. In 1927, Aschheim and Zondak found that the urine of pregnant females (rat, human, etc.) contained a hormone called the *chorionic gonadotrophin*. It is formed by syncytiotrophoblast cells of the placenta immediately after the implantation of the fertilized ovum.
2. Urine from one pregnant female, when injected into the non-pregnant female of another species, produces luteinizing and luteotrophic changes, *i.e.* formation and development of *corpus luteum*. This is used as a test for pregnancy.
3. **Principle of pregnancy diagnostic tests**. These are all based on the presence of *human chorionic gonadotrophin (HCG)* in urine, which can be detected as early as 14 days after conception with the test accuracy of 99%. The sensitivity of these tests varies, but usually a HCG concentration of about 2500 IU/L of urine is required to obtain a positive result. This will normally occur about 10-12 days after the first missed period.

II. PROCEDURE

The detection of HCG in the urine permits an early diagnosis of pregnancy. These tests are classified into: *(A) Biological tests, (b) Immunological tests and (C) Miscellaneous tests.*

(A) Biological Tests

1. *Aschheim-Zondak Test.* 2 ml of urine is given subcutaneously to immature mice over 2 days and the ovaries examined on the fifth day. The presence of haemorrhagic and luteinizing follicles indicates that the urine contains chorionic gonadotrophin.
2. *Kuppermann Test.* Here 2 ml of urine is injected subcutaneously into three immature female rats, which are killed six hours later. If the injected urine contains HCG, a marked hyperaemia of the ovaries is observed. Alternatively, response may be read after 2 hours following intra-peritoneal administration of the hormone.
3. *Friedman Test.* This depends on the release of ova (*i.e. ovulation*) from the ovaries in the mature rabbit following the intravenous injection of 10 to 15 ml of urine. The ovaries are examined after 24 to 48 hours later.
4. *Hogben Test.* A mature female South African clawed toad (*xenopus laevis*) is isolated for 3-4 days. Therefore, no sperms are present due to mating, and a concentrate, prepared from 20 to 30 ml of urine, is injected into the dorsal lymph sac. If the urine contains HCG, ovulation follows between 6 and 12 hours later.
5. *Galli-Mainini Test.* This is based on the ability of HCG in the urine of pregnant subject, when injected into male frogs or toads to induce the release of sperms. The sperms can be detected in the urine taken from the cloaca of the test animal, three hours after urine injection.

(B) Immunological Tests

(1) Gravindex Test

Principle: Antibodies to HCG can easily be induced in rabbits (by injecting HCG) and the antiserum so produced can be used to detect the presence of HCG in urine or serum from the pregnant women by means of complement fixation, haemagglutination or precipitation tests.

Procedure: The presence of HCG is demonstrated by an immunochemical reaction between HCG absorbed on to **latex particles** and HCG antiserum. The steps involved in the reaction are (Fig. 3.14.1):

(*i*) A drop of urine of *non-pregnant* women (*contains no HCG*) + A drop of HCG antiserum (contains HCG antibodies) causes no neutralization of HCG antiserum, therefore it will produce **agglutination** when mixed with HCG-coated latex (which contains HCG).

(*ii*) A drop of urine of *pregnant* women (*contains HCG*) + A drop of HCG antiserum causes neutralization of HCG antiserum. Therefore, it will produce

1. Place one drop of water onto the green latex dot.

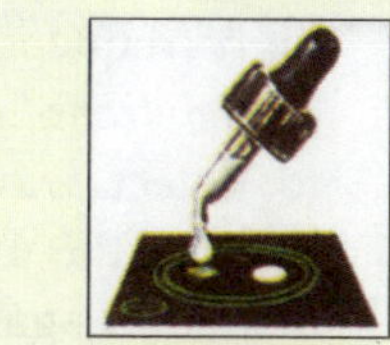

2. Draw up the urine sample.

3. Squeeze one free-falling drop of urine onto the colourless antiserum dot; mix the urine and antiserum thoroughly. Then rock the slide for 30 seonds.

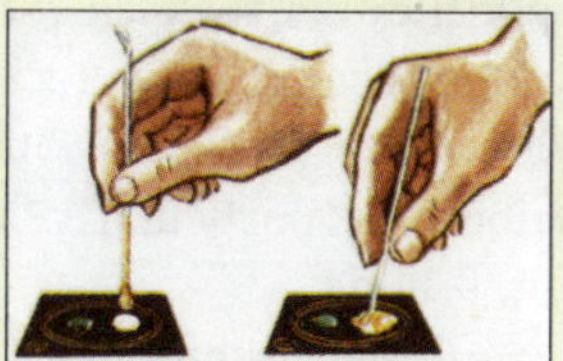

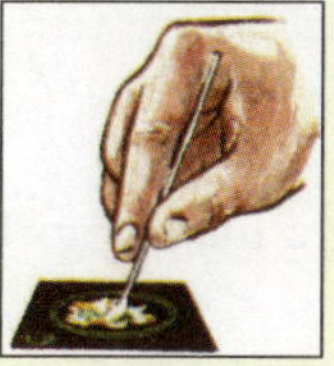

4. After this 30-second period, using the same dispenstir mix the drop of dissolved antiserum and the drop of resuspended latex particles together.

5. Rock the slide (or slide holder) back and forth gently in a "figure 8" motion for two minutes so that the liquid may slowly flow over the entire encircled area.

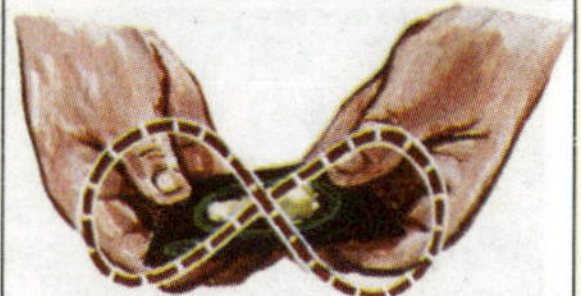

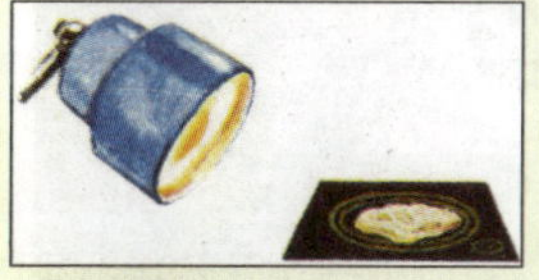

6. Read the result under a strong glare-free light at the end of two minutes while still gently rocking the slide.

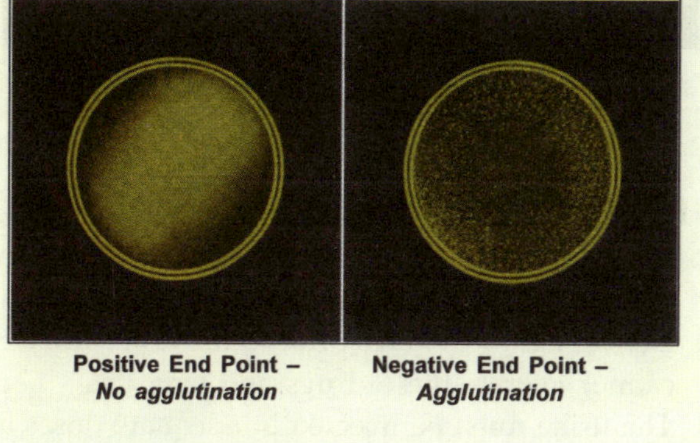

Fig. 3.14.1 Gravindex Test–Steps

no agglutination when mixed with HCG-coated latex.

In this test, the reaction is carried out on a glass slide with a black background.

> **Important Note:** If the urine HCG is low, a **false negative** result will occur; also **false positive** results can occur either at the menopause or ovulation due to increased secretion of LH.

(2) Radioimmunoassay (RIA)

RIA is a more sensitive test for the quantitation of antigens or antibodies.

Principle: This test is based on competition for a fixed amount of specific antibody between a known radiolabelled antigen and an unknown unlabelled (*test*) antigen (Fig. 3.14.2). This competition is determined by the level of the *test* antigen present in the reacting system. After antigen-antibody reaction, the antigen is separated into the *'free'* and *'bound'* fractions and their radioactivity is measured. The concentration of *test* (unlabelled) antigen is calculated from the ratio of the bound and total antigen labels, using a reference curve (Fig. 3.14.3).

The *standard* dose response (or *reference curve*) has to be prepared for calculations. The ratio of bound to total labels (*B:T ratio*) plotted against the unlabelled antigen concentrations gives the standard (reference) curve.

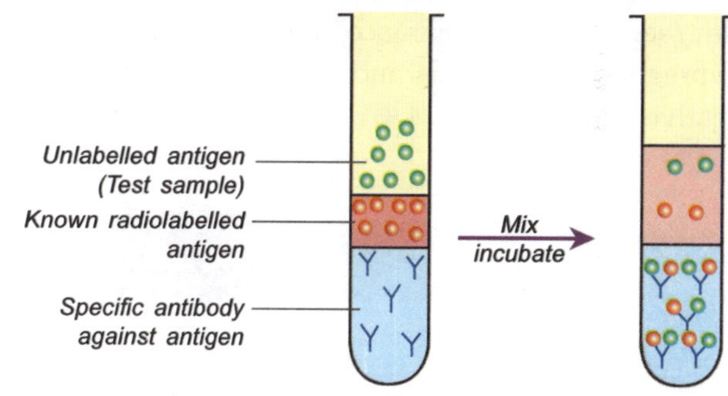

Fig. 3.14.2 Radioimmunoassay

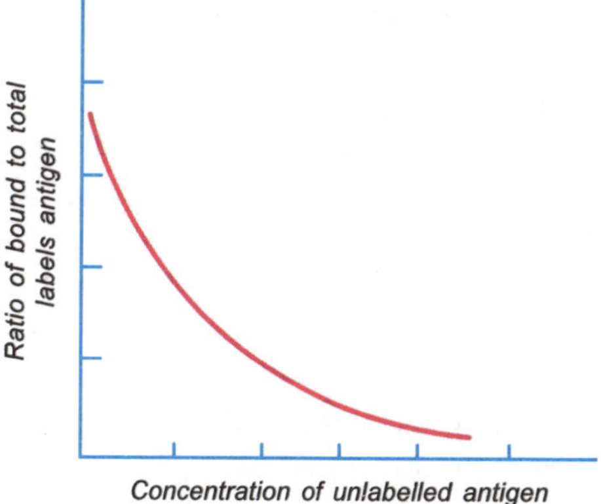

Fig. 3.14.3 Standard (Reference) curve

Procedure:

(i) Here HCG is radiolabelled with iodine (I^{125}). The known amount of this radiolabelled Iodo HCG (Radio ligand) is mixed with the fixed amount of antibodies raised against HCG and sample (urine/serum) containing HCG antigen.

(ii) The *labelled* and *unlabelled* antigen compete for limited binding sites on the antibody. The *free* and *bound* Iodo HCG are separated.

(iii) The radioactivity of bound form is measured and from the *standard curve,* HCG value is determined.

(3) Elisa-Enzyme Linked Immunosorbent Assay

Elisa has been applied widely for the detection of a variety of antibodies and antigens. It is simple and as sensitive as radioimmunoassay. It requires only very small quantities (microlitre) of test reagents.

Principle: The principle of elisa is almost the same as that of radioimmunoassay, the only difference being, an *enzyme* is used instead of a radioactive substance. The enzyme acts on substrate to produce a colour in a positive test.

Procedure: In this test a *monoclonal antibody based* visual enzyme *immunoassay* is used to detect HCG in urine/serum. The appearance of a *blue* colour is positive for pregnancy diagnosis and a *colourless* response as a negative result. (Fig. 3.14.4)

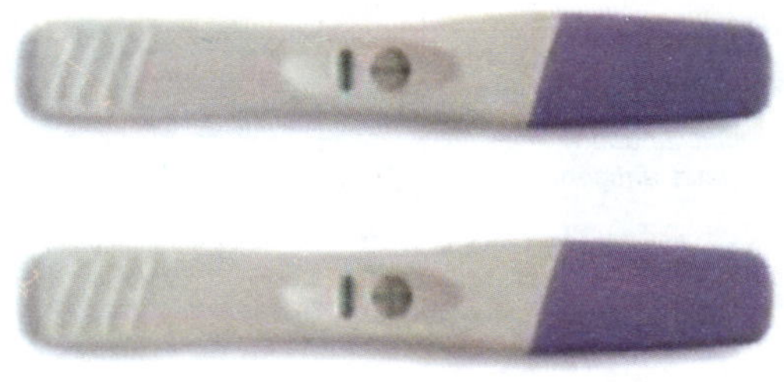

Fig. 3.14.4 Elisa for pregnancy diagnosis

(C) Miscellaneous Tests

(1) Hormone withdrawal bleeding test

High doses of progesterone and oestrogen are given orally or by injection for **three** consecutive days:

(i) If withdrawal bleeding occurs 4-5 days after last dose, this indicates that **amenorrhoea** (cessation of period) may be due to other hormonal imbalance; such bleeding usually rules out conception.

(ii) If no withdrawal bleeding occurs, amenorrhoea may be due to pregnancy.

(2) Radiological investigations

(i) *Lateral X-ray pelvimetry:* Radiologically foetal skeleton can be made out by 16-18 weeks of pregnancy and is a conclusive evidence. However, due to the realisation of hazards of the radiations in pregnancy its use is restricted.

(ii) *Ultrasound – Sonography*

In sonography, the pulses of ultrasonic waves at high frequency are generated from a *piezo-electric crystal transducer* that also functions as a receiver to detect waves reflected back from the various parts of the uterus. Reflected waves (*i.e. echoes*) are displaced against time on an oscilloscope to obtain a record of the size of the object scanned.

Ultrasonics by the pulse echosonar method is now being widely used (rather misused) for the diagnosis of pregnancy as well as for sex determination purposes. By the use of this technique, the ***gestation ring*** is evident as early as 5th weeks of pregnancy. The method is particularly useful in the assessment of: (Fig. 3.14.5)

(i) gestational age
(ii) presence of foetal abnormalities
(iii) multiple pregnancy
(iv) the site of the placenta
(v) size and relationships of pelvic masses to the viscera.

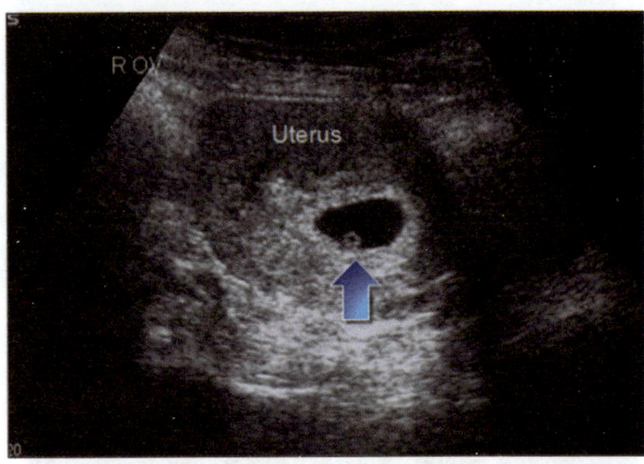

Fig. 3.14.5 Sonography showing gestational ring (Arrow)

III. PRECAUTIONS

1. The female to be tested must abstain all drugs (especially sleeping pills, aspirin, LSD, barbiturates, etc.), at least 7-10 days prior to the test, since a frog cannot tolerate these drugs and may die.
2. The urine must be injected in adequate doses and, if necessary, even concentrated urine may be used after centrifugation.

IV. UTILITY OF PREGNANCY DIAGNOSTIC TESTS

1. Important to diagnose pregnancy
2. Helps assess and determine the course of action in cases of disturbed pregnancy.
3. Tests are also positive in cases of **hydatidiform mole** or **vesicular mole** (*i.e.* benign tumour of placenta). How? In normal pregnancy HCG in

urine peak lasts for about 10 days but in a mole, a peak continues to exist and the level of HCG remains at a level higher than 4000 I.U./day.

4. The levels of HCG are strongly positive in cases of chorio-carcinomas, *i.e.* malignant tumour of placenta; where even urine dilution to 1 : 5000 may show positive test.

IMPORTANT VIVA-VOCE QUESTIONS

Q.1. *What is amenorrhoea?*

Ans. Page 202.

Q.2. *Mention the source of HCG and its action.*

Ans. Page 200.

Q.3. *Give one condition each where false positive and false negative results are obtained by gravindex test.*

Ans. Page 201.

Q.4. *Give the physiological basis of immunological tests to diagnose pregnancy?*

Ans. Page 200.

Q.5. *Give the principle and advantages of ultrasound.*

Ans. Page 202.

Q.6. *Name the most reliable test to diagnose pregnancy.*

Ans. Ultrasonography is the most reliable of all the pregnancy diagnostic tests; it is accurate, cost-effective and least time-consuming.

Q.7. *Give an account of the utility of pregnancy diagnostic tests.*

Ans. See above.

STUDY NOTES

OBSERVATIONS, RESULTS AND DISCUSSION

....

....

....

....

....

....

....

....

....

....

....

....

....

....

....

....

Date: ....

15 *Perimetry*: Mapping Out of the Visual Field

I. APPARATUS

Subject, perimeter, perimetric chart, test object of different colours

Perimeter: Priestley-Smith Model

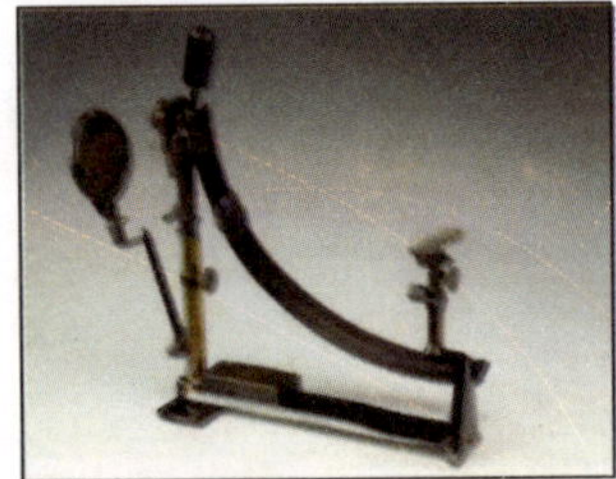

The perimeter is an instrument for the accurate charting of the field of vision. It consists of: (Fig. 3.15.1)

1. **A vertical stand** on which a metallic arc is pivoted. It also bears a circular black disc to read the meridian in which the metallic arc is brought.
2. **The metallic arc**
   (i) It is a concave arc in the shape of a semicircle with radius 330 mm; the concavity faces the subject.
   (ii) The arc can be rotated in any direction and can also be fixed at any position with the help of a tightening screw. When rotated, it describes a hollow sphere so that all points on it may be equidistant from the retina.
   (iii) The arc is graduated from 0° to 90°, the 'zero' being at the centre and the 90° at the periphery.

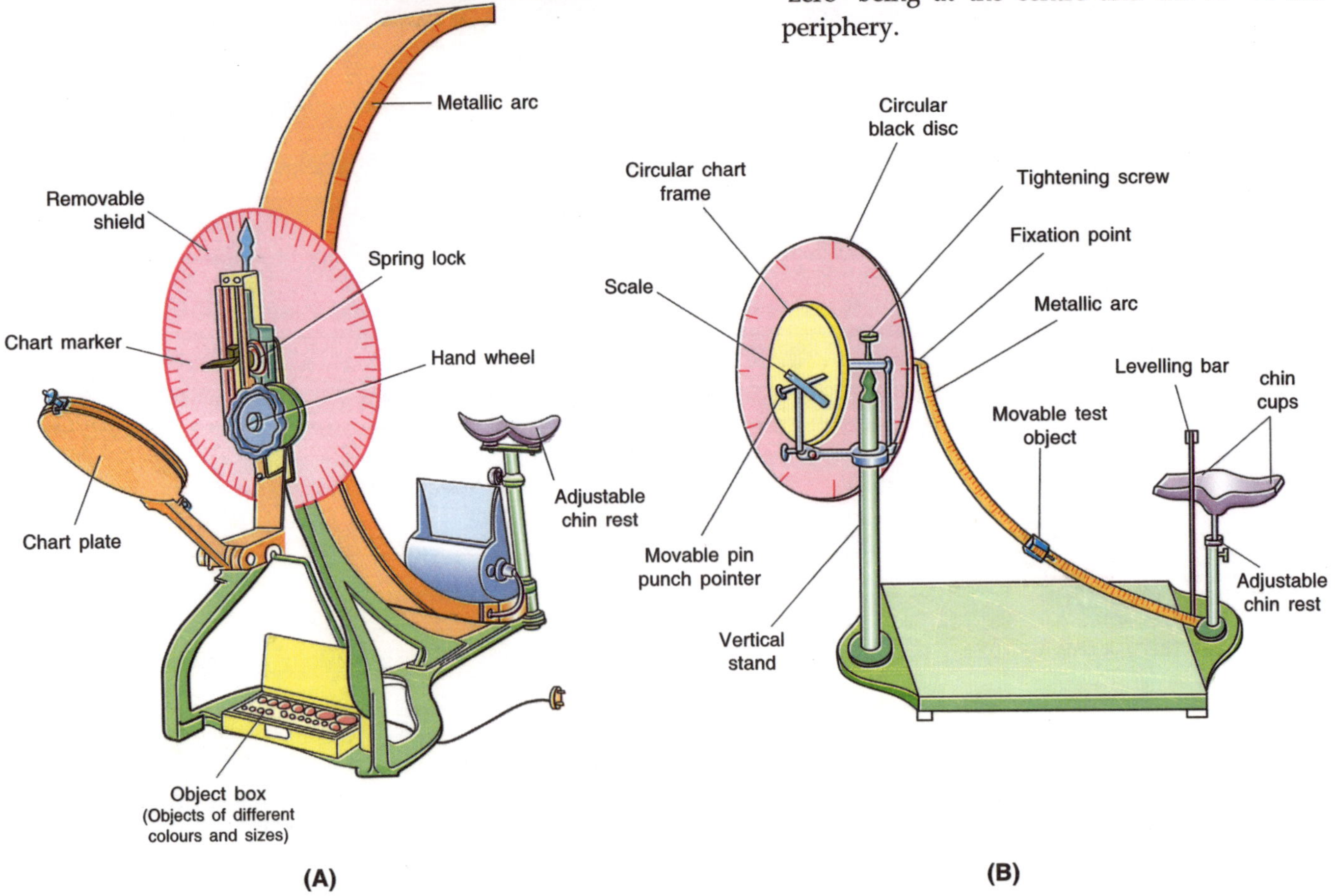

(A) (B)

Fig. 3.15.1 A perimeter: (A) Lister Model and (B) Priestley-Smith Model

(iv) The centre of the arc, *i.e.* point of pivot, is occupied by a **fixation point**, which is a circular (5 mm diameter) white spot. The subject is asked to fix the *gaze* at it while the field of vision is being mapped out.

(v) The arc bears a moveable **test object**, which is a white colour spot, of size 10 mm diameter painted on a circular disc. It can be moved along the length of the arc from its periphery to the centre.

Note: For plotting the field of vision, the test objects of different colours and sizes can be used.

3. **An adjustable chin rest** and a detachable **levelling bar** is fixed in front of the metallic arc, near the centre of curvature.

   (i) The chin rest has two *chin cups*, the right **chin cup** is to be used for mapping the visual field of the left eye and vice versa.

   (ii) The chin rest is to be adjusted with the help of a levelling bar so that the central fixation point, the tip of the levelling bar and the eye may be in the same horizontal plane. Therefore, the visual axis of the eye coincides with the axis of the rotation of the eye.

4. **Scale and chart frame**. A circular chart frame to hold the chart paper in position is provided at the back of the black circular disc. To this a metallic graduated scale with a movable **pin-punch** pointer is fixed to mark latitude degrees on the perimeter chart paper.

5. **Perimetric chart** (Fig. 3.15.2)

   (i) The central point of the chart corresponds with the visual axis; the concentric circles/lines are drawn around it at 10° intervals. Each concentric line denotes a point of equal visual

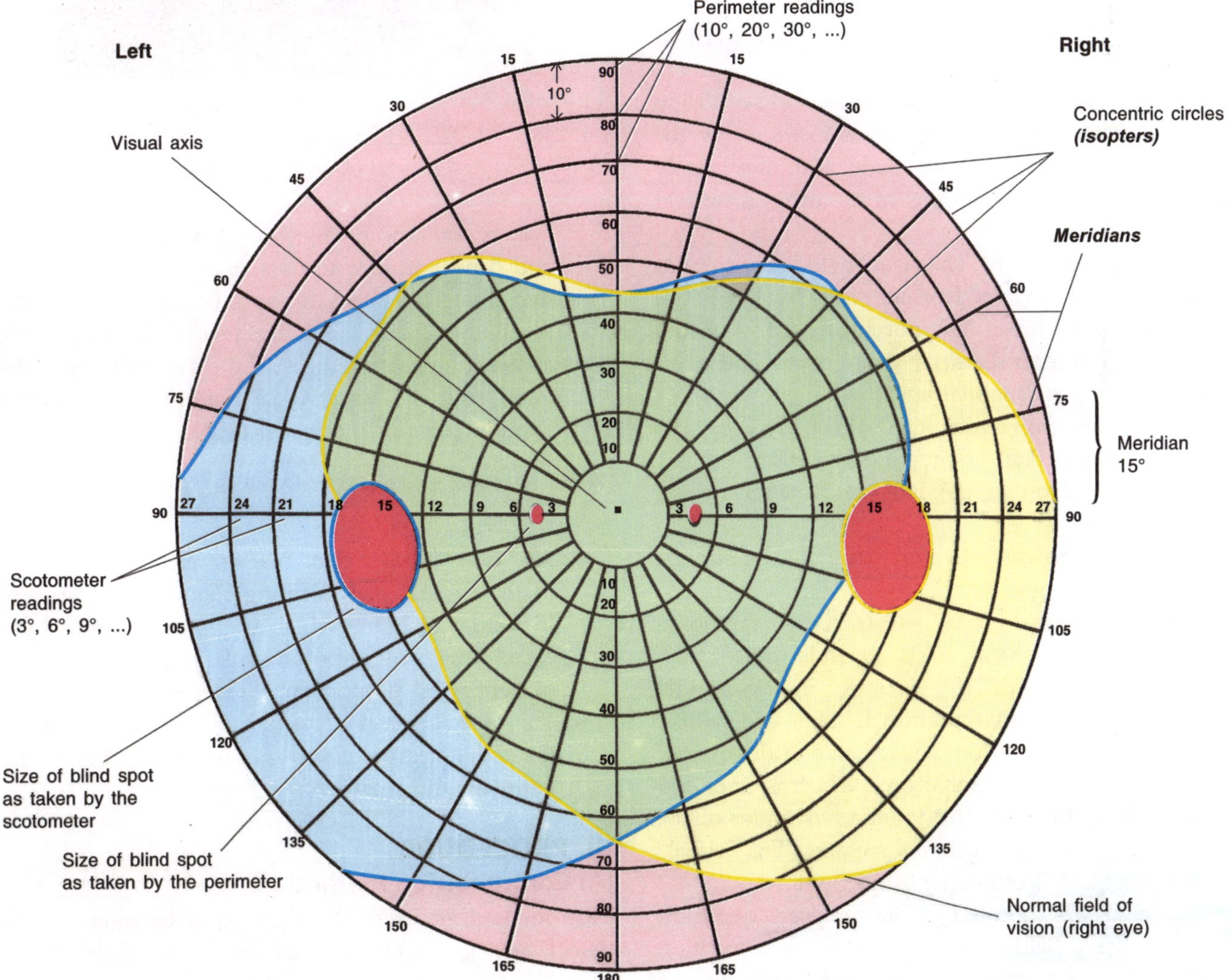

Fig. 3.15.2 The perimetric chart

acuity, called **isopters**; therefore, all the points on a particular concentric line subtend the same visual angle with the visual axis at the nodal point of the eye.

(ii) The radii of the circles are marked at 15° intervals, which denote the various **meridians**.

(iii) For ready comparison, the normal limits of the field of vision of both the eyes are drawn on the chart. A small oval black dot marked on the horizontal meridian, 15° on either side of the central fixation point represents the area of the normal **blind spot**.

(iv) The chart is attached to the back of the perimeter and it rotates with the arc.

II. THEORY

1. When we fix the eye upon an object, we see not only the object but also a number of objects in the neighbourhood more or less distinctly. The sum of the objects that form images upon the retina while the ***gaze*** (*i.e.* eye is looking steadily for some time) is fixed at a particular point, called the **field of vision**.
2. It should be noted that although the field of vision differs with each different act of fixation, yet the peripheral limits are the same and are largely determined by the margins of the orbit, nose and cheek.
3. **Extent of visual field**. The visual field is not circular because it is restricted on all sides by the bones of the orbital fossa. The normal extent of visual field with 10 mm diameter white object and good illustration *for monocular vision* is:
   (i) Superior (upwards): 60° - restricted by the superior orbital margin and brows.
   (ii) Temporal (outwards): 100° - restricted by orbital margin.
   (iii) Inferior (downwards): 75° - restricted by inferior orbital margin.
   (iv) Medial (inwards): 60° - restricted by the nose.
   For Binocular Vision. Field extends more than 200° laterally, and 140° vertically in the middle of what is a circular portion to each eye with a diameter of about 120°; on each side of this paired area is a lateral semilunar area which is unpaired (*monocular*), this accounts for the remainder of the field. It is called the *temporal crescent.* (Fig. 3.15.3)
4. **Physiological Scotoma** or **Blind Spot**
   This is an area located in the temporal quadrant of the visual field in which there is no perception of light. This corresponds to the **optic disc,** *i.e.* the small area of retina where optic nerve leaves the eye. It contains no light sensitive receptors (rods and cones) as a result, vision is not possible over this area. Therefore, this spot is called *blind spot.* As the optic disc lies 3 mm medial to and slightly above the posterior pole of the eye ball hence the blind spot lies approx. 15° lateral to the central fixation point of the visual field.

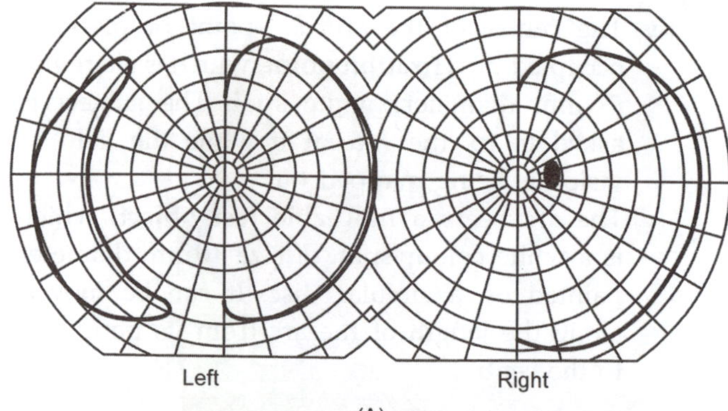

(A)

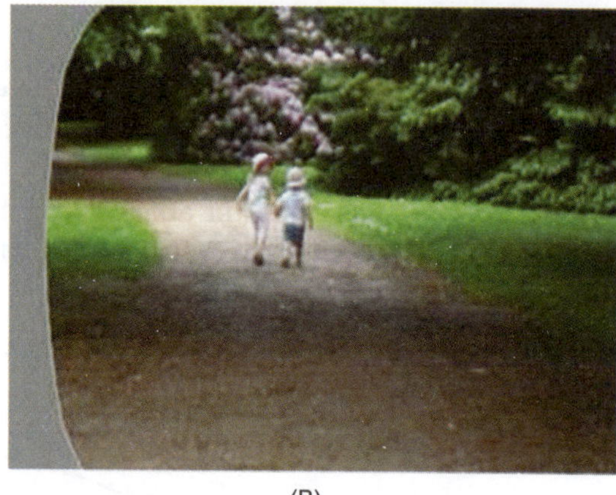

(B)

Fig. 3.15.3 (A) Monocular temporal crescent
(B) An actual view of figure above

Note: *Blind spot measures about 7.5° in height and 5.5° in width.*

5. The two visual fields, one for each eye, overlap in the medial part forming the so-called area of **binocular vision** in which an object is seen by both eyes. It plays an important role in the appreciation of depth and proportion of objects.
6. The mapping out of visual field is important for the diagnosis of: glaucoma, lesions in the visual pathway and retina.

III. PROCEDURE

(A) Confrontation method

This method is used clinically as a bedside test to detect any gross changes in the visual field. *Steps:* (Fig. 3.15.4)

1. Each eye must be examined separately.

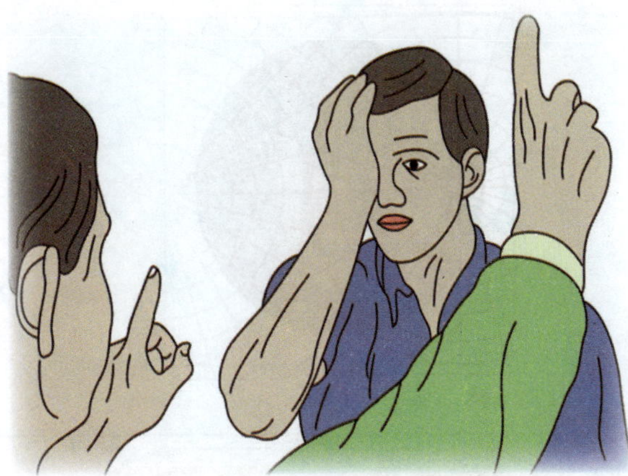

Fig. 3.15.4 Examination of visual field by confrontation method

2. The subject sits with his back to the light and facing the examiner at a distance of about 1/2 metre.
3. If his right eye is to be tested, ask him to place his hand on his left and look steadily at your own left eye. Look steadily yourself at the subject's right eye, your own right eye being closed. This is to maintain both eyes in the same straight line.
4. Hold up your left hand in a plane midway between his face and your own, and at first at almost full arm's length to the side. Keep moving the fingers of the hand, bringing it nearer until you yourself can just 'with the tail of your eye' catch the movements of the fingers.
5. Then ask the patient whether he sees them, telling him meanwhile to be sure not to take his own eye off yours. If he fails to see the fingers, keep bringing the hand until he sees them.
6. Test the field in this fashion in every direction, upwards, downwards to right, and to left, using the extent of your own field for the purpose of comparison.

Note: Do not cross the hand, *i.e.* for the left half, use the left hand and for the right half, use the right hand.

(B) Perimetry

1. **Fixing the perimeter chart.** Place the metallic arc in the horizontal position (90° meridian) on the right of the subject. The chart paper is then fixed at the back of the perimeter so that its centre may correspond with the visual axis. Finally adjust the chart paper so that the 90° meridian on it may correspond with the metallic arc.
2. Ensure illumination is adequate and if the subject wears spectacles, they should be removed; else its frame will restrict the visual field.

Note: Contact lenses need not be removed.

3. Make the subject comfortably seated in front of the apparatus; ask him to rest his chin on the appropriate chin rest (use the right chin rest for testing the left eye and vice versa).
4. Adjust the level of the head of the subject so that the lower lid of the eye under test may touch the tip of the levelling bar. This brings the eye in line with the fixation point. Fix the chin in this position.
5. The other eye is covered by placing the hand on it. Ask the subject to fix his gaze of test eye on the central fixation object. Instruct him not to shift his gaze from the point.
6. The metallic arc is adjusted in a particular meridian. The field of vision is first tested with a white object, 5 mm in diameter. Put the target object at the farthest point on the arc and gradually bring it forward by means of the rod. Instruct the subject to indicate point at which he just sees the object. This reading in degrees on the arc is marked on the perimetric chart for that particular meridian.

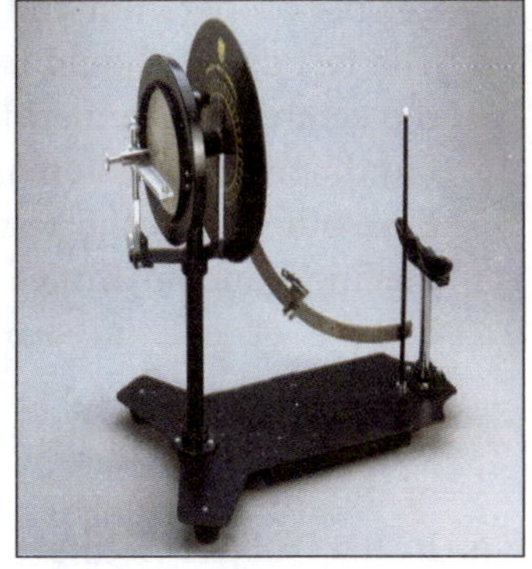

7. Move the target object further throughout the length of the arc up to the fixation point in order to detect any blind spot within the field of vision.
8. Repeat the whole procedure at an interval of 15 degrees (12 meridians) till the field of vision is marked in four quadrants.
9. All the points in different meridians joined together give the limit of the field of vision for that eye. This is **monocular field of vision**. Similarly, test the other eye; use different marks.
10. **Mapping of blind spot**. Fix the metallic arc in the horizontal meridian in the temporal quadrant. Repeat the whole procedure (step 6); at a certain point, the target object (white spot in the black circle) will disappear, but will reappear when the object is moved further towards the fixation point. By marking the points at which the spot disappears and reappears, the location of the blind spot is found.
11. Label the chart paper properly indicating:
    (i) Name, age and sex of the subject
    (ii) Date and time
    (iii) Size (in mm) and colour of the test object
    (iv) Type of illumination in the room (natural/artificial), whether adequate or inadequate

(v) The subject's cooperation and reliability of the response; whether good, fair or poor.

> **Important Note:** Map the visual field for coloured test objects, red, green and blue; and also of a colourblind subject and compare with a normal subject.

IV. PRECAUTIONS

1. Illumination should be adequate.
2. The fixation of the eye to be rigidly maintained while testing.
3. Explain the procedure to the subject beforehand to get his cooperation and confidence.
4. The test object should be moved from periphery to the centre in each meridian; this helps to detect the blind spot and scotoma.
5. Eye, other than the test eye, should be closed by placing hand in front of it and not by voluntary closure of eye lid; care should be taken while covering the other eye with hand; it should not project in front of the nose and obstruct the field of the other eye.
6. If the subject wears spectacles, they should be removed.
7. Keep the colour, size and illumination of the object constant for any one reading.
8. The healthy eye should always be tested first to get an idea of the normal field of vision of the subject.

V. PHYSIOLOGICAL SIGNIFICANCE

A. Size of field of vision varies with:

1. The size of the test object: the extent of visual field is directly related to the size of the object.
2. The colour of the object.
   (i) In general, the field of vision for the blue object is the largest, followed by yellow, red and green in that order.
   (ii) The field of vision for blue and yellow is roughly 10° less in each direction than that for white, and for red and green another 10°.
   (Colour is a poor stimulus for light sensitive receptors as compared to 'white' which contains the wavelength of all spectral colours.)
3. The contrast of the test object with background
4. The state of the adaptation of the eye
5. Whether the object is stationary or moving. Moving stimuli are best perceived in the peripheral field since the specialized movement sensitive receptor cells are located mainly in the peripheral parts of the retina.
6. Illumination: visual field directly proportional to the intensity of illumination.

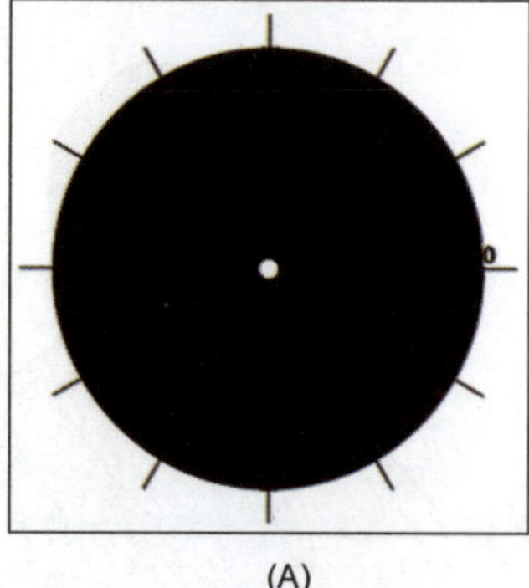

(A)

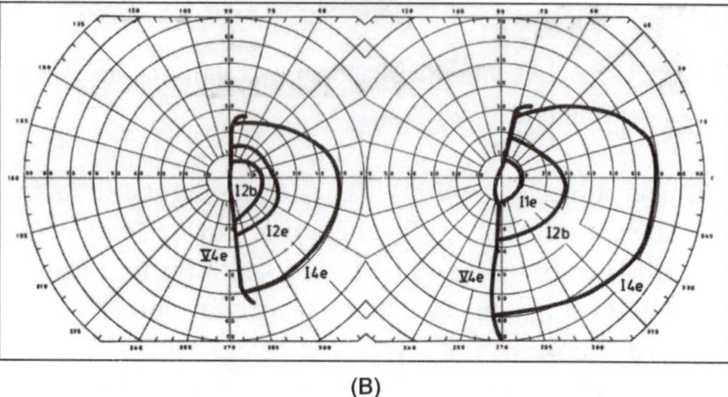

(B)

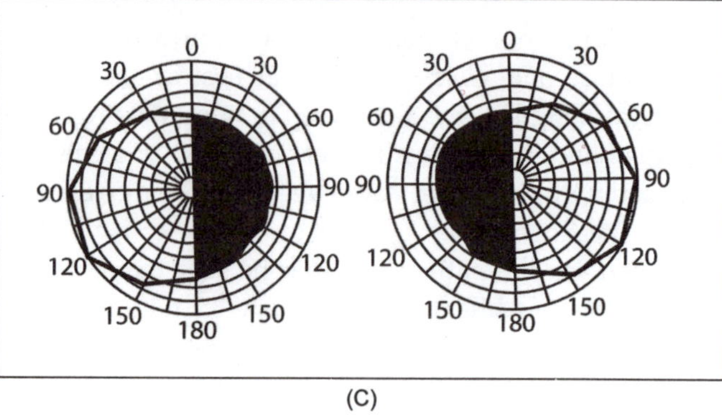

(C)

Fig. 3.15.5 Some common defects in the field of vision
(A) Complete Anopia with macular sparing
(B) Right homonymous hemianopia
(C) Heteronymous hemianopia (Binasal)

B. The effects of the lesions of the visual pathways are described in terms of the field of vision. Some common defects found in the field of vision are: (Fig. 3.15.5)

1. **Anopia**; complete loss of visual field, *i.e.* blindness, seen following an injury to the optic nerve.
2. **Hemianopia**; blindness of half of the visual field; it is further divided into:
   (i) *Homonymous hemianopia* – when the same halves of the field of vision in both eyes are lost; for example, loss of right or left halves of the field of vision in both the eyes, seen in lesion of the optic tract.
   (ii) *Heteronymous hemianopia* – when different halves of the visual field are lost in two eyes.

For example, loss of right half of visual field in one eye and loss of left half of visual field in the other eye. Therefore, it is of two types either **bitemporal** or **binasal**; seen in the lesions of outer margins of the optic chiasma (binasal hemianopia) or lesion of optic chaisma (bitemporal hemianopia).

IMPORTANT VIVA-VOCE QUESTIONS

Q.1. *Give the normal extent of the field of vision.*

Ans. Page 206.

Q.2. *Give the position and extent of the blind spot.*

Ans. Page 206.

Q.3. *How will you map out the area of the blind spot?*

Ans. Page 207.

Q.4. *Define: optical axis, nodal point, visual axis, isopter, scotoma.*

Ans. (i) The line joining the anterior pole to the posterior pole of the eyeball is called the **optical axis** while the line joining the fixation point to fovea centralis is the **visual axis**.

(ii) The centre point of the lens is called **nodal point**.

(iii) Isopter (page 206).

(iv) Scotoma - area in the visual field where no perception of light occurs.

Q.5. *Enumerate the factors influencing the field of vision.*

Ans. Page 208.

Q.6. *Why should the field of vision not be mapped with spectacles on?*

Ans. Page 207.

Q.7. *What is the relevance of doing perimetry in a person suffering from glaucoma?*

Ans. Glaucoma by increasing intraocular tension may produce various defects in the field of vision (page 208).

Q.8. *Mention the precautions for performing perimetry.*

Ans. Page 208.

Q.9. *Give some causes of scotoma.*

Ans. (i) Unilateral scotoma seen in: demyelination of optic nerve; glaucoma.

(ii) bilateral scotoma causes are: alcoholism, vitamin B_{12} deficiency, lesion in visual cortex.

Q.10. *What type of defect in the visual field will be produced in the lesion of occipital cortex?*

Ans. Its lesion produces only discrete quandrantic (1/4th) visual field defects because of the specific anatomic arrangement of the optic nerve fibres in the occipital cortex.

STUDY NOTES

RESULTS AND DISCUSSION

....

....

....

....

....

....

....

....

....

....

Date: ....

16 Retinoscopy; Ophthalmoscopy

Retinoscopy

I. APPARATUS

Subject, dark room, light source, retinoscope

II. PROCEDURE

Retinoscopy is an objective method of assessing the refractive state of the eye. It is usually performed in a dark room after instilling Homatropine 0.5 to 2% in the subject's eye. Homatropine is pupillary dilator and also paralyses the accommodation power. The retinoscope is a plane mirror with a central perforation mounted on a handle (Fig. 3.16.1).

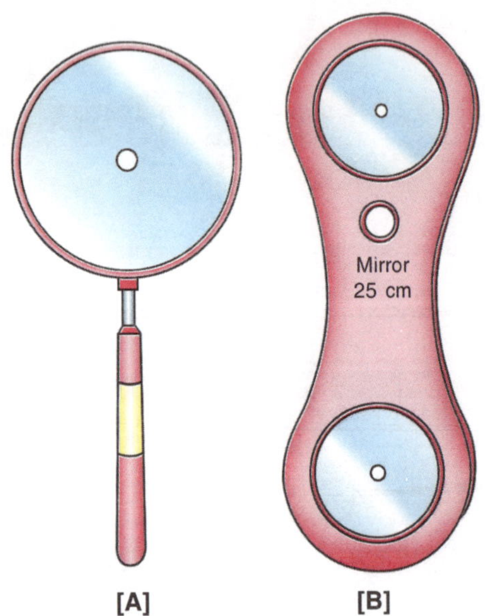

Fig. 3.16.1 Retinoscope: (A) Plane mirror and (B) Priestley-Smith mirror

Steps in Retinoscopy

1. In a dark room, the examiner sits at a distance of 1 meter from the subject.
2. Using a plane mirror retinoscope, a reflected beam of light is thrown into the subject's eye.

Note: In the self-illuminating retinoscope, a source of light is provided in the instrument itself.

3. The examiner then looks through the central perforation into the subject's eye and observes a **red reflex** or **glow** at the pupillary level. At one border of the illuminated reflex, a black crescentric shadow/image can be seen. This is the edge of the illuminated glow. (Fig. 3.16.2 A and B)

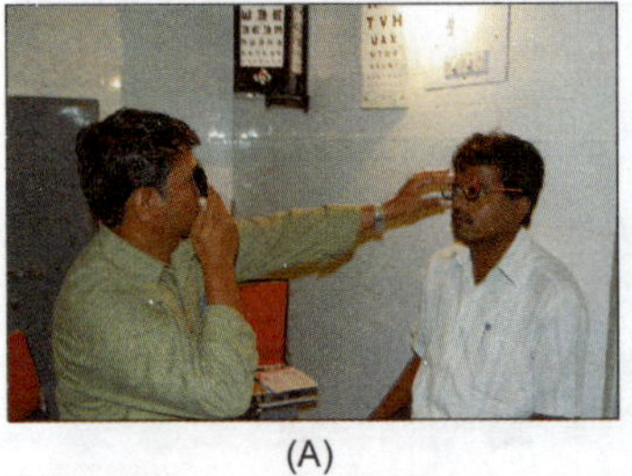

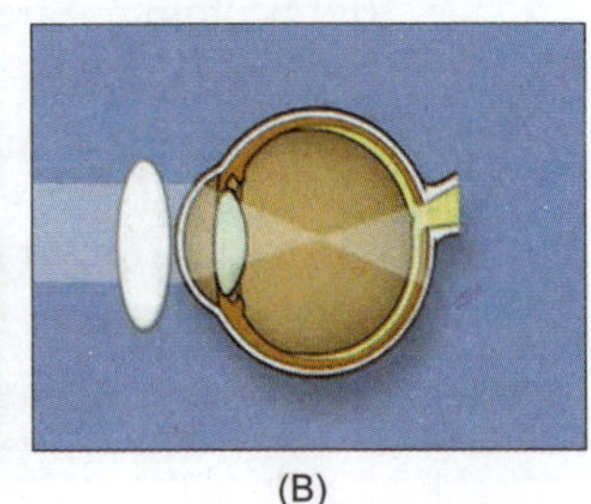

(A) (B)

Fig. 3.16.2 Retinoscopy (A) procedure and (B) optical principle

4. Keeping the glow in view, the mirror is tilted in horizontal, vertical and oblique axes. The direction of the movements of the shadow/image is noted while the mirror is tilted.
   (i) *If the shadow/image moves in the same direction* as the tilt of the mirror, the subject's eye shows either emmetropia, hypermetropia or myopia of less than 1D (diopter). To find out the actual refractive state of the eye, the procedure is repeated by using in a trial frame, convex lenses of increasing power in front of the subject's eye, till the shadow/image moves in the opposite direction. Note the refractive power of the convex lens in diopter that first reversed the direction of the image. To this observation, a correction factor of minus 1D has to be added. If the convex lens of +0.5D reverses the movement of the image then the subject has a refractive error of +0.5 – 1.0D = –0.5D (**Myopia**).

(ii) *If the shadow/image moves in a direction opposite to that of the tilt,* the eye shows myopia of more than 1D. Using concave lenses, in front of the subject's eye, the lens required to reverse the original movement is noted. If the concave lens of - 0.5D is required for reversal, the subject has myopia of -1.5D (-0.5D - 1.0D) in that eye.

III. CLINICAL SIGNIFICANCE

Retinoscopy is used to determine:

1. The refractive state of the eye: emmetropia (normal), hypermetropia or myopia.
2. Opacities in the media of the eye (cornea, anterior chamber, lens, vitreous humor) will appear as black lines against the red reflex (or glow) of the fundus.

IMPORTANT VIVA-VOCE QUESTIONS

Q.1. *Derive the refractive state of the eye if the lenses required to reverse the original movement of the images are: (i) +1.0D, (ii) +2.0D, (iii) -2.0D (the correction factor is 1.0D).*

Ans. (i) +1.0D - 1.0D = 0.0D (Emmetropia)
(ii) +2.0D - 1.0D = +1.0D (Hypermetropia)
(iii) -2.0D - 1.0D = -3.0D (Myopia)

Ophthalmoscopy

1. APPARATUS

Subject, ophthalmoscope, dark room, light source

The Ophthalmoscope (invented by Hermann von Helmholtz in 1950)

An ophthalmoscope consists of the following components: (Fig. 3.16.3)

1. **The Handle**. It possesses three mirrors and also serves as a case for dry cells.
2. The three mirrors are: two concave (one large and one small) and one plane.
   (i) The **large concave** mirror is used for indirect ophthalmoscopy and the **smaller** one for direct ophthalmoscopy.
   (ii) The plane mirror is used for retinoscopy.
   (iii) Each mirror is having a **central aperture**, called **sight hole** or **viewing aperture**. It is placed just above a system of prisms which reflects a parallel beam of light from a low voltage bulb. The aperture is divided into two parts:

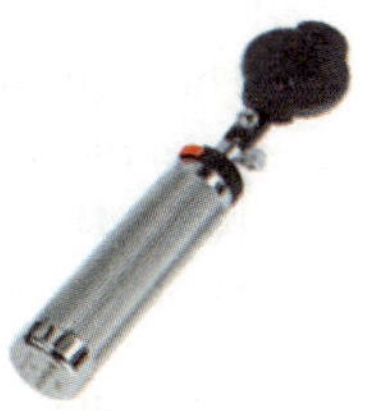

   (a) lower half for throwing light into the subject's eye, and
   (b) upper half for the examiner's observation.
3. **Serrated (or notched) disc**. It contains a series of lenses. The disc can be rotated to move the desired lens against the viewing aperture. The diopteric power of the lens in use is indicated on the back of the instrument.
4. **On/Off switch**. By rotating this ring, the amount of light being directed into the subject's eye can be controlled.

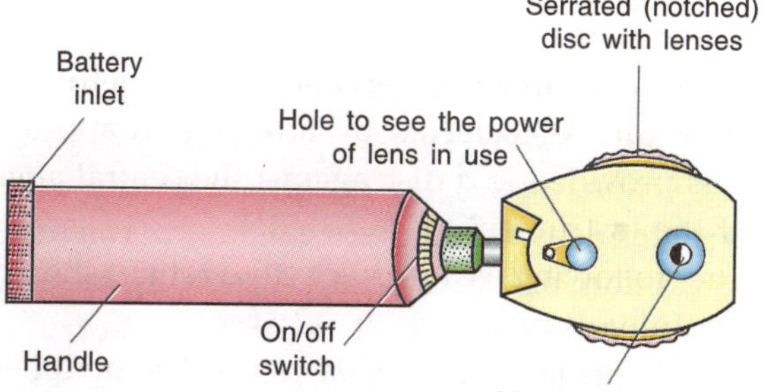

Fig. 3.16.3 An ophthalmoscope

Important Note: If the examiner himself has any refractive error, he should use his glasses while using the ophthalmoscope.

II. PROCEDURE

Ophthalmoscopy is the procedure to study the retina of the eye with the ophthalmoscope. This procedure is based on the principle of illuminating a part of the retina and seeing a magnified image of the retina with the aid of an instrument called ophthalmoscope.

Steps in ophthamoscopy

A. Indirect Ophthalmoscopy

1. Prepare the subject as already described (page 210); in a dark room the subject sits at a distance of one meter in front of the examiner. Using the **large concave mirror**, hold the ophthalmoscope in the right hand and reflect the light into the subject's eye. An illuminated and ill-defined fundus glow (**red reflex**), in the pupil of the subject's eye, can be seen by the examiner through the aperture of the instrument. (Fig. 3.16.4 A and B)

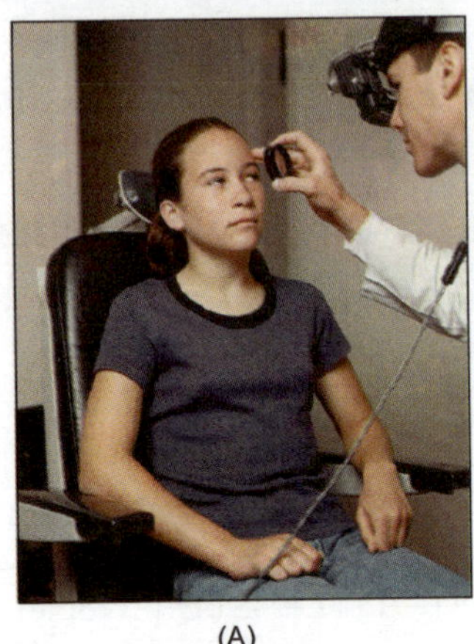

(A)

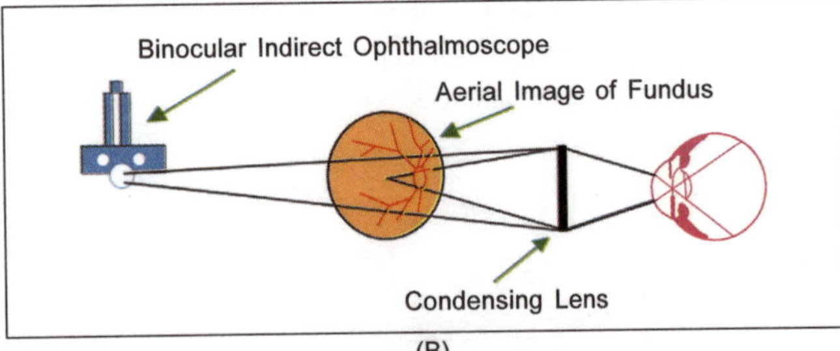

(B)

Fig. 3.16.4 Indirect ophthalmoscopy (A) Proceedure and (B) Optical principle

2. A convex lens (+13D) is now interposed between the subject's eye and the examiner. By adjusting the distance of the lens, a real, inverted, magnified image of the retina is observed between the lens and the examiner's eye.
3. Carefully examine the fundus occuli and look for: (Fig. 3.16.6 A)
   (i) *Optic disc:* The subject must look in the direction of the examiner's right ear.
   (ii) *Macular region:* The subject must look into the mirror.
   (iii) *Periphery of the fundus:* Direct the subject to look upwards, downwards, to the right and to the left.
4. This procedure helps in the study of the large portions of the retina. However, the magnification of the image is low (approx. five times). The method can be very useful when the subject has gross errors of refraction.

B. Direct Ophthalmoscopy

In this, a virtual, erect (upright) and much more magnified (**about fifteen times**) retinal image can be seen by the direct observation of the interior of the eye.

1. The same as point (1) of indirect ophthalmoscopy
2. While examining the right eye of the subject, the examiner stands on the right side of the subject, using the **small concave mirror**, holds the instrument in his right hand and uses his right eye.
3. Keeping his eye against the aperture, the light is thrown on the subject's eye from the side. A pale red glow is observed in the subject's eye. This is the ill-defined image of the retina. (Fig. 3.16.5 A and B)

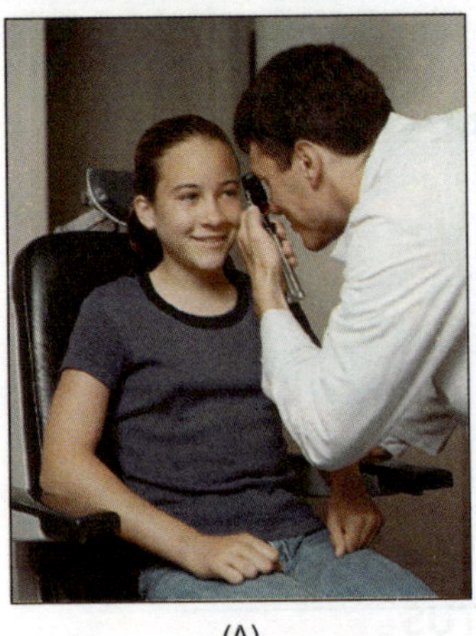

(A)

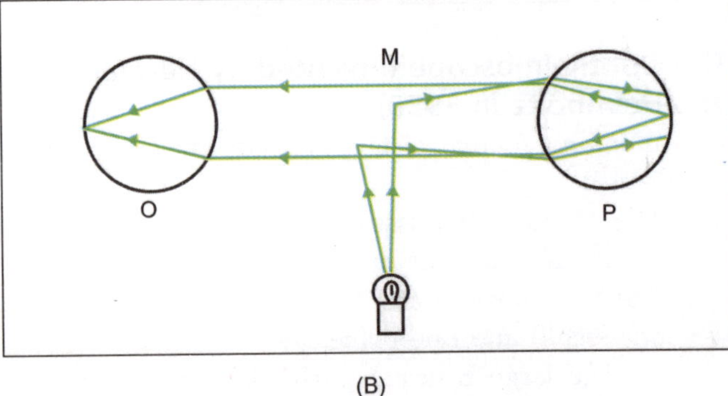

(B)

Fig. 3.16.5 Direct ophthalmoscopy (A) Procedure and (B) Optical principle

4. The ophthalmoscope is then moved as near as possible to the subject's eye keeping in view the **red reflex** till a well-defined portion of the retina is observed.

> **Note:** A distinct appearance of blood vessels coursing over a pinkish or brick red retina indicates that the examiner now obtained a well-defined view of the retina.

5. If the eye under observation is emmetropic, the error can be corrected by bringing an appropriate lens provided in a disc against the central aperture of the instrument.
6. The following features of the retina should be carefully examined: (Fig. 3.16.6-B)
   (i) *The peripheral part of the retina.* The periphery of the retina is seen lighter than the central area; occasional irregularities of pigmentation and lighter areas may be seen.

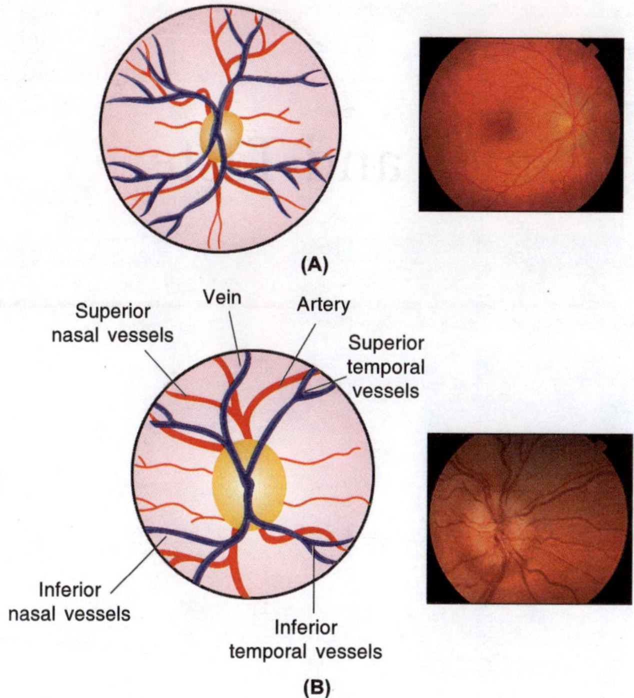

Fig. 3.16.6 Optic disc and vessels as seen by the ophthalmoscope (A) by indirect method; (B) by direct method (**Inset:** An actual view)

(ii) *The optic disc*

(a) *Shape:* round or slightly oval; diameter 1.5 to 1.7 mm.

(b) ***Physiological cup:*** In its central part, there is usually a depression in the disc, the physiological cup. The cup is paler than the surrounding disc, and from it the retinal vessels enter and leave the eye.

(c) *Edge of the disc:* well defined.

(iii) *Position and appearance of the fovea centralis (macular region).* This is situated 1.5 disc diameter from the temporal border of the optic disc. It is darker in colour than the surrounding fundus with glistering appearance.

(iv) *The retinal blood vessels.* These radiate from the disc, dividing abruptly into many branches as they pass towards the periphery of the retina. The retinal arteries are narrower (about 1/3rd) than the veins; brighter red in colour and have a brighter longitudinal lines.

IMPORTANT VIVA-VOCE QUESTIONS

Q.1. *Give the differences between indirect and direct ophthalmoscopy.*

Ans. Page 211.

Q.2. *What information can be obtained by ophthalmoscopy?*

Ans. Valuable information which can be obtained by ophthalmoscopy is:

(i) The state of the optic nerve and of the arteries and veins of the retina

(ii) The detection of local ophthalmic disorders

Q.3. *What is physiological cup?*

Ans. See above.

Q.4. *Describe the ophthalmoscopic features of the retina.*

Ans. See above.

STUDY NOTES

RESULTS AND DISCUSSION

....

....

....

....

....

....

....

....

Date: ....

17 Tests of Hearing, Smell and Taste

TESTS FOR HEARING

Refer to page 251.

TESTS FOR SMELL

Refer to page 240.

TESTS FOR TASTE

Refer to page 249.

Date: ....

18 An Introduction to Clinical Examination

A good clinical examination requires a cooperative subject and a quite warm and well-lighted room. It includes **general physical examination,** *i.e.* examination of the general state of the patient, and detailed examination of different systems (**systemic examination**).

Pre-requisites for clinical examination

The following conditions should be fulfilled before the start of any clinical exmaination.

1. Presence of natural sunlight. Daylight is better than artificial light because the latter may mask changes in skin colour. For example:
   (i) the faint yellow tinge of slight jaundice, or
   (ii) the bluish colouration of cyanosis, or
   (iii) the pallor due to anaemia
2. Every attempt should be made to reassure and relax the subject. This can be achieved by:
   (i) putting him at ease and encouraging him to talk freely, and
   (ii) explaining the test procedure beforehand which is to be carried out on him; impress upon the subject that you will be as gentle as possible.
3. Ideally, a relative or a female attendant should be present when a male doctor is examining a female subject. This is essential, both to reassure the subject and to protect the doctor for subsequent accusation of improper conduct.
4. Complete exposure of the body parts to be examined of the subject. For a thorough examination, the subject should be asked to take off all his clothes and should then be covered by a dressing gown or bed sheet.
5. Always stand on the right-hand side of the subject. It is helpful for a right-handed doctor, especially when, the physical examination of the subject begins.

THE GENERAL PHYSICAL EXAMINATION

The general physical examination is the minimum necessary requirement before any systemic examination is to be carried out in the subject. This provides much useful information which serves to remind the doctor of any omissions. Such a routine form of examination has to be modified according to the need of the subject. For example, a complete examination of the respiratory system in a patient with breathing signs and symptoms. This kind of examination should be carried out as gently as possible. During the performance of general physical examination the following points should be observed.

1. General appearance

(i) Does the subject look healthy, unwell or ill? His facial expressions may indicate his real feelings better than his words.
(ii) Is his appearance consistent with his age? Much can be learnt from the subject's physique (height and weight).
(iii) The gait, *i.e.* the way he walks. The gait should be observed in persons able to walk. It is of major importance in the diagnosis of many brain disorders.

2. Intelligence

Bizarre (awkward) behaviour may be a sign of subnormal intelligence.

3. Mental and emotional state

An over-anxious person may be restless, with wide palpebral fissures and sweating palms.

4. Speech/expression

Does the person speak at all or is he silent? If so, is this deliberate, organic or hysterical?

5. Skin

The major important abnormalities in skin examination are pallor, yellowness, pigmentation, cyanosis and cutaneous eruption.

(i) *Pallor:* As a rule, it is caused by a condition of anaemia. The pallor of skin, mucous membranes of mouth/conjunctivae and creases of palms give a better indication of anaemia than skin colour, as anaemia is to be judged by the colour of the blood rather than that of the subject.

(ii) *Yellowness:* The yellow discolouration of the skin may be due to:
   (a) jaundice
   (b) hypercarotenemia, or
   (c) tobacco stains

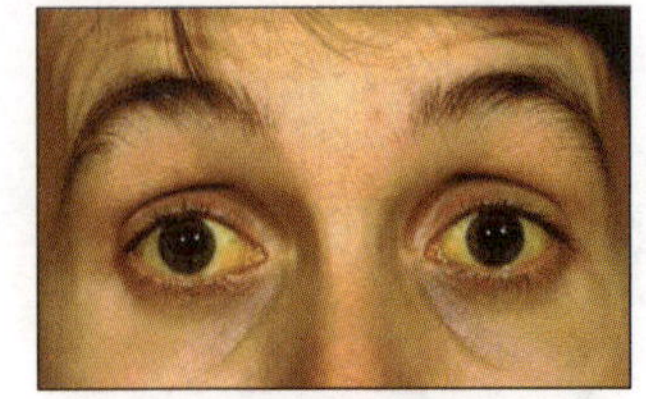

Fig. 3.18.1 Yellow discolouration of sclera in jaundice

The first site where jaundice is clinically detected is the sclera (Fig. 3.18.1).

(iii) *Cyanosis:* The bluish discolouration of skin and/or mucous membrane due to presence of at least 5 gm of reduced haemoglobin per 100 ml of blood in the capillaries is called cyanosis. It is commonly seen at sites where the skin is thin, for example (Fig. 3.18.2):
   (a) The mucous membrane of the under surface of tongue
   (b) lips
   (c) ear lobes
   (d) nail beds, and
   (e) tip of nose

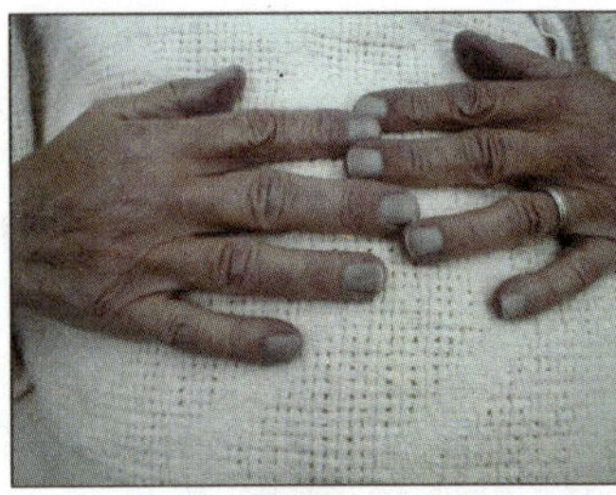

(A)

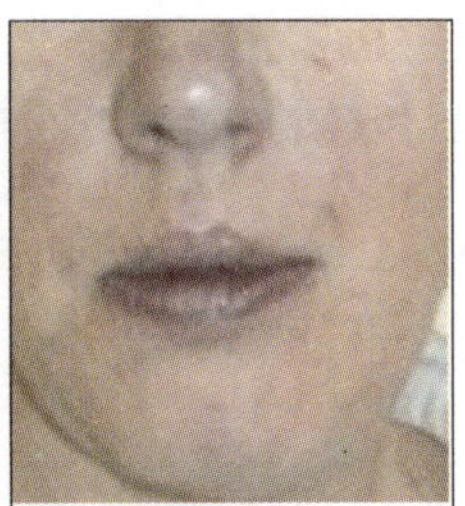

(B)

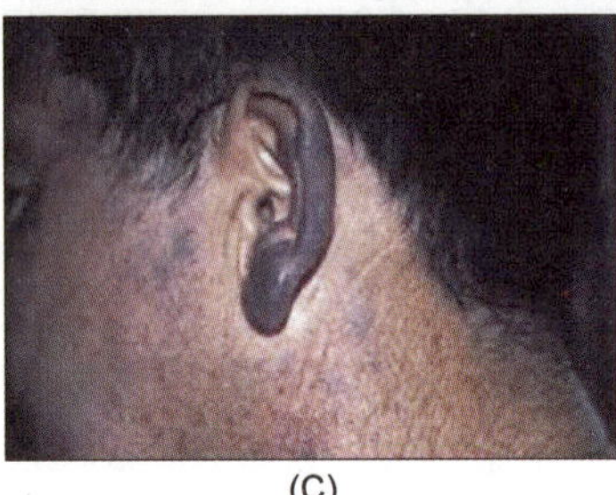

(C)

Fig. 3.18.2 Common sites of cyanosis (A) Nail beds (B) Lips and tip of nose (C) Ear lobe

6. Temperature

While taking the temperature, remember the following points:

(i) The thermometer must be accurate and must be kept in position for 1-2 minutes to allow the mercury to reach body temperature
(ii) In conscious adults, the temperature is taken in the mouth or in the axilla.
(iii) In young children, the thermometer should be placed in the fold of the groin, and the thigh flexed on the abdomen, or it may be inserted into the rectum.

Note: The temperature of the mouth and rectum is generally at least 0.5°C higher than that of the groin or axilla.

(iv) Normal temperature range is: 36.3–37.1°C, *i.e.* 97.3–98.8°F.

7. Pulse rate

(i) Count the pulse for a full minute. The pulse rate in a healthy person varies from 60-80 beats/minute.
(ii) The common causes of:
   (a) *rapid pulse* are immediately after exercise, excitement, anxiety, bleeding, fever and thyrotoxicosis;
   (b) *slow pulse* are regular exercise/sports, hypothyroidism and complete heart block.

(For details, refer to page 233)

8. Respiration

Count the respiration for a full minute by looking at the subject's abdominal movements when his attention is distracted from the breathing. The normal rate in an adult is 12 to 16 respirations/minute.

9. Eyes

Look for : jaundice (Fig. 3.18.1), pallor, exophthalmos (bulging eyes) (Fig. 3.18.3).

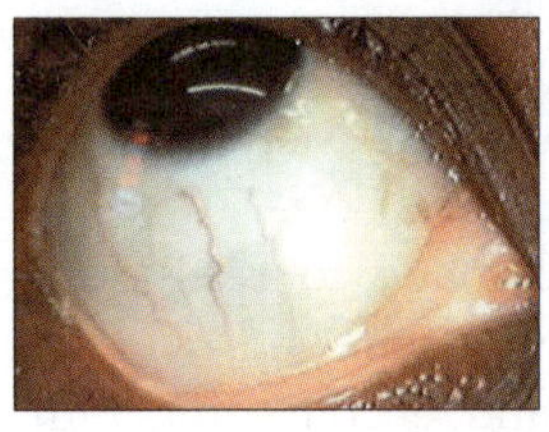

(A)

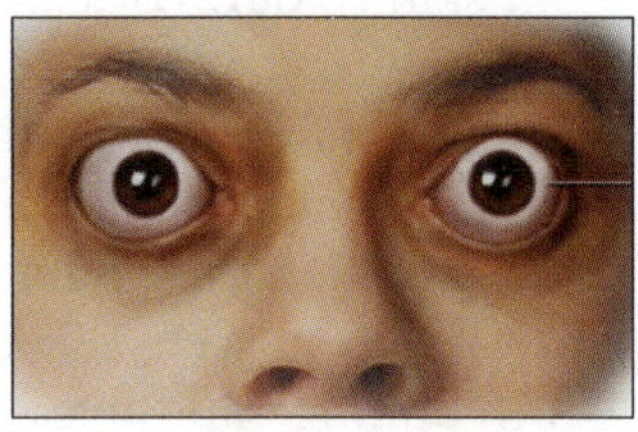

(B)

Fig. 3.18.3 Eyes: (A) Pale (B) Bulging eyes

10. Neck

Look for the enlargement of lymph nodes and thyroid gland; venous distension, pulsations of carotid vessels, position of trachea and jugular venous pressure.

THE SYSTEMIC EXAMINATION

A common approach is being followed clinically for all systemic examinations. It is helpful to have a logical sequence to follow and if this is done as a matter of routine then no important points will be omitted. The suggested sequence is: *Inspection, palpation, percussion and auscultation.*

(A) Inspection

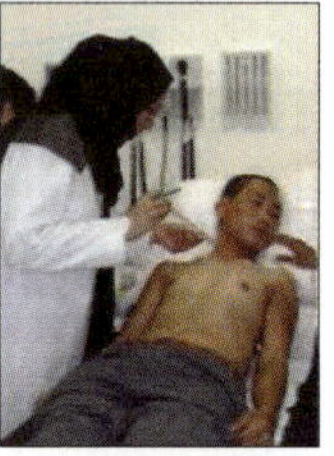

It means the art of observing. The following conditions should be taken care of before an inspection is carried out on a subject:

1. The examination should be done ideally in a good daylight and the warm room.

2. The subject should be at ease and fully relaxed.
3. Completely expose the part of the body to be examined.
4. Observe the part from different positions before a decision is made.

(B) Palpation

It means examination by the flat surface of fingers or palm.

Requirements

1. Stand on the subject's right side and explain the test procedure to him beforehand.
2. Ensure your hands are warm and that you will be as gentle as possible.
3. Tell the subject to relax as best as he can.

Method (Fig. 3.18.4)

Start by placing the right hand flat on the part to be palpated with the wrist and forearm in the same horizontal plane, where possible. The art is to 'mould' the relaxed right hand to the body surface, and not to hold it rigid. The best movement is gentle but with firm pressure with the finger held almost straight with slight, flexion at the metacarpophalangeal joints.

Important Note: At all costs, avoid poking with the fingertips.

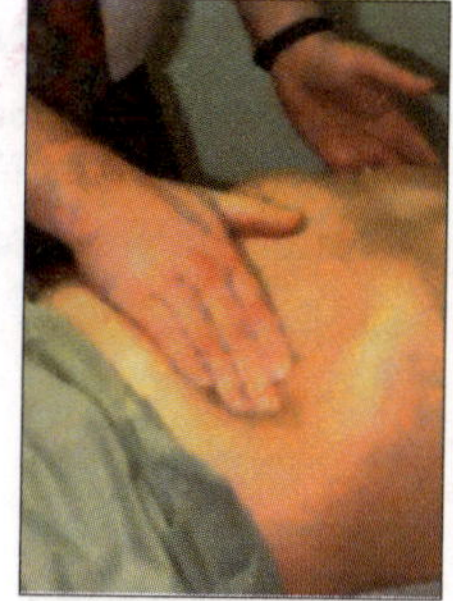

(A) The hand is held flat and relaxed and moulded to the abdominal wall

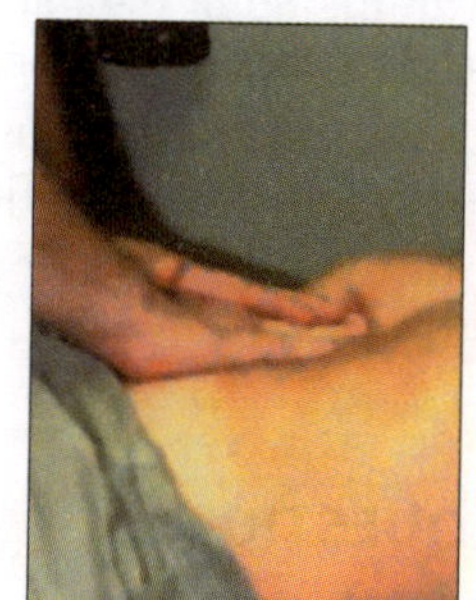

(B) The hand is held rigid and mostly **not** in contact with the abdominal wall

Fig. 3.18.4 (A) Correct and (B) incorrect method of palpation of abdomen

(C) Percussion

It means tapping or giving an impact.

Requirements

As already described above.

Method

How to percuss? Steps:

1. Place the middle finger (pleximeter finger) of the left hand firmly on the part to be percussed; other fingers should be well separated apart and should not touch the surface (Fig. 3.18.5 A).
2. The back of the middle phalanx of pleximeter finger is then struck with the tip of the middle finger of the right hand in a perpendicular direction.
3. The percussion movement should be carried out by flexion and extension at the wrist joint rather than the elbow.
4. As soon as the percussion stroke has been given, the striking finger must be lifted up, else it will damp the vibrations set up (Fig. 3.18.5 B).

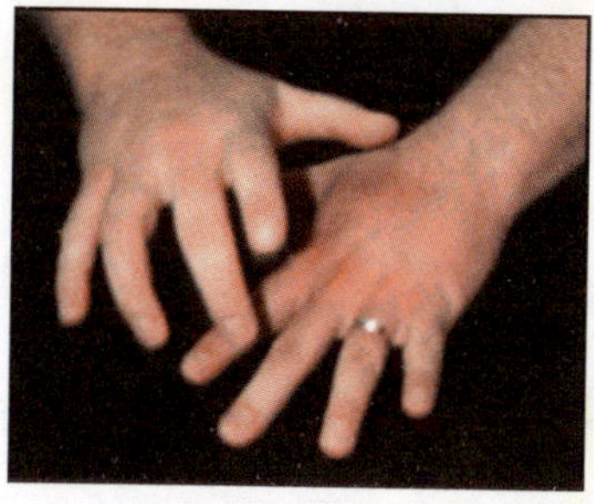

(A)

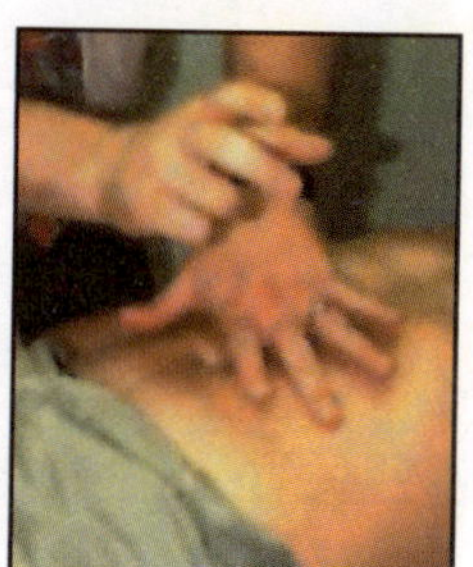

(B)

Fig. 3.18.5 Percussion steps A and B (Refer to text for details)

Note: Repeated heavy blows which may cause discomfort to the subject should not be given. At first, it is worth practising on yourself or on colleagues.

Character of sound produced

Depending on the body parts percussed, the characteristic percussion sounds (**Notes**) produced vary qualitatively and quantitatively. They are classified into three categories:

1. Hollow viscera containing a gas gives a *note* (sound), which is described as a ***Tympanic***. It is of a musical character.
2. A viscus like lungs in which air is trapped in tiny compartments gives a *note* described as ***Resonant***. It is of a low pitch and clear in character.
3. Solid viscera containing no air and made up of soft fleshy material or fluid gives a *note* which is described as ***dull***. It is of a high pitch, of a short duration and can be heard only in close surrounding.

Important Note: Percussion is always carried out from a resonant or tympanic area towards the dull area.

(D) Auscultation

It means listening with the help of a stethoscope.

Working of a stethoscope. It consists of two ear pieces (or ear knobs) which are joined together with the help of *metallic tubes* to a *Y-shaped* rubber tube. The other end of the rubber tube combines both a *bell type chest piece* and a *diaphragm* (Fig. 3.18.6).

(i) The *diaphragm* is suitable for the auscultation of high pitch and sharp sounds, such as heart sounds and breath sounds in adults.

(ii) The *bell* is suitable for the auscultation of low pitch and loud sounds such as the third and fourth heart sounds and breath sounds in children.

Note: Because of the thin chest wall, breath sounds are louder in children than in adults.

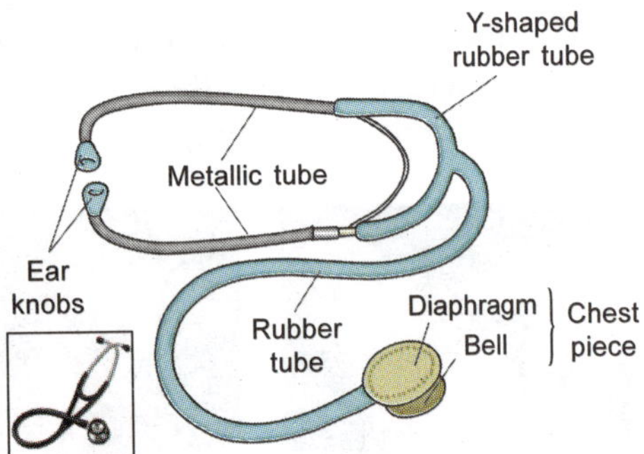

Fig. 3.18.6 The stethoscope (Littman's type)

Method

The **diaphragm** of the stethoscope should be placed lightly on one place and kept there until sounds are heard. It should not be moved from place to place. One must listen for several minutes before coming to any conclusion. Therefore, skill in auscultation depends on the ability to concentrate over one portion of the sound at a time.

Precautions

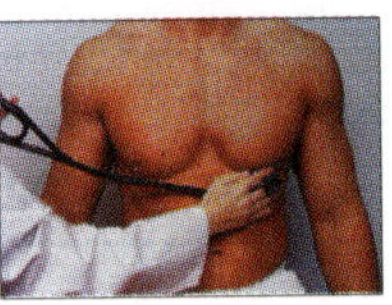

1. The ear piece should fit comfortably into the ears and exclude external sounds almost completely. They should be directed forward and medially into the ears along the direction of the ear canals.
2. Check for the normal functioning of the diaphragm by lightly tapping its diaphragm with a finger.

Important Note: Before making an attempt to examine the affected part, always first examine the normal counterpart on the opposite side. This will provide you with a good deal of information for comparison.

(For detailed systemic examination, refer to the individual system examination on the following pages).

OSPE

Aim: To percuss the abdomen or chest of the subject chart provided.

Procedure steps: Refer to page 217.

Checklist

1. Stands on the subject's right side and explains the test procedure. **(Yes/No)**
2. Ensures that his hands are warm. **(Yes/No)**
3. Exposes the part to be percussed. **(Yes/No)**
4. Places the middle finger of the left hand firmly on the abdomen or chest with other fingers well separated apart and not touching the surface. **(Yes/No)**
5. Strikes the miiddle phallanx of the left-hand finger firmly with the tip of the middle finger of the right hand in a perpendicular direction. **(Yes/No)**
6. Carries out the percussion movement of flexion and extension at the wrist joint. **(Yes/No)**
7. Lifts the striking finger immediately after the precussion stroke has been given. **(Yes/No)**

IMPORTANT VIVA-VOCE QUESTIONS

Q.1. *What conditions should be fulfilled before you proceed for doing a clinical examination on a subject?*

Ans. Page 215.

Q.2. *Why is natural light preferred over artificial light for doing a clinical examination?*

Ans. As the natural sunlight contains the wavelengths of all spectral colours, the different colours can be made out easily, hence any change in skin colour will not be masked.

Q.3. *What is the clinical significance of the general physical examination?*

Ans. General physical examination by providing much useful information, serves to remind the examiner of any omissions.

Q.4. *What will happen if palpation is carried out with a cold hand?*

Ans. Palpation, when carried out with a cold hand, results in the contraction of underlying muscles; now it will be difficult for the examiner to gain optimal information from the palpation of a poorly relaxed portion.

Q.5. *What is percussion? Give the basis of percussion 'notes'.*

Ans. Page 217.

Q.6. *Why should percussion always be carried out from resonant or tympanic area towards the dull area?*

Ans. This is because the resonant and tympanic sounds are clear sounds which can be heard from a distance; on the other hand, a dull sound is of a short duration and can only be heard in a close surrounding.

Q.7. *What are the components and functions of a stethoscope?*

Ans. Page 217.

Q.8. *What should be the direction of the 'ear knobs' while putting them into the ears?*

Ans. See above

STUDY NOTES

OBSERVATIONS, COMMENTS AND DISCUSSION

Date: ....

19 Clinical Examination of the Abdomen

Clinically, the examination of the abdomen of a subject is carried out by using a standard sequence of examination: *inspection, palpation, percussion and auscultation.* For the purposes of convenience, clinically whole abdomen is divided into nine regions by two lateral vertical planes and two horizontal planes (Fig. 3.19.1).

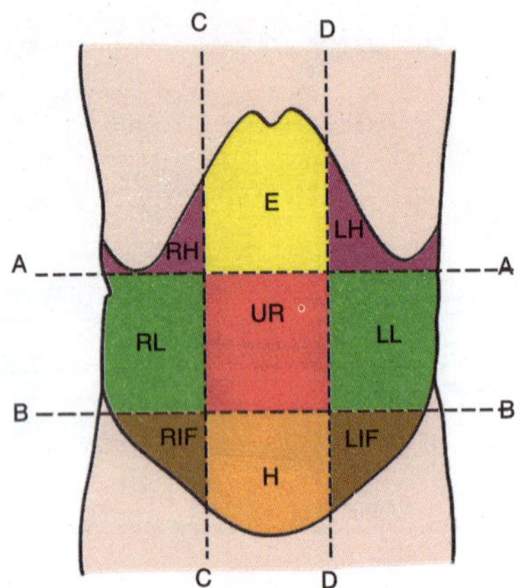

Fig. 3.19.1 Regions of the abdomen

RH and LH: right and left hypochondrium; E: epigastrium; RL and LL: right and left lumbar; UR: umbilical; RIF and LIF: right and left iliac fossa; H: hypogastrium (or supra pubic).
A-A: upper horizontal plane (to connect lowest points on costal margins; B-B: lower horizontal plane (to connect two tubercles of the iliac crests; C-C and D-D: right and left lateral vertical plane (to connect tip of 9th costal cartilage and femoral artery respectively).

I. INSPECTION (*Also refer to* page 216)

Make the subject to lie flat comfortably on his back with arms by his side and neck supported by pillows, on a firm couch or an examination table. Make sure there is good light and the room is warm. Stand on the subject's right side and ensure your hands are warm. The abdomen is fully exposed up to just above the xiphisternum and note the following features.

1. **Shape**. Look for normal abdominal contour (*i.e.* flat) and presence of sunken, fullness or distension. (Fig. 3.19.2)
   (i) A *sunken (scaphoid)* abdomen is seen in:

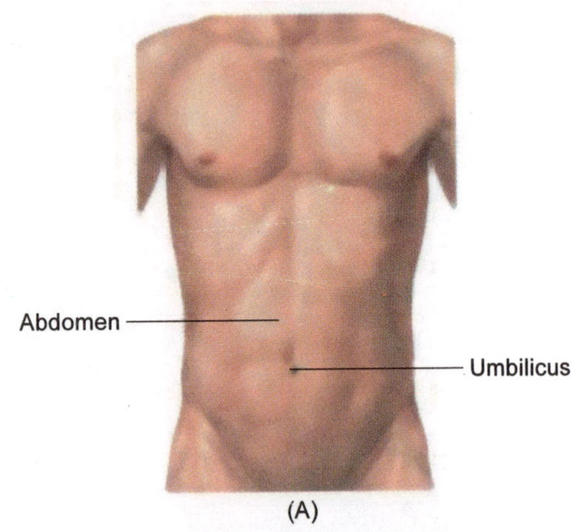

(A)

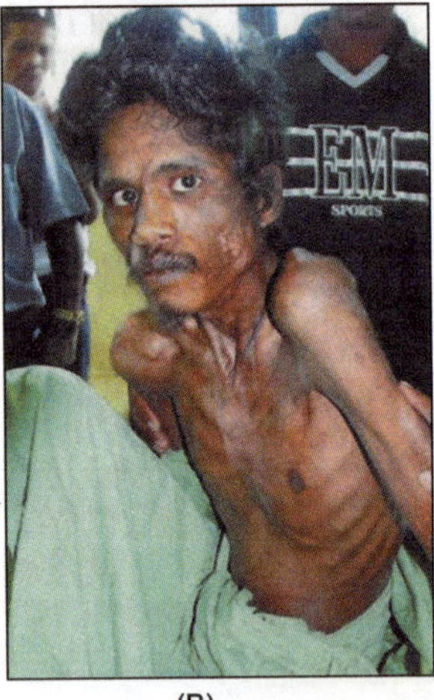

(B)

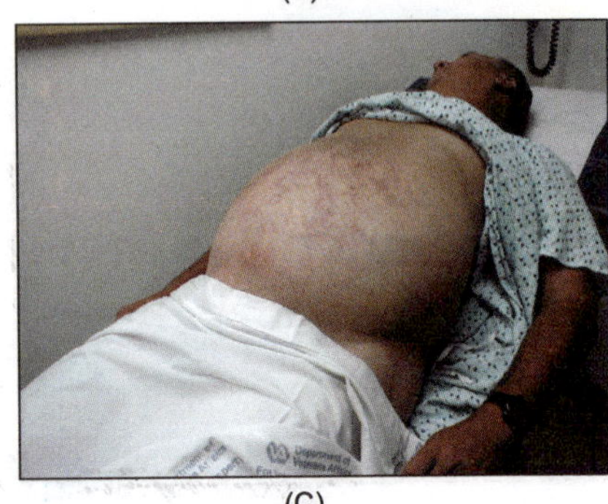

(C)

Fig. 3.19.2 Slope of Abdomen (A) Normal (flat) (B) Sunken (scaphoid) and (C) Distended

(a) severe malnutrition,
(b) starvation, and
(c) malignant diseases – carcinoma of the oesophagus and stomach.

(ii) *Generalized fullness* or *distension* may be due to fat, fluid, flatus, faeces or foetus (*Five 'Fs'*).

(iii) *Localized distension* may be due to the gross enlargement of the liver, spleen or any other organ.

2. **The Umbilicus**. Normally the umbilicus is slightly retracted and inverted. If it is everted then an umbilical hernia may be present. (Fig. 3.19.3)

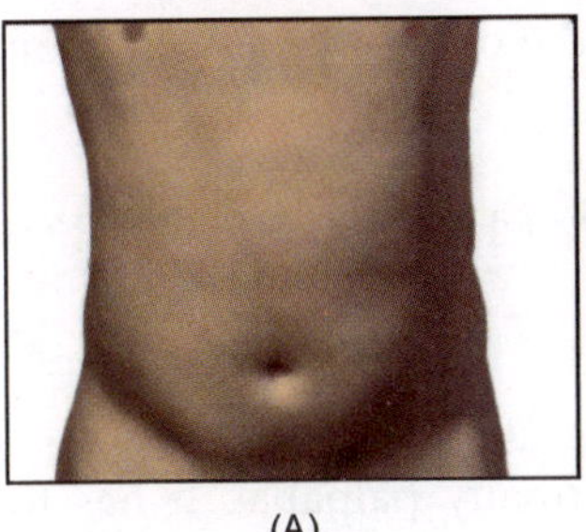

(A)

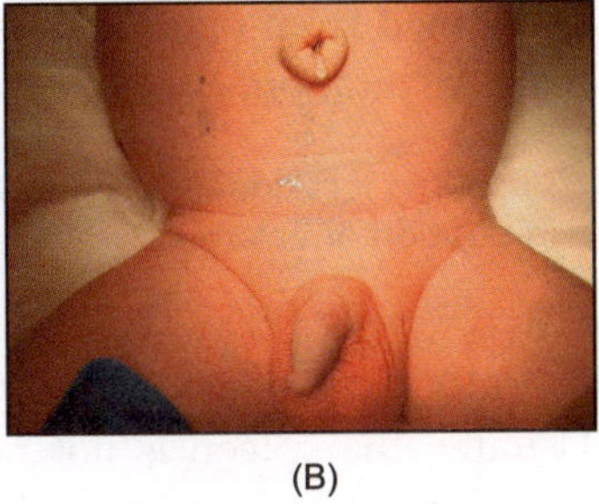

(B)

Fig. 3.19.3 (A) Normal retracted and inverted umbilicus
(B) Everted umbilicus

3. **Movements of the abdominal wall**
   (i) Normally there is a gentle rise in the abdominal wall during inspiration and a fall during expiration; the opposite occurs in the paralysis of the diaphragm.
   (ii) The movement should be free and equal on both sides; it is absent or markedly decreased in generalized peritonitis.
4. **Presence of any visible pulsations**
   (i) The *visible pulsation* of the abdominal aorta in the epigastrium is a frequent finding in nervous thin patients.
   (ii) The *visible peristalsis* of the stomach or small intestine may be observed in three conditions:
   (a) As *a normal finding* in very thin, elderly patients with lax abdominal muscles.
   (b) *Obstruction at the pylorus*. Peristalsis will be seen as a slow wave either passing across the upper abdomen from left to right hypochondria or passing down to the suprapubic region and ascending to terminate in the epigastrium.
   (c) *Obstruction in the distal small bowel*. Peristalsis will be seen locally along with the distended coils of small bowel.
5. **Skin and surface of the abdomen**
   (i) In marked distension, the skin is *smooth and shiny*.
   (ii) *White or pink wrinkled linear marks* on the abdominal skin are produced by the gross stretching of the skin with the rupture of the elastic fibres. This indicates a recent change in the size of the abdomen, such as is found in: pregnancy, ascites, wasting disease, severe dieting, excessive steroid treatment or Cushing's syndrome. (Fig. 3.19.4)

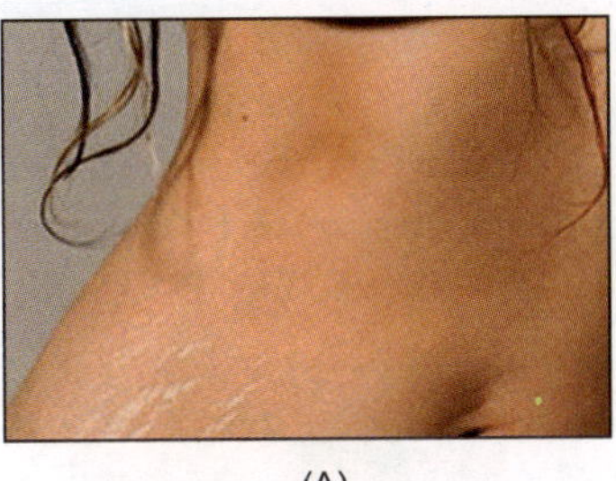

(A)

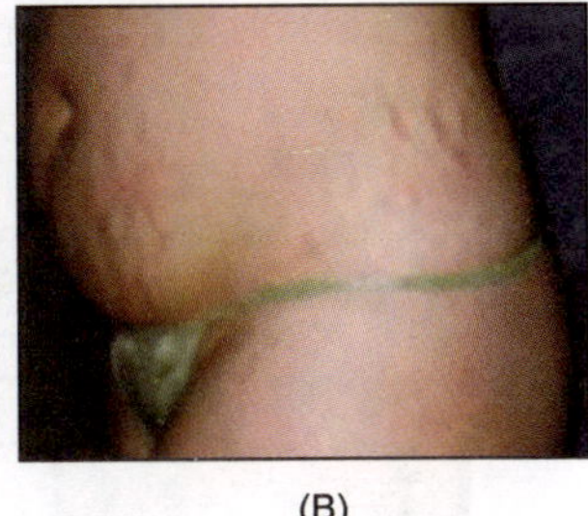

(B)

Fig. 3.19.4 Stretch marks over abdomen: (A) White marks after delivery and (B) Pink marks in Cushing syndrome

   (iii) Note for any scars present, their site; whether they are old (white) or recent (red/pink), linear or stretched.
   (iv) *Distribution of hair*. Hair colour and texture are genetically determined. Secondary sexual hair begins to appear at puberty and has characteristic male and female patterns. Pattern of public hair: *Males* – triangle with apex up *Females* – concave upwards/flat-topped (Fig. 3.19.5).

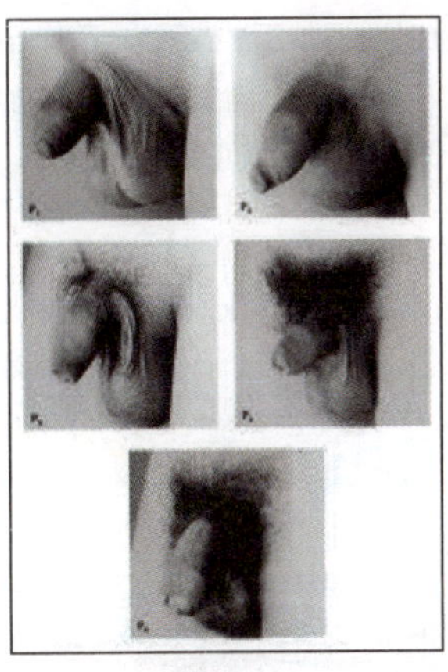

(A)

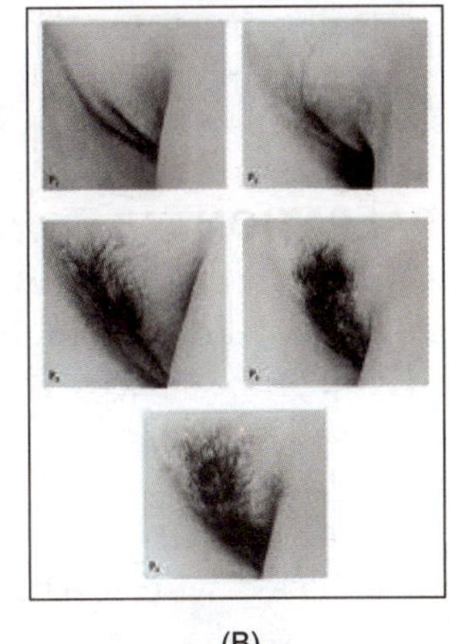

(B)

Fig. 3.19.5 Pubic hair (A) Male pattern (B) Female pattern

Note: The absence of hair after the attainment of puberty suggests hypopituitarism or hypogonadism.

   (v) *Pigmentation* of the abdominal wall may be seen in the midline below the umbilicus, where it forms the *linea nigra* and is a sign of pregnancy.

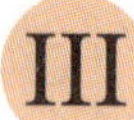

6. **Presence of prominent veins**
   (i) Small, thin veins over the subcostal margins are a common finding in thin individuals.
   (ii) Distended veins around the umbilicus (*caput medusae*) signify portal hypertension. They represent the opening up of anastomoses between portal and systemic veins (Fig. 3.19.6 A).
   (iii) Distended veins on the abdominal wall and chest wall appear in patients with obstruction to inferior vena cava. They represent dilated anastomotic channels between the superficial epigastric and circumflex iliac veins below, and the lateral thoracic veins above (Fig. 3.19.6 B).

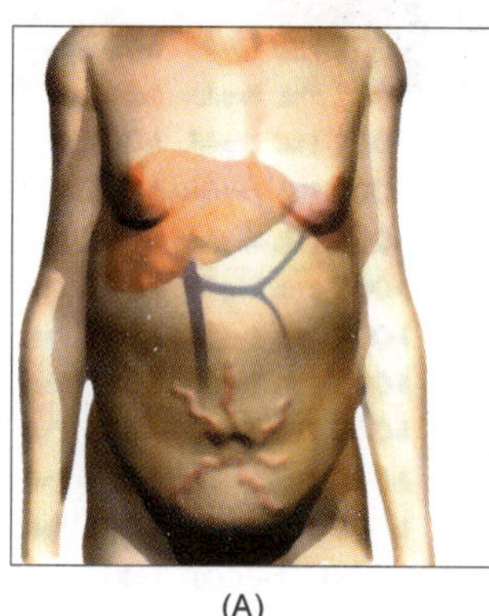
(A)

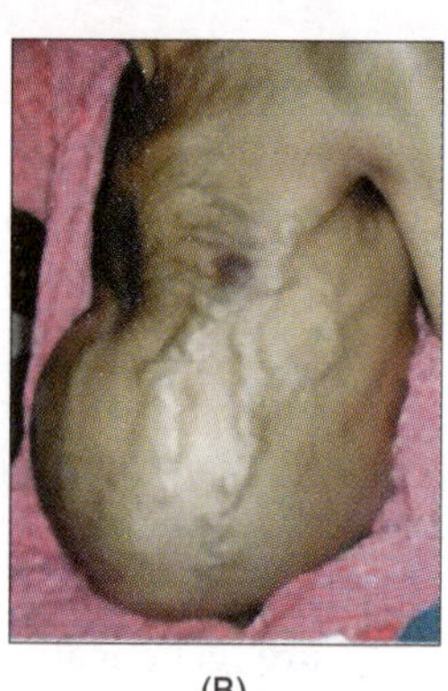
(B)

Fig. 3.19.6 Veins on the abdominal wall : (A) Caput medusae in portal hypertension (B) In a patient with IVC obstruction

7. Finally, inspect both groins, and the penis and scrotum of a male, for any swelling and to ensure that both testes are in their normal position.

II. PALPATION *(Also refer to page 217)*

The subject should lie flat on his back, and breathe quietly; the examiner sits or kneels besides the right-hand side of the subject. To gain the maximum amount of information a logical sequence should be followed as described below.

Start in the left iliac region palpating lightly and work anti-clockwise to end in the suprapubic region. Try and visualise the normal anatomical structures beneath the examining hand, and gently palpate each quadrant of the abdomen noting any area of tenderness or localized rigidity. Peritonitis produces rigidity from a reflex contraction of the muscles of the abdominal wall. *Normally,* the palpation of abdomen is painless and gives an elastic or doughy feeling.

1. Palpation of the kidneys

To feel for the kidneys, **bimanual palpation** is carried out. How? (Fig. 3.19.7)

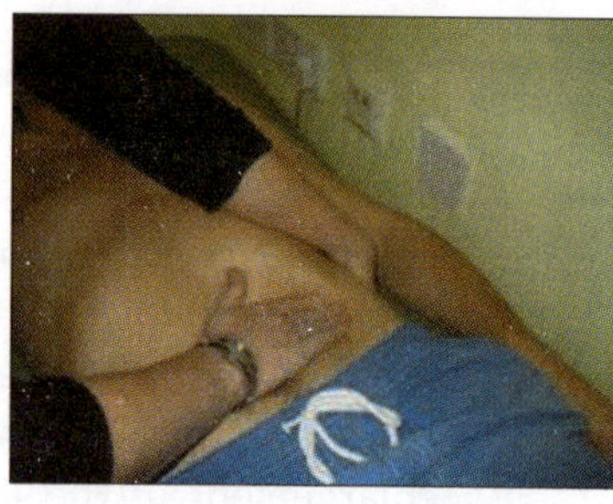
Fig. 3.19.7 Palpation of the left kidney (Bimanual palpation)

The right hand is placed anteriorly in the lumbar region while the left hand is placed posteriorly in the loin. Ask the subject to take a deep breath in, press the left hand forwards, and the right hand upwards and inwards. The kidney is not usually palpable except its lower pole is felt as a smooth, rounded firm swelling between both the right and left hands, *i.e. bimanually palpable.* It can be pushed from one hand to the other and descends on deep inspiration.

> **Note:** The left kidney is *not* usually palpable unless either low in position or enlarged.

2. Palpation of the spleen

Usually, the spleen is not normally palpable. It has to be enlarged two or three times its usual size before it becomes so and then is felt under the left subcostal margin. The direction of enlargement is downwards and towards the right iliac fossa (Fig. 3.19.8-inset).

(i) Place the flat of the left hand over the lowermost rib cage posterolaterally, and the right hand beneath the costal margin (Fig. 3.19.8). Ask the subject to breathe in deeply, press in deeply with the fingers of the right hand beneath the costal margin, at the same time exerting pressure medially and downwards with the left hand.

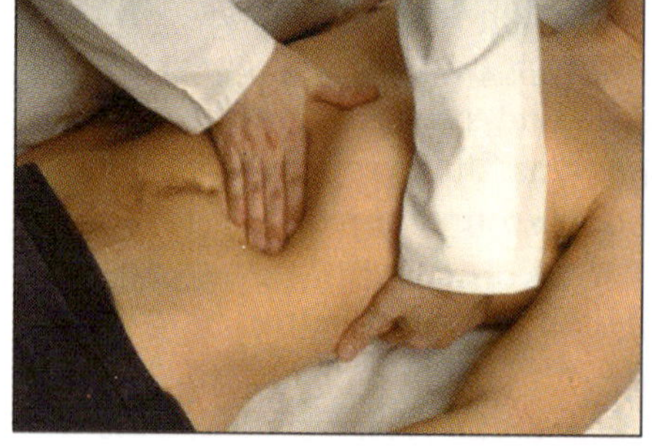

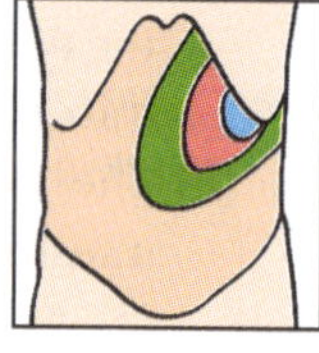

Fig. 3.19.8 Palpation of the spleen (Inset: the direction of its enlargement)

(ii) Repeat this procedure with the right hand being moving more medially beneath the costal margin on each occasion.

(iii) If the enlargement of the spleen is suspected and it is still not palpable, turn the subject onto his right side and repeat the whole procedure.

3. Palpation of the liver

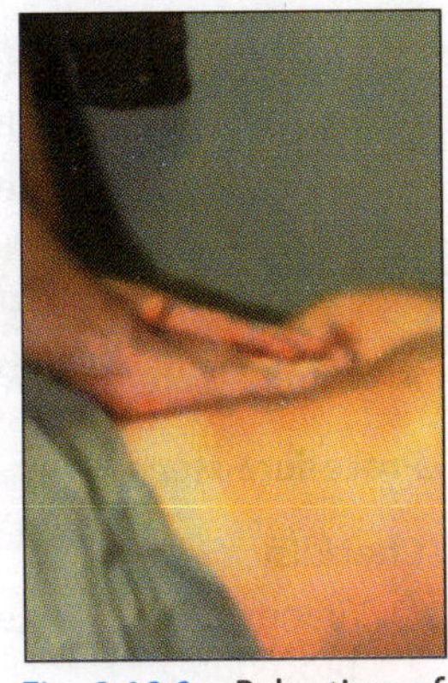

Fig. 3.19.9 Palpation of the liver

(i) Sit beside the right-hand side of the subject and place both hands side by side flat on the abdomen in the right subcostal region lateral to the rectus with the fingers pointing towards the ribs (Fig. 3.19.9). If resistance is felt, move the hands further down until the resistance disappears.

(ii) Ask the subject to breathe in deeply and at the height of inspiration press the fingers firmly inwards and upwards.

(iii) Normally, the liver is not palpable in health; if palpable, it will be felt as a sharp regular border which slides beneath the fingers.

(iv) The enlargement of the liver (***hepatomegaly***) is described as being so many centimetres palpable below the right costal margin in the midclavicular line.

III. PERCUSSION *(for details, refer to page 217)*

In the abdomen, only light percussion is necessary – a **tympanic** note is heard throughout except over the liver, where the note is dull.

Defining the boundaries of abdominal organs

1. *Liver* (Fig. 3.19.10)
   (i) The upper and lower borders of the right lobe of the liver can be defined accurately by percussion. Start anteriorly, at the fourth intercostal space, where the note will be resonant over the lungs, and work vertically downwards.
   (ii) In the normal liver, the upper border is at about the fifth intercostal space, where the note will become dull; this dullness extends down to the lower border found at just below the right subcostal margin.
   (iii) The normal dullness over the upper part of the liver is reduced in:
   (a) severe emphysema
   (b) large pneumothorax
   (c) presence of gas or air in the peritoneal cavity
2. *Spleen.* Its dullness extends from the left lower ribs into the left hypochondrium and left lumbar region.

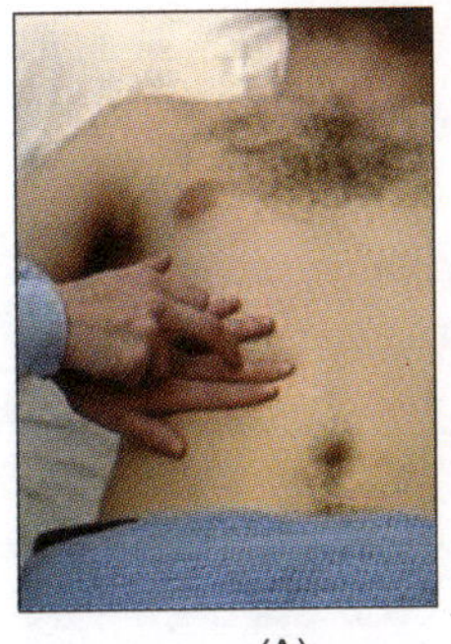

(A)

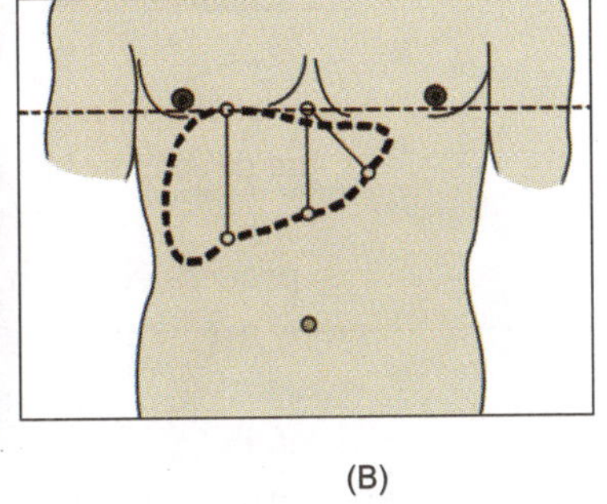

(B)

Fig. 3.19.10 Defining the boundaries of liver by percussion (A) Procedure and (B) Extent of liver

Clinical significance

The percussion of abdomen provides a rapid confirmation of presence of free fluid (*ascites*) in the peritoneal cavity. It is difficult to diagnose *ascites* unless there is sufficient free fluid present to give the generalized enlargement of the abdomen. The presence of any one of the *two signs: shifting dullness* and a *fluid thrill* either singly or together, makes the diagnosis of ascites certain.

1. *To elicit shifting dullness.* Lie the subject supine and percuss laterally from the midline, keeping your fingers in the longitudinal axis, until dullness is detected (Fig. 3.19.11 A). In normal individuals, dullness is detected only over the lateral abdominal structures. Then, keeping your hand on the abdomen, ask the subject to roll away from you, onto the left side. Percuss again in this new position; if the previous dull note has now become resonant then ascitic fluid is probably present. To confirm, repeat the procedure on the left side of the abdomen.
2. To elicit a *fluid thrill,* the subject is lain on his back. Place one hand flat over the lumbar region of one side, get an assistant to put the side of his hand firmly in the midline of the abdomen, and then flick or tap the opposite lumbar region. A fluid thrill or wave is felt as a definite impulse by the detecting hand held flat in the lumbar region (Fig. 3.19.11 B).

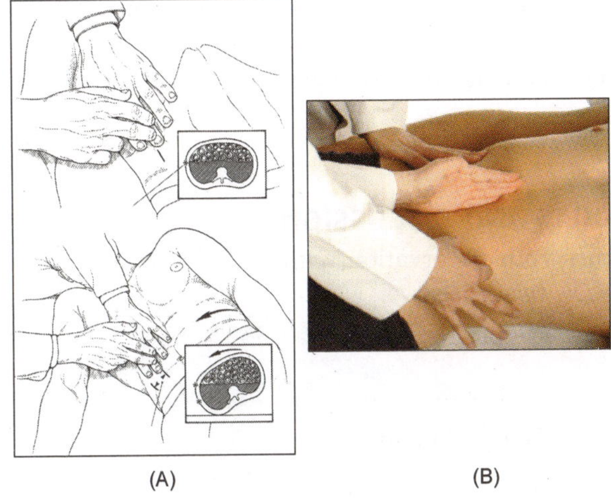

(A) (B)

Fig. 3.19.11 Technique for testing : (A) Shifting dullness and (B) Fluid thrill

Note: The purpose of the assistant's hand is to dampen any impulse that may be transmitted through the fat of the abdominal wall.

IV. AUSCULTATION *(Also, see page 217)*

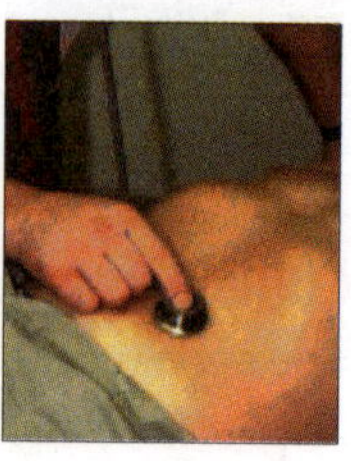

Auscultation is a useful way of listening for bowel sounds. One must listen for several minutes before being certain that such sounds occur. The stethoscope should be placed on one portion on the abdominal wall and kept there until sounds are heard. It should not be moved from place to place.

1. Normal bowel sounds are heard as intermittent low- or medium-pitched gurgles interspersed with an occasional high-pitched noise or tinkle.
2. In *simple acute mechanical obstruction of the small bowel,* the bowel sounds are excessive and exaggerated. Frequent loud low-pitched gurgles (***borborygmi***) are heard, often rising to a peak of high-pitched tinkles and occurring in a rhythmic pattern with peristaltic activity.
3. In *generalized peritonitis* bowel activity rapidly disappears and the abdomen is **silent,** *i.e.* no bowel sounds can be heard.

OSPE

Aim: To palpate the liver of the subject provided

Procedure steps: Refer to page 223.

Checklist

1. Stands on the subject's right side and explains the test procedure. **(Yes/No)**
2. Ensures that his own hands are warm. **(Yes/No)**
3. Asks the subject to lie flat on his back and breathe quietly. **(Yes/No)**
4. Places his both hands side by side flat on the abdomen of the subject in the right subcostal region with fingers pointing towards the ribs. **(Yes/No)**
5. Asks the subject to breathe in deeply and at the height of inspiration presses the finger firmly inwards and upwards. **(Yes/No)**

Note: The palpation of spleen may be asked as a separate OSPE

IMPORTANT VIVA-VOCE QUESTIONS

Q.1. *Describe the different steps of clinical examination of the abdomen.*

Ans. Page 220.

Q.2. *Mark the anatomical planes of the abdomen and name them.*

Ans. Page 220.

Q.3. *Give the physio-clinical significance of prominent veins on the surface of the abdomen.*

Ans. Page 222.

Q.4. *Is a palpable liver or spleen pathological?*

Ans. Usually, the liver or spleen is not normally palpable unless the subject is extremely thin with lax abdominal musculature.

Q.5. *How big does a spleen have to get before it can be palpable?*

Ans. Page 222.

Q.6. *What are the signs indicating fluid accumulation in the peritoneal cavity?*

Ans. Page 223.

Q.7. *Define ascites.*

Ans. The accumulation of abnormally large amounts of fluid in the abdominal cavity is called ascites.

Q.8. *Give some common causes of presence of the visible pulsations in the abdomen.*

Ans. Page 223.

Q.9. *Why should palpation be carried out with warm hands?*

Ans. Palpation with cold hands will result in the contraction of abdominal muscles and many vital signs may be missed.

STUDY NOTES

RESULTS AND DISCUSSION

Discuss your observation with the table teacher.

I. *On Inspection*

1. Shape

....

2. The umbilicus

....

3. Movements of the abdominal wall

....

4. Presence of any visible pulsations

....

5. Skin and surface of the abdomen

....

6. Presence of prominent veins

....

7. Genitalia examination

....

II. *On Palpation*

1. Feeling

....

2. Tender or non-tender

....

3. Feel for the kidneys

....

4. Feel for the spleen

....

5. Feel for the liver

....

III. *On Percussion*

1. Extent of tympanic note

....

2. Boundaries of abdominal organs:

(i) liver ....

(ii) spleen ....

(iii) presence of free fluid. ....

IV. *On Auscultation*

1. Character and intensity of bowel sounds

....

2. Any other sound heard

....

COMMENTS AND DISCUSSION

....

....

....

Date: ....

20 Clinical Examination of the Respiratory System

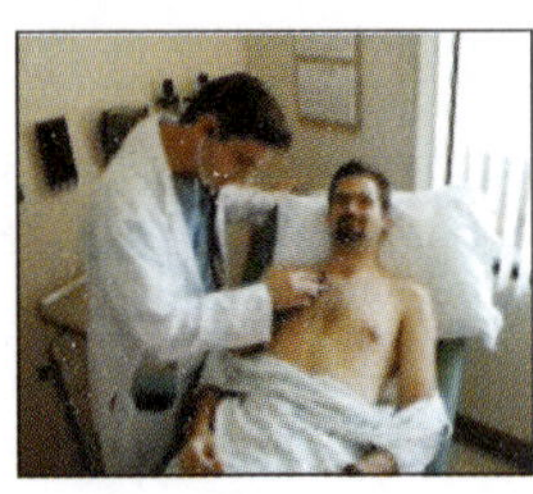

The clinical examination of the respiratory system is ideally done with the subject comfortably resting on a bed, sitting at an angle of 45° and supported by pillows. It is carried out under the following heads: *inspection, palpation, percussion and auscultation.*

I. INSPECTION (*Also, refer to* page 216)

During the inspection of the respiratory system, look for the shape and movement of the chest.

A. Shape of the chest

The normal chest is bilaterally symmetrical and elliptical in cross-section. It may become asymmetrical by a disease of the lungs or of the bony cage (ribs or spinal vertebrae). Some common abnormal forms of the chest are described as under: (Fig. 3.20.1)

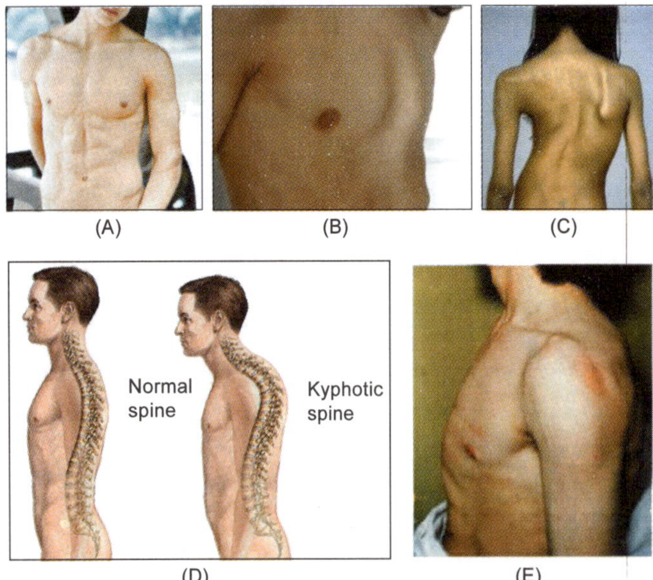

Fig. 3.20.1 Shape of the chest : (A) Normal (B) Pigeon (C) Scoliosis (D) Kyphosis and (E) Barrel-shaped

1. **Pigeon-shaped chest,** *i.e.* chest is elliptical in shape with prominent sternum. It is seen in children with *Rickets.*
2. **Scoliosis** or lateral bending of the vertebral column, *i.e.* prominence of front of the chest on one side with flattening on the other side. This is associated with the prominence of scapula on the side of the convexity with hip prominence on the other side.
3. **Kyphosis** or forward bending of the vertebral column, *i.e.* shortening of the chest with prominent sternum.

   (2) and (3) are together called as *kypho-scoliosis* and is a common finding of tubercular spine.
4. **Barrel-shaped chest.** In this condition the antero-posterior diameter of chest increases; sternum becomes arched and chest fixed as in full inspiration position. It is seen in chronic airway diseases like emphysema, bronchial asthma, fibrosis or collapse of lungs.

B. Movements of the chest

Observe whether these are similar or different on the two sides and make a note of the following points:

1. ***Rate of respiration.*** Count the frequency of breathing by observing abdominal wall movements for a full minute. The rate of respiration for a relaxed normal adult is 12-16 breaths/minute.
   (i) Causes of fast and shallow breathing (*tachypnoea*) are: exercise, nervousness, hysterical, fever, cardiac or pulmonary conditions causing hypoxia.
   (ii) Causes of slow breathing are: cerebral disturbances, brain damage, etc.
2. ***Depth of respiration.*** Look whether the breathing is shallow (as in bronchial asthma) or deep (as in brain damage or uremia).
3. ***Rhythm.*** It varies in health greatly, particularly if breathing is performed consciously. Irregular breathing occurs in:

(i) Obstruction in the respiratory passage (obstructive airway disease).
(ii) Alternating periods of apnoea and hyperventilation (*Cheyne-Stokes respiration*) seen in left ventricular failure, brain damage, voluntary hyperventilation, high altitude and in some normal individual during sleep.

4. ***Expansion of the chest.*** Note whether it is expansile and symmetrical. Chest expansion can be measured using a measuring tape around the chest at the level of the nipples. In healthy adults, the chest may expand 5-8 cm. Diminished or asymetrical expansion may occur when the underlying lung is abnormal, such as in emphysema, pleural effusion, pneumothorax, collapse, consolidation or fibrosis.

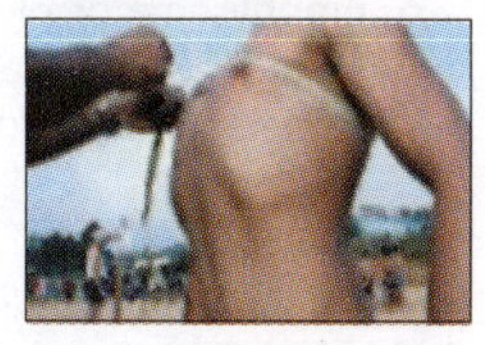

5. ***Type of respiration.*** See whether it is abdominal or thoracic. Normally, it is abdominal. Thoracic type of respiration occurs during pregnancy and the tumours of the GIT.

II. PALPATION *(Also, see page 217)*

1. ***Position of the trachea.*** Feel for the trachea using 3 fingers in the suprasternal notch and decide whether it is central or deviated to one side by its relation to the suprasternal notch and the insertion of the sternomastoids. A slight deviation of the trachea to the right may be found in healthy people.
   (i) The trachea may be *pushed away* from the affected side by: pleural effusion or pneumothorax; or
   (ii) The trachea may be *pulled towards* the affected side by fibrosis or collapse of the lung.
2. ***Position of the apex beat.*** Feel and locate the apex beat of the heart (normal location, page 232). It may be displaced due to: scoliosis, enlargement of left ventricle, displacement of the mediastinum by disease of the lungs or pleura.
3. ***Expansion of the chest.*** The asymmetrical expansion of the chest, as observed during inspection, may be further confirmed by palpation. How? (Fig. 3.20.2)

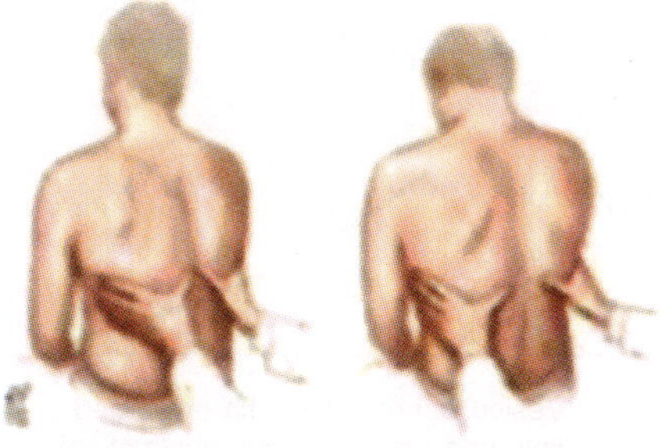

Fig. 3.20.2 Chest expansion assessment by palpation

If one faces the subject and places the fingertips of both hands on either side of the lower rib cage, so that the tips of the thumbs may meet in the midline in front of but not touching the chest, then a deep breath by the subject will increase the distance between the thumb and indicate the degree of expansion. If one thumb remains closer to the midline, this is the confirmation of decreased expansion of that side.

4. ***Vocal Fremitus.*** *Vocal* means pertaining to voice, *fremitus* means a vibratory sensation perceived by palpation. Vibration may thus be detected by palpation either with the palm or ulnar border of the hand placed flat on the chest. The subject is then asked to repeat something like "1, 2, 3 or Ram-Ram" in a clear normal voice. The examining hand perceives distinct vibrations. This is called *Vocal Fremitus* (VF) (Fig. 3.20.3).

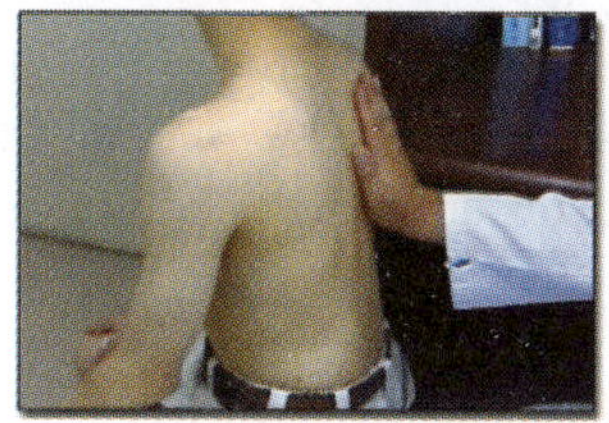

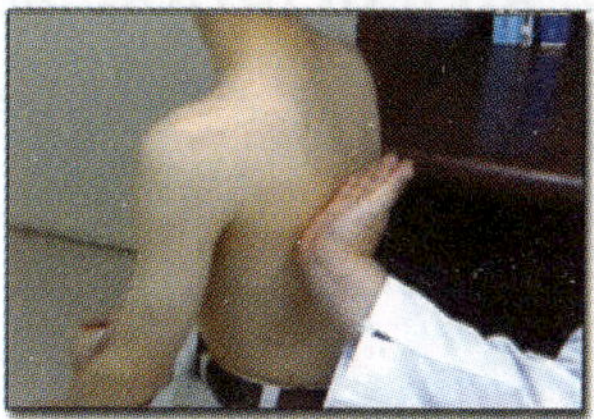

Fig. 3.20.3 Assessment for vocal fremitus

Determine whether the vibrations in corresponding areas on the two sides of the chest are approximately equal in intensity or not.

(i) VF is **increased** when the lung is consolidated or contains a large cavity near the surface.
(ii) VF is **decreased** when the corresponding bronchi are obstructed.
(iii) VF is **totally absent** when the lung is separated from the chest wall by pleural effusion or pneumothorax.

III. PERCUSSION *(for details, refer to page 217)*

Notes
1. One should systemically compare the percussion note on two equivalent sides of the chest.
2. The normal degree of resonance varies from individual to individual and in different parts of the chest in the same individual, being most resonant below the clavicles and scapulae where the muscles are relatively thin, and least resonant over the scapulae.

(A) The lower limits of lung resonance should be determined by percussing from above downwards with pleximeter finger parallel to the diaphragm.

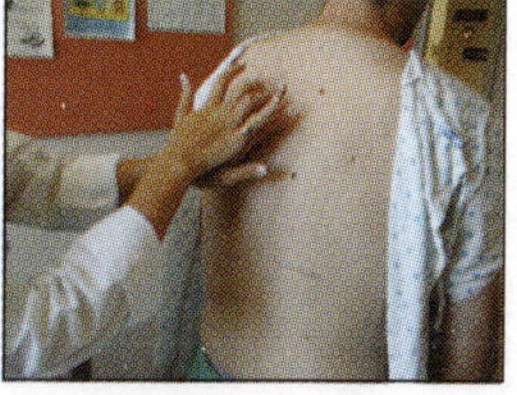

(B) The lower border of the *right lung* lies in the mammary line at the sixth rib, in the mid-axillary line at the eighth rib and in the scapular line at the tenth rib.

(C) The lower border of the *left lung* overlaps the stomach, so there is a change from lung resonance to tympanic stomach resonance. Posteriorly, besides the splenic dullness, the sounds resemble those found on the right.

1. An **increase in resonance** (or *hyperresonance*) is seen in pneumothorax in which the pleural cavity contains air and the lung is collapsed towards the hilum.
2. **Reduction in resonance** (dullness to percussion) occurs when:
   (i) pleura is thickened;
   (ii) pleural cavity contains fluid (*stony dullness*).

IV. AUSCULTATION *(Also, see page 217)*

For good auscultation, the subject should breathe with his mouth open, regularly, slightly deeper and faster than normal. The following observations should be made:

A. Character and intensity of breath sounds

Two main types of breath sounds can normally be heard over the chest: **vesicular** and **bronchial**. The main differentiating features between the two are given in Table 3.20.1.

Notes:
1. Breath sounds will be of **normal** intensity when the lung is inflating normally.
2. Breath sounds are **reduced** if there is localized airway narrowing, or lungs are extensively damaged as in emphysema or pleural thickening or pleural effusion.
3. Breath sounds may be of **increased** intensity in very thin subjects and children or when they become bronchial in character.

B. Vocal Resonance

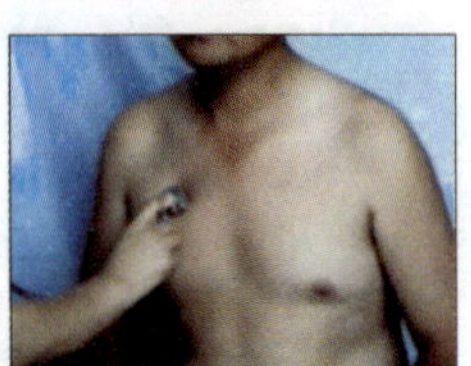

It is the sound of the whispering voice heard on the auscultation of the chest. Therefore, when the subject repeats '1, 2, 3 or Ram-Ram', the ear perceives not only the distinct syllables but also a resonant sound. The intensity of this sound depends on the loudness and depth of the subject's voice and the conductivity of the lungs. The nearer the stethoscope is to a large bronchus, the more intense is the sound.

1. The vocal resonance (VR) of **normal** intensity generally conveys the impression of being produced just at the chest piece of the stethoscope.
2. VR is **increased** if it seems to be nearer the ear than the chest piece of the stethoscope.

Table 3.20.1 Vesicular and bronchial breath sounds compared

	Vesicular breath sounds	Bronchial breath sounds
1. Origin	In the larger airways but when the normal healthy lung is present between the airways and the chest wall.	It also originates from the same larger airways but when the lung between these airways and the chest wall is airless (as in consolidation, fibrosis, cavity or collapse of lungs).
2. Character	(i) Low pitch rustling (ii) (a) There is no gap/pause between the end of inspiration and the beginning of expiration. (b) Inspiration sound is fairly intense and heard twice as long as the expiratory sound (Fig. 3.20.4).	(i) High frequency and harsh. (ii) (a) There is gap between the end of inspiration and the beginning of expiration. (b) The expiratory sound has more sibilant (whistling) character than inspiratory one; it lasts for most of the expiratory phase and of the same duration as of the inspiration sound (Fig. 3.20.4).
3. Sites	It is heard all over the healthy lungs and most typically in the axillary and infra scapular regions.	It is heard over the trachea, and portion of the lungs where bronchus is patent and air is not entering the alveoli (such cases are given above).

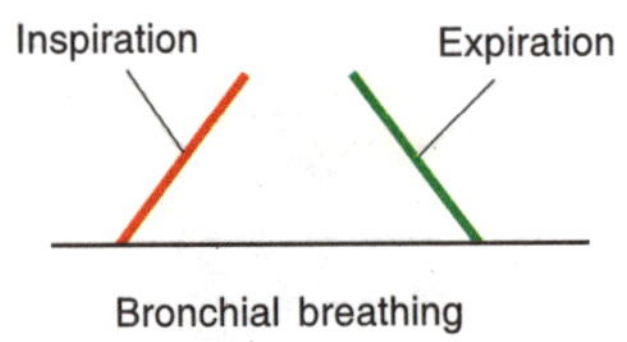

Bronchial breathing

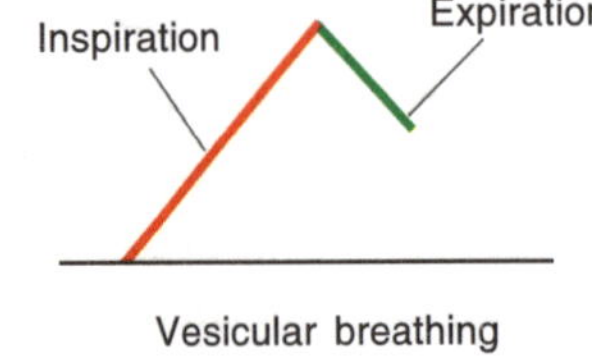

Vesicular breathing

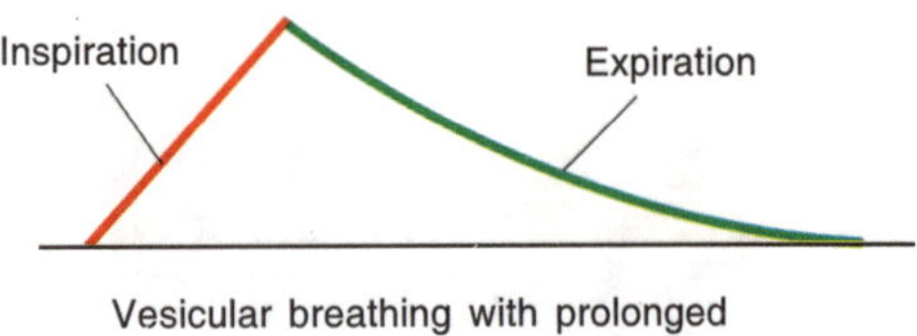

Vesicular breathing with prolonged expiration (as in airways obstruction)

Fig. 3.20.4 Breath sounds

3. VR is **markedly increased** when it appears to be near the earpiece of the stethoscope. This is described as ***bronchophony***.
4. **Further increase in VR**, if the words become clear and seem to be spoken right into the listener's ear. This is described as ***whispering pectoriloquy***. This occurs in:
   (i) in the proximity of the trachea and large bronchi;
   (ii) consolidation;
   (iii) cavity in the lungs.
5. VR is either abolished or much **diminished** in cases of:
   (i) pleural effusion
   (ii) pneumothorax
   (iii) thickened pleura, and
   (iv) emphysema.

Important Note: Each point examined on one side of the chest should be at once compared with corresponding point on the other side.

C. Added Sounds

In addition to vesicular and bronchial breath sounds, added sounds may arise in the lung or in the pleura.

1. ***The pleural rub***. This is characteristic of pleural inflammation. It has a creaking or rubbing character as produced by the movement of the stethoscope on the subject's smooth skin.
2. ***Rhonchi or wheeze***. These are prolonged uninterrupted musical sounds associated with airway narrowing and are particularly heard during expiration. These sounds are characteristic of bronchial asthma and bronchitis.
3. ***Crepitations or crackles***. These are short, explosive sounds often described as bubbling or clicking noises, as produced by the stethoscope rubbing over hairy skin. Crepitations are produced by sudden change in gas pressure related to the sudden opening of previously closed small airways. They may be heard both during expiration and inspiration, and are common in patients with pneumonia, tuberculosis, bronchitis, bronchiectasis. They may be *fine or coarse*.

IMPORTANT VIVA-VOCE QUESTIONS

Q.1. *Describe your observations of the clinical examination of the respiratory system.*

Ans. See below

Q.2. *Demonstrate*

(i) How will you count the respiration frequency?
(ii) Expansion of the chest
(iii) Position of the trachea
(iv) Vocal fremitus
(v) Vocal resonance

Ans. Refer to the procedure above.

Q.3. *How will you identify normal breath sounds? Describe their characteristic features.*

Ans. Page 228.

Q.4. *What are the types of added breath sounds and their characteristics?*

Ans. See above.

Q.5. *Define Cheyne-Stokes breathing. Give some physiological conditions in which it occurs.*

Ans. Page 227.

Q.6. *Name the sites from where you can normally listen to vesicular and bronchial breath sounds.*

Ans. Page 228.

Q.7. *How are the* **Rhonchi** *produced? Give their types.*

Ans. Rhonchi arise in the bronchi and are due to the partial obstruction of their lumen either by swelling of the mucosa or by viscid secretion or by the constriction of bronchial smooth muscle. They are often associated with turbulent air-flow within the lumen. They may be high-pitched (**sibilant**) or low-pitched (**sonorous**).

V. RESULTS AND DISCUSSION

Discuss with the table teacher.

I. *On inspection*

1. Shape and symmetry of the chest

....

2. Movements of the chest:
   (i) Rate of respiration

....

(ii) Depth of respiration

....

(iii) Rhythm

....

(iv) Expansion of the chest

....

(v) Type of respiration

....

II. *On palpation*

1. Position of trachea

....

2. Position of apex beat

....

3. Expansion of the chest

....

4. Vocal fremitus

....

III. *On percussion*

1. Type of percussion note and its intensity

....

2. Increased or decreased

....

IV. *On auscultation*

1. Breath sounds:

(i) Types/character

....

(ii) Increased or decreased or impaired

....

2. Vocal resonance

....

3. Added sounds (if any)

....

COMMENTS AND DISCUSSION

....

....

....

Date: ....

21 Clinical Examination of the Cardiovascular System (CVS)

The examination of cardio-vascular system includes:

1. Examination of precordium;
2. Examination of radial pulse;
3. Examination of venous pulse; and
4. Measurement of blood pressure

EXAMINATION OF THE PRECORDIUM

Precordium is the portion of the anterior aspect of the chest wall which overlies the heart. Its examination is carried out under four headings: *Inspection, Palpation, Percussion and Auscultation.*

I. Inspection (*Also, refer to* page 216)

It should be carried out when the subject is lying or ideally at 45° with neck muscles relaxed and the clothing removed up to the waist. Make a careful note of the following points:

1. **Dyspnoea,** *i.e.* difficulty in breathing. (Make a note of the movement of the chest, page 226)
2. **Cyanosis,** *i.e.* blue colouration of the skin or mucous membrane or both
3. **Shape and form of the chest**. Shape varies with the build of the individual being:
   (i) short, broad and deep in thick set; and
   (ii) long, flat and narrow in thin set
   In healthy individuals, it is bilaterally symmetrical.
4. **The neck veins**. The external jugular veins can be seen on the surface in the posterior triangle of the neck (Fig. 3.21.1). They communicate directly with the right atrium. Therefore, the level of pressure in these veins can be regarded as an increase of right atrial pressure, *i.e. central venous pressure* (as all the body veins open directly into the right atrium).
   In a healthy individual, in whatever position the subject may be (sitting, standing or lying), the external jugular veins get filled up to the level of manubrium sterni only (Fig. 3.21.2). If veins are filled higher than this, it indicates the presence of increased central venous pressure. This is seen in:
   (i) pregnancy, due to increase in circulating blood volume;
   (ii) right heart failure;
   (iii) obstruction to superior vena cava, and
   (iv) acute nephritis

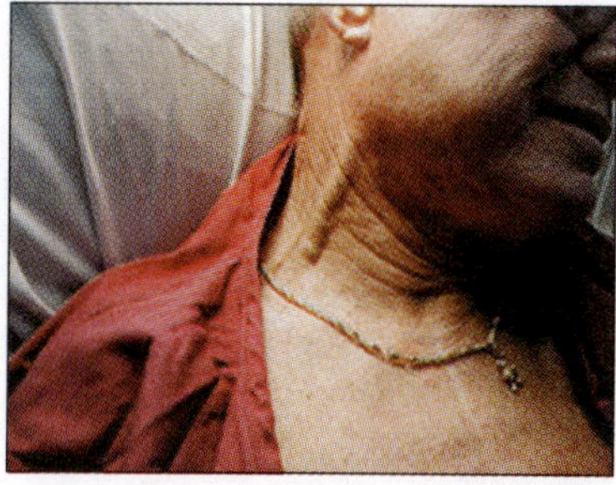

Fig. 3.21.1 Position of external jugular vein in the neck

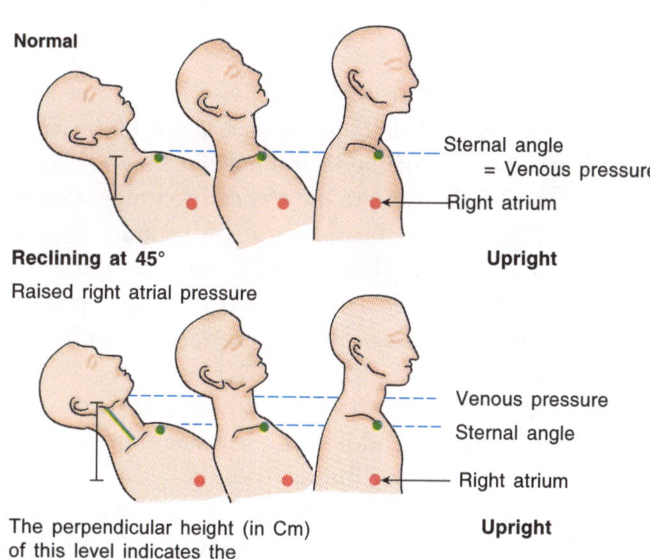

Fig. 3.21.2 Clinical assessment of right atrial pressure, *i.e.* central venous pressure

5. **Veins on the chest wall**. Normally, full and prominent veins are not seen in healthy individuals. If seen, the

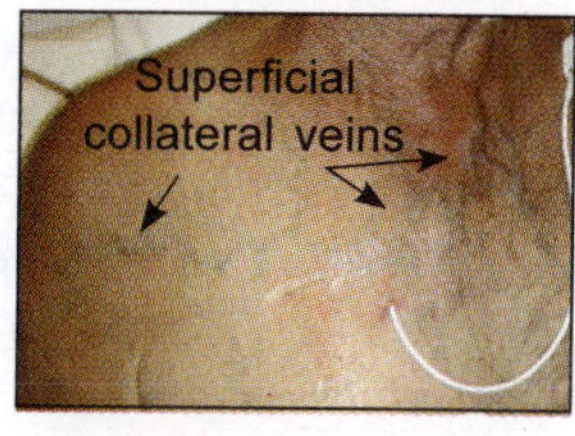

causes are:

(i) Subject with skin unusually transparent shows thin and tiny veins.
(ii) Intrathoracic growth with aneurysm obstructs the venous return.
(iii) Secondary to portal obstruction or obstruction to inferior vena cava.

6. **Cardiac impulse**. It refers to movements occurring due to the impact of the heart against the chest wall during the systole. The area over which the impact is seen is a circular area having a diameter of about 2.5 cm. Count the heart beat by counting the number of impacts per minute.
   The lowest and outermost point of definite cardiac impulse, where it is seen/felt most forcibly, is called the ***Apex Beat***. Normally it lies 9 cm from the midline (or 1 cm internal to the mid-clavicular line) in the left 5th intercostal space.
   Apex beat may not be seen due to:
   (i) obesity (thick chest wall);
   (ii) if lying behind a rib;
   (iii) dextrocardia; it will be seen on the right side;
   (iv) after deep inspiration (when lungs cover the heart);
   (v) deformity of rib cage e.g. scoliosis
   Apex beat becomes *prominent* due to: anxiety, nervousness, after exercise.
7. **Other pulsations**
   (i) *In the neck*. Carotid artery pulsations are visible on either side in the anterior triangle of the neck by the side of the sternomastoid muscle. They are diffuse and are the transmitted movements of the carotid pulse. They are prominent and never absent. *These arterial pulsations differ from the venous pulsations in respect that they are more sinous, easily palpable and thrusting (expansile) in character.*
   (ii) *Over the precordium*. In thin slender subjects, especially in children, the cardiac impulse can be seen all over the precordium.
   (iii) *In the epigastrium*. Normally, no pulsations are seen. If present, these can be due to: nervousness or excitement (in a thin person), right ventricular hypertrophy (RVH), aneurysm of abdominal aorta.

II. Palpation (*Also, see* page 217)

Collect the following information by doing palpation:

1. Feel for the *temperature*.
2. Feel for the *texture of skin*.
3. Feel for *cardiac impulse and apex beat*. Confirm the findings obtained by inspection with respect to its location, extent, repetition, rate and rhythm.

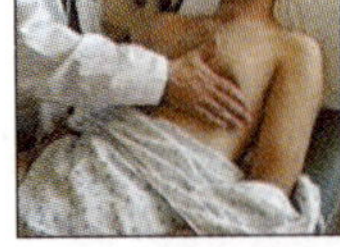

4. Feel for *carotid pulsations*.
5. *Veins in the neck*. Find the direction of blood flow and inability to feel the venous pulsations.
6. Feel for a ***thrill***. Any sound or *murmur* which is loud and low-pitched will be palpable like a worm moving under the hand. These palpable vibrations are called a thrill.

III. Percussion (*Also, refer to* page 217)

1. By percussing the fourth intercostal space from the left lung towards the heart it is possible to define the left border more or less precisely. It is found about 1.5 cm internal to mid-clavicular line.
2. The right border of the heart is just to the right of sternum at the level of the fourth rib. It is difficult to define since the sternum acts as a sounding board.
3. The upper border of the heart cannot be defined accurately as the dullness of the heart tissue continues with the dullness of the big vessels.
4. Similarly, the lower border of the heart cannot be defined as it lies in relation with the diaphragm and the left lobe of the liver below it.

Clinical Significance

1. The area of pericardial dullness *increases* due to large pericardial effusion and aortic aneurysm.
2. The area of pericardial dullness is either *absent or decreases* due to emphysema.

IV. Auscultation (*Also, see* page 217)

The heart sounds produced by the closure of heart valves can be heard all over the precordium but are heard best over four ***cardiac areas*** *on the chest wall* (Fig. 3.21.3). The areas chosen are such that in each of the valvular region, its

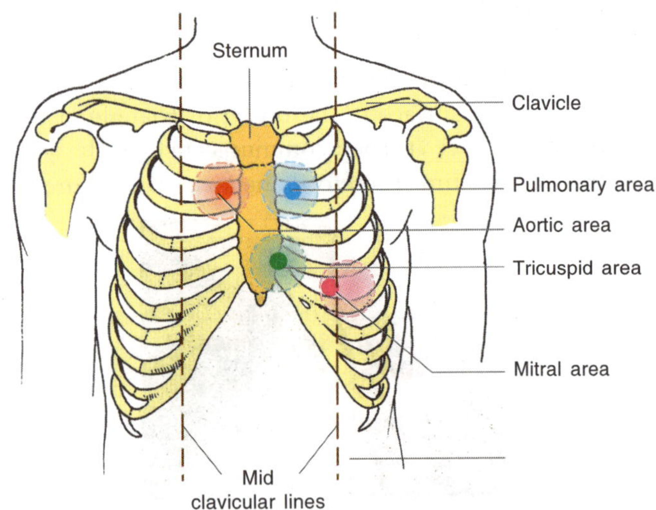

Fig. 3.21.3 Location of cardiac areas over the chest

own sounds are conducted best. The areas are:

1. *Mitral area* – lies over the apex beat, *i.e.* left fifth intercostal space in mid-clavicular line.
2. *Tricuspid area* – lies just to the left in the fifth intercostal space at the lower end of sternum.
3. *Aortic area* – lies in the right second intercostal space about 2 cm away from the sternum.
4. *Pulmonary area* – lies in the left second intercostal space about 2 cm away from the sternum.

Mainly two heart sounds are heard. The major differences between the two are given in Table 3.21.1.

1. **Third heart sound (HS_3)** occurs in early diastole due to the sudden filling of both the ventricles. Its presence otherwise indicates abnormal left ventricular filling (such as in left ventricular failure or mitral regurgitation).
2. **Fourth heart sound (HS_4)** occurs due to ventricular filling as a result of atrial contraction.

Important Note: HS_3 and HS_4 are usually inaudible and are of low-frequency sounds caused by abnormal filling patterns in the ventricles. These sounds are best heard with the bell of the stethoscope.

EXAMINATION OF RADIAL PULSE

Radial pulse is best felt with the tips of three middle fingers slightly compressing the vessel against the underlying bone. The subject's forearm should be pronated and the wrist slightly flexed (Fig. 3.21.4). The following observations should be made systematically.

1. Rate
2. Rhythm
3. Character or form
4. Volume
5. Condition of the vessel wall
6. Equality on both the sides

1. Rate

The Rate of pulse is expressed as so many beats per minute. In a healthy individual, it indicates the true rate of ventricular contraction. *Count the beats for full one minute.* It is counted **not** when the fingers are first laid upon the pulse but only when it has resumed to normal rate. This is to avoid quickening due to nervousness in the subject.

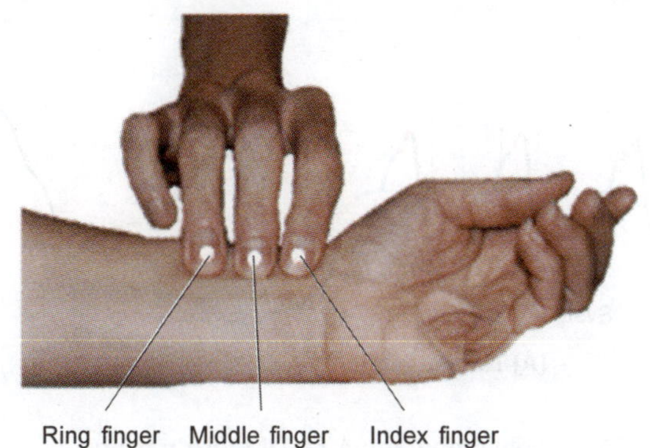

Fig. 3.21.4 Examination of the radial pulse

Causes of increase in pulse rate: Exercise, anxiety, excitement, fever, thyrotoxicosis, arrythmias, shock (e.g. haemorrhage).

Causes of decrease in pulse rate: Athletes (regular training), myxoedema, complete heart block.

2. Rhythm

Normally the pulse beat at regular interval, decide whether the rhythm is regular or irregular. If irregular, whether it is *regularly irregular* (due to extra systole) or completely/*irregularly irregular* (due to atrial fibrillation).

3. Character or Form

By feeling alone the contours of the pulse cannot be appreciated, for this record needs to be done using **sphygmograph**. It is characterized by the following waves (Fig. 3.21.5).

(i) **P**: *percussion wave* due to the left ventricular contraction.
(ii) **t**: *tidal wave* (predicrotic wave) due to the elasticity of aorta.

Table 3.21.1 Main differentiating features between the first and second heart sounds

	First heard sound (HS_1)	Second heart sound (HS_2)
1. Cause	It is due to the closure of A-V valves and marks the onset of ventricular systole.	It is due to the closure of semilunar valves and marks the onset of ventricular diastole.
2. Character	**Low pitch**; frequency 30-80 Hz (cycles per second), producing **loud sound**. It sounds like the syllable L-U-B-B.	**High pitch**; frequency 150-200 Hz producing **sharp sound**. It sounds like the syllable D-U-P.
3. Duration	Longer: 0.1-0.17 sec.	Shorter: 0.1-0.14 sec.
4. Site	Best heard over the mitral and tricuspid areas.	Best heard over the pulmonary and aortic areas.
5. Correlation	It is synchronous with the carotid artery pulsation and coincides with the R-wave of the E.C.G.	It follows the carotid artery pulsation and coincides with the end of the T-wave of the E.C.G.

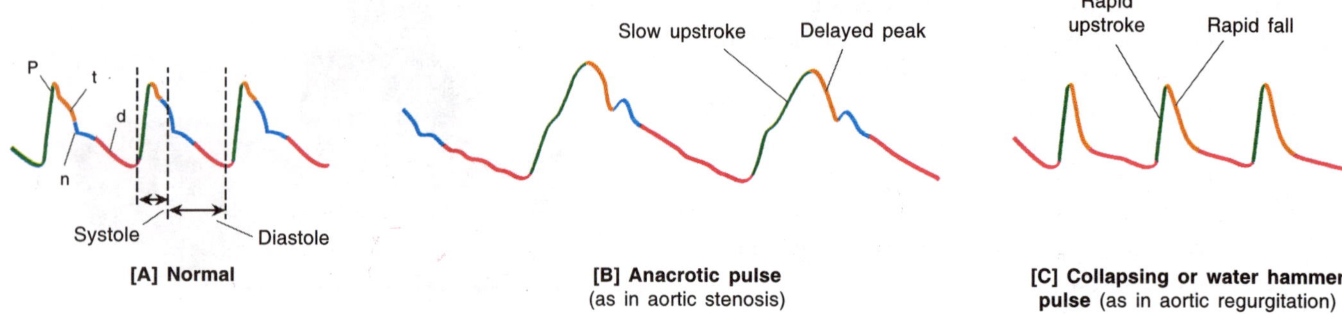

Fig. 3.21.5 Sphygmogram: A radial pulse tracing

(iii) **n**: *aortic notch* due to the regurgitation of blood towards the left ventricle from aorta at the beginning of diastole.

(iv) **d**: *dicrotic wave* caused by the return of the same blood volume being reflected back by closed semilunar valves.

Types or abnormal character of the arterial pulse wave:

(i) ***Anacrotic Pulse*** means two upbeats. This is seen in aortic stenosis which results in the slow ejection of blood from left ventricle. The pulse is typically of 'small volume' with slow rising characteristic, *i.e.* peak is delayed compared with normal pulse.

(ii) ***Collapsing or Water Hammer Pulse***. It is characterized by rapid upstroke and rapid descent of pulse wave. The collapsing character is due to the regurgitation of blood from aorta back into the left ventricle or due to abnormal leak from the arterial system. This is seen in aortic valve incompetence (AR), patent ductus arteriosus, arterio-venous fistula etc.

(iii) ***Bisferiens Pulse***. Combination of (i) and (ii), *i.e.* combination of slow rising and collapsing pulses. It is seen in combined aortic stenosis and aortic regurgitation.

(iv) ***Pulsus Paradoxus***. In this condition, pulse becomes smaller or even disappears at the end of deep inspiration. It is called 'paradoxus' because heart sounds may still be heard on auscultation over the precordium at a time when no pulse is palpable at the radial artery. It is commonly seen in:
 (a) large pericardial effusion (also called **cardiac tamponade**),
 (b) constrictive pericarditis.

(v) ***Pulsus Alternans***. Here arterial pulses typically show alternate large and small beats. It is seen when the left ventricle is severely damaged (such as during myocardial infarction) so as to develop alternate strong and weak contractions.

4. Volume

This refers to the amplitude of the movement of the vessel wall during the passage of pulse wave. This is a measure of:
 (i) amount of blood flowing with every beat; and
 (ii) pulse pressure.

Causes of the abnormal volume of pulse are:
 (i) pulse is weak and thready in shock, and
 (ii) pulse is strong and high volume during exercise, in old subjects (due to widened pulse pressure).

5. Condition of the vessel wall

To assess this sufficient pressure should be exerted on the brachial artery to abolish pulsation in the radial vessel which should then be rolled beneath the fingers against the underlying bone:
 (i) arterial wall cannot be felt or it is soft in young subjects;
 (ii) arterial wall becomes tortuous, easily palpable and felt like whip cord due to arteriosclerosis in old persons.

6. Equality on both the sides

Compare each of the above-mentioned features with the other side. Normally in a healthy individual, all features should be the same.

Important Note: The presence or absence of the other main peripheral arterial pulses: the brachial, carotid, femoral, popliteal, posterior tibial, and dorsalis pedis pulse, should be noted. The volume of each is compared with the other side.

EXAMINATION OF VENOUS PULSE

Refer to the examination of the neck veins, page 232.

The venous pulse record *or* jugular venous pressure (JVP) record

A venous pulse record, such as recorded from the jugular vein in the neck, has three positive waves: *a, c and v waves and two negative waves or descents: x and y* (Fig. 3.21.6).

1. The **a wave** is due to atrial contraction.
2. The **c wave** coincides with the onset of ventricular systole and results from the bulging of the tricuspid valve ring into the right atrium as the right ventricular pressure rises during isovolumetric ventricular contraction phase.
3. The **v wave** indicates a passive rise in pressure as venous return to the atrium continues during ventricular systole while the tricuspid valve is closed.
4. The **x descent** results from the return of tricuspid valve ring back to original position with the opening of the pulmonary valve.
5. The **y descent** results from the lowering of right atrial pressure due to the opening of tricuspid valve.

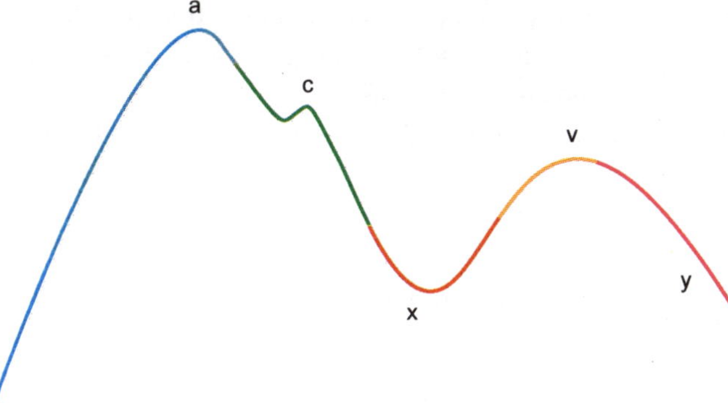

Fig. 3.21.6 The normal venous pulse (abbreviation as in the text)

MEASUREMENT OF THE BLOOD PRESSURE

Refer to page 151.

OSPE-I

Aim: To locate the apex beat of the subject provided

Procedure steps: Refer to page 232.

Check list

1. Stands on the subject's right side and explains the test procedure. **(Yes/No)**
2. Exposes the subjects' chest completely. **(Yes/No)**
3. Ensures that his own hands are warm. **(Yes/No)**
4. Marks mid-clavicular line and locates the 5th intercostal space by proper counting of the ribs. **(Yes/No)**
5. Defines the cardiac impulse area and feels for the apex beat. **(Yes/No)**

OSPE-II

Aim: To examine the radial pulse of the subject provided

Procedure steps: Refer to page 233.

Checklist

1. Stands on the subject's right side and explains the test procedure. **(Yes/No)**
2. Places the subject's forearm in semi-pronated position with the wrist slightly flexed. **(Yes/No)**
3. Feels for the radial pulse with the tip of his three middle fingers slightly compressing the vessel against the underlying bone. **(Yes/No)**
4. Counts the radial pulse for full one minute only when it has resumed to normal rate. **(Yes/No)**
5. Assess the pulse also for rhythm, character, volume and condition of the vessel wall. **(Yes/No)**
6. Feels for the equality of pulse on both the sides. **(Yes/No)**

OSPE-III

Aim: Auscultate the chest for heart sounds of the subject provided.

Procedure steps: Refer to page 232.

Check list

1. Stands on the subject's right side and explains the test procedure. **(Yes/No)**
2. Checks for the normal functioning of the stethoscope. **(Yes/No)**
3. Exposes the subject's chest completely. **(Yes/No)**
4. Places the diaphragm of the stethoscope on any one of the heart areas after the proper counting of intercostal spaces. **(Yes/No)**
5. Places the ear piece comfortably into the ears along the direction of the ear canals. **(Yes/No)**
6. Listens to one heart sound for several minutes before coming to any conclusion. **(Yes/No)**

IMPORTANT VIVA-VOCE QUESTIONS

Q.1. *How will you assess for raised jugular venous pressure in an individual?*

Ans. Page 231.

Q.2. *Name the condition in which apex beat cannot be visualised. What is dextrocardia?*

Ans. Page 232.

Q.3. *How will you differentiate between the arterial and venous pulsations?*

Ans. Page 232.

Q.4. *Define a thrill.*

Ans. Page 232.

Q.5. *Name cardiac areas. Give their significance.*

Ans. Page 232.

Q.6. *Differentiate between the first and second heart sounds.*

Ans. Page 233.

Q.7. *Why are the heart sounds produced only by the closure of valves?*

Ans. The closure of heart valves is a sudden phenomenon which causes the surrounding blood to become turbulent; the turbulent blood-flow is noisy flow. On the other hand, the opening of heart valves is a slowly developing process and the blood-flow remains silent, a characteristic of streamline (or laminar) flow.

Q.8. *Give the method of counting ribs and intercostal spaces.*

Ans. In order to count the ribs, feel for the ridge which marks the junction of the manubrium with the body of the sternum, known as the angle of Louis or sternal angle (Fig. 3.21.7). Now, run the finger outwards until it reaches the second costal cartilage, which articulates with the sternum at this level. The space immediately above this is the first intercostal space. The space should then be counted downward well away from the sternum, as they are more easily felt there.

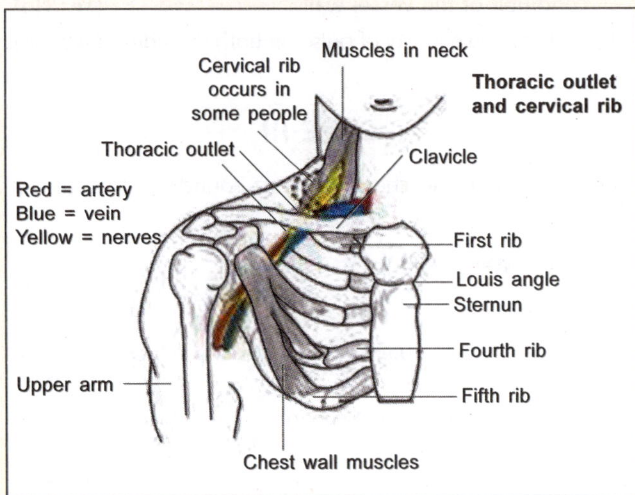

Fig 3.21.7 Method of counting ribs and intercostal spaces

Q.9. *What precautions should be observed while examining the radial pulse?*

Ans.
- (i) The arm should be properly positioned.
- (ii) Count the pulse for full one minute.
- (iii) Never count the pulse when the fingers are first laid on the pulse.
- (iv) Consideration should be given to all the factors which may affect a pulse.

Q.10. *After what duration of peak ventricular contraction, is the pulse felt at the wrist?*

Ans. After a gap of 0.1 second.

Q.11. *Describe the pulse of a normal old-aged individual.*

Ans. In old age due to atherosclerosis, pulse pressure increases (systolic increases more than diastolic pressure); this results in a high-volume pulse and pulse wave moves faster.

Q.12. *How many extrasystoles are regarded as normal? Give its causes.*

Ans. 2-4 extrasystoles/minute are regarded as normal. (For causes, see page 120)

Q.13. *Give abnormal forms (or character) of the arterial pulse wave.*

Ans. Page 234.

Q.14. *Describe the pulse of an individual presented with haemorrhagic shock.*

Ans. During shock, sympathetic activity increases which results in tachycardia; this along with hypotension produces rapid thready (low-volume) pulse, which is non-collapsing in character.

Q.15. *Give two physiological causes of a high-volume pulse.*

Ans. Exercise and in old age.

Q.16. *What is pulse deficit? Give its causes.*

Ans. The difference between the heart rate and pulse rate is referred as pulse deficit. It is seen in atrial and/or ventricular fibrillations.

STUDY NOTES

OBSERVATIONS, COMMENTS AND DISCUSSION

....

....

....

....

....

....

Date: ....

22 Clinical Examination of the Nervous System

A routine examination of the whole nervous system is carried out in a sequential manner in order to exclude any major neurological disability. A scheme for a quick routine neurological examination, which is followed in clinical practice, is as follows:

1. *Examination of higher functions*
2. *Examination of cranial nerves*
3. *Examination of motor system (including reflexes)*
4. *Examination of sensory system*
5. *Examination of autonomic nervous system*

Important Note: In clinical practice, the order of examination outlined above should not be rigidly adhered to. For example, if a person presents with complaint concerned with sensory dysfunction, it is appropriate to begin with sensory system examination, or if concerned with difficulty in performing movements, then begin with motor system examination.

(A) Examination of Higher Functions

The higher functions of the nervous system include: mental state, memory and language (speech).

1. In general, the higher functions of the nervous system in humans depend on one cerebral hemisphere than on the other. This hemisphere is concerned with categorization and symbolization and has often been called the **Dominant** or **Categorical hemisphere**. However, other hemisphere is not simply less developed or non-dominant; instead it is specialized in the area of *spatio-temporal relations* such as with the recognition of faces, identification of objects by their form, etc. This hemisphere is called **Representational hemisphere.**
2. Hemisphere specialization is related to *handedness,* which appears to be genetically determined. In right-handed individuals, who constitute about 90% of the human population, the left hemisphere is the dominant or categorical hemisphere. In about 30% of left-handed individuals, the right hemisphere is the categorical hemisphere; however, in the remaining 70%, left hemisphere is the categorical hemisphere.

I. MENTAL STATE

Much useful information regarding the mental state of a subject can be obtained during history-taking and physical examination. To assess the mental state, the following aspects should be carefully looked for:

1. Appearance and Behaviour

(i) Important points to look for include: dress, personal hygiene and general grooming.

(ii) Any inappropriate behaviour should be noted such as facial tics, verbal or physical aggression, etc.

2. Emotional State

(i) It is important to note his mood; facial expression is one of the outward signs of the subject's mood; the abnormal mood includes: depression, mania, anxiety, schizophrenia, etc.

(ii) Inquire about sleep and dreams; *insomnia* is likely to be due to psychological disorders such as mania or depression. Dreams are frequent and sleep-disturbing in the anxiety states.

3. Delusions and Hallucinations

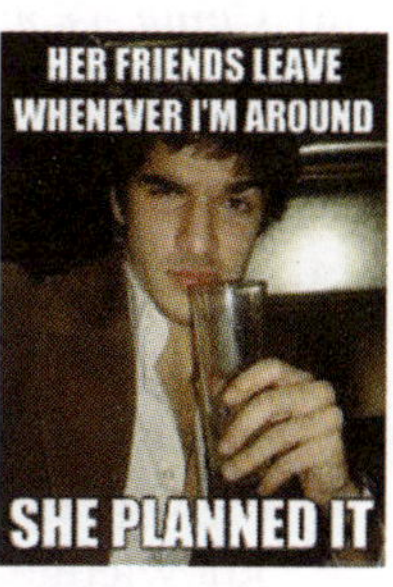

(i) **Delusions** are false and unshakeable beliefs which continue to be held despite evidence to the contrary such as:

(a) *Misinterpretations.* A person feels that others are laughing behind his back (this is commonly seen in sensitive people) or his nose is too long.

(b) *Suspicion* e.g. a person is usually jealous of his

wife, and is convinced that she is having an extramarital affair.

(ii) **Hallucinations** are false impressions referred to the organs of special sense (hearing, smell, vision, etc.) for which no cause can be found. For example:

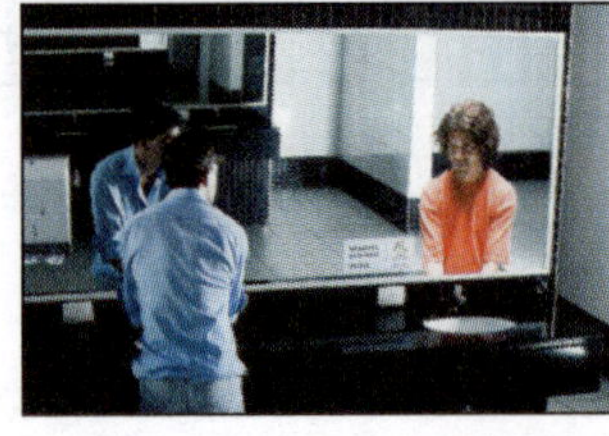

(a) *Visual hallucination.* A person may complain of seeing ghost figures.

(b) *Auditory hallucination.* A person may complain of hearing voices and he may talk back to the voice, or he may appear to be listening to them intently. In some cases, the voices direct the person to certain actions which he may feel duty-bound to follow.

(c) Some persons complain that, when alone, they feel the presence of someone else beside them.

4. Orientation in Place and Time

This should be assessed by direct questioning. Ask his name and address; ask about the day, date, month, year and time of the day. He should know where he is, e.g. home or hospital or college and where it is situated e.g. in what part of the town.

Disorientation is an important sign of organic brain disease, but may also occur in schizophrenics and in hysterical states.

5. Level of Consciousness

Note whether there is any disturbance of consciousness such as confusion, stupor or coma.

(i) In ***dementia*** (loss of memory), the person is confused in time, place and person and shows impaired abstractional abilities, but is awake and alert.

(ii) In ***stupor***, the person, although inaccessible, does show some response, for instance to pain stimuli.

(iii) ***Coma*** is a state in which the person makes no psychologically meaningful response to external stimulus or to inner need.

6. Intelligence

(i) An approximate assessment of intelligence can be obtained from the educational and occupational history and from an assessment of his general knowledge.

(ii) Alternatively, this can be tested more formally.

(a) See whether the person is able to solve simple mathematical problems, specially related to daily activities e.g. shopping. Ask him to substract 5 from 13.

(b) Tests in which the person is asked: What would you do if you see a house on fire?

(c) Ask him to copy a complex figure e.g. a house.

(iii) The people of relatively low intelligence can often give the month of the year parrot-fashion but not which month comes before or after a particular month.

II. MEMORY

Memory is the ability to recall past events at the conscious or unconscious level. It is the relatively permanent storage form of the learnt information. Depending on how long a memory lasts, it is divided broadly into two major types:

1. **Recent or short-term memory**. It involves mechanisms mediating an *immediate* recall of events that occurred seconds to hours before. It is lost in individuals with certain neurological disorders.
2. **Remote or long-term memory**. It involves mechanisms mediating memory of the *remote* past. It is remarkably resistant and persists in the presence of severe brain damage or psychiatric disorders.
3. The degree to which recent or short-term memory is lost is an index of the severity of organic brain disorder.
   (i) Ask the person to recall what he has read in the paper or seen on television or to repeat a name and address immediately and again after about 5 minutes or to repeat seven digits backwards without distraction.
   (ii) It is characteristically impaired in: vitamin B deficiency following poor nutrition and in persons with Alzheimer-type dementia.
4. There is frequently a loss of memory for the events immediately before brain concussion or electroshock therapy. This phenomenon is termed as ***retrograde amnesia***, which persists from a few hours to even a year, but remote memory is not affected. (*Concussion* means transient loss of consciousness resulting from a head injury.)

III. LANGUAGE or SPEECH

To understand the spoken and printed words and to express ideas in speech and writing is called **language**. It is an example of skilled voluntary movements.

Speech disorders

1. Aphasias

This means the abnormalities of language (speech) function that are not due to the defects of vision or hearing or motor paralysis. It is of three types: *sensory, motor* and *global aphasia.*

(i) **Sensory** or **fluent aphasia**. This condition is produced due to lesion in the Wernicke's area (*i.e.* area 22, sensory speech centre). It is located in the region at the posterior end of the superior temporal gyrus in the dominant hemisphere. It is concerned with the comprehension of auditory and visual informations, *i.e.* interpretation and understanding. It is *characterized by*:
   (a) speech is not disturbed but the person talks excessively that makes little sense;
   (b) the person fails to understand the meaning of spoken or written words (*pure word blindness* or *anomic aphasia*).

(ii) **Motor or Non-fluent aphasia**. It is due to lesion in the Broca's area (*i.e.* area 44, motor speech centre). It is located in the inferior frontal gyrus in the dominant hemisphere. It processes the information received from Wernicke's area into a detailed and coordinated pattern for vocalization. This pattern then projected to the motor cortex which initiates the appropriate movements of the lips, tongue and larynx to produce speech. It is *characterized by*:
   (a) loss of articulate speech or inability to write or both;
   (b) the person is dumb, and the speech is slow; and
   (c) words are hard to come by (*i.e.* limited to 2 or 3 words).
   Thus the person frequently uses automatic words, such as days of week, etc.

(iii) **Global aphasia**. This condition is produced as a result of loss of both Wernicke's and Broca's area; therefore, all the functions of speech are involved.

2. Dysarthria

In this condition, there is difficulty in spoken speech, *i.e.* imperfect vocalization. Since muscle for expressing the speech cannot be used effectively, the main defect lies in the motor areas (area 4, 6 and 8) and their connections.

Types of dysarthria:

(i) ***Stammering***. It is a developmental disorder, more common in boys than girls. It is only very rarely due to organic brain diseases.

(ii) ***Lalling or baby speech***. In this condition, all the difficult consonants are dropped; the person speaks like a baby. Lalling in adults is usually the result of congenital or infantile deafness. Speech is usually louder than normal.

IMPORTANT VIVA-VOCE QUESTIONS

Q.1. *Name the headings under which the examination of nervous system is carried out.*
Ans. Page 237.

Q.2. *Describe your observations of the higher functions of the nervous system on the subject.*
Ans. Refer to the text.

Q.3. *How does the dominant hemisphere differ from representational one?*
Ans. Page 237.

Q.4. *Differentiate between:*
(i) delusions and hallucinations;
(ii) recent and remote memory;
(iii) Fluent and non-fluent aphasia.
Ans. Page 238.

Q.5. *How will you judge the general intelligence of a person?*
Ans. Page 238.

Q.6. *What is retrograde amnesia? When does it occur?*
Ans. Page 238.

Q.7. *What is Hieroglyphics?*
Ans. This means words written in sacred symbol, *i.e.* inability to understand the written words. A condition seen in persons suffering from sensory aphasia (See above).

(B) Examination of the Cranial Nerves

These nerves have their cell bodies in the brain. There are twelve pairs of the cranial nerves. Some are *afferent (sensory)*, some are *efferent (motor)* and those containing both of these components are called *mixed* nerves. The essential points indicating its functions, the clinical disorders resulting from lesions affecting it, and the method for the examination of each cranial nerve are described.

FIRST NERVE: THE OLFACTORY NERVE

Origin

From the olfactory epithelium

Function

It is a *pure sensory* nerve and is concerned with olfaction (smell).

Effect of paralysis

Complete loss of sense of smell, called *Anosmia* on the affected side

How to test

Apply the clove oil or other substances which are not irritating such as oil of peppermint or tincture of asafoetid to each nostril separately, and ask the subject if he recognises it or not.

Notes: Each nerve should be tested separately.

Notes

(1) Exclude local changes in the nose itself e.g. common cold before labelling it as neurological disorder.

(2) Irritating substances such as ammonium chloride which acts partially through trigeminal nerve, should be avoided. It may lead to difficulty in recognising the smell.

IMPORTANT VIVA-VOCE QUESTIONS

Q.1. *Define anosmia, parosmia and hyposmia.*

Ans. **Anosmia** is a complete absence of smell; **parosmia** is alteration in the character of smell; **hyposmia** is the reduction of the sense of smell. All these conditions usually develop due to *bilateral* damage to the olfactory mucosa or olfactory pathways by trauma or diseases.

Q.2. *Name a condition in which the sense of smell is greatly increased.*

Ans. The persons with adrenal insufficiency have greatly increased sensitivity for smell.

Q.3. *Mention a few unique features associated with the sense of smell.*

Ans. (i) All other sensations (general or special) pass through the thalamus and project to the neocortex, whereas the smell pathways have no relay in the thalamus and there is no neocortical projection area for olfaction.

(ii) Its receptor neurons are in direct contact with the external environment.

(iii) The smell receptors are distant receptors (telereceptors) as well as chemoreceptors; their adaptation is early and rapid.

Q.4. *What is olfactory fatigue? How can it be measured?*

Ans. Adaptation to the smell of odoriferous substances is called olfactory fatigue. It develops within seconds or minutes, depending on the nature of the substance. The degree of adaptation can be measured by the rise in threshold concentration required to excite the sense of smell.

Q.5. *What are macrosmatic and microsmatic animals?*

Ans. The olfactory sense is highly developed in the rabbit and the dog, which are called **macrosmatic**, but is much less in man, apes, monkeys (primates), which are called **microsmatic**. This is due to the fact that the total area of the olfactory mucous membrane is much larger in dogs and rabbits as compared to primates.

SECOND NERVE: THE OPTIC NERVE

Origin

From the retina

Function

It is a *pure sensory* nerve concerned with the transmission of various visual sensations to the brain.

How to test

Each eye should be examined separately for the following:

1. Visual acuity
2. Field of vision
3. Colour vision, and
4. Examination of fundus by ophthalmoscope (*Ophthalmoscopy*).

Visual Acuity

1. It is the degree to which the details and contours of objects are perceived. It is expressed in terms of *visual angle.* We can resolve two points or parallel lines and recognise them as two only when the visual angle is 1 minute (1° = 60 minutes).
2. It is usually defined in terms of *minimum separable, i.e.* the shortest distance by which two lines can be separated and still can be perceived as two lines or power determining the shape, outline, etc. of surroundings.
3. Clinically, visual acuity is tested separately for near and distant vision.
   (i) *Test for near vision.* Ask the subject to read the ***Jaeger's chart*** at the ordinary reading distance at which he is used to read in a well-lighted room without glasses (Fig. 3.22.1-B). The chart consists of reading *test types* of varying sizes, the notation being based on the 'printers' point system. The smallest print is N6. The near vision is recorded as the smallest type which the subject can read comfortably.

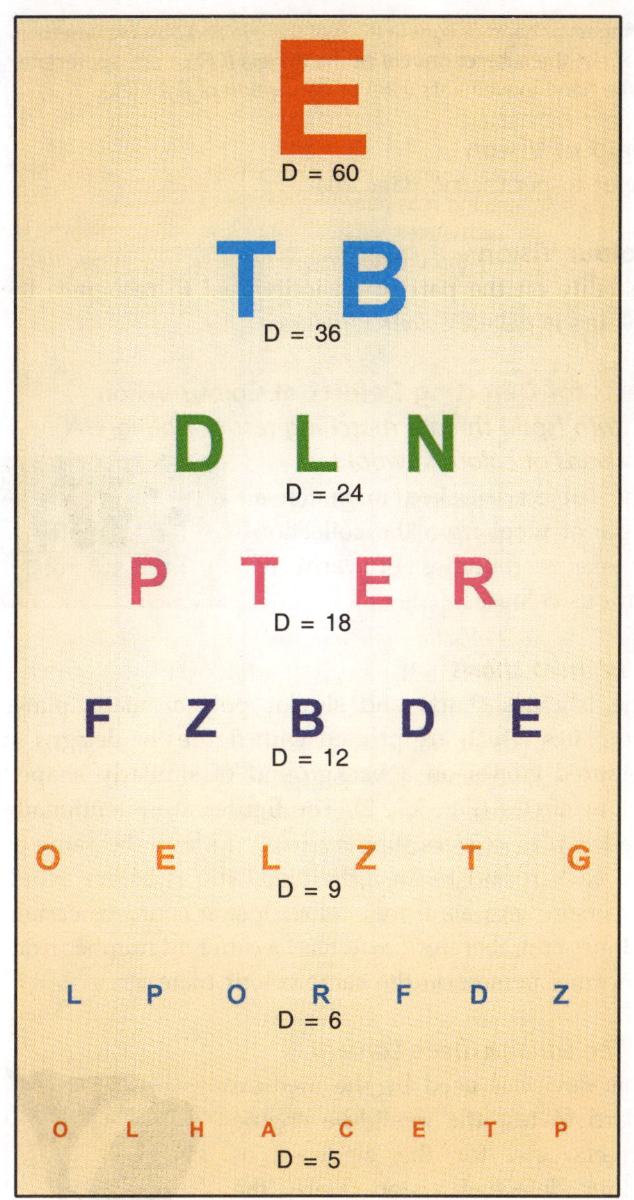

[A] (60% reduction, from the original chart, D = distance in metres)

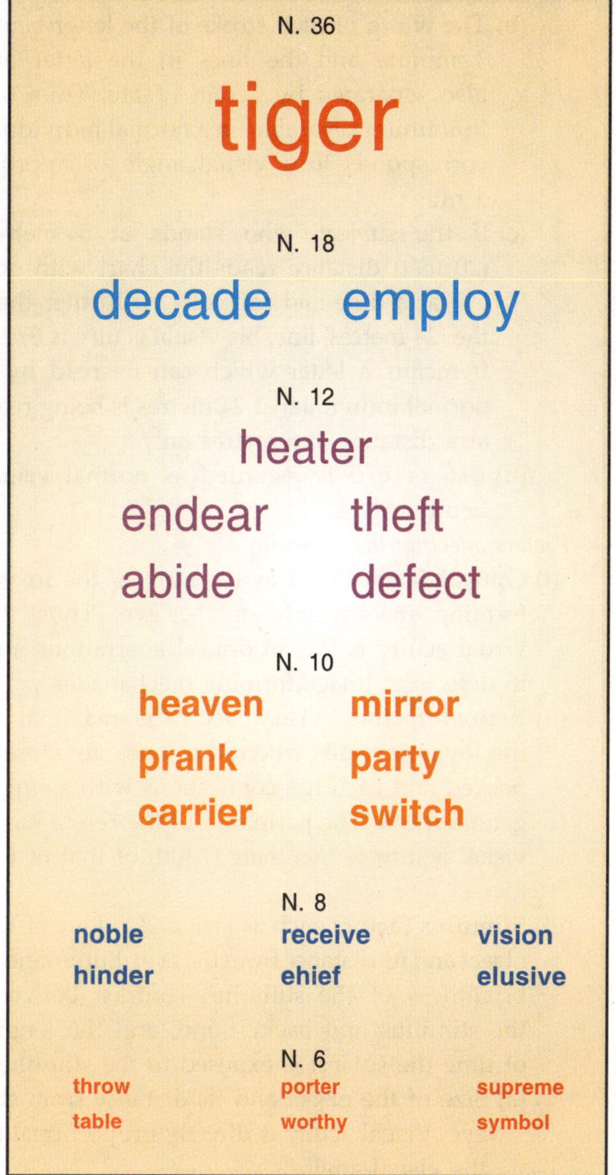

[B]

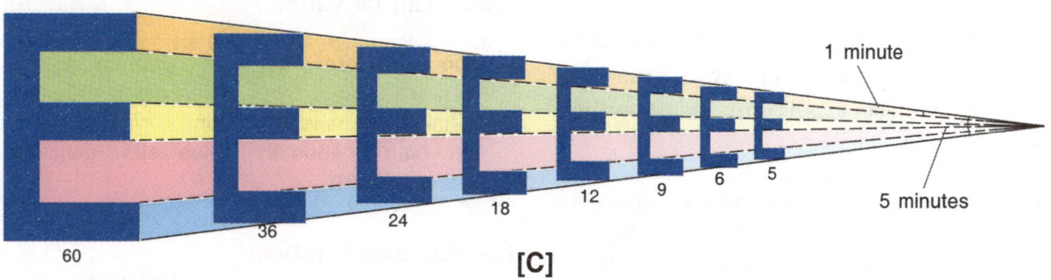

[C]

Fig. 3.22.1 (A) Snellen's and (B) Jaeger's charts for testing the visual acuity and (C) basis of designing the 'test' letters

(ii) *Test for distant vision.* This is tested with the help of ***Snellen's Chart*** by the ability of the subject to recognise *test letters* when illuminated suitably (Fig. 3.22.1-A).

(a) The test 'block' letters which are black on a white background are of different sizes. Each line of letters has a figure of 60, 36, 24, 18, 12, 9, 6 and 5 metres noted beside it. The chart is so designed that each letter a normal individual can read at a required distance, subtends a visual angle of 5 minutes. (Fig. 3.22.1-C)

(b) The width of each stroke of the letter being 1 minute and the lines in the letter are also separated by 1 min of arc. Thus the 'minimum separable' in a normal individual corresponds to a visual angle of approx. 1 min.

(c) If the subject, who stands at 6 metres (20 feet) distance reads the chart with one eye at a time and can read no further than the '24 metres' line, his visual acuity is 6/24. It means a letter which can be read by a normal individual at 24 metres is being read at a distance of 6 metres only.

(d) 6/6 or 6/5 is regarded as normal visual acuity.

4. *Factors affecting visual acuity*

(i) **Optical factors** such as the state of the image forming mechanisms of the eye. Thus the visual acuity is low in optical aberrations and in defects of image forming mechanisms.

(ii) **Retinal factors**. Visual acuity is maximal at the fovea centralis where the cones are closely packed and each has connections with a single ganglion cell. The periphery of the retina has a visual acuity of less than 1/30th of that of the fovea.

(iii) **Stimulus factors** such as size and colour of the object and its distance from the eye; illumination, brightness of the stimulus, contrast between the stimulus and background, and the length of time the subject is exposed to the stimulus.

(a) Size of the object and its distance from the eye. Visual acuity is directly proportional to the visual angle.

$$\text{Visual angle} = \frac{\text{Size of the object}}{\text{distance of the object from the eye}}$$

(b) Colour of the object. Coloured object means a weak stimulus. Visual acuity is thus less for coloured objects as compared to white objects.

Important Note: The visual acuity of less than 1/60 is recorded as: (i) counting fingers (CF), (ii) hand movements (HM), (iii) perception of light (PL) or (iv) no perception of light (no PL). This is done in the gross impairment of vision. Show the fingers or hand or light in front of the eye and observe whether or not the subject can count the fingers (CF) or can appreciate the hand movements (HM) or perception of light (PL).

Field of Vision

Refer to perimetry, page 204.

Colour Vision

Inability on the part of an individual to recognise the colours is called *Colour Blindness.*

Tests for Detecting Defects of Colour Vision

1. Yarn (spun thread) matching test or Holmgren's skeins of coloured wool test

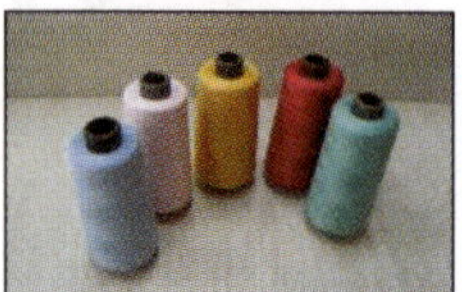

The subject is asked to match a piece of wool from the collection of skeins (bundles of yarn) of various colours.

2. Ishihara charts

The Ishihara charts and similar polychromatic plates are plates which are printed with figures or designs in coloured circles on a background of similarly shaped colour circles (Fig. 3.22.2). The figures are intentionally made up of colours that are likely to look the same as the background to an individual who is colour blind. A person with abnormal colour vision confuses certain colours and, therefore, will read a different number from a normal person on the same colour plate.

3. The Edridge Green Lantern

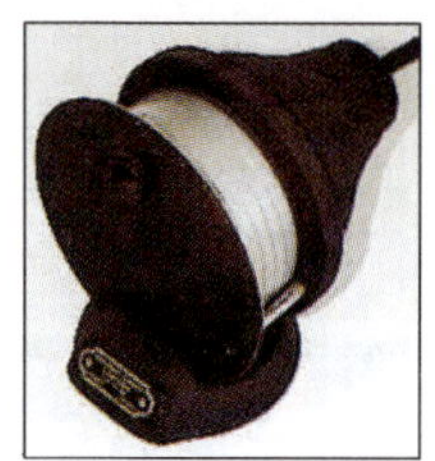

This device is used by the medical board to test the would-be engine drivers, etc. for the evidence of colour defective vision. Here, the subject has to identify the colour of a small illuminated area, the size of which can be varied.

Important Note: The most common anomalies of colour vision are various types of red-green deficiency, inherited as sex-linked recessive conditions (*incidence*, male:female :: 16:1). Next common anomaly is blue-yellow deficiency. Total colour blindness is rare.

Fundus examination

Ophthalmoscopy (refer to page 211).

IMPORTANT VIVA-VOCE QUESTIONS

Q.1. *Define: nodal point, visual angle, minimum separable, visual acuity, far and near point of vision.*

Ans. (i) *Nodal point:* the centre point of a lens is known as its optical centre or nodal point; a ray of light passing through it does not suffer any refraction and goes straight.

(ii) *Visual angle:* the angle subtended by any object on the nodal point of the eye is called visual angle.

(iii) *Minimum separable,* page 240.

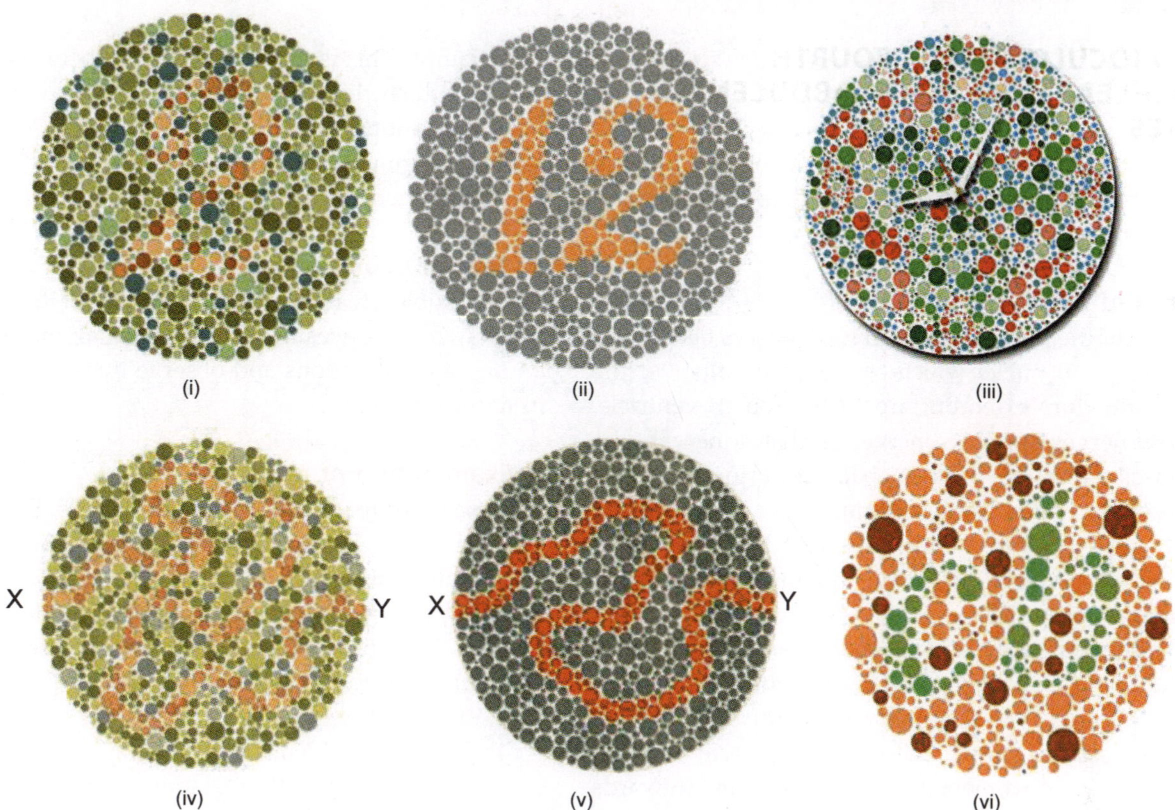

The plates are designed to be appreciated when held 75 cm from the subject in natural daylight. The numbers or pictures which are seen on plates (i), (ii) and (iii) are stated and each answer should be given without more than three seconds' delay. If the subject is unable to read the numbers, plates (iv) and (v) are used and the winding lines between the two X's are traced with a brush. Each tracing should be completed within ten seconds.

Fig. 3.22.2 Ishihara's series of Plates designed as a test for Colour blindness

(iv) *Visual acuity*, page 240.

(v) *Far point of vision:* Under resting condition (*i.e.* when the eye is adapted for distant vision, the ciliary muscle is relaxed) parallel light rays from distant object (more than 6 metres) are brought to a focus on the retina. In this state, the resting power of the eye is 59 Dioptres which is taken as 'zero' and the position of the object is referred as the *far point of vision*.

(vi) *Near point of vision.* When a person focuses clearly on a near object in addition to this resting power, an extra amount of refractive power is required to focus the image on the retina. Thus the nearest point to the eye at which object can be clearly seen with maximum accommodation is called the *near point of vision*. It increases with age. (At the age of 10 years, near point of vision in 9 cm.)

Q.2. *Explain the basis of designing the 'test' letters of Snellen chart.*

Ans. Page 241.

Q.3. *Name the factors influencing the visual acuity.*

Ans. Page 242.

Q.4. *What are primary and complementary colours?*

Ans. Red, green and blue are called primary colours. When two colours are mixed in appropriate amounts, it leads to the cancellation of colour sensation producing the sensation of white. Therefore, for any colour, there is a complementary colour that, when properly mixed with it, produces a sensation of white.

Q.5. *What does a blind eye see?*

Ans. A blind eye sees nothing, not even black.

Q.6. *Define: Mono, di and tri-chromats.*

Ans. Monochromats are individuals with only one cone system present, whereas dichromats have two cone systems present and trichromats have all the three cone systems but one may be weak.

Q.7. *Give an example of physiological dichromatic vision.*

Ans. The example of physiological dichromatic vision is at fovea centralis where only blue and red cones are present.

Q.8. *Give the reason behind the traffic lights.*

Ans. The common defects of colour blindness, in order of occurrence, are: deuteranomaly, deutranopia, protanopia, protanomaly, tritanomaly. *Pro, deuter* and *trit* refer to red, green and blue colour defected cone system, whereas *anomaly* is colour weakness and *anopia* is colour blindness. This explains the reason behind the traffic lights.

THIRD (OCULOMOTOR), FOURTH (TROCHLEAR) AND SIXTH (ABDUCENT) NERVES

All these nerves are described together for convenience as they innervate the extraocular muscles which move the eyeball.

Origin and function

The fibres of the third, fourth and sixth nerves take origin from a series of nuclei which begins in the floor of the sylvian aqueduct extending up to the fourth ventricle. All these nerves are *mixed* nerves as they innervate the eye muscles that move the eyeball and bring sensation from proprioceptors in the eye muscle.

The eye is moved within the orbit by six external muscles of the eye to bring about the following movements: (Fig. 3.22.3)

1. Abduction, *i.e.* horizontal movement outwards
2. Adduction, *i.e.* horizontal movement inwards
3. Elevation, *i.e.* vertical movement upwards
4. Depression, *i.e.* vertical movement downwards
5. Rotatory movements: *Internal rotation* (towards the nose) or *external rotation* (away from the nose) occurs by the cooperative action of various extraocular muscles.

Normally, the movements of the two eyes are symmetrical so that the visual axes may meet at the point at which the eyes are looking. This is called as *conjugate* movement of the eyes.

The ***innervation, action and effect of the paralysis*** of these nerves are summarized in Table 3.22.1.

How to test

1. Look for the following:

(i) Presence of ptosis, *i.e.* drooping (hanging) of upper eyelid

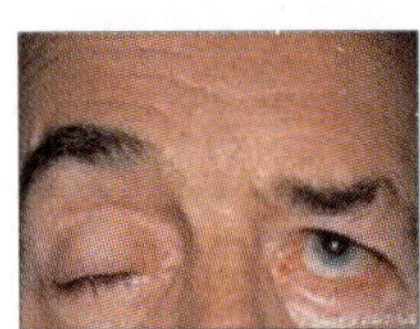

(ii) Squint. This is an abnormality of ocular movement in which the visual axes do not meet at the point of fixation.

(iii) Nystagmus, *i.e.* involuntary rhythmic to-and-fro movement of the eyeball.

2. Test for ocular movements

Ask the subject to follow the movements of the examiner's fingers with his eyes in superior, medial, inferior, lateral and oblique directions and observe if an error is present in any direction.

3. Examination of pupil

(i) *Size.* Compare the size of two pupils. Even a slight inequality of pupils may be present in perfectly healthy subjects.

(ii) *Shape.* Note whether the pupil is circular in outline (as it normally is) or its contour is irregular (as in *iritis* due to adhesion of the iris to the lens).

(iii) ***Visual reflexes***

(a) *PUPILLARY LIGHT REFLEX*

Direct light reflex: Examine each eye separately. The subject sits opposite a bright light (indirectly illuminated); ask him to look at a distant object (to be sure his accommodation is relaxed). Shine a bright light into one eye with a torch, the pupil in the same eye should contract almost immediately. When the light is switched off, the pupil will rapidly dilate to its previous diameter.

Indirect (consensual) light reflex: It should be tested by covering one eye while the other eye is tested. Showing the bright light into the test eye with a torch causes the constriction of pupil in both the eyes. If light is shut off from one eye, both pupils dilate slightly.

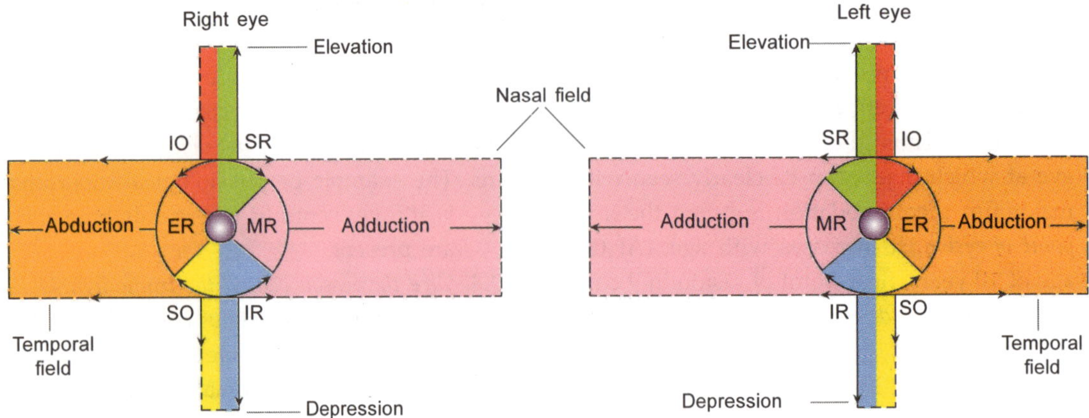

Fig. 3.22.3 Movement of the eyeball induced by contraction of the individual extraocular muscles (IO: inferior oblique; ER: external (lateral) rectus; MR: medial (internal) rectus; SR: superior rectus; SO: superior oblique; IR: inferior rectus)

Table 3.22.1 Innervation, action and effect of the paralysis of extraocular muscles (Fig. 3.22.4)

Cranial nerve and its type	Innervation (or supply)	Action/function	Effect of paralysis
1. Third (oculomotor)	(i) Ciliary muscle	Helps in accommodation	Loss of power of accommodation
	(ii) Iris (sphincter) pupillae	Constricts the pupil	Pupil usually gets dilated and fixed
	(iii) Levator palpebrae superioris	Elevator of upper eyelid	Ptosis, *i.e.* drooping of upper eyelid
	(iv) All extraocular muscles except superior oblique and external (or lateral) rectus:		
	(a) medial rectus	Rotate eyeball medially (adduction)	Lateral deviation of eye due to the unopposed action of lateral rectus
	(b) Inferior oblique	Rolls the eye outwards and pulls it upwards	The paralysis of an individual muscle is rare; however, these muscles get involved during the lesion of the third nerve; as a result eye is displaced downward and outward.
	(c) Superior rectus	Upward movement of the eye with adduction	
	(d) Inferior rectus	Downward movement of the eye with adduction	
2. Fourth (Trochlear)	Superior oblique	Pulls the eyeball downwards, outwards and rotates it inwards	(i) A person cannot move the eye downwards and suffers *diplopia*; the eyeball gets rotated outwards. (ii) Visible squint (rare)
3. Sixth (Abducent)	External (or lateral) rectus	Rotate the eyeball laterally (abduction)	(i) Inability to move the eye outwards (ii) *Diplopia* (double vision) on looking in that direction

Important Notes:

1. Formula for remembering the innervation of external ocular muscles: $ER_6(SO_4)_3$. External (lateral) rectus (supplied by VI); SO_4 is superior oblique (supplied by IV) and remaining all eye muscles (by III nerve).
2. Recti acts as elevators and depressors alone when the eye is in abduction; and obliques act similarly when the eye is in adduction. Therefore, the function of extraocular muscles are easily assessed by testing the movements of elevation and depression in both full adduction and full abduction (and not simply testing them in the mid-position of the gaze).

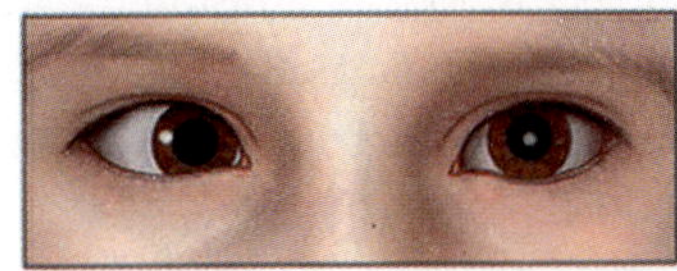

Esotropia (*Eso* inwards, *trope* a turning)

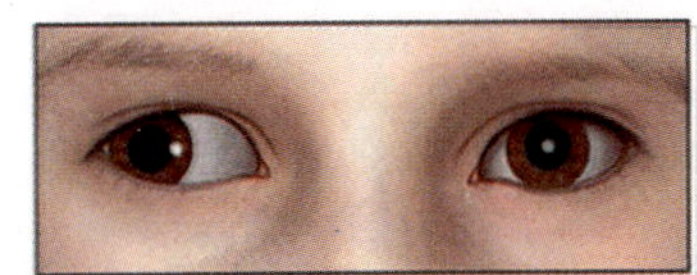

Exotropia (*Exo* outwards, *trope* a turning)

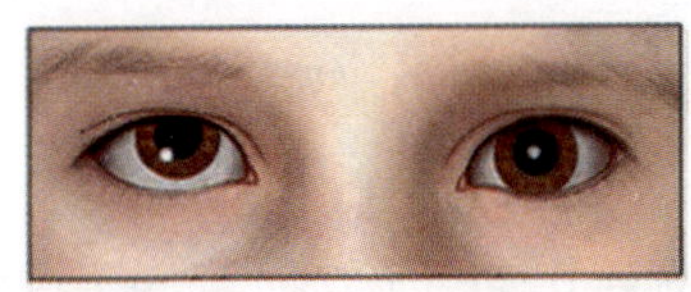

Hypertropia (*Hyper* above, *trope* a turning)

Fig. 3.22.4 Effect of the paralysis of the extraocular muscles

Pathway for light reflex : (Fig. 3.22.5)

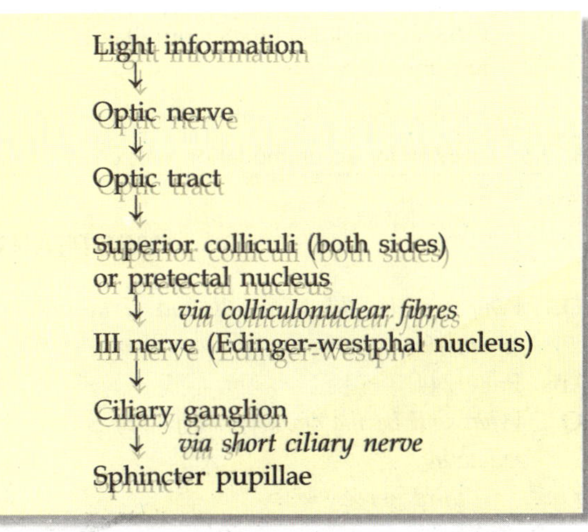

Fig. 3.22.5 Pathway for light reflex (direct and consensual)

(b) *ACCOMMODATION REFLEX*

Accommodation is a process by which the images of the near object are focused on the retina by increasing the curvature of anterior surface of the lens.

Hold up one finger close to the subject's nose, ask him to look away at a distant object and then ask him to look suddenly at your finger. The *reaction to accommodation* (accommodation reflex) is comprised of the following components:

- *Contraction of ciliary muscle* via III nerve. As a result, the anterior curvature of lens increases (see above).
- *Constriction of pupil* due to the contraction of sphincter pupillae. This allows the light to fall only on the centre of the lens in which the accommodation changes are maximum. The constriction of pupils also helps:
  - to decrease spherical and chromatic aberrations;
  - to decrease the intensity of light entering into the eye; and
  - to increase the depth of focus.
- The *convergence of visual axes* due to the contraction of medial rectus muscle. This helps focus the image of an object on fovea centralis. If the convergence of visual axes fails, diplopia (double vision) occurs.

Pathway for Accomodation reflex : (Fig. 3.22.6)

Visual information
↓ *via visual pathway*
Primary visual area, area 17
↓
Frontal eye field, area 8
↓ *via corticonuclear fibers*
III nerve (Edinger-westphal nucleus)
↓
Ciliary muscle; sphincter pupillae and medial rectus

Fig. 3.22.6 Pathway for accommodation reflex

Important Note: Accommodation reflex is bilateral, *i.e.* if we close one eye and look at the near object with the other eye, both the eyes show the constriction of the pupil.

OSPE-I

Aim: To check for the light reflex in the subject provided.

Procedure steps: Refer to page 244.

Checklist

1. Explains the test procedure to the subject. **(Yes/No)**
2. Checks for the functioning of the torch. **(Yes/No)**
3. Sits opposite a bright light source and asks the subject to look at a distant object. **(Yes/No)**
4. Covers the subject's one eye and shines a bright light into the other eye with a torch. **(Yes/No)**
5. Looks for the constriction of pupil in the eye in which light has been shone. **(Yes/No)**
6. Repeats the above steps 4 and 5 in the other eye as well. **(Yes/No)**
7. Looks for the indirect light reflex as well. **(Yes/No)**

OSPE-II

Aim: To demonstrate the accommodation reflex in the subject provided.

Procedure steps: See above.

Checklist

1. Explains the test procedure to the subject. **(Yes/No)**
2. Sits opposite a bright light source and holds one finger close to the subject's nose. **(Yes/No)**
3. Asks the subject to look at a distant object. **(Yes/No)**
4. Asks the subject to look suddenly at his finger. **(Yes/No)**
5. Repeats the whole procedure with the subject's other eye as well. **(Yes/No)**

IMPORTANT VIVA-VOCE QUESTIONS

Q.1. *Why are the third, fourth and sixth nerves tested together?*

Ans. Page 244.

Q.2. *What will be the effect of the paralysis of each of the following?*

(i) third nerve

(ii) fourth nerve

(iii) sixth nerve

Ans. Page 245.

Q.3. *How will you test for the paralysis of the third cranial nerve?*

Ans. Page 244.

Q.4. *Give the pathways for: (i) light reflex and (ii) accommodation reflex.*

Ans. Pages 244 and 245.

Q.5. *What is Argyll-Robertson pupil and Reverse Argyll-Robertson pupil?*

Ans. (i) *Argyll-Robertson pupil*

In this condition, pupillary constriction in response to a light stimulus is absent or decreased while the response to accommodation is present. It is associated clinically with lesions in or near the aqueduct of Sylvii and the superior colliculi which interrupt the pathway of light reflex only. This sign is very frequently found in the syphilis of CNS which affects this region.

(ii) *Reverse Argyll-Robertson pupil*

This is the reverse of (i) above; here pupillary constriction in response to light is present while the response to accommodation is absent. This is due to the bilateral damage of frontal lobe or damage of its descending fibres to the III nerve nucleus.

Q.6. *What is near response?*

Ans. Reaction to accommodation is a three-part response. Therefore, accommodation reflex is also called near response.

Q.7. *What is an amplitude of accommodation?*

Ans. This is the difference in the refractive power of the eye between the two states, complete relaxation and maximal accommodation.

FIFTH NERVE: THE TRIGEMINAL NERVE

Origin

From the lateral surface of pons at about its middle

Function

It is a *mixed* nerve with sensory, motor and secreto-motor components. The nerve separates into three divisions:

1. *First or ophthalmic division*
   (i) It supplies the conjunctival surface of the upper lid only; the lacrimal gland;
   (ii) The skin of the medial part of nose as far as its tip, the upper eyelids, the forehead, and the scalp as far as the vertex (Fig. 3.22.7).

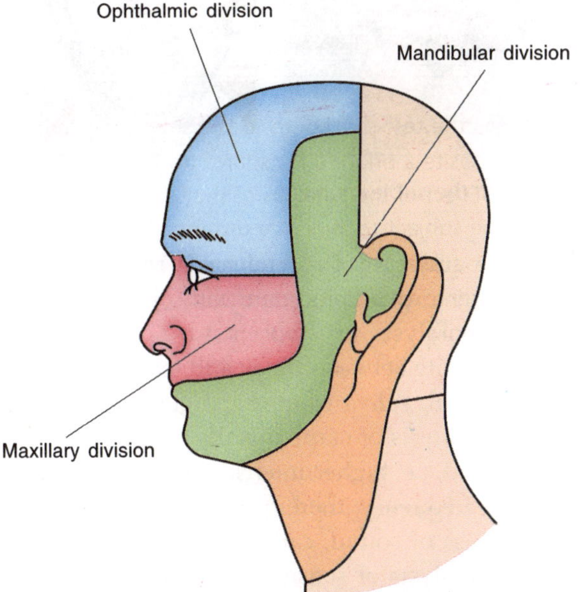

Fig. 3.22.7 Lateral view of the face skin area supplied by the fifth (trigeminal) nerve

2. *Second or maxillary division*
   (i) It supplies the cheek, the front of the temple, the lower eyelid and its conjunctival surface, the sides of the nose, the upper lip, the upper teeth;
   (ii) The mucous membrane of: the nose, upper part of the pharynx, the roof of mouth, parts of soft palate, tonsils and medial-inferior portion of cornea.
3. *Third or mandibular division*
   (i) It supplies the lower part of the face, the lower lip, the ear, the tongue and the lower teeth;
   (ii) It also supplies parasympathetic fibres to the salivary glands.
   (iii) It is joined by the *motor root* and innervates all the muscles of mastication **except** buccinator which is supplied by the seventh (facial) nerve.

Effect of paralysis

1. Lesion of ophthalmic division results in:
   (i) loss of cutaneous sensibility in the area supplied by it;
   (ii) loss of corneal reflex with inflammatory changes (*neuropathic keratitis*)
2. Lesion of maxillary division results in:
   (i) loss of sensation in the area supplied by it;
   (ii) loss of palatal reflex
3. Lesion of mandibular division results in:
   (i) loss of sensation in the area supplied by it;
   (ii) the salivary and buccal sensations may be decreased;
   (iii) trophic ulcers may develop in the mouth, nose and cornea;
   (iv) weakness of the muscles of mastication

Important Note: The lesion of whole trigeminal nerve results in all above features. The loss of oral sensations may cause subjective impairment in *taste sensation* but it is not lost completely.

How to Test

(A) Test for sensory functions

1. *Test for various sensations* (touch, pain, pressure, temperature) over the skin and mucous membrane

of face by all the three branches of trigeminal nerve (for details, refer to page 268).

2. *Testing the corneal reflex.* Ask the subject to look at some distant object, then lightly touch the lateral edge of the cornea at its conjunctival margin with a cotton wool. If reflex is present, the subject blinks; compare the reflex on the opposite side as well. (Also, refer to page 265)

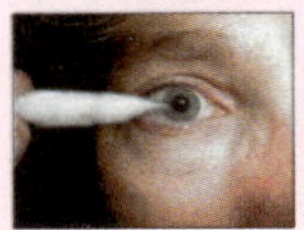

Note: The centre of cornea should never be touched, as it carries the risk of corneal ulceration and subsequent visual impairment.

(B) Test for motor functions: *Muscles of mastication*

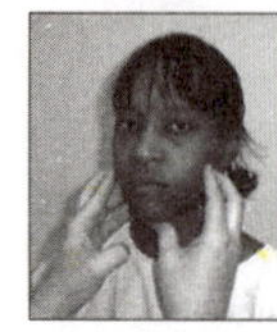

1. Ask the subject to clench his teeth; the temporalis and masseter muscles should stand out with equal prominence on each side; confirm this by palpation. If there is paralysis on one side, the muscle on that side will fail to become prominent.
2. Ask the subject to open his mouth; on opening the mouth, the jaw will deviate towards the paralysed side, being pushed over by the healthy external pterygoid muscle.

IMPORTANT VIVA-VOCE QUESTIONS

Q.1. *Give the division and functions of trigeminal nerve.*
Ans. Page 247.
Q.2. *What are the effects of the paralysis of the fifth nerve?*
Ans. Page 247.
Q.3. *Name the muscles of mastication.*
Ans. The muscles of mastication are: Masseter, temporalis, internal and external pterygoid and buccinator.
Q.4. *What precautions should you observe while eliciting corneal reflex?*
Ans. Refer to note above.

SEVENTH NERVE: THE FACIAL NERVE

Origin

From the pons, lateral to that of the sixth nerve nucleus

Function

It is a *mixed* nerve, consisting of three sets of fibres:

1. *Motor fibre supplies:*
   (i) All the muscles of face and scalp except levator palpebrae superioris
   (ii) Stylohyoid muscle
   (iii) Buccinator muscle
   (iv) Stapedius muscle
2. *Sensory fibres.* It brings taste sensation from anterior 2/3rd of tongue (salt, sour, sweet).
3. *Secreto-motor fibres.* It supplies lacrimal gland, sublingual and submandibular salivary glands (*i.e.* all salivary glands except the parotid gland).

Effect of paralysis on the affected side

1. The paralysis of the muscles of face and scalp results in (Fig. 3.22.8):
   (i) Loss of facial expression, asymmetry of face.
   (ii) Furrows over forehead and nasolabial folds disappear or smoothen out.
   (iii) Ala nasi muscle does not function properly during respiration.
   (iv) The angle of mouth is drawn upwards and deviated to the opposite side.
   (v) Eyes are wide open due to the paralysis of orbicularis oculi muscle; eyebrows droop down.

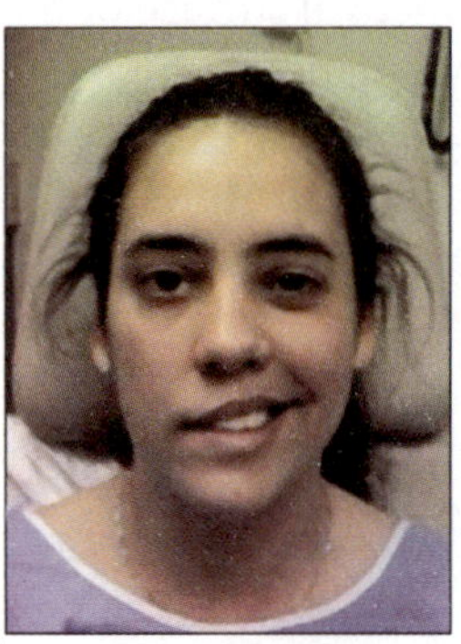
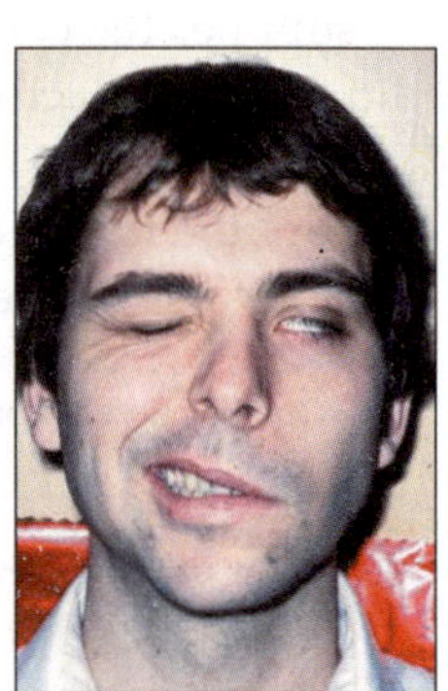

Fig. 3.22.8 Effect of the paralysis of the facial nerve

2. The paralysis of stylohyoid muscle; clinically difficult to detect its paralysis.
3. The paralysis of buccinator causes food to accumulate between cheek and teeth and it dribbles along with saliva from the angle of the mouth.
4. The paralysis of stapedius. Its function is damping of sound, *i.e.* higher intensity sounds are turned to lower frequency; therefore, the subject complains of loudness of sound, called **Hyperacusis**.
5. The paralysis of sensory fibres leads to the loss of taste sensations from anterior 2/3rd of tongue. The effect is better appreciated in bilateral paralysis.
6. The paralysis of secreto-motor fibres produces:
   (i) Decrease in tear formation which results in the dryness of conjuntiva, called **Xerosis** or **Xerophthalmia**.

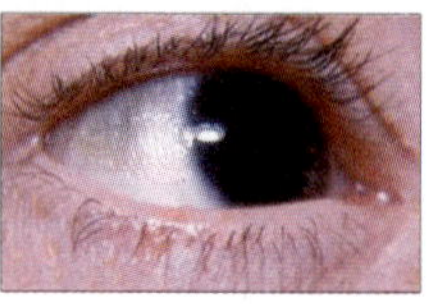

(ii) Decrease in salivary secretion resulting in difficulty in the swallowing of food.

How to test

1. Tests for the muscles of face and scalp
   (i) Look for
   (a) facial expression
   (b) symmetry of the face
   (c) Furrows over forehead
   (d) Nasolabial folds and its movement with deep breathing
   (e) Angle of mouth
   (f) Width of palperal fissure
   (g) Position of eyebrows

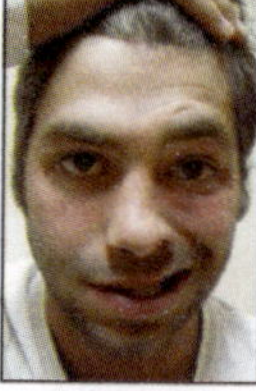

   (ii) Ask the subject to show upper teeth or to smile; the angle of mouth gets deviated to the healthy side due to the unopposed action of facial muscles.
   (iii) Ask the subject to close his eyes as tightly as he can.
   (a) In case of a complete paralysis of orbicularis oculi muscle he would not be able to close his eyes. In an attempt to do so, the eyeballs roll upwards (**Bell's Phenomenon**). (Fig. 3.22.9)

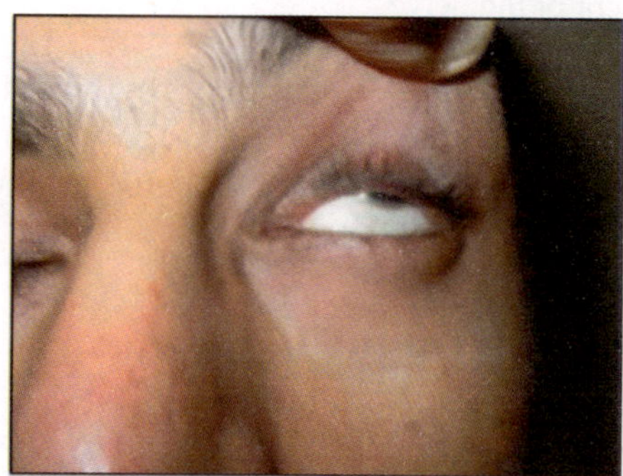

Fig. 3.22.9 Bell's phenomenon

   (b) In partial paralysis, very little resistance is required to open the eye while the subject attempts to keep it closed.
   (c) In normal healthy individuals, it should be almost impossible to open it against the subject's effort.

Note: Bilateral facial weakness is difficult to recognise.

2. *Tests for Buccinator muscles*
   (i) Ask the subject to whistle; even if one side is paralysed, he cannot whistle.
   (ii) **Inflation Test**: Ask the subject to inflate his mouth with air and blow out his cheeks; tap with the finger in turn on each inflated cheek; on paralysed side, air can be made to escape easily from the mouth.
3. *Test for stapedius muscle.* Ask for the loudness of sound heard in any one of the ears.
4. *Test for taste sensations.* To test the sense of taste, use strong solutions of sugar (for sweet) and common salt (for salt), and weak solutions of citric acid (for sour) and quinine (for bitter). These are applied with the help of a glass rod to the surface of the protruded tongue, and if the taste is recognised, the subject should write down accordingly (sweet, salt, sour or bitter) without withdrawing the tongue or should indicate by raising one, two, three or four fingers as instructed beforehand. After each test, the mouth must be rinsed. The quinine test should be applied last as its effect is more lasting than that of the others. Both the anterior and posterior parts of the right and left halves of the tongue should be tested separately.

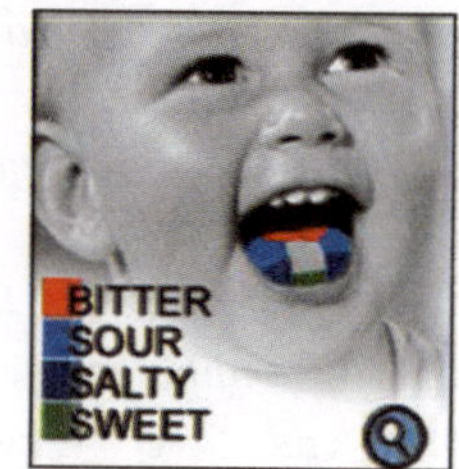

5. *Test for lacrimation*: **Schirmer's Test**. Take two strips of filter paper of the same size and length and hang them from lower eyelids of both the eyes. Ask the subject to smell a lacrimating stimulant, such as ammonium chloride. Little or no moistening of the filter paper occurs on the paralysed size.

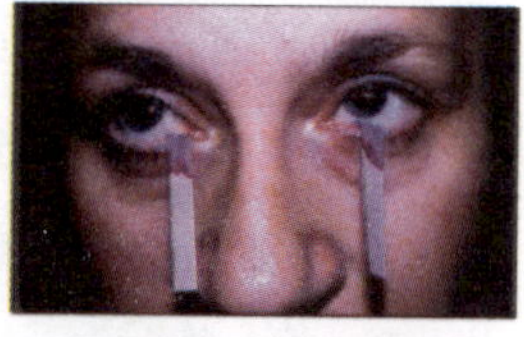

OSPE

Aim: Test for the muscles of face and scalp of the subject provided

Checklist

1. Explains the test procedure to the subject. **(Yes/No)**
2. Looks for: Facial symmetry, nasolabial folds and furrows over forehead. **(Yes/No)**
3. Looks for: Eyebrows, angle of mouth and width of palperal fissure. **(Yes/No)**
4. Asks the subject to show upper teeth or to smile. **(Yes/No)**
5. Asks the subject to close his eyes as tightly as he can. Tries to open them passively. **(Yes/No)**

IMPORTANT VIVA-VOCE QUESTIONS

Q.1. *Give the functions and effect of the paralysis of the seventh nerve.*

Ans. Page 248.

Q.2. *Define: Hyperacusis, xerosis.*

Ans. Page 248 and 249.

Q.3. *What is Bell's phenomenon? When is it seen?*

Ans. Page 249.

Q.4. *How will you test for lacrimation?*

Ans. Page 249.

Q.5. *What are the types of facial palsies? How will you differentiate between them?*

Ans. Two types of facial palsies are identified (Fig. 3.22.10):

(i) Lesions within or distal to the facial nucleus cause *infra nuclear facial palsy or lower motor neuron paralysis*. This results in the paralysis of both upper and lower parts of the face with the atrophy of the facial muscles. It also causes the loss of taste in anterior 2/3rd portion of the tongue and sounds on the affected side unusually loud (*hyperacusis*).

(ii) Lesions above the facial nucleus cause *supra-nuclear facial palsy or upper motor neuron paralysis*. This mainly results in the paralysis of the lower half of face because the muscles of the upper part of the face have double (bilateral) innervation. It does not produce the atrophy of facial muscles and taste is not affected in anterior 2/3rd portion of the tongue.

Q.6. *What precautions must be observed for testing the taste sensation?*

Ans. The subject should not withdraw the tongue into his mouth; rather he should indicate the sensation felt either in writing or pre-directed signals.

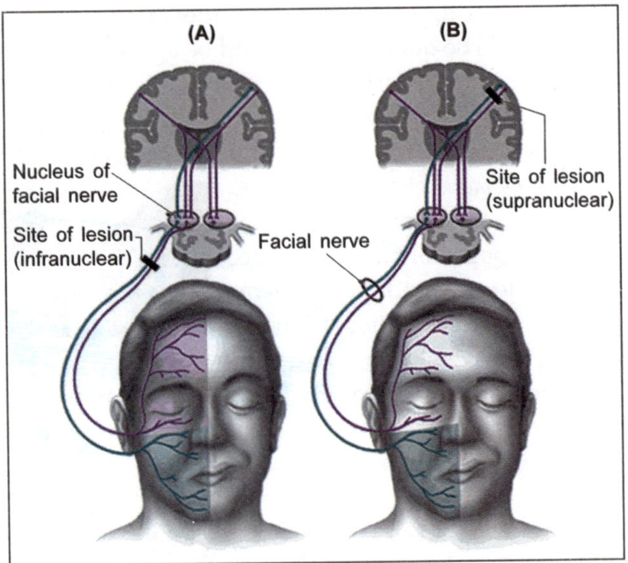

Fig. 3.22.10 Facial palsy: (A) infranuclear and (B) supranuclear

EIGHTH NERVE: AUDITORY (or VESTIBULOCOCHLEAR) NERVE

Origin

From the groove in between the junction of the pons and the medulla

Function

It is a *pure sensory nerve* consisting of two sets of fibres:

(i) One set supplies the vestibule and semicircular canals and is concerned with the maintenance of equilibrium, balance and sensation of bodily displacement.

(ii) Other set supplies the cochlea and is concerned with hearing.

Effect of paralysis

1. The lesion of vestibular nerve results in:
   (i) *Vertigo, i.e.* a sense of instability, often with a sensation of rotation; Therefore, the person complains of a feeling of giddiness or dizziness.

   Note: This becomes more prominent with the bilateral involvement of the nerve.

   (ii) *Nystagmus, i.e.* involuntary rhythmic to-and-fro movement of the eyeball
2. Lesion of cochlear nerve results in the loss of hearing on the affected side.

How to test

(A) Test for the vestibular functions

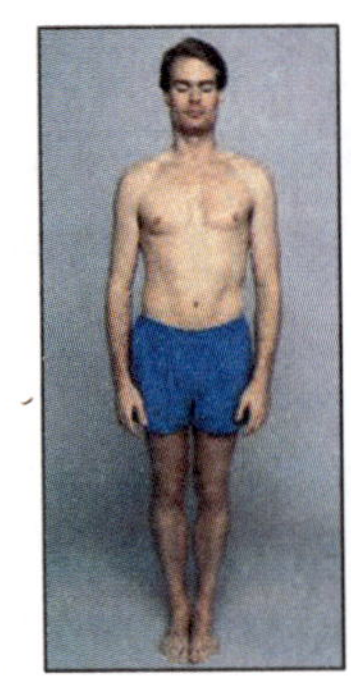

1. Ask if there is any history of vertigo or nystagmus.
2. ***Romberg's Sign***. The person is asked to stand with his feet close together, and if he can do this, then ask him to close his eyes. If Romberg's sign is present, as soon as his eyes are closed, he begins to sway about or may even fall. This is a test for the loss of position sense (*sensory ataxia*).

Note: In cerebellar ataxia, the person is ataxic whether the eyes are closed or not.

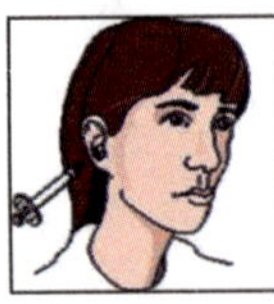

3. ***Barany's Caloric Test***. The semicircular canals can be stimulated by introducing water at 30°C or 44°C (7°C above and below the normal

body temperature) into the external auditory meatus. The temperature difference sets up convection currents in the endolymph; as a result, cupula is set into motion. This technique of *caloric stimulation* is used clinically for diagnostic purposes. It causes some nystagmus, vertigo and nausea.

> **Important Note:** While irrigating the ear canals in the treatment of ear infections, it is important to be sure that the fluid used is at body temperature so that the above mentioned symptoms may be avoided.

(B) Tests for Cochlear function: Hearing tests

Hearing tests, besides determining whether hearing is present or absent, also help assess the type of deafness in an individual. These are broadly divied into:

1. Watch test
2. Tuning fork tests, and
3. Audiometry

1. Watch Test

Steps:

(i) Ask the subject to close the eyes.
(ii) Stand behind the subject and plug one ear.
(iii) Slowly bring a watch from a distance and note the distance at which its tickling is heard.
(iv) Repeat the observation on the opposite ear.
(v) Compare the results of the two ears and with that of other subjects.
(vi) This test helps detect the impairment of hearing (deafness) in either one or both ears.

Alternatively, the test can be performed using tuning forks of different frequencies or instructing the subject to repeat the words, when whispered from a distance (*speech test*).

2. Tuning Fork Tests

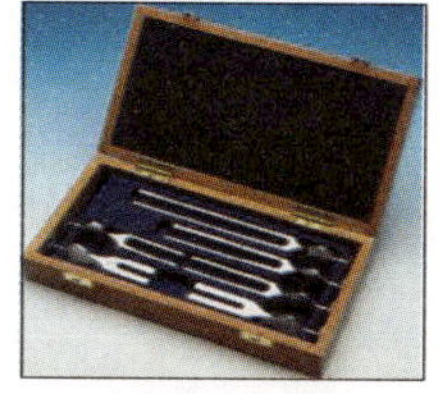

These tests are used to differentiate the type of deafness: conduction deafness or nerve deafness. These tests are performed using a tuning fork vibrating at 256 or 512 Hz (cps), since the apex of the cochlea contains the units which respond to the lower octaves (16-32-64-128-256-512-1024). The *pure tones* up to 2000 Hz produce clear synchronous volleys of action potentials in the eighth nerve (*volley principle of pitch discrimination*).

(i) ***Rinne's Test.*** In this, each ear is examined separately to compare the ability to hear through the bone (*bone conduction*) and through the air (*air conduction*) (Fig. 3.22.11).

(a) Occlude the subject's external auditory meatus of other ear with the thumb.

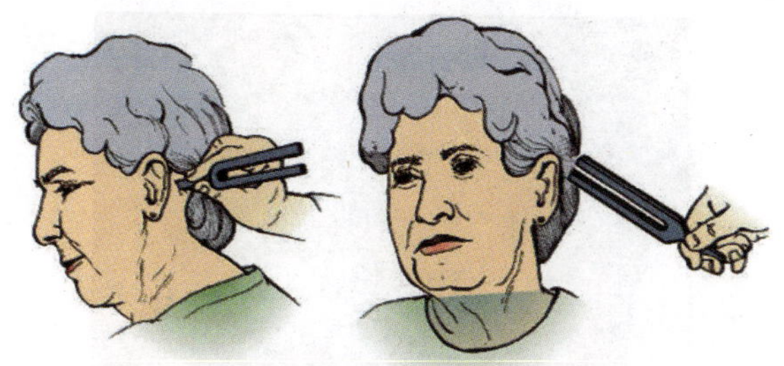

Fig. 3.22.11 Rinne's Test

(b) Set the tuning fork vibrating and press the base of the fork over the mastoid process behind the ear.
(c) Instruct the subject to indicate when he can no longer hear it (bone conduction).
(d) Immediately transfer the still vibrating tuning fork to the side of the head close to the ear.
(e) If the hearing is *normal,* the subject will hear the vibrating fork by air conduction even after he has ceased hearing by bone conduction, *i.e. in a healthy individual air conduction is better than bone conduction.* This is referred as **Rinne test positive.**
(f) In *conductive deafness,* vibrations in air are not heard after bone conduction is over, *i.e.* bone conduction is better than air conduction. This is referred as **Rinne test negative.**
(g) In total or complete **nerve deafness,** no sound is heard either by way of air or bone conduction.

(ii) ***Weber's Test.*** In this, only bone conduction is tested in both the ears simultaneously. Place the base of the vibrating tuning fork on the forehead and ask the subject to indicate whether the sound is heard equally in both ears or is better heard in one of the ears (Fig. 3.22.12).

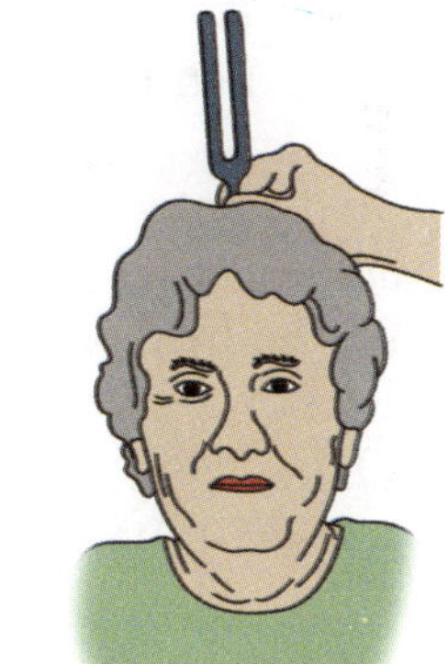

Fig. 3.22.12 Weber's Test

(a) In a healthy individual, both the ears 'hear' the sound equally well.
(b) If the sound is heard better by the defective (*deaf*) ear, the defect is due to *conduction deafness.* This is because the masking effect of environment noise is absent on the affected side.
(c) If the sound is better heard in the normal ear, the so-called sound is **lateralised to the normal ear**; then hearing loss in the defective ear is due to *nerve deafness.*

(iii) ***Schwabach Test.*** In this, the bone conduction of the subject is compared to that of the normal subject (examiner) (Fig. 3.22.13).

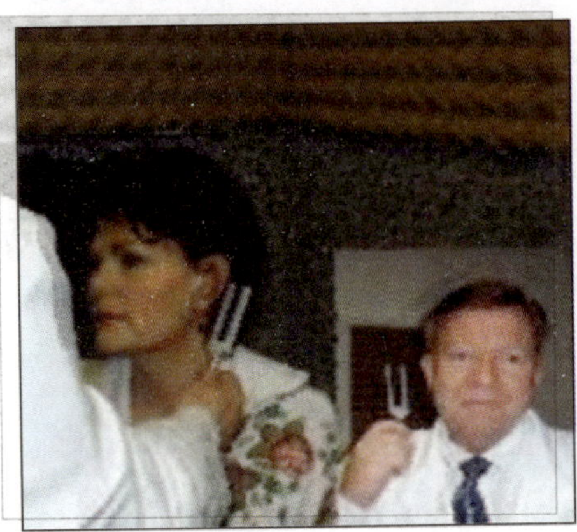

Fig. 3.22.13 Schwabach Test

(a) Place a vibrating tuning fork over the subject's mastoid process. When he indicates that he is unable to hear it any more, transfer it to your (examiner's) mastoid process.

(b) If you can still hear it, the subject's hearing loss is due to *nerve deafness*, since his bone conduction is impaired.

(c) If the examiner cannot hear it, repeat the whole procedure by testing the examiner's first. In *conduction deafness*, the subject's bone conduction is longer than that of the examiner.

(iv) ***Absolute Bone Conduction (ABC) Test.*** It is a modification of Schwabach test and is more reliable. Here the external auditory meatus of both the subject and the examiner is occluded and the test is carried as for Schwabach test.

3. Audiometry

Auditory acuity(sharpness of hearing) can be measured with the help of an *audiometer*. The device consists of the following parts (Fig. 3.22.14 A):

(i) Electronic oscillator, it can differentiate various sound frequencies.

(ii) Intensity dial, it helps to adjust the threshold intensity of hearing for each tone.

(iii) A headphone.

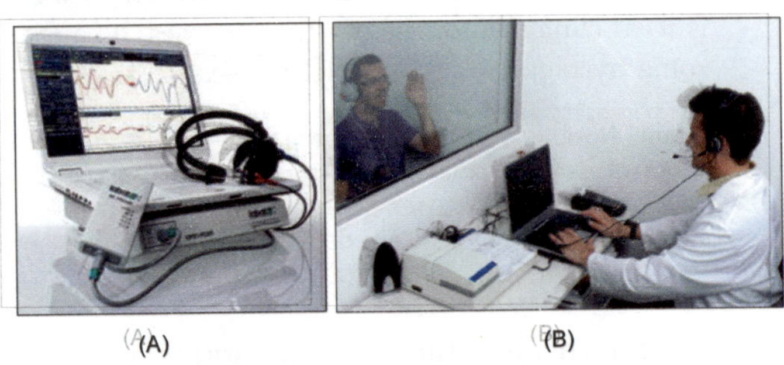

(A) (B)

Fig. 3.22.14 (A)Audiometer and (B) Audiometry, *i.e.* prodedure

Procedure (Fig. 3.22.14 B)

(i) The test is conducted in a sound-proof room. Each ear is tested separately. The subject wears a headphone. This device presents the subject with the pure tones of various frequencies through the headphone. He flashes a light whenever he hears the sounds. At each frequency, the threshold intensity is determined and plotted on a graph as a percentage of normal hearing. This provides an objective measurement of the degree of deafness and a picture of the tonal range most affected (Fig. 3.22.15).

(ii) **Hearing loss** is determined by increasing the intensity until threshold audibility is achieved for each tone tested; the corresponding dB increase on the intensity dial is noted.

Significance of the test

(i) To assess the degree of the deafness, and

(ii) To assess the frequency range in which deafness is most affected. Thus *hearing aids* can be designed to overcome some of the hearing problems of the individual patient.

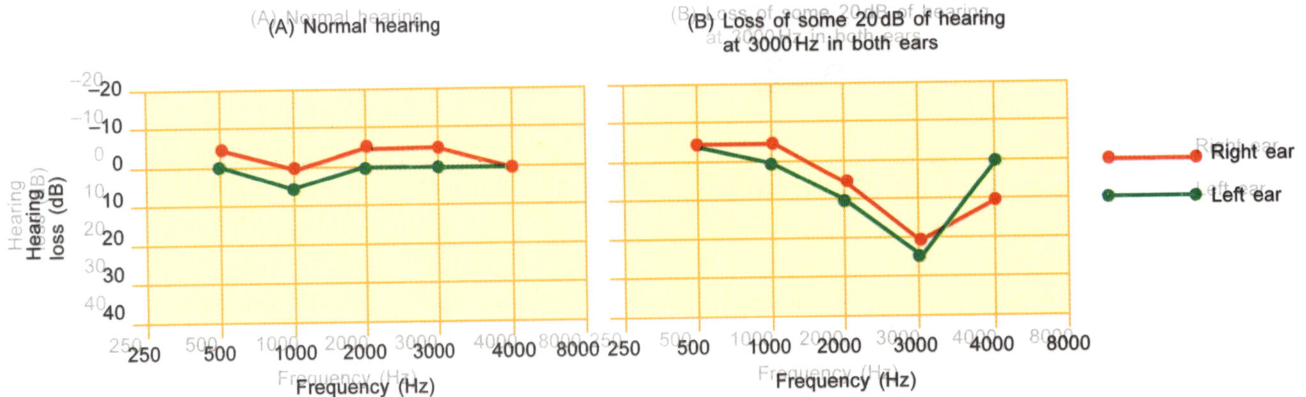

Fig. 3.22.15 Audiograms showing hearing loss against frequency. A hearing loss of 'zero' dB implies normality (standard used in the calibration). A negative loss (above zero line) indicates an auditory threshold lower than normal.

OSPE

Aim: To demonstrate the Rinne's test on the subject provided

Checklist

1. Explains the test procedure and gives proper instructions to the subject. **(Yes/No)**
2. Selects either 256 or 512 Hz tuning fork. **(Yes/No)**
3. Occludes the subject's external auditory meatus of one of the ears with his thumb. **(Yes/No)**
4. Sets the tunning fork vibrating and presses the base of the fork over the mastoid process behind the ear taking care not to touch the prongs. **(Yes/No)**
5. Instructs the subject to indicate by raising his finger when he can no longer hear the sound. **(Yes/No)**
6. Immediately transfers the still vibrating tuning fork to the side of the subject's head close to the ear. **(Yes/No)**
7. Asks the subject whether he could still hear the vibrating fork by air conduction even after he had ceased hearing via bone conduction. **(Yes/No)**

IMPORTANT VIVA-VOCE QUESTIONS

Q.1. *What is masking? Give its physiological significance.*

Ans. Masking (means a covering). It represents the inability of the *auditory mechanism* to separate the total stimulation into the separate components. Masking tends to be greater for the tones of approximately similar frequency than for tones widely different in frequency. Low-frequency tones mask high-frequency tones more easily than the reverse.

Q.2. *How are the sound waves conducted into the ear?*

Ans. (i) The main pathway for normal hearing, *i.e.* conduction of sound waves to the fluid of the inner ear via the tympanic membrane and the ear ossicles is called *Air or Ossicular Conduction.*

(ii) The transmission of the vibrations of the bones of the skull to the fluid of the inner ear is called *Bone Conduction.* Considerable bone conduction occurs when tuning forks or other vibrating objects are applied directly to the skull. This route also plays a role in the transmission of extremely loud sounds.

Q.3. *Define the term 'deafness'. List the causes of conduction and nerve deafness.*

Ans. Deafness literally means inability on a part of an individual to hear either wholly or partly. Deafness is of two main types: conduction and nerve deafness.

(i) **Conduction deafness.** It is due to sound transmission defect either in the external or middle ear. Therefore, it is characterised by the partial loss of hearing. The hearing loss is fairly uniform throughout the frequency range but it is never complete. It is because the skull bones themselves conduct sound to the cochlea (*bone conduction*) and the basilar membrane can be set into vibration.

Causes

(a) Wax or foreign bodies in the external ear
(b) Thickening of the tympanic membrane due to repeated infections; therefore, its vibrations decrease.
(c) Otitis media, *i.e.* middle ear inflammatory disorders which damage the tympanic membrane and/or the ear ossicles.
(d) Otosclerosis (ear ossicles sclerosis), *i.e.* pathological fixation of the foot plate of stapes in the oval window
(e) Blockage of the eustachian tube

(ii) **Nerve Deafness.** It is due to either defect of the internal ear (hair cells) or damage of neural pathways. Therefore, it is characterized by a complete loss of hearing.

Causes

(a) Hereditary
(b) Injury to the VIII nerve (acoustic trauma)
(c) Hazards of industrial noises (prolonged exposure to noise damages the hair cells, initially, it manifests as the loss of the sensitivity of hearing in 300-3000 Hz range resulting in the impairment of the subject's understanding of conversation).
(d) Toxic degeneration of the VIII nerve such as due to streptomycin injection, quinine, measles, meningitis, etc.
(e) Tumours of the VIII nerve (acoustic neuroma)
(f) Vascular damage in medulla which leads to the destruction of the auditory pathways.

Q.4. *Give the normal range of frequencies and intensities of sound for the human ear.*

Ans. The human ear can perceive the pitch (frequency) of sound between 16-20,000 cps (or Hz) with maximally sensitive to pitch variations in the 1000-3000 Hz range. The range of sound intensity, which can be heard without any damage, is from zero to 120 decibel (dB).

Q.5. *Mention the precautions taken while testing for the hearing test using a tuning fork?*

Ans. (i) Exclude the presence of wax in the external ear.
(ii) The other ear should be plugged.
(iii) The correct frequency of the tuning fork should be used.
(iv) The room should be noise-free.

NINTH NERVE: THE GLOSSOPHARYNGEAL NERVE

Origin

It is attached by five to six rootlets to upper part of the medulla oblongata.

Function

It is a *mixed nerve* consisting of three set of fibres:

1. *Motor fibres* supply stylopharyngeous muscle (inferior constrictor of the pharynx which helps swallow).
2. *Sensory fibres* bring taste from posterior 1/3rd of tongue and mucous membrane of pharynx (bitter taste sensibility).
3. *Secreto-motor fibres* supply the parotid gland.

Effect of paralysis

1. Deglutition is not much affected because superior and medial constrictor of pharynx are intact. These are supplied by the tenth (vagus) nerve.
2. The loss of taste (bitter sensations) from posterior 1/3rd portion of the tongue (better appreciated in bilateral paralysis).
3. Decrease in salivary secretion, this may result in difficulty in swallowing.

How to test?

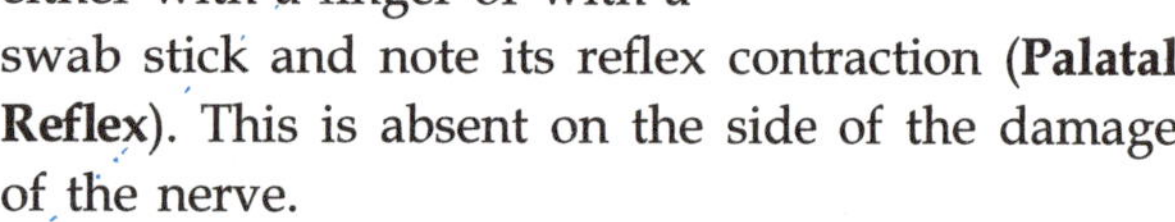

1. Test for taste sensation in posterior 1/3rd portion of the tongue (refer to page 249).
2. Tickle at the back of pharynx, either with a finger or with a swab stick and note its reflex contraction (**Palatal Reflex**). This is absent on the side of the damage of the nerve.

IMPORTANT VIVA-VOCE QUESTIONS

Q.1. *What will be the effects of the paralysis of the ninth nerve?*

Ans. See above.

Q.2. *Describe the pathway of palatal reflex.*

Ans. Afferent travel in the IXth nerve and efferents (motor) component is mediated via the Xth (vagus) nerve.

TENTH NERVE: THE VAGUS NERVE

Origin

It is attached by 8-10 rootlets to the lateral aspect of medulla oblongata below the origin of the ninth nerve.

Function

It is a *mixed nerve* and consists of two sets of fibres: *Motor* and *Sensory*.

1. Motor fibres supply:
   (i) The involuntary muscles of respiration, heart and GIT (up to right 2/3rd of transverse colon).
   (ii) Voluntary muscles:
      (a) all constrictor muscles of pharynx;
      (b) all intrinsic muscles of larynx; and
      (c) muscles of soft palate.
2. Sensory fibres are distributed to:
   (i) The mucous membrane of GIT up to right 2/3rd of transverse colon.
   (ii) The mucous membrane of larynx, pharynx and soft palate.

Effect of paralysis

1. The subject complains of the *regurgitation of fluids* through the nose during swallowing due to the defective elevation of the soft palate.
2. The defective pronouncing of words which require a complete closure of naso-pharynx. This results in *nasal tone* in the voice. Therefore, 'rub' is pronounced as 'rum', 'egg' as 'eng'. This effect is more pronounced with bilateral paralysis.
3. *Voice becomes hoarse and deep,* because vocal cords get relaxed. Therefore, the utterance of high notes is impossible. This is specially seen with bilateral paralysis.

How to test

1. *For the palate*
   (i) Ask the subject about any history of regurgitation of fluids through nose during swallowing.
   (ii) Observe for any nasal twang.
   (iii) *Palatal reflex* (see above).
   (iv) Examine the soft palate movements during phonation. Ask the subject to say 'Ah' and observe the movements of both sides of palatal arch (Fig. 3.22.16).

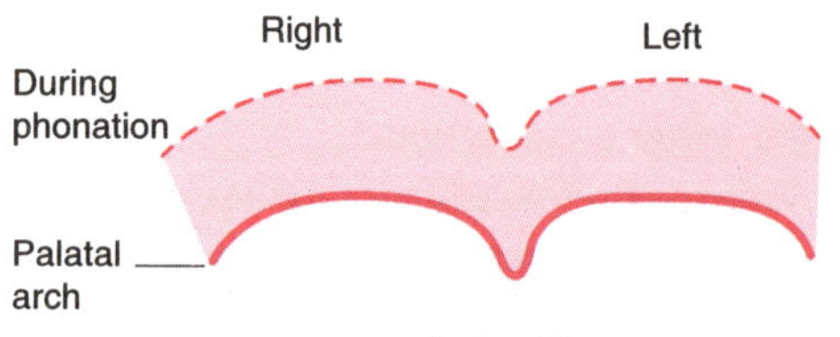

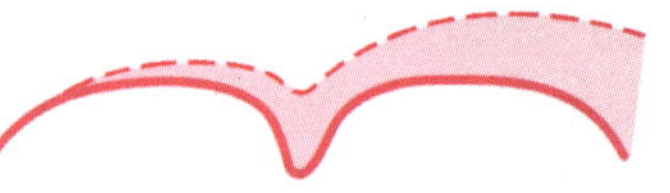

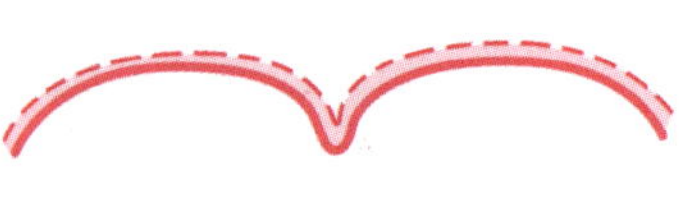

Fig. 3.22.16 Examination of soft palate movements during phonation

(a) In a healthy individual, both palatal arches should raise upwards normally with uvula (median raphe) remaining in the midline.
(b) If one side is paralysed, that side will remain flat and immobile and the median raphe will be pulled towards the healthy side.
(c) In bilateral paralysis, the whole of the soft palate remains motionless.

2. *For the larynx:* **Laryngoscopy,** *i.e.* direct visualisation of larynx (vocal cords) with the help of laryngoscope. The subject is asked to say the vowel 'ee'; this brings the vocal cords together to meet in the midline; the vocal cords remain immobilized on the side of nerve involvement.

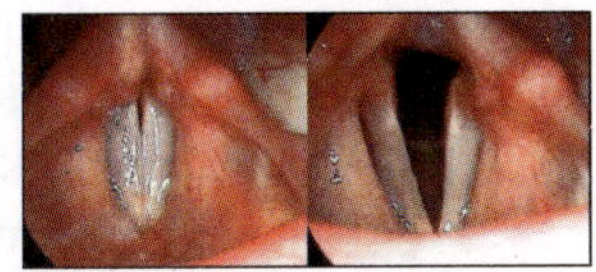

IMPORTANT VIVA-VOCE QUESTIONS

Q.1. *Mention the presenting complaints of a person with the involvement of the vagus nerve.*

Ans. Page 254.

Q.2. *What type of soft palate movements occur during bilateral tenth nerve palsy.*

Ans. Page 254.

Q.3. *What precautions should you observe during laryngoscopy?*

Ans. The instrument should be cleaned and warmed (at body temperature); if cold, it may trigger the reflex contraction of the larynx.

Q.4. *Give the physiological basis of the regurgitation of fluids through nose and nasal twang in the tenth nerve palsy.*

Ans. Page 254.

ELEVENTH NERVE: THE SPINAL ACCESSORY NERVE

Origin

It originates from two separate locations (Fig. 3.22.18).

1. **Cranial part** arises from the medulla below the origin of the vagus nerve. Its fibres get distributed along with the motor branches of the vagus nerve to the larynx and pharynx.
2. **Spinal part** arises from the spinal nucleus of the lateral part of anterior grey column of the spinal cord extending up to the fifth cervical segment.

XI Spinal Accessory
Cranial nerve X
Cranial part XI
Spinal part XI

Fig. 3.22.17 Origin of the XIth cranial nerve

Function

It is a *pure motor* nerve and supplies two muscles: sterno (cleido) mastoid and trapezius.

How to test

1. **Test for sterno (cleido) mastoid muscle** (Fig. 3.22.18)
   (i) When both sides of sternomastoid act together, the head is flexed. Ask the subject to flex the head while the examiner applies passive resistance from below; if the muscle is paralysed, it will not be possible for the subject to flex the head (Fig. 3.22.18 A).
   (ii) When only one muscle acts alone, chin is rotated to the other/opposite side. The paralysis can be assessed by applying passive resistance from the other side while the subject tries to rotate the chin. If paralysed, the rotation of chin towards the opposite side is not possible (Fig. 3.22.18 B).

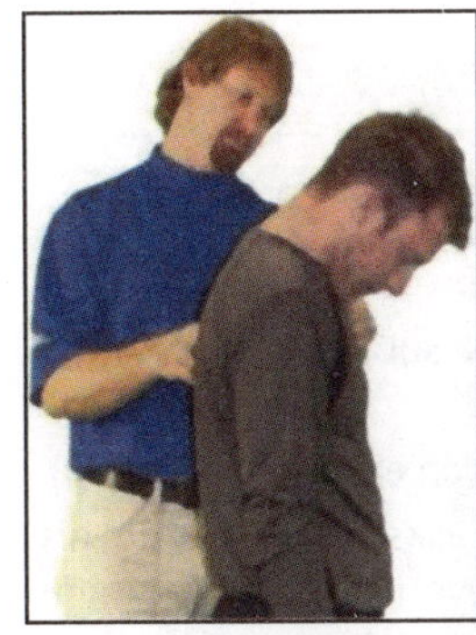

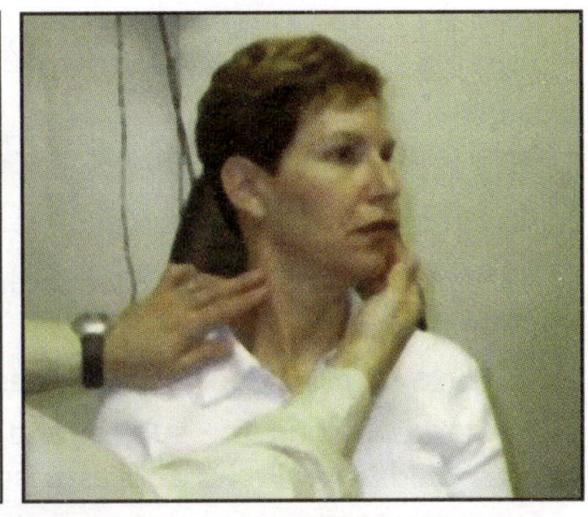

Fig. 3.22.18 Test for sterno (cleido) mastoid muscle (A) when both sides act together (B) when only one muscle acts alone

2. **Test for trapezius muscle**
   (i) Look for the drooping of shoulder on the affected side.
   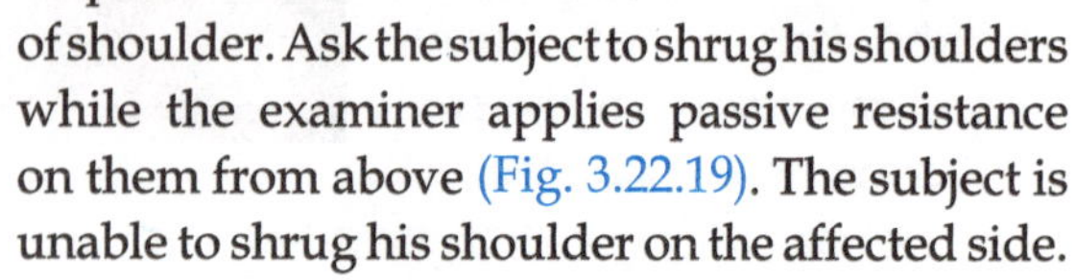
   (ii) Trapezius along with levator scapulae causes the elevation of shoulder. Ask the subject to shrug his shoulders while the examiner applies passive resistance on them from above (Fig. 3.22.19). The subject is unable to shrug his shoulder on the affected side.

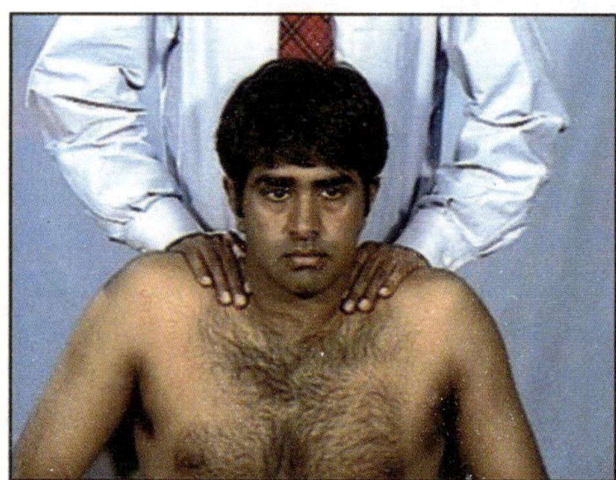

Fig. 3.22.19 Test for trapezius muscles

OSPE-I

Aim: Test for the sternocleidomastoid muscle of the subject provided.

Checklist

1. Explains the test procedure to the subject and gives proper instructions. (Yes/No)
2. Asks the subject to flex the head while he applies passive resistance from below. (Yes/No)
3. Asks the subject to rotate the chin to right while he applies passive resistance from the left side. (Yes/No)
4. Repeats the whole procedure by applying passive resistance from the right side and now asks the subject to rotate the chin to left. (Yes/No)

OSPE-II

Aim: Test for trapezius muscle of the subject provided

Check list

1. Explains the test procedure to the subject and gives the proper instructions. (Yes/No)
2. Looks for the drooping of shoulder on either side. (Yes/No)
3. Stands behind the subject and asks him to shrug his shoulders while he applies passive resistance on them from above. (Yes/No)

IMPORTANT VIVA-VOCE QUESTIONS

Q.1. *How will you test for sternomastoid muscle when:*
(i) only one muscle is acting,
(ii) both muscles are acting together.

Ans. See above.

Q.2. *What precautions must you take while examining the trapezius muscle.*

Ans. Always stand behind the subject, while he is sitting on a stool and then apply passive resistance on the muscle from above.

TWELFTH NERVE: THE HYPOGLOSSAL NERVE

Origin

It takes origin from the lowermost part of the medulla oblongata.

Function

It is a *pure motor* nerve and supplies all the muscles of the tongue. This helps in the articulation of tongue during speech and proper mixing of food with the saliva.

Effect of paralysis

The effects are observed only in bilateral paralysis; if so, it results in:

1. Defective articulation and improper mixing of food.
2. No atrophy of tongue muscles is seen because blood supply is intact.

How to test

1. Ask the subject to protrude (put out) his tongue as far as possible.
   (i) In *unilateral* paralysis, the tongue will deviate *towards* the paralysed side. This is because right hypoglossal nerve supplies muscles of the left side of tongue and this causes the movement of the tongue towards the left side and vice versa. (Fig. 3.22.20)

   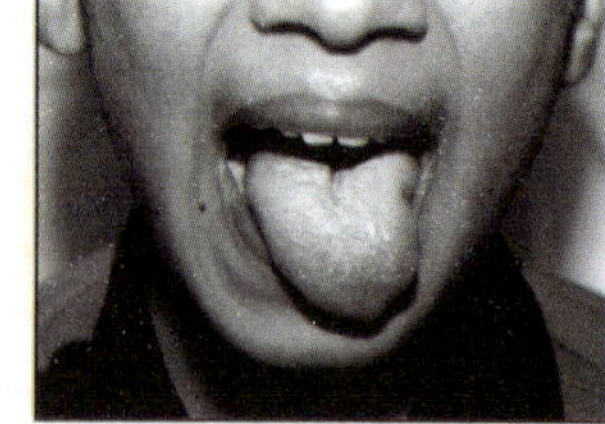

   Fig. 3.22.20 Left XII cranial nerve palsy. **Note :** Wasting of left half the tongue

   (ii) In bilateral paralysis, the person will not be able to protude out his tongue at all.
2. Ask the subject to move his tongue from side to side, and to lick each cheek with it. Observe whether he can do so freely or not.

OSPE

Aim: To test for the functioning of the XII cranial nerve of the subject provided.

Checklist

1. Explains the test procedure to the subject. **(Yes/No)**
2. Asks the subject to protrude out his tongue as far as possible. **(Yes/No)**
3. Asks the subject to move his tongue from side to side and to lick each cheek with it. **(Yes/No)**
4. Observes whether he can do so freely or not. **(Yes/No)**

IMPORTANT VIVA-VOCE QUESTIONS

Q.1. *What will be the person's complaints in the paralysis of the twelfth nerve?*

Ans. See above.

Q.2. *How will you test the functions of the hypoglossal nerve?*

Ans. See above.

(C) Examination of the Motor System

The examination of the motor system includes:

1. *Bulk of muscles*
2. *Tone of muscles*
3. *Strength (or power) of muscles*
4. *Reflexes*
5. *Co-ordination of movements*
6. *Gait*
7. *Presence or absence of involuntary movements*

BULK OF MUSCLES

1. This is estimated by inspection and palpation. Measure the circumference of the arm, forearm, thigh and leg at an identical level on both sides. The level should be decided in relation to some fixed, subcutaneous bony landmark; judgement regarding the presence of muscular wasting or otherwise depends most often on a comparison of the two sides.

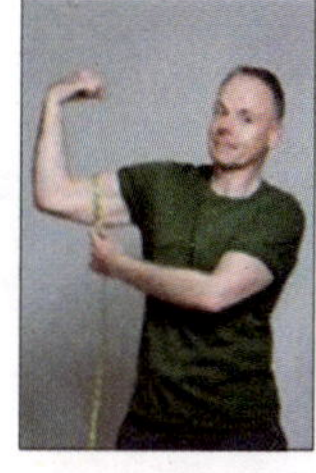

Note: Occasionally, both sides may show wasting. Therefore, common sense about what should be normal muscle mass for a given person should also be employed.

2. **Wasted** or **Atrophic** muscles are smaller, softer and more flabby (loose) than normal when they are contracted.
3. Muscle wasting associated with fibrosis is called **contracture**. The muscle feels hard, inelastic and shortened; therefore, it is not possible to stretch them passively to a normal degree.

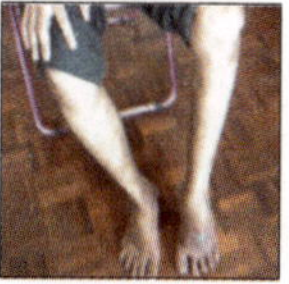

4. The bulk of muscle **decreases** in:
   (i) injury or disease of a muscle/joint, such as inflammed muscles or during prolonged hypertonia in a group of muscles;
   (ii) neurological disorders;
   (iii) cachexia of any cause
5. The bulk of muscle **increases** in: following atheletic training, continued excessive workload in certain occupations like carpenters, labourers, etc. myotonic disorders.

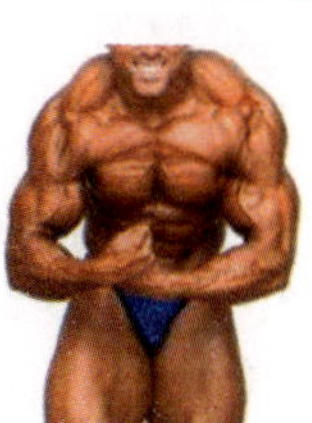

TONE OF MUSCLES

1. **Definition**: Certain amount of tension present in the resting muscle due to *low frequency* and *asynchronous* discharge of γ-motor neuron which produces the resistance of a muscle to stretch (or lengthening); this is referred as the 'tone' of a muscle. It is a partial tetanus. It depends on the integrity of stretch reflex which is under the control of higher centres.
2. **How to assess muscle tone** Clinically, muscle tone is assessed by moving the muscles passively at their various joints and feel for resistance offered by a moving muscle. This comes by experience, whether such resistance is normal, low or high.
3. **Hypotonia,** *i.e.* decrease in resting muscle tone. Such muscles offer little or no resistance to stretching. Causes are:
   (i) During sleep
   (ii) Lower motor neuron lesion, *i.e.* destruction of local reflex arc anywhere in its pathway. For example,
      (a) destruction of efferent (motor) nerve to a muscle by injury or poliomyelitis;
      (b) destruction of afferent (sensory) nerve as seen in syphilis (*tabes dorsalis*).
4. **Hypertonia,** *i.e.* increase in resting muscle tone. Such muscles offer high resistance to stretch. It is commonly seen in upper motor neuron lesion.
   In brain diseases, which cause increase in muscle tone, if hypertonia is confined to only one group of muscles, it is called ***spasticity***; however, when hypertonia involves both groups of muscles,

extensor as well as flexor, equally, it is referred to as ***rigidity***. For example, the lesions of internal capsule produce spasticity, whereas basal ganglia lesions lead to rigidity (Fig. 3.22.21).

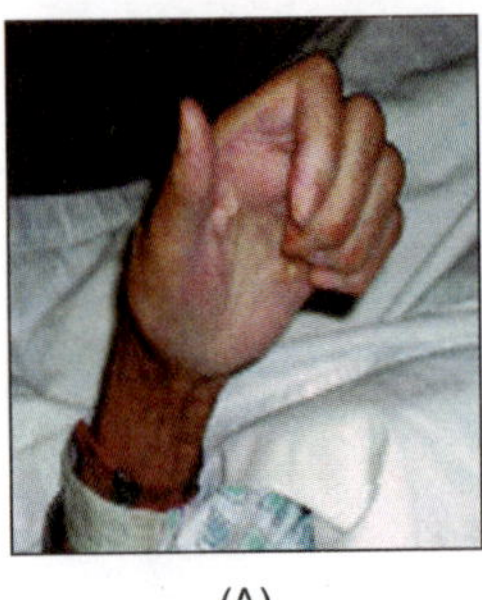
(A)

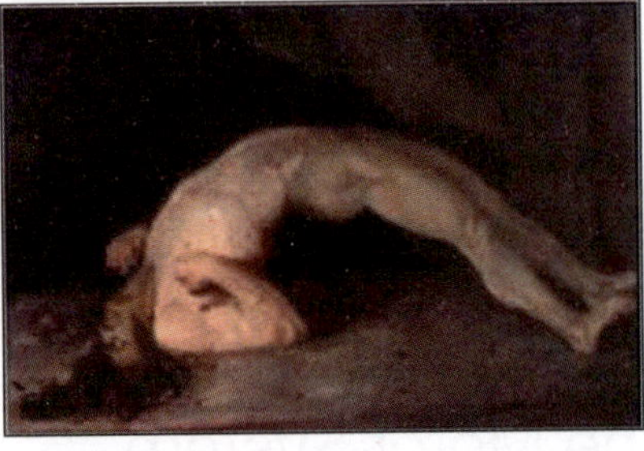
(B)

Fig 3.22.21 (A) Spasticity and (B) Rigidity

STRENGTH (or POWER) OF MUSCLES

1. How to test

(i) The strength of muscles varies with the build of the subject and its assessment requires practice and experience. The ***general rule*** is to ask the subject to throw into action the particular muscle or group of muscles which one wishes to test while the examiner offers passive resistance to that action. The muscle, if healthy, will be seen and felt to stand out prominently.

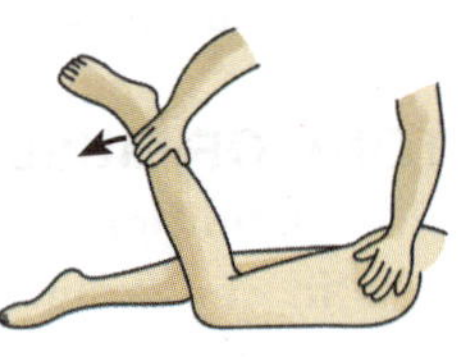

(ii) Each movement made during this assessment is tested by comparison with the examiner's own strength or by comparison with what he judges to be normal in a person of comparable build to the patient.

2. Testing for the strength of individual muscle

Muscles of upper limb

(i) *Abductor pollicis brevis.* Ask the subject to abduct his thumb in a plane at right angles to the palmar aspect of the index finger, against the resistance of the examiner's own thumb. The muscle can be seen and felt to contract.

(ii) *Interossei and lumbricals.* Test the subject's ability to flex his metacarpophalangeal joint and to extend the distal inter-phalangeal joints.

> Note: Interossei also adduct and abduct the fingers. This action should also be tested.

(iii) *Flexors of the fingers.* Ask the subject to squeeze your fingers.

(iv) *Flexors of the wrist.* Ask the subject to bring the tips of his fingers towards the front of the forearm.

(v) *Extensors of the wrist.* Ask the subject to make a fist (this results in a firm contraction of both the flexors and extensors of the wrist), and try forcibly to flex the wrist against his effort to maintain his posture.

(vi) *Brachioradialis.* Place the subject's forearm in mid-prone position and then ask him to flex it against resistance.

(vii) *Biceps.* Place the subject's forearm in full supination and then ask him to flex it against resistance. The muscle will stand out clearly.

(viii) *Triceps.* Place the subject's forearm fully flexed against the chest and then ask him to straighten it out against resistance.

(ix) *Supraspinatus and deltoid.* Ask the subject to lift his arm straight out at right angles to his side against resistance. The first 30° of this movement is carried out by the supraspinatus; the remaining 60° is produced by the deltoid. (Fig. 3.22.22).

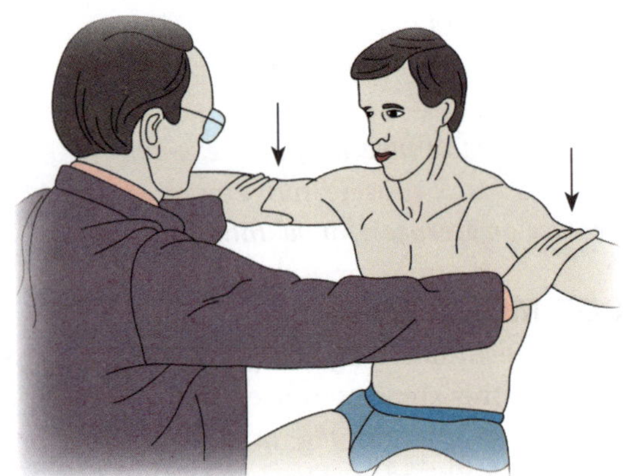

Fig 3.22.2 Testing for deltoid muscle power

Muscles of the trunk

(i) *Muscles of the abdomen:* ***Babinski's rising up sign.*** The weakness of these muscles is shown by the subject's inability to sit up in bed from the supine position without the aid of his arms.

(ii) *Diaphragm.* In a healthy individual, inspiration is associated with bulging and expiration with the fall of abdominal wall; opposite occurs in the paralysis of the diaphragm.

(iii) *Trapezius*

(a) Upper part. Ask the subject to shrug his shoulders against the examiner's resistance (Page 256).

(b) Lower part. Ask him to approximate the shoulder blades.

Muscles of the lower limb

(i) *Dorsiflexion and plantar flexion of the feet and toes.* Ask the subject to elevate or depress the part against resistance.

(ii) *Extensors of the knee.* Ask the subject to flex his knee and then, pressing with your hand on his shin, ask him to try to straighten it out again.

(iii) *Flexors of the knee.* Raise the leg up from the bed, supporting the thigh with your left hand and holding the ankle with your right hand; then ask the subject to bend his knee.
Using the general principle (page 258), test the flexors and extensors of the hip and adductors, abductors and rotators of the thigh.

3. Grading of the muscle strength

Grade 0 : Complete paralysis (*flaccid muscle*)
Grade 1 : Muscle just shows a flicker of contraction only.
Grade 2 : Muscle movement is possible only when the *force of gravity is excluded* by appropriate postural adjustment.
Grade 3 : Muscle movement is possible *against the force of gravity,* therefore, a limb can be held against the force of gravity but not against the examiner's resistance.
Grade 4 : Muscle movements are possible *against a variable degree of examiner's resistance,* and muscle movement is described as poor, fair or of moderate strength.
Grade 5 : Normal muscle strength (power) is present; therefore, muscle action can be made against the examiner's passive resistance.

REFLEXES

Refer to page 262.

CO-ORDINATION OF MOVEMENTS

1. *Definition.* This means the smooth recruitment, interaction and cooperation of separate muscles or group of muscles in order to perform a definite motor act.
2. The coordination of muscle movement depends on:
   (i) sense of position of a limb (via muscle spindle) or joint (via joint receptors);
   (ii) cerebellar functions; and
   (iii) the state of tone of muscles
3. A disturbance in the coordination of muscle movement is called **Ataxia**. It is of two types:
   (i) *Sensory ataxia.* This results from defective sensory information and is usually found in the injury or disease of the dorsal column such as tabes dorsalis.
   (ii) *Cerebellar ataxia.* This results due to cerebellum dysfunctions.
4. The sensory ataxia may be compensated for by vision; therefore, the disturbance of movements may become apparent only when the eyes are closed or the person is in the dark.

Tests for Coordination of Movements

In the upper limb

1. ***Finger-nose test***. Ask the subject to touch first his nose with his own index finger and then the examiner's index finger. If he performs these movements without making errors, coordination is normal. He is then asked to perform the same action with his eyes closed; irregularity indicates the impairment of position sense in the limb. (Fig. 3.22.23)

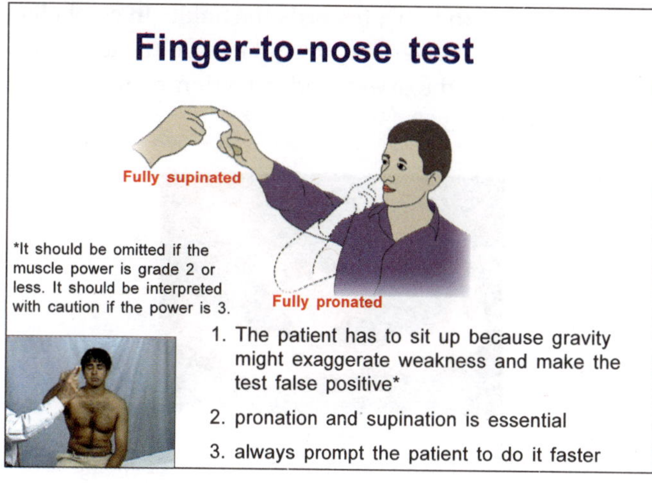

Fig. 3.22.23 Coordination of muscle movement in the upper limb : ***Finger-Nose Test***

2. Ask the person to describe a circle in the air with his index finger, first with eyes open and then with eyes closed. All normal persons can draw a circle smoothly and accurately whether the eyes are open or closed.
3. ***Adiadochokinesia***. The person is unable to carry out rapidly alternate and opposite movements. For example, rapid supination and pronation of the forearm. This is because they cannot start or stop movements quickly or easily and their motions are slow and irregular. This is a special and very useful sign of cerebellar ataxia. All normal persons can do this very rapidly (Fig. 3.22.24).

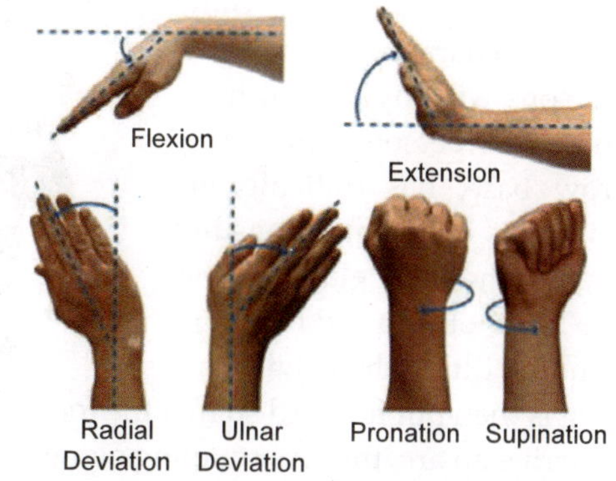

Fig. 3.22.24 Demonstration for Adiadochokinesia

Note: When the movements are slow, incomplete with irregular rhythm, and often become impossible after a few attempts, this is referred as **Dysdiadochokinesia**.

In the lower limb

1. *If the person is able to walk,* ask him to walk along a straight line; if incoordination is present, he will soon deviate to one side or the other .
2. *If he cannot walk,* perform *Heel-Knee Test* with the eyes open. Ask him to place the heel of his leg on the opposite knee and then to slide the heel along the shin of the tibia towards the ankle. In cerebellar ataxia, a characteristic, irregular, side-to-side series of errors in the speed and direction of movement occurs (Fig. 3.22.25).

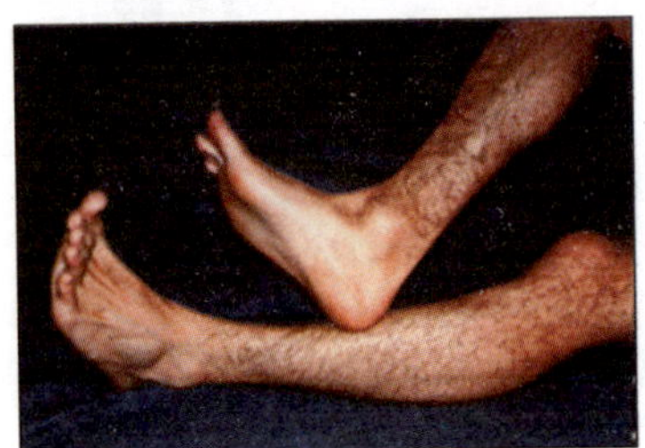

Fig. 3.22.25 Coordination of muscle movement in the lower limb : ***Heel-Knee Test***

3. *Romberg's Sign.* Refer to page 250.

GAIT

Gait means the manner of walking. Certain requirements should be fulfilled before examining the gait of a person. These are:

1. The legs should be fully exposed.
2. The feet should be bare.
3. Examine the bone and joints to exclude local diseases like the osteoarthritis of the hip; local injury (or pain) in the knee, leg or pelvis.

Gait is of major importance in diagnosis. Some common abnormal types of gait recognised are described as under:

1. **Spastic (or Hemiplegic) Gait.** This is a characteristic feature of persons with pyramidal tract lesions. The person walks on a narrow base, has difficulty in bending his knees and drags his feet as if they are glued to the floor. The foot is raised from the ground by tilting the pelvis, and the leg is then put forward so that the foot may tend to describe an arc, the toes scraping along the floor.

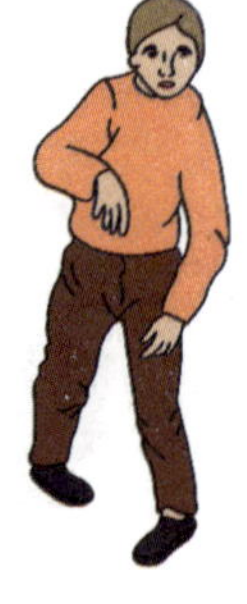

2. **Stamping Gait.** *Stamping* means to strike the ground heavily with the sole of the foot. This is characteristic of a person with sensory ataxia. The person raises his feet very suddenly, often abnormally high, and then jerks them forward, bringing them to the ground again with a stamp, and often heels first. If he watches the ground, he may be fairly steady, as he can use his eyes in place of his position sense. However, the person becomes severely ataxic when his eyes are closed or if he walks in the dark.

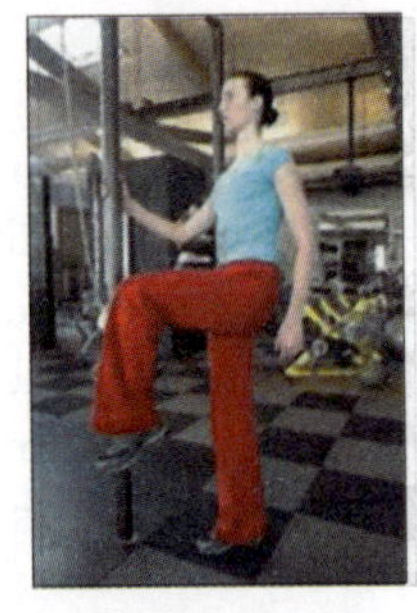

3. **Drunken (or Reeling) Gait.** *Reeling* means frame on which thread is wound. This is seen typically in person with cerebellar lesion. The person walks awkwardly (in clumsy manner), with the feet well apart (wide base). They have such difficulty in maintaining balance that their gait appears drunken, called *drunken gait.* The person walks in a *zigzag* line and deviates to the affected side due to hypotonia. The ataxia is equally severe whether eyes are open or closed.
4. **Festinant Gait.** This is characteristic of Parkinson's disease (extrapyramidal tract lesion). The person bends forward, and walks quickly with short steps as if trying to catch up centre of gravity or preventing himself from falling down. If he is suddenly pulled backwards, he begins to walk backwards and is unable to stop himself.

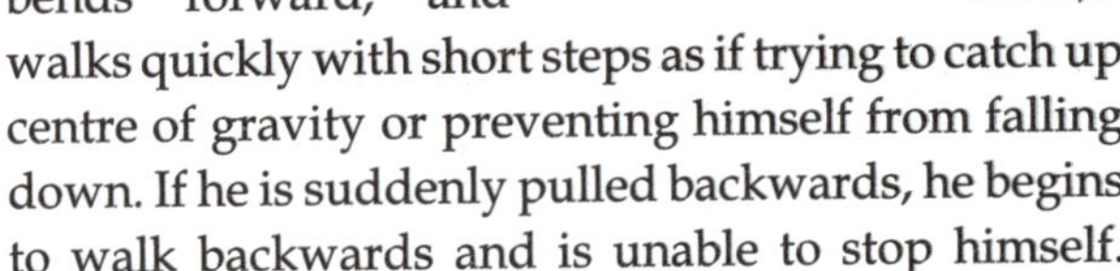

5. **Waddling Gait.** *Waddling* means to walk with short steps like the gait of a duck. This is typically seen in persons with proximal muscular weakness (myopathies, muscular dystrophies). Thus there is difficulty in maintaining trunk and pelvic posture. The body is lifted backwards (Lumbar lordosis). The feet are planted widely apart and the body sways from side to side as each step is taken. The heel and toes tend to be brought down simultaneously.

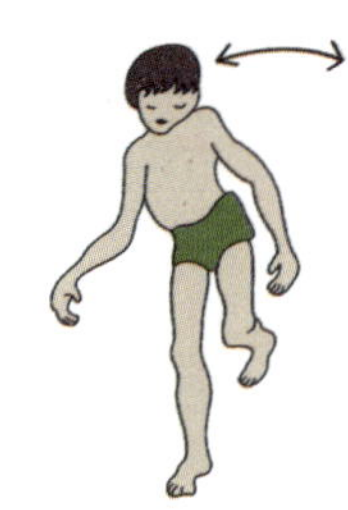

INVOLUNTARY MOVEMENTS

1. Epilepsy

(i) An involuntary movement is limited to one side of the body or to one limb. *Aura* precedes the generalised convulsions.

(ii) Movement is usually complex, repetitive and stereotyped which lasts only for a short duration.

(iii) It may be increased by arousal or by handling or touching the limb.

2. Tremors

Definition: Regular or irregular distal movements having an oscillatory (vibrating) character are referred as tremors. Clinically, they are classified as:

(i) Fine and rapid tremors. This is seen in anxiety, thyrotoxicosis.

(ii) Coarse and irregular tremors; typically occur in awkward (difficult) postures; examples include:

(a) Senile tremors; present both at rest and during movements

(b) Hysterical tremors; increased by the examiner's attempt to control it.

(iii) Resting tremors of Parkinson disease. It consists of regular, rhythmic, alternate contraction of antagonist and agonist muscles @ 6-8 times/sec. Its frequent presence can be seen as *pill-rolling movements, i.e.* rhythmic contraction of thumb over first two fingers. (Fig. 3.22.26 A and B)

Common sites: fingers, hand, lips or tongue, and often it causes the movements of pronation and supination.

It is present at rest but disappears during activity, therefore, popularly called as *resting (static) tremors.*

(iv) Intentional tremors of cerebellar dysfunction. The tremors are coarse which occur @ 4-6 times/sec. and can clearly be seen when the part is used in voluntary movement (Fig. 3.22.26 C).

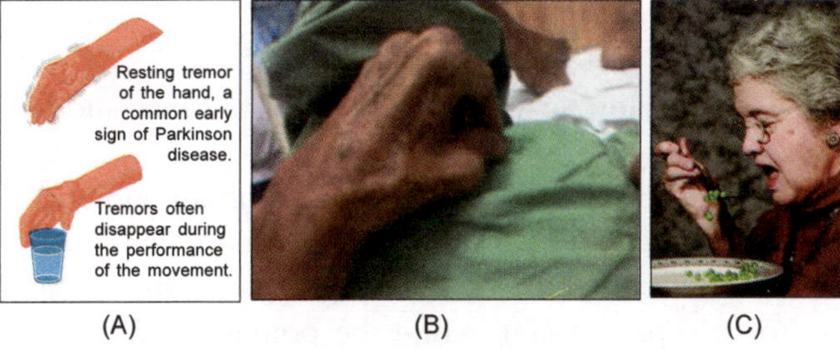

Fig. 3.22.26 (A) Resting tremors and
(B) Pill rolling movements of the hand of Parkinson disease
(C) Intentional tremors of cerebellar dysfunction

3. Athetosis

It is primarily due to the lesion of the lenticular nucleus and is characterized by continuous, slow-twisting movements (one phase of movement getting merged with the next).

4. Chorea

It is mainly due to the involvement of caudate nucleus and is characterized by: rapid, irregular involuntary movements of short duration and is associated with decreased muscle tone and muscular weakness.

Note: Chorea is seen frequently in children as the complication of rheumatic fever.

5. Tics

These are simple, normal movements which become repeated unnecessarily to the point that they become an embarrassment or a source of, or reaction to, psychiatric problem. It commonly involves the face and shoulders and usually develops early in life, also called *habit spasm.* For example, head nodding, blinking, cheek/lips/nail biting, laryngeal tic, etc.

OSPE-I

Aim: To assess the tone of muscles in the upper arm of the subject provided

Check list

1. Explains the test procedure to the subject. **(Yes/No)**
2. Makes the subject comfortably seated. **(Yes/No)**
3. Assess the muscles passively at their various joints and feels for the resistance offered by moving muscles. **(Yes/No)**
4. Compares the muscle tone in the similar fashion on the opposite side for the individual muscle. **(Yes/No)**

OSPE-II

Aim: To assess the strength of muscles in the upper arm of the subject provided

Checklist

1. Explains the test procedure to the subject. **(Yes/No)**
2. Makes the subject comfortably seated. **(Yes/No)**
3. Asks the subject to throw into action the particular muscle/group of muscles and he applies passive resistance to that action.
4. Compares the movement/strength of each muscle on the opposite side or with his own muscle strength.

Note: OSPE can be asked for an individual muscle or group of muscles in any of the limbs or for trunk muscles.

OSPE-III

Aim: To test for the coordination of movements in the upper or lower limbs of the subject provided

Check list

1. Makes the subject comfortably seated in a chair. **(Yes/No)**
2. Explains the test procedure to the subject. **(Yes/No)**
3. Watches for any error in the movements performed first with eyes open and then with eyes closed. **(Yes/No)**

In upper limb	*In lower limb*
(i) Finger-nose test	(i) Heel-knee test
(ii) Describing a circle in the air with his index finger	(ii) Walking along a straight line
(iii) Carrying out rapidly alternate and opposite movements	(iii) Romberg's sign

IMPORTANT VIVA-VOCE QUESTIONS

Q.1. *Give the causes where the bulk of the muscles gets altered.*
Ans. Page 257.
Q.2. *How will you assess the bulk of muscles?*
Ans. Page 257.
Q.3. *Mention the sequence under which the examination of motor system is carried out.*
Ans. Page 257.
Q.4. *Give the higher control of stretch reflex.*
Ans. Brain areas which facilitate the stretch reflex are: facilitatory reticular formation and vestibular nucleus, and areas which inhibit the stretch reflex are: inhibitory reticular formation, cerebral cortex, basal ganglia and cerebellum.
Q.5. *Enumerate the two major differences between spasticity and rigidity.*
Ans. Page 257.
Q.6. *What general principle is commonly employed to assess the strength of muscles?*
Ans. Page 258.
Q.7. *How will you test the muscle power in fingers?*
Ans. Page 258.
Q.8. *Define the coordination of muscle movements. Name the factors on which it depends.*
Ans. Page 259.
Q.9. *Differentiate between: (i) sensory and cerebellar ataxia; (ii) Adiadochokinesia and dysdiadochokinesia; (iii) resting and intentional tremors; (iv) chorea and athetosis.*
Ans. (i) Page 259; (ii) Page 259; (iii) Page 261; (iv) Page 261.
Q.10. *What is Romberg's sign? Give its clinical significance.*
Ans. Page 250.
Q.11. *Mention some varieties of the involuntary movements of clinical significance.*
Ans. Page 260.
Q.12. *How can 'gait' be of any importance in diagnosis.*
Ans. Page 260.

(D) The Reflexes

Reflex is an involuntary (automatic) response to a stimulus which depends on the integrity of a particular nervous pathway, *i.e.* the reflex arc:

APPARATUS

Patellar (or knee) hammer, examination couch, subject, torch

Patellar (or knee) hammer

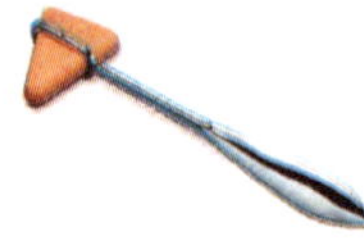

It derives its name from its invention as an instrument for eliciting knee (or patellar) reflex; the first tendon reflex to become a regular part of the neurological examination.

1. It consists of a **long metallic handle** at one end of which a triangular shaped soft **rubber piece** is attached (Fig. 3.22.27). This piece is used to provide a sharp blow to a tendon, in order to cause sudden stretching of its muscle.
2. The **rubber piece** has two ends: a broad end and a pointed end. The broader end is used when muscle tendon belly is broad and thin (as of the tendon of triceps muscle), while the pointed end is used when the tendon is stout and narrow (as of biceps muscle).

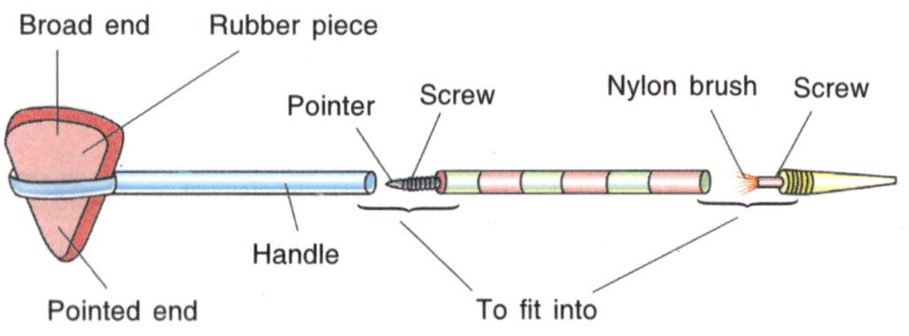

Fig. 3.22.27 A patellar (or knee) hammer

3. The body of the handle is also provided with a **brush** with nylon hair and a **pointer**. These are used for the sensory component of neurological examination.

TYPES OF REFLEXES

Reflexes are broadly divided into 3 major heads:

A. The superficial reflexes
B. The deep or tendon reflexes
C. The organic or sphincteric reflexes

(A) The Superficial Reflexes

1. If a stimulus is applied to the superficial structures of the body like skin or mucous membrane, it results in the contraction of underlying muscle. For example, *plantar and abdominal reflexes.* These are polysynaptic reflexes, *i.e.* many synaptic connections are present between afferent and efferent neurons.
2. *Pathway.* Information from the superficial structures runs in sensory nerve fibres to reach first in the grey matter of spinal cord, then travel up to the higher centre in brain stem or forebrain, and descends down via descending tracts in motor nerve fibre, finally to the underlying muscle of skin or mucous membrane. (Fig. 3.22.28)

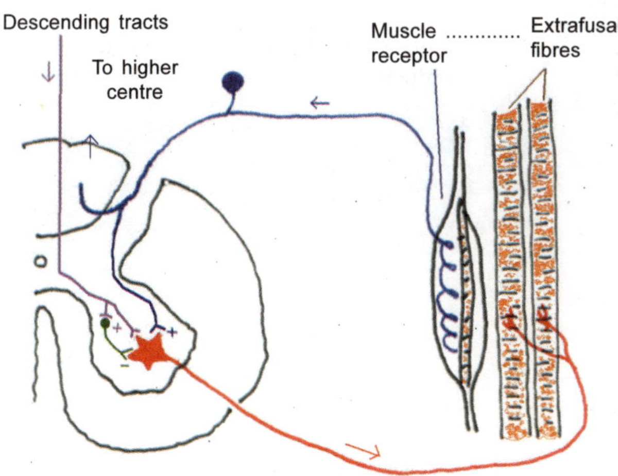

Fig. 3.22.28 Pathway for superficial reflex

3. *Main characteristic features*
   (i) The reflex excitability varies with the subject.
   (ii) These reflexes are of significance in unilateral lesions, when healthy side can be taken as standard for comparison purposes.
   (iii) In hemiplegia, these reflexes are disturbed on the paralysed side, because they are mediated by the pyramidal tracts.
4. The superficial reflexes are broadly divided into two major types:
   (i) *reflexes based on spinal nerves* and
   (ii) *reflexes based on cranial nerves*
   (Table 3.22.2.)

(B) Deep (or Tendon) Reflexes

Pre-requisites

1. Make sure the subject is warm and comfortable.
2. Explain the test procedure to the subject beforehand, in order to make him relax, reassure and decrease anxiety and apprehension associated with the test.
3. The subject should be completely relaxed with the attention diverted.
4. *Pathway*: Refer to (Fig. 3.22.29)

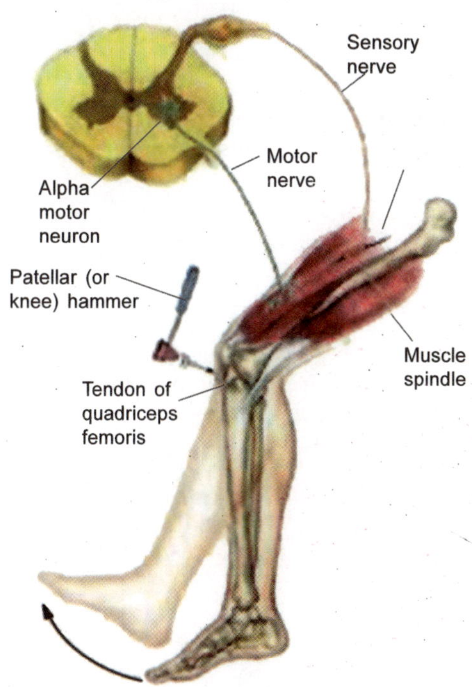

Fig. 3.22.29 Pathway for deep reflex (Example : Knee jerk)

The chief deep or tendon reflexes are described in Table 3.22.3 on page 266.

Grading of Reflexes

Grade 0 : Absent
Grade 1 : Present (as a normal ankle jerk)
Grade 2 : Brisk (as a normal knee jerk)
Grade 3 : Very brisk
Grade 4 : *Clonus* (it is a sign of increased reflex activity characterised by repetitive muscular contraction produced by stretch).

Table 3.22.2 The superficial reflexes

Reflex	How to elicit	Response	Level of spinal cord involved
Reflexes based on spinal nerves			
1. Plantar reflex (to elicit it, the sole should be warm and clean with leg completely relaxed)	Gently scratch the outer edge of the foot with a blunt object (say, key) from the heel towards the little toe and then medially across the metatarsals 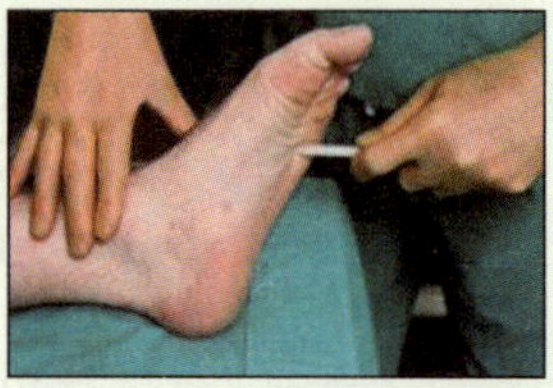	Plantar flexion (downward movement) of all the toes. (Also, see important note page 250)	L_5S_1
2. Abdominal reflex	Subject lying supine and relaxed with abdomen uncovered; stroking abdominal wall with key parallel to costal margin and inguinal ligament 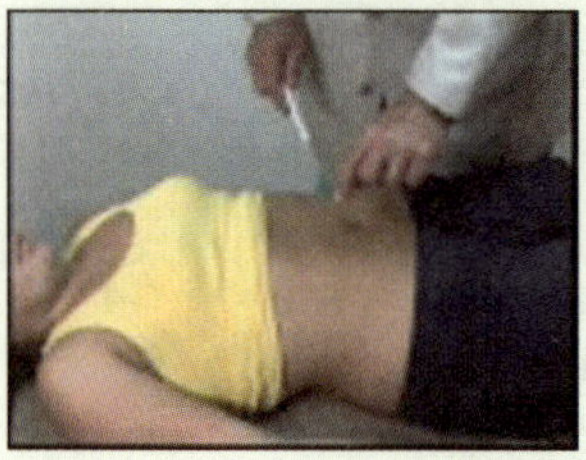	A ripple of contraction of underlying abdominal muscles. (It is usually difficult to obtain this reflex in anxious persons, elderly, obese and multipara women.)	T_{7-12}
3. Scapular reflex	Stroking skin in interscapular region 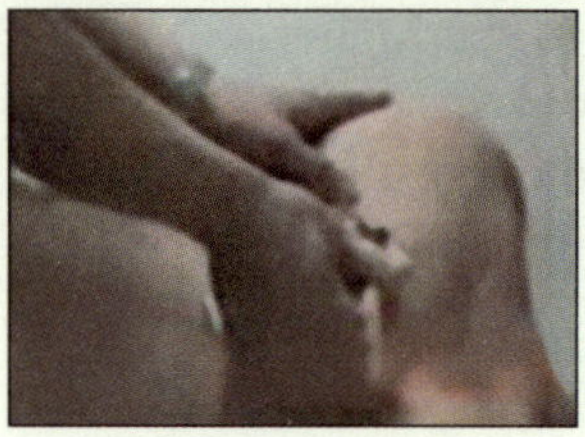	Contraction of scapular muscles (supra and infra-spinatus).	C_5 to T_1
4. Anal reflex	Stroking or scratching the skin near the anus 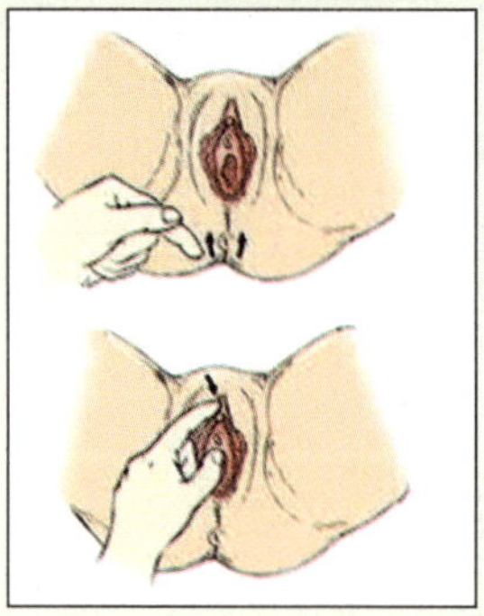	Contraction of anal sphincter	S_{3-4}
5. Cremasteric reflex	Stroking skin at upper and inner part of thigh 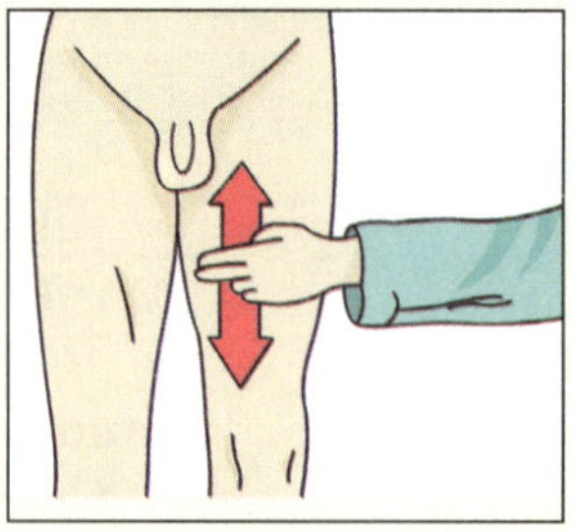	Drawing upwards (ascend) of testicles due to the contraction of cremasteric muscle	L_{1-2}
6. Bulbo-cavernous reflex	Pinching dorsum of glans penis 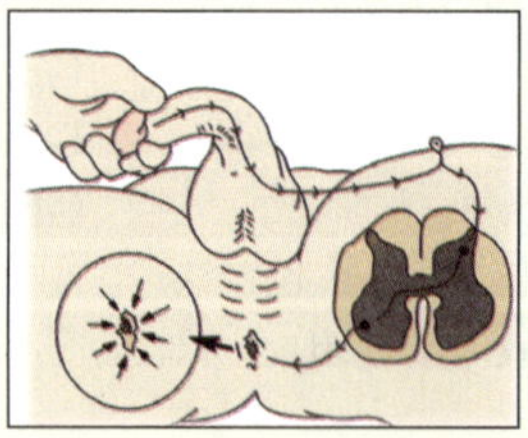	Contraction of bulbo-cavernous muscle	S_{3-4}

Reflexes based on cranial nerves			
1. Conjunctival reflex	Touch the conjunctiva with a cotton wool swab.	Contraction of orbicularis oculi resulting in rapid closure of eye lid	Afferent: Vth nerve Efferent: VIIth nerve
2. Corneal reflex	Lighty touch the lateral edge of the cornea at its conjuctival margin with a cotton wool swab.	Contraction of orbicularis oculi resulting in rapid closure of eye lid	-do-
	Important Note: The centre of cornea should ***never*** be touched, as it carries the risk of corneal ulceration and subsequent visual impairment.		
3. Visual reflexes (i) Pupillary light reflex (direct/ indirect) (ii) Accommodation reflex	Refer to page 244. Refer to page 246.		Afferent: IInd nerve Efferent: IIIrd nerve -do-
4. Palatal reflex	Refer to page 254.		Afferent: Vth and IXth nerve Efferent: Xth nerve

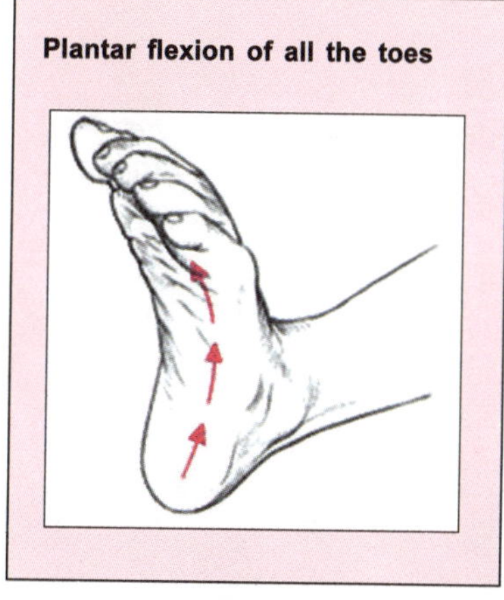

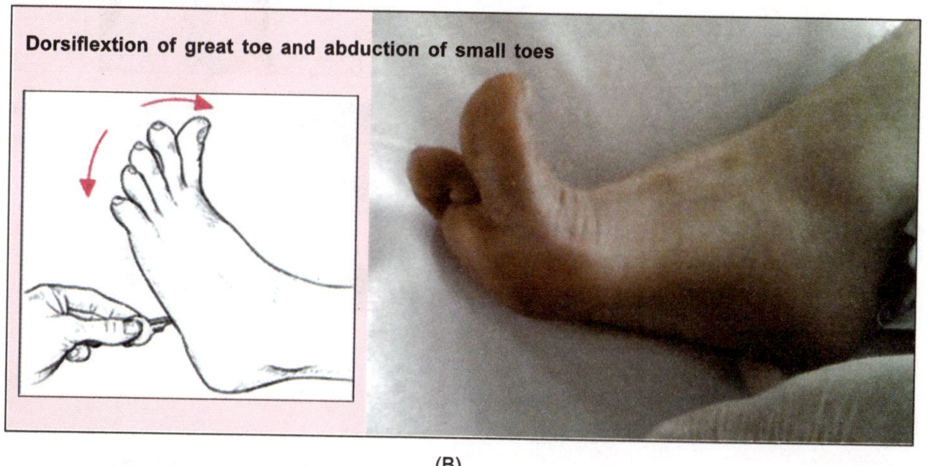

Fig. 3.22.30 Plantar reflex (A) Normal and (B) Abnormal (Babinski sign)

* **Important Note:** In upper motor neuron lesion, the same stimulus causes dorsiflexion (upward movement) of great toe and abduction (fanning out) of small toe and even withdrawal of the limb. This is referred as ***Babinski Sign*** (*Abnormal*). Physiologically, this is a flexor (withdrawl) plantar reflex, as all the muscles which contract during a flexor response are called physiological flexors. (Fig. 3.22.30)

Table 3.22.3 The deep (or tendon) reflexes

Reflex	How to elicit		Response	Level of spinal cord involved
1. Knee (or patellar) jerk or quadriceps femoris jerk	(i) The subject either supine or sitting (ii) The examiner's hand is passed under the knee to be tested and placed on the opposite knee. (iii) The test knee rests on the dorsum of the examiner's wrist. (iv) Strike the patellar tendon midway between its origin and insertion. 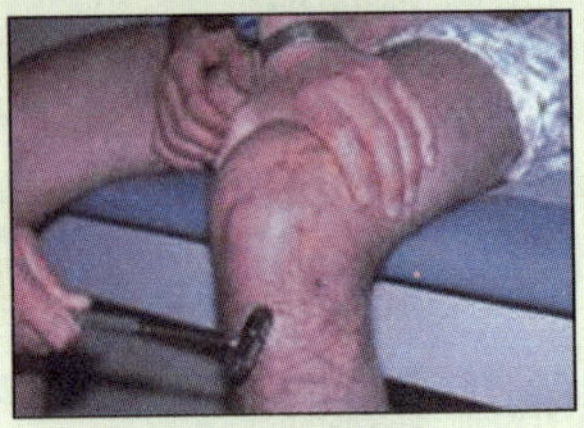	*Alternately,* it can also be more easily elicited with the subject sitting up, the leg hanging freely over the other knee or the edge of the bed.	A brief contraction of the quadriceps femoris muscle results in the extension of the knee. (If unable to elicit, apply reinforcement; Jendrassik's Manoeuvre, page 268)	$L_{2,3,4}$ (Femoral nerve)
2. Ankle jerk or gastrocnemius and soleus jerk	(i) Place the lower limb in everted and slightly flexed position; then with one hand, slightly dorsiflex the foot so as to stretch it. (ii) With the other hand, strike the tendon on its posterior surface. 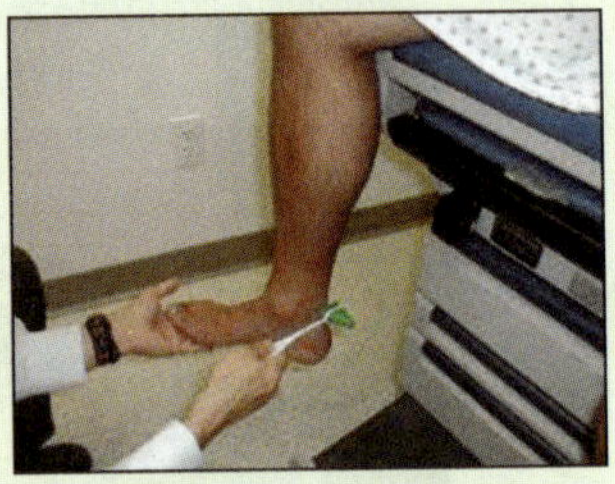		A sharp contraction of calf muscle (gastrocnemius) is seen.	$S_{1,2}$ (Tibial nerve)
3. Triceps jerk	(i) Flex the elbow and allow the forearm to rest across the subject's chest. (ii) Tap the triceps tendon with a patellar hammer (broad end) 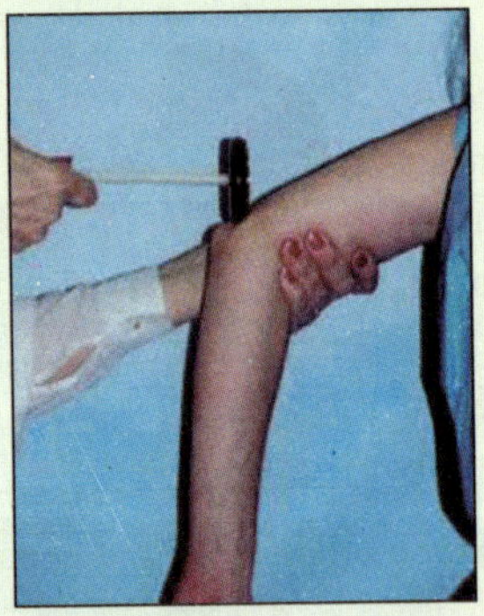		Contraction of triceps muscle	$C_{6,7}$ (Radial nerve)
4. Biceps jerk	(i) The elbow is flexed to a right angle and the forearm is placed in a semiprone position. (ii) The examiner then places his thumb or index finger on the biceps tendon and strike it with the patellar hammer (pointed end). 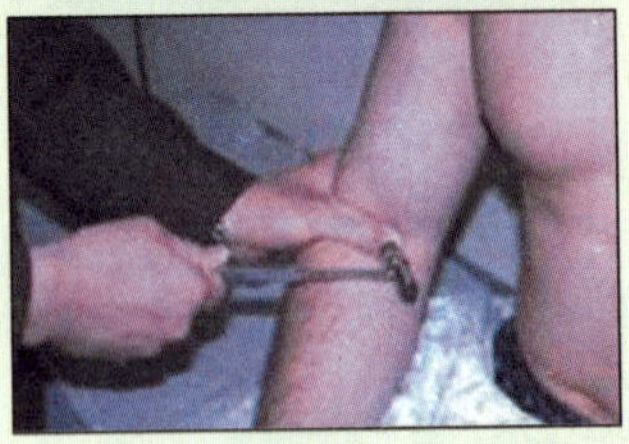		Contraction of biceps muscle	$C_{5,6}$ (Musculo-cutaneous nerve)
5. Supinator jerk or brachioradialis jerk	(i) Same as 4(i). (ii) Tap the Brachioradialis tendon upon the styloid process of radius 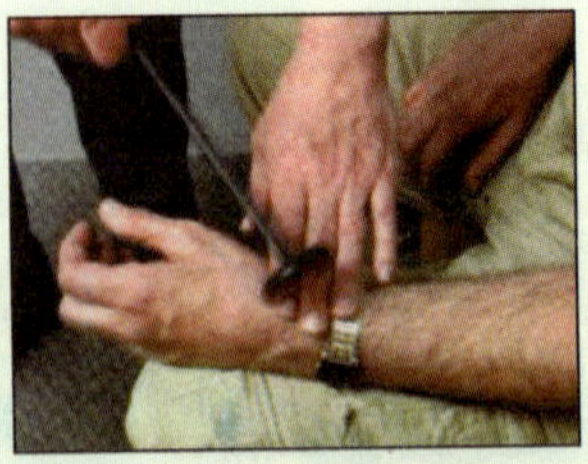		Contraction of Brachioradialis muscle with the supination of elbow	$C_{5,6}$ (Radial nerve)

Reflex	How to elicit	Response	Level of spinal cord involved
6. Jaw jerk	(i) Ask the subject to open his mouth but not too widely. (ii) Place one finger firmly on his chin and then tap it suddenly either with the patellar hammer *or* with the other hand (as in percussion).	Contraction of masseter muscle resulting in the closure of the jaw (this jerk is sometimes absent in a healthy individual).	Fifth cranial nerve nuclei

Abnormal tendon reflexes

1. Tendon reflexes are diminished or absent:
   (i) during sleep;
   (ii) if the subject watches it;
   (iii) lower motor neuron lesion (LMNL).
2. Tendon reflexes become exaggerated (hyperactive) in:
   (i) anxiety or nervousness;
   (ii) upper motor neuron lesion (UMNL);
   (iii) thyrotoxicosis;
   (iv) tetanus.
3. Pendular reflex is seen in the persons with cerebellar lesions.

(C) The Organic or Sphincteric Reflexes

These are reflexes concerned with such processes as respiration, deglutition (swallowing), micturition and defecation. They depend upon complex muscular movements excited by increased tension in the wall of the viscus concerned. They involve both skeletal and smooth muscles, and their integrity is mainly ascertained by the interrogation of the person.

1. ***Deglutition (swallowing) reflex.*** A person with neurological disorder complains of difficulty in swallowing (*dysphagia*) liquids, whereas those with mechanical obstruction to the oesophagus or pharynx cannot swallow solids.
2. ***Defecation reflex or anal sphincter reflex.*** The reflex action of the voluntary anal sphincter may be tested by introducing the lubricated gloved finger into the anus and noting whether the contraction of the sphincter occurs with normal force, whether the sphincter is weak or paralysed, or whether any spasm is excited.

Note: The anal sphincter normally contracts briskly in response to sudden cough – *the cough reflex.*

3. ***Micturition reflex***
   (i) Make a note of retention, incontinence or urgency of micturition.
   (ii) Incontinence in neurological disorders may be due to:
      (a) Overflow from an *atonic* distended bladder in which sensation has been lost.
      (b) *Reflex micturition,* occurring either at regular intervals as the bladder fills, or precipitated by and unexpectedly in response to a sudden noise, to movement or to exposure to cold (unstable, urge incontinence).

OSPE-I

Aim: To elicit knee jerk on the subject provided

Checklist

1. Makes the subject confortably seated in a chair or lying supine in the bed. **(Yes/No)**
2. Explains the proper instructions of test procedure to the subject. **(Yes/No)**
3. Makes the subject completely relaxed with attention diverted. **(Yes/No)**
4. Places the knee to be tested of the subject to rest on the dorsum of the examiner's wrist. **(Yes/No)**
5. Locates the patellar tendon. **(Yes/No)**
6. Strikes gently, by flexing the wrist joint with the broader end of the hammer, the patellar tendon mid-way between its orgin and insertion. **(Yes/No)**
7. Looks/feels for the contraction of the quadriceps femoris or extension of the knee. **(Yes/No)**

Note: On similar lines, OSPE can also be framed for other deep reflexes; for detailed procedure steps, refer to Table 3.22.3.

OSPE-II

Aim: To elicit plantar reflex on the subject provided

Checklist

1. Makes the subject comfortably seated on a chair or lying supine in the bed. **(Yes/No)**
2. Explains the test procedure to the subject. **(Yes/No)**
3. Checks that the sole of the subject's test foot is warm and clean with leg completely relaxed. **(Yes/No)**
4. Gently scratches the outer edge of the subject's foot with a blunt object from heel towards the little toe and medially across the metatarsals. **(Yes/No)**
5. Watches for the toe movements of the subject. **(Yes/No)**

Note: OSPE for other superficial reflexes are also framed similarly. The student should learn the detailed procedure steps, refer to Table 3.22.2.

IMPORTANT VIVA-VOCE QUESTIONS

Q.1. *Define stretch reflex and give its characteristic features.*

Ans. When a skeletal muscle with an intact nerve supply is stretched, it contracts. This response is called the stretch reflex. Features are:

(i)It is a monosynaptic reflex.

(ii)It is a fundamental reflex which plays an important role in the control of body posture.

(iii)It is highly developed in antigravity muscles, *i.e.* muscles which oppose the force of gravity. *Examples:* the extensor group of muscles of legs, flexor group of muscles of arms and muscles of the back.

Q.2. *Give the components of a reflex arc.*

Ans. The components are: a receptor (muscle spindle); an afferent neuron, an efferent neuron and an effector organ.

Q.3. *Give the significance of deep (or tendon) reflexes.*

Ans. It offers a reliable and reproducible method of the assessment of integrity of the reflex arc and its higher connections.

Q.4. *What is reinforcement and how does it work?*

Ans. The reinforcement or **Jendrassik's manoeuvre** is done by asking the individual to hook the fingers of the two hands together and then to pull them against one another as hard as possible or to make a clenched fist with the ipsilateral hand. It acts by increasing the excitability of α-motor neurons and by increasing the sensitivity of the muscle spindle primary sensory endings to stretch (by increased γ-efferent drive).

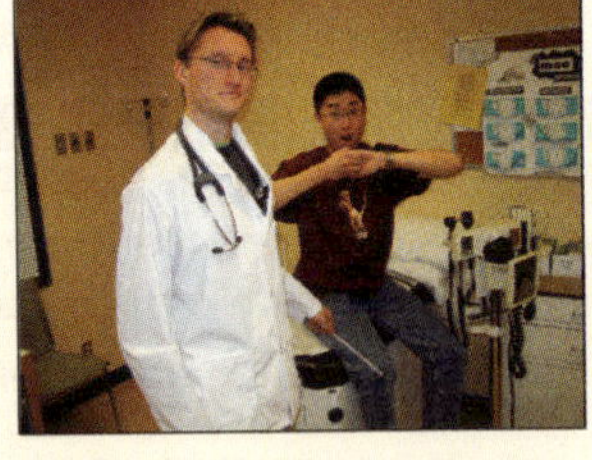

Q.5. *Give the grading of reflexes.*

Ans. Page 263.

Q.6. *What is myotonic reflex?*

Ans. In myxoedema, both the contraction and relaxation phases of the tendon reflex may be prolonged. This is called myotonic reflex. It is also found in hypothermic patients.

Q.7. *Give the pathway of impulse in a superficial reflex.*

Ans. Page 263.

Q.8. *What happens to superficial and deep reflexes in upper and lower motor neuron lesions?*

Ans. (i) In upper motor neuron lesion, initially during the **stage of shock,** all reflexes are lost; however, some 2-3 weeks later (**stage of recovery**), deep (or tendon) reflexes are hyperactive (exaggerated) and are more sustained, *i.e.* relaxation is still further prolonged, and all superficial reflexes are lost (usually abdominal, cremasteric and anal reflexes are lost).

(ii) In lower motor neuron lesion, both superficial and deep reflexes are lost as the reflex path is damaged.

Q.9. *Give the causes of abnormal Babinski sign.*

Ans. (i) Infants below 1 year of age, as the pyramidal tracts are not developed till a child starts walking.

(ii) During deep sleep

(iii) Inhibition of pyramidal tracts

(iv) Cheyne-Stokes respiration due to hypoxia

(E) Examination of the Sensory System

The examination of the sensory system includes the testing of various forms of sensations as described under:

1. *Tactile sensibility, i.e.* sensation of light touch, pressure, tactile localization and discrimination
2. *Pain*
3. *Temperature*
4. *Sense of position*
5. *Vibration sense*
6. *Recognition of the size, shape, weight and form of objects*
7. *Presence of any abnormal sensations*

Before starting the examination, explain the nature of the test to be performed to the subject to get his full cooperation. Ask the subject to close his eyes or turn the face to the other side and test the different forms of sensations; always compare corresponding points on both sides of the body. The location of major ascending tracts in the spinal cord and various sensations they convey are shown in Fig. 3.22.31.

TACTILE SENSIBILITY

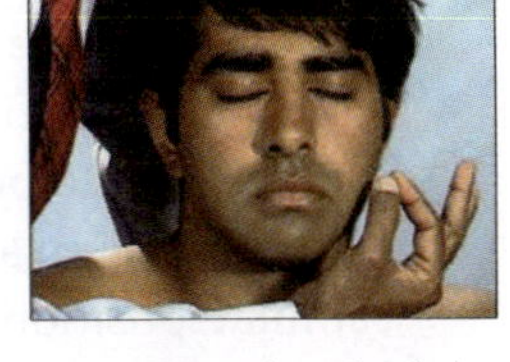

1. ***Light Touch.*** Touch with low threshold.
   (i) Use a wisp of cotton wool and test from different parts of the body; ask the subject to say 'yes' every time he feels a touch.
   (ii) Complete absence of touch sensibility is called *anaesthesia;* its partial loss, called *Hypoaesthesia* and exaggerated (increased) sensibility to touch, is called *Hyperaesthesia*.

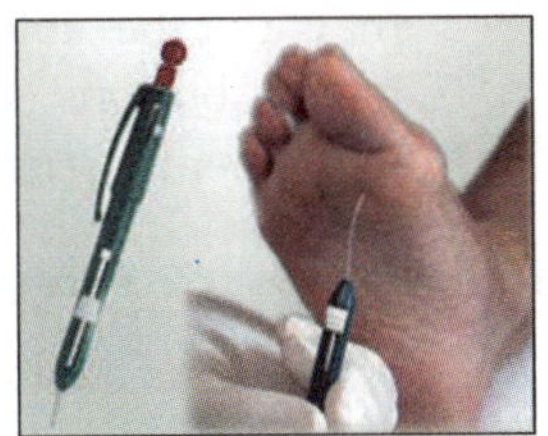

2. ***Pressure Sense.*** Pressure is *sustained touch* sensation. Repeat the above test using a blunt object (it should be at body temperature); note any disturbance in its perception over the different portions on the body.
3. ***Tactile Localization,*** *i.e.* the ability to tell precisely (exactly) the portion of body part touched. Repeat the above procedure 1(i) and ask the subject to localise it.

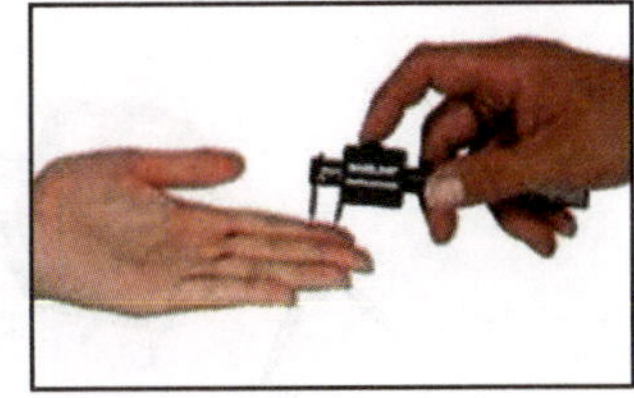

4. ***Tactile Discrimination,*** *i.e.* the ability to distinguish between two adjacent touch stimuli to the skin. It is greater on the thumb, fingers and lips, where the sensory units are small and overlap considerably, than on the back, where the sensory units are large and widely spaced.
   It depends upon the intactness of touch sensibility and parietal lobe. Normally, 2-3 mm of separation of the points can be recognised as two separate stimuli on fingertips, whereas two points on the back must be separated by 65 mm or more before they can be distinguished as separate points.
   The tactile discrimination is tested by the use of *compass aesthesiometer* (Fig. 3.22.32), the two limbs of the instrument are separated and the subject's skin is touched by both points; ask whether he is being touched with one or both the points.

PAIN SENSIBILITY

Pain may be produced either by a cutaneous stimulus such as the prick of a pin (*superficial pain*) or by pressure

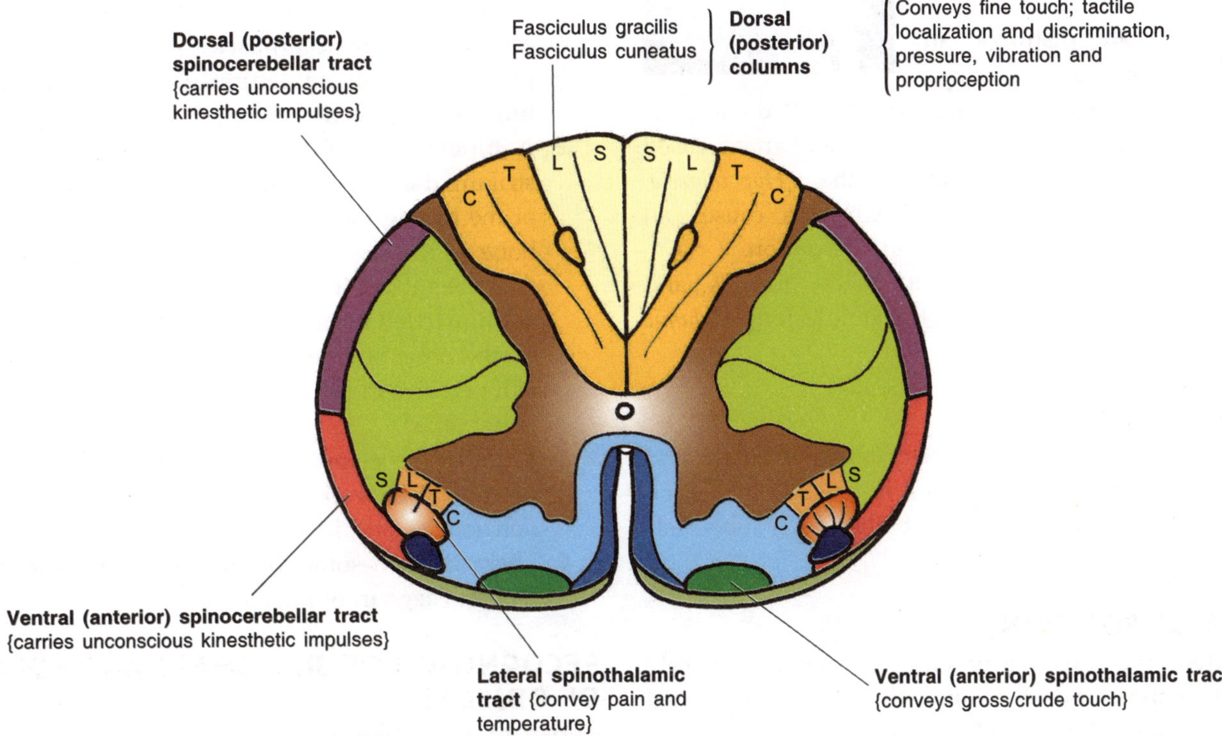

Fig. 3.22.31 A cross-section of the spinal cord showing the location of major ascending tracts and various sensations they carry (S-sacral; L-lumbar; T-thoracic and C-cervical)

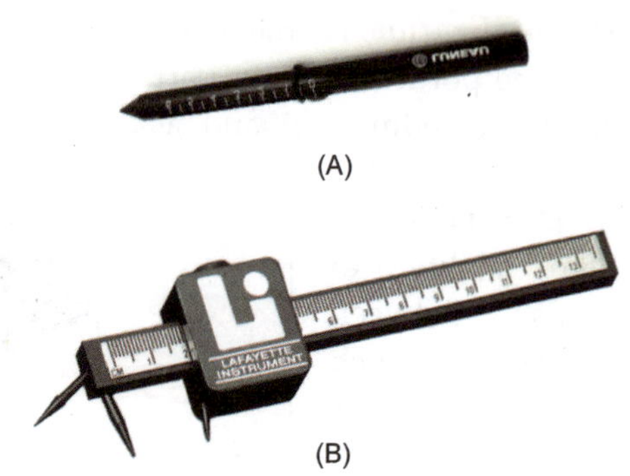

(A)

(B)

Fig. 3.22.32 An aesthesiometer: (A) simple; (B) compass

on deeper structure, such as muscles or bone (*deep* or *pressure pain*).

1. ***Superficial pain.*** Use the point of an ordinary domestic pin (a hypodermic needle which is designed to cut skin relatively painlessly is not suitable) and using the same technique as used for touch, ask the subject to distinguish between the *sharpness* of the point (*i.e.* its relative size) and the *pain,* which the prick produces.

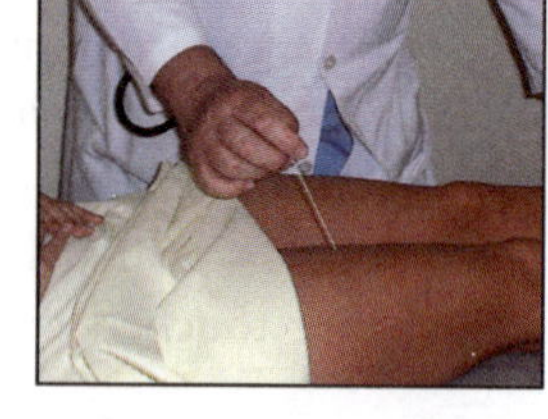

2. ***Deep or pressure pain.*** This is tested by squeezing the muscle or the tendo-achilles; this sensation is particularly disturbed in tabes dorsalis.

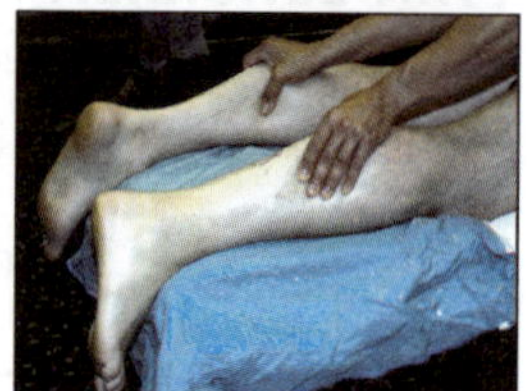

   (i) The absence of pain sensibility is called *Analgesia.* Its partial loss, the *Hypoalgesia,* and an increased (exaggerated) response, the *Hyperalgesia,* therefore, even a mild stimulus causes an unnatural degree of painful sensation.
   (ii) Hyperalgesia occurs in tabes dorsalis and deep-seated parietal or thalamic lesions (*thalamic pain*).

THERMAL SENSE

This is tested by using test tubes containing warm and cold water. The part to be tested is touched with each in turn, and the person says whether each tube feels hot or cold.

SENSE OF POSITION

The extent and direction of joint movements is closely related to the sense of position that can be examined accurately with the person's eyes closed.

1. Ask the subject to look away, explain the procedure to the subject, then move his finger (or toe or elbow) up or down and ask him to tell you which way it has been moved. He should be able to recognize the movements of only a few degrees (less than 10°) at all joints, including knee, ankle, elbow, wrist, finger and toes.

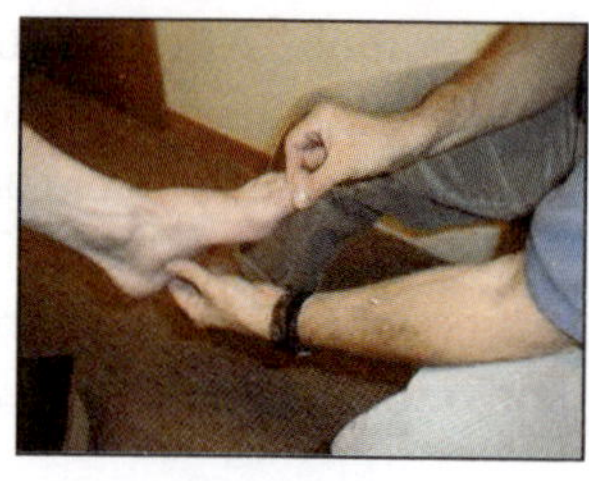

2. Hold one of the subject's limbs and move it about in various directions through the air, finally leaving in some definite position, say semiflexed or extended; then ask him to put the corresponding limb in a similar position.

Important Note: While testing the sense of position, do not allow the part tested to touch any other skin surface, otherwise the subject will be able to appreciate its position by information derived from his sense of touch.

3. The persons with the defective sense of position may not be able to manipulate small objects or fasten buttons without visually observing their movements (*sensory ataxia*).

VIBRATION SENSE

1. If the foot of a vibrating tuning fork is placed on the surface of the body, the vibrations can be felt. The sensation is most marked over bones; the *receptors* involved are touch-pressure receptors, especially pacinian corpuscles. A pattern of rhythmic pressure stimuli is interpreted as vibration and the impulses are carried in the dorsal column.

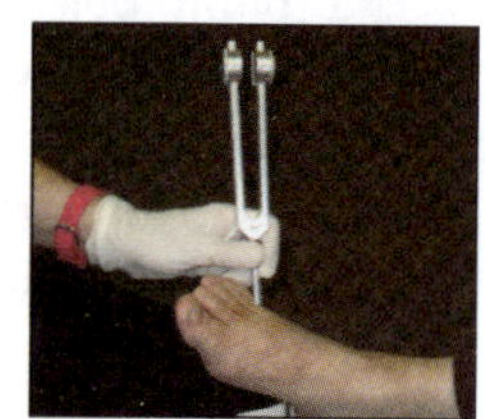

2. A tuning fork of 128 Hz is made to vibrate by striking the prongs gently on a firm object. The foot of the tuning fork is placed on some subcutaneous bone in the region to be tested (say shin of tibia). Ask the subject if he perceives the vibrations; if so, ask him to tell when he ceases to feel them. Compare on the other side. *Alternatively,* if the examiner can still perceive it, the person's perception of vibration is impaired.
3. Vibration sensibility is lost in tabes dorsalis, peripheral neuropathies, such as diabetes, vitamin deficiencies and in posterior column disorders.
4. There is often some loss of vibration sense in the feet and legs in old age.

RECOGNITION OF SIZE, SHAPE AND FORM OF OBJECTS

Sense of Stereognosis

1. The ability to recognise *familiar objects,* such as coins, a pencil, pen, scissors, etc. by handling

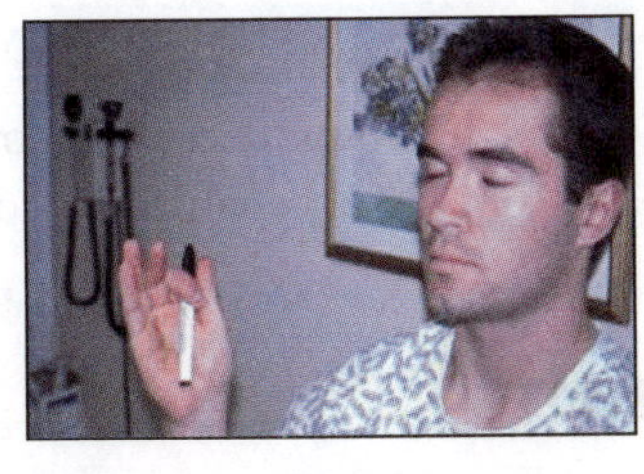

them without looking at them, is called *stereognosis*. It depends upon intact touch-pressure sensation, but cerebral cortex plays a major role.

2. These sensations can be tested most accurately in the hands with the eyes closed:
   (i) **To test the size**, place in the subject's palm, objects of the same shape, but of different sizes. For example, small balls or matchsticks of different lengths. Ask him to say which is the larger. The objects should be given consecutively.
   (ii) **To test the recognition of shape**, familiar objects are placed in the hand, and the subject is asked to identify them or describe their forms.
3. Loss of stereognosis (*astereognosis*) is an early sign of damage to the parietal lobe when touch-pressure sensation is normal.

PRESENCE OF ANY ABNORMAL SENSATIONS

The presence of abnormal sensations over the body is referred to as **paraesthesias**. This consists of various sensations experienced by the person in the absence of any outside stimulus. For example, feeling of 'pins and needles', of numbness, of pressure, of tightness, of itching or a feeling as if an insect is crawling over the body (**formication**). This phenomenn is called *sensory inattention* and is sometimes found in persons with parietal lobe lesions.

OSPE

Aim: Test for any one sensory modality on the subject provided

Checklist

1. Makes the subject comfortably seated on a chair or lying supine in the bed. **(Yes/No)**
2. Explains the test procedure to the subject. **(Yes/No)**
3. Makes the subject completely relaxed with attention diverted. **(Yes/No)**
4. Checks for different sensations separately on both sides of the subject for comparison purposes. **(Yes/No)**

Note: Students should learn the detailed procedure steps with precautions for each sensibility viz.: Tactile localization and discrimination; pain, thermal sense, vibration sense and sense of stereognosis (refer to pages 269 to 271).

IMPORTANT VIVA-VOCE QUESTIONS

Q.1. *Give the neural pathway of various somatic sensations.*

Ans. Page 269.

Q.2. *Which sensations get affected if (i) dorsal columns get destroyed, and (ii) lateral spinothalamic tracts are destroyed?*

Ans. (i) Dorsal column involvement causes the loss of fine touch, tactile localization and discrimination, pressure, vibration and propioception.
(ii) The involvement of lateral spinothalamic tracts causes the loss of pain and temperature.

Q.3. *Differentiate between fine and crude touch.*

Ans. Fine touch is the touch with low threshold and is carried by dorsal columns, whereas crude touch is the touch with high threshold of excitation and is conveyed by ventral (anterior) spinothalamic tracts.

Q.4. *Define pain. How does it differ from the other sensations?*

Ans. The *psychical* (pertaining to mind) adjunct (= joined to) of an imperative (= urgent) protective reflex is pain, *i.e.* pain is a sensation which draws the attention of an individual as a whole. It differs from other sensations in respect that it is associated with emotions, withdrawl response and autonomic changes such as alteration in the heart rate, BP, respiration, etc.

Q.6. *What is paradoxical cold fibre discharge?*

Ans. The maximal frequency of the steady discharge by a cold fibre occurs at a tissue temperature of 25-30°C. However, it also discharges at an increasing rate at the tissue temperature of 45°C producing a mixed sensation of cold and pain. This is referred to as paradoxical response of a cold fibre.

Q.5. *Differentiate between superficial and deep pain.*

Ans.

Superficial (cutaneous) pain	Deep pain
(i) It involves skin and subcutaneous tissue.	(i) It involves muscles and hollow viscera.
(ii) It is sharp in character and well localised.	(ii) It is dull and poorly localised.
(iii) It usually does not radiate.	(iii) It is local and radiates to the distant site.
(iv) It leads to reflex withdrawl movement, increase in heart rate, BP and respiration.	(iv) It produces faintness, nausea, vomiting, sweating, fall in heart rate and BP.

Q.7. *Can tuning fork with high frequencies (above 256 Hz) be used to test vibration sense?*

Ans. No, because the vibrations of higher frequencies are more difficult to perceive.

Q.8. *Which part of the brain is concerned with the perception of the sense of position?*

Ans. The angular gyrus of parietal lobe is concerned with the perception of position sense.

STUDY NOTES

RESULTS AND DISCUSSION

(A) EXAMINATION OF HIGHER FUNCTIONS

1. Mental state ....

2. Memory ....

3. Speech ....

(B) EXAMINATION OF CRANIAL NERVES

I. ***Olfactory Nerve***

Smell sensibility:

On right side – Present/absent ....

On left side – Present/absent ....

II. ***Optic Nerve***

The following observations were made on the given subject:

1. *Visual acuity*
   (i) for near vision, tested with the help of
      (a) Right eye ....
      (b) Left eye ....
   (ii) for distant vision, tested with the help of
      (a) Right eye ....
      (b) Left eye ....
2. *Field of vision* as tested by confrontation method.
   (i) Right eye ....
   (ii) Left eye ....
3. *Colour vision*

   ....
4. *Fundus examination* (whether done or not; if yes, give findings).
   (i) Right eye ....
   (ii) Left eye ....

III. ***(Oculomotor), IV: (Trochlear) and VI: (Abducent) Nerves***

Present/absent

1. Ptosis ....
2. Squint ....
3. Nystagmus ....

4. Ocular movement
   (i) upward gaze ....
   (ii) temporal gaze ....
   (iii) downward gaze ....
   (iv) nasal gaze ....
5. Pupil: size and shape ....
6. Visual reflexes
   (i) Pupillary Light reflex
      (a) direct ....
      (b) indirect ....
   (ii) Accommodation reflex ....

V. ***Trigeminal Nerve***
1. Cutaneous sensibility over skin and mucous membrane: Present/absent (if absent, specify the area involved)
2. Corneal reflex
   (i) On right side Present/absent
   (ii) On left side Present/absent
3. Muscles of mastication
   (i) On right side ....
   (ii) On left side ....
4. Deviation of jaw on opening the mouth: Present/absent

VII. ***Facial Nerve***
1. Tests for the muscles of face and scalp
2. Tests for buccinator muscle
3. Tests for stapedius muscle
4. Tests for taste sensation

	Anterior part		Posterior part	
	Right side	Left side	Right side	Left side
(i) Sweet				
(ii) Salt				
(iii) Sour				
(iv) Bitter				

5. Tests for Lacrimation

VIII. ***Vestibulo-cochlear Nerve***

A. Tests for vestibular functions

B. Tests for cochlear function

IX. ***Glossopharyngeal Nerve***

1. Taste sensations in the posterior 1/3rd of tongue:
   - (i) On right side present/absent
   - (ii) On left side present/absent
2. Palatal reflex:
   - (i) On right side present/absent
   - (ii) On left side present/absent

X. ***Vagus Nerve***

1. History of the regurgitation of fluids through nose present/absent
2. Nasal twang present/absent
3. Palatal reflex present/absent
4. Soft palate movements during phonation:
   - (i) on right side
   - (ii) on left side
5. Laryngoscopy examination findings (if done):

XI. ***Spinal Accessory Nerve***

1. Flexion of the head against examiner's passive resistance.

   ....

   ....
2. Rotation of chin
   - (i) towards right ....
   - (ii) towards left ....
3. Shrugging off the shoulder
   - (i) right side ....
   - (ii) left side ....

XII. ***Hypoglossal Nerve***

....

....

(C) EXAMINATION OF MOTOR SYSTEM

Tabulate your results in the Table.

	Upper limb		Trunk		Lower Limb	
	Right	Left	Right	Left	Right	Left
1. Bulk of muscles						
2. Tone of muscles						
3. Coordination of movements						
4. Strength (or power) of muscle						
5. Gait						
6. Involuntary movements						

(D) REFLEXES

Tabulate your results as under:

	Right	Left
The superficial reflexes		
1. Plantar		
2. Abdominal		
3. Scapular		
4. Anal		
5. Cremasteric		
6. Bulbocavernous		
7. Conjunctival/Corneal		
8. Pupillary (i) direct (light) (ii) indirect (light) (iii) accommodation		
9. Palatal		
The deep (or tendon) reflexes		
1. Knee (or patellar)		
2. Ankle		
3. Triceps		
4. Biceps		
5. Supinator		
6. Jaw		
The organic (or sphincteric) reflexes)		
1. Deglutition (swallowing)		
2. Defecation		

	Right	Left
3. Micturition		

(E) EXAMINATION OF THE SENSORY SYSTEM

Tabulate your results as under.

	Right side of body	Left side of body
1. Tactile sensibility (i) Light touch (ii) Pressure sense (iii) Tactile localization (iv) Tactile discrimination		
2. Pain sensibility (i) Superficial pain (ii) Deep (or pressure) pain		
3. Thermal sense		
4. Sense of position		
5. Vibration sense		
6. Stereognosis sense		
7. Any abnormal sensation		

Date: ....

23 Reaction Time (*Visual and Auditory*) and Reflex Time

I. APPARATUS

Two tapping keys, a signal marker, short circuiting key, a bulb, 6 volts mains, kymograph with drum, patellar hammer enveloped with tin foil, tuning fork, thread, tin foil sheath, mercury key

II. THEORY: *REACTION TIME VERSUS REFLEX TIME*

A. Reaction time

1. Reaction time is the interval of time between the application of a stimulus and appearance of appropriate *voluntary* response in a subject.
2. Being voluntary in nature, the response is primarily governed by the ability of an individual to concentrate and to establish a muscular attitude of readiness. The reaction time thus indicates the time lost between the application of a stimulus and the appearance of its end effect.
3. Different types of stimulus can be tried to elicit a particular response such as touch, cold, sound, heat, light, pain, etc.
4. It varies with the complexity of the reflex and the inter-related sensory pathways associated with the course of the impulse as it travels to the centre. For example, the factors which:
   (i) *facilitate* (speed up) the reaction time are: alertness, training, concentration; and
   (ii) *inhibit* (prolong) the reaction time are: advancing age, distraction, muscular weakness, etc.

B. Reflex time

1. Reflex time is the time interval between the application of an adequate stimulus and appearance of *reflex (involuntary) response.* For example, reflex time for a stretch reflex, such as knee jerk, is 19-24 m/sec.
2. The reflex activity is stereotyped (fixed) and specific in terms of both the stimulus and the response. Therefore, a particular stimulus produces a particular response. As the receptors respond maximally only when an appropriate specific stimulus is applied; likewise, the stimulus that produces a reflex is very precise and is called the *adequate stimulus* for the particular reflex.

III. PROCEDURE

A. Visual reaction time

1. Make the circuit using two tapping keys, signal marker and short circuiting key; all connected in series with low voltage mains (6 volts). Drum is not included in the circuit (Fig. 3.23.1-A).
2. The subject whose reaction time is to be determined operates the key marked 'A', the subject's partner operates key 'B'.
3. Keep the short circuiting key open with a bulb connected to its two central terminals (which are meant for muscle electrodes in amphibian experiments). Therefore, when both the subject as well as and his partner close their keys, the circuit is complete and bulb will glow; simultaneously, the signal marker will draw the writing point down.
4. Ask the subject to press on key 'A' (his own key) and release it off as soon as he sees the bulb glowing. The glowing of bulb is controlled by the subject's partner via key 'B'.
5. Rotate the drum at the fastest speed of 640 mm/sec and record the baseline (while only subject's key 'A' is pressed).
6. The subject's partner completes the circuit by pressing his key 'B':
   (i) The moment the partner presses his key, the bulb glows and the signal marker goes down. This marks the point of stimulus on the drum which is indicated by depression of the straight line.
   (ii) As soon as the subject releases his key 'A' (on seeing the bulb glowing), there will be break in the continuity of the straight line, which is marked by its elevation.

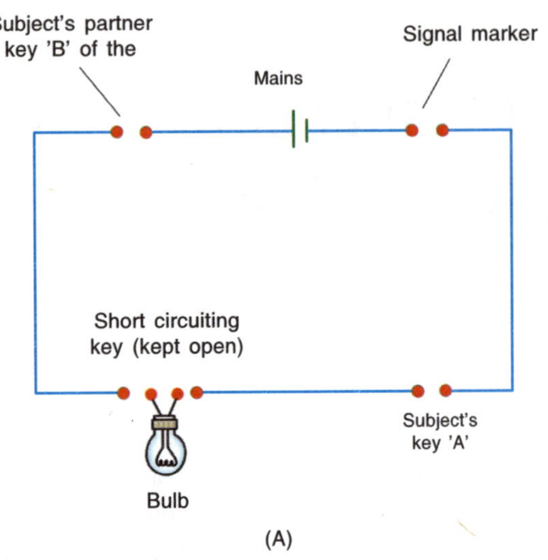

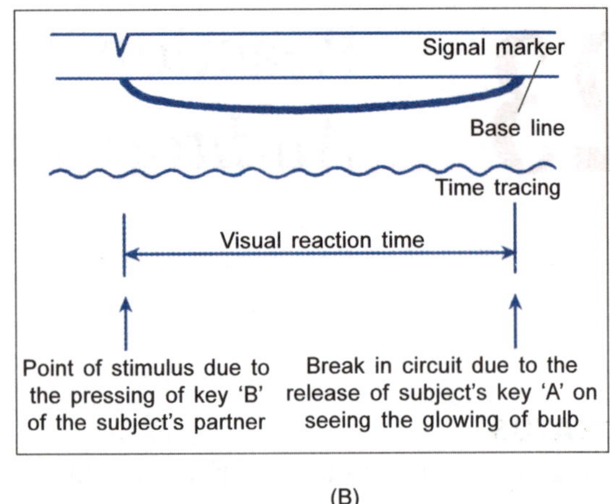

Fig. 3.23.1 Visual reaction time. (A) circuit diagram; (B) an actual record

7. Take the time tracing with the help of a vibrating tuning fork of 100 Hz frequency below the record.
8. Calculate the visual reaciton time for the duration of break in the straight line (Fig. 3.23.1-B).

B. Auditory reaction time

1. Similarly, instead of light signal, auditory signal can be used. The mere 'tap' of the key will do.
2. In order to avoid making circuit again, the same set up, as above, can be used with the exception that the bulb and secondary key is taken out from the circuit.
3. The procedure is the same as above except that this time the subject immediately releases his key (A) on hearing the tapping sound of his partner's key (B).
4. The auditory time is measured by means of a time tracing taken with the help of a vibrating tuning fork.

IV. PRECAUTIONS

1. The subject should not be facing his partner (the operator) as he should respond to the visual and auditory stimuli and not to the movements of his partner.
2. The subject partner (operator) should tap his own key gently so as to produce no noise during the recording of the visual reaction time.

C. Reflex Time - Knee Jerk (Monosynaptic Reflex)

1. Make two independent circuits with drum not included in the circuit: (Fig. 3.23.2)
   (i) In one circuit, include low-voltage mains, patellar hammer enveloped with tin foil, patellar metallic plate and signal marker. Therefore, when the patellar plate is struck

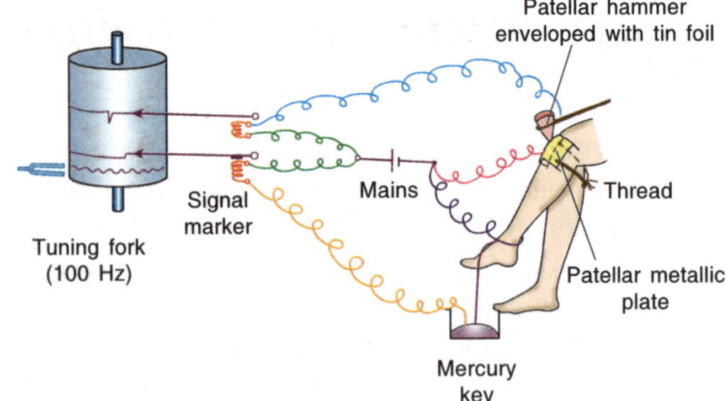

Fig. 3.23.2 Circuit diagram for recording knee reflex time

   with the patellar hammer, circuit is closed and pointer marks on the drum.
   (ii) In the second circuit, include the signal marker, low-voltage mains and mercury key taking one wire around ankle and letting it dip in mercury. Therefore, during the extension of leg, contact will be broken and signal marker will indicate on the fast-moving drum.
2. Arrange the two signal markers in alignment over the recording drum.
3. Make the subject comfortably seated on a stool with crossed legs.
   (i) Adjust the height of the wire and the ankle in such a way that the slightest extension of the leg results in the breaking of the circuit.
   (ii) Position the patellar metallic plate on the patellar tendon with the help of a thread.
4. Rotate the drum at the fastest speed of 640 mm/sec, and strike a sharp blow on the patellar tendon to produce the brisk contraction of the extensors of the leg.

5. Take time tracings with the help of a vibrating tuning fork of 100 Hz below the record.
6. Calculate the time interval between the application of a sharp blow on patellar tendon and the onset of extensor movement of leg and find out reflex time for monosynaptic reflex.

IMPORTANT VIVA-VOCE QUESTIONS

Q.1. *How does 'reaction time' differ from 'reflex time'? Explain.*

Ans. Page 277.

Q.2. *What are the conditions in which reaction time is increased or decreased?*

Ans. Conditions which increase the reaction time are:

(i) lack of concentration
(ii) advanced age
(iii) distraction
(iv) muscular weakness
(v) Person performing for the first time.

Conditions in which reaction time is decreased:

(i) alertness
(ii) training/repetitions (learning)
(iii) introspection (subject concentrates his attention)

Q.3. *Give the normal values for visual and auditory reaction time.*

Ans. (i) Normal auditory reaction time is 100-200 msec.
(ii) Normal visual reaction time is 200-400 msec. (It is more because it involves the chemical changes in its occurrence.)

Q.4. *Define discrimination time and recognition time.*

Ans. (i) Discrimination time - differences in the visual reaction time to different colours.
(ii) Recognition time - this is the time in excess of initial observation. For example, having measured the visual reaction time to white light, next find the additional time lost when some other coloured light (say red or green) is flashed at random.

Q.5. *Give the normal value of monosynaptic reflex time.*

Ans. Normal knee jerk time is 19-24 msec.

STUDY NOTES

RESULTS

(A) Calculate the ***visual and auditory reaction time*** from the graph obtained and express the results in the table as follows:

	Reading (in msec)			
	1st	2nd	3rd	Best of 3
1. Visual Reaction Time				
2. Auditory Reaction Time				

(B) ***Reflex Time***: knee jerk

COMMENTS AND DISCUSSION

....

....

....

....

....

....

....

....

Date: ....

24 Electroencephalogram: *EEG*

I. APPARATUS

Subject, EEG machine or student physiograph, EEG jelly (or paste), EEG electrodes, photo stimulator

EEG machine

A 16-channel EEG machine (Grass model-8) consists of the following parts: (Fig. 3.24.1)

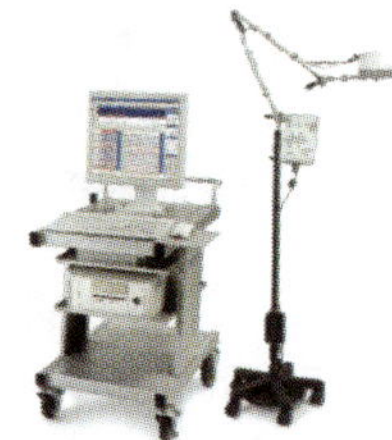

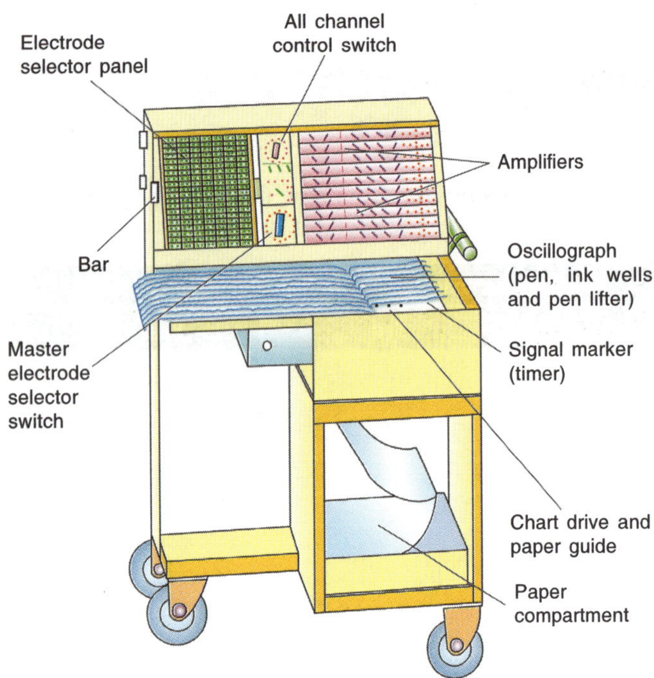

Fig. 3.24.1 An EEG machine (Grass model-8)

1. **Manual push button electrode selector panel**. It is coded for international system (on left half panel) and numerical system (on right half panel) of electrode placement. It permits the manual selection of electrode pairs. The bar to the left of selector panel simultaneously depresses the CAL NEG or CAL POS buttons for calibration. The bar on right permits ALL CHANNELS transfer to the master electrode selector switch.
2. **Master electrode selector switch**. It should be kept at CAL position for the calibration of all 16 channels with master selection button on the right of selector panel depressed. At BIOCAL position all channels record EEG from the same pair of electrodes.

> **Note:** This switch also has preset programming of electrodes to record EEG in eleven different montages.

3. **All channel controls switch**. It contains the circuit for all channels to be operated at the same setting with reference to:
   (i) control of sensitivity
   (ii) high, low and 50 Hz filter
   (iii) calibration of the instrument

   Components

   (i) **Calibrator**. It is provided with two push buttons (G_1 NEG and G_2) and a switch for calibrating the instrument in the desired range 2 µV to 10 mV per mm (*for ideal record, it should be kept at 50 µV/mm*).
   The calibration of instrument is done by depressing PUSH G_1 NEG button, which introduces a negative signal to G_1 and a positive signal to G_2; this results in the positive deflection of the pen record.

   (ii) **Electrode test** to verify the electrode impedence of any pair of electrodes. It is used when the sensitivity controls of channels are on ALL CHANNEL CONTROL. It is used for verification during cerebral death recording. It should not be left in ON position when not in use.
4. **Amplifier**. There is one full line for each channel on the right side of the front panel to increase the amplitude of small electrical signal from any selected pair of electrodes.
5. **Oscillograph, pen and ink wells, pen lifter**. The electrode signals from the amplifier output drives

the galvanometer. Its deflection can be recorded on the moving chart with the help of ink pens. *Ink wells* are reservoir for the ink fed to the pens by capillary action. The *pen-lifter* lifts the pens simultaneously from the writer surface.

6. **Chart drive and paper guide**. It is provided with 12 speeds (1.5, 3, 6, 15, 30 and 60 mm/sec or mm/min). Press a particular push button chart drive button to run the paper at a desired speed (*for normal record, usual speed is 30 mm/sec*).
   The *paper guide* and *rubber pressure roller* assure that the paper moves along a straight path.
7. **Signal marker/timer**. It gives an upward or a downward mark to signify an event.
8. **Writer switch** determines whether the chart moves or the chart and pen move.
9. **Paper compartment and paper tray**, for collecting the folded paper after recording, it can hold three packets of chart paper.

EEG electrodes

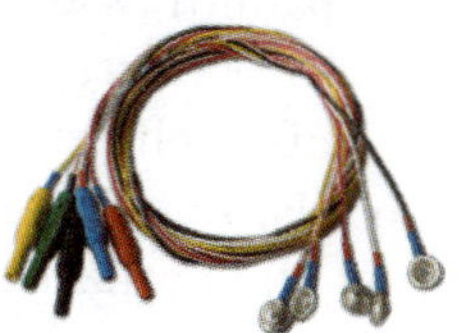

These are gold plated discs (or cups) to be placed on the scalp with the help of EEG paste. These can be cleaned with normal saline or warm water or NaOH solution; alternatively, they can be kept overnight in any one of them.

EEG jelly (or paste)

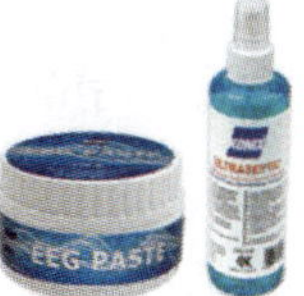

It is BENTONITE paste, prepared by thoroughly mixing 100 gm of bentonite powder with 130 ml normal saline and by adding glycerine gradually. It decreases the resistance between scalp and the electrodes.

II. THEORY

1. The record of electrical activity of the brain (cerebrum) is called *Electroencephalogram (EEG).* It can be recorded by placing two electrodes on the scalp and connecting them via a suitable amplifier to a cathode ray oscilloscope (CRO). This method of EEG recording was first introduced by German psychiatrist, *Hans Berger.* A similar record resembling EEG may be obtained by placing the electrodes directly on the exposed surface of the cerebral hemispheres - is termed the *Electrocorticogram (ECoG).*
2. **Source of the EEG**. The activity recorded in the EEG is that of rhythmically discharging cell bodies in the most superficial layers of the cortical grey matter. The EEG is due to graded potentials which are *summed* postsynaptic potentials in the brain neurons. The potential changes in the EEG are due to current flow in the fluctuating *dipoles* formed on the dendrites of the cortical cells and the cell bodies. The dendrites are the site of *non-propagated* hypo- and hyperpolarizing local potential changes. The cell-dendrite relationship is, therefore, that of a constantly shifting dipole. Current flow in this dipole produces wave-like potential fluctuations in a volume conductor. When it is positive, the cell is hyperpolarized and less excitable.
3. **Normal EEG**. The EEG can be recorded by using two methods: *Bipolar* and *Unipolar.*
   Bipolar method. It is a record of potential difference between two cortical electrodes. For example, frontal area, occipital area, temporal area or parietal area.
   Unipolar method. It is a record of potential difference between an active cortical electrode and an indifferent electrode applied on some part of the body distant from the cortex such as ear lobe.
   If an EEG record is taken in a normal subject who abstains from mental activity and keeps his eye closed, the usual pattern of electrical activity consists of the sequence of *rhythmic* waves (Fig. 3.24.2). The waves are classified according to their *frequency* and *voltage* (amplitude) (Table 3.24.1).

Important Notes

(i) Each EEG tracing is a complex rhythmic wave which *never repeats* itself precisely.

(ii) In general, lower EEG frequencies indicate less responsive behaviour, such as sleep, whereas higher frequencies indicate arousal.

Table 3.24.1 Main features of normal EEG rhythm

EEG Rhythm	Frequency (Hz)	Amplitude (μV)	Associated features
1. Alpha (α)	8-12	50	Present maximally in the *occipital* and *parieto-occipital* areas.
2. Beta (β)	14-30	5-10	Generally seen in *frontal* region; commonly seen in infants.
3. Theta (θ)	4-7	10	Often found over the *parietal* and *temporal* areas.
4. Delta (δ)	1-4	20-200	Usually appear during sleep; can be produced by overbreathing or organic brain disease.

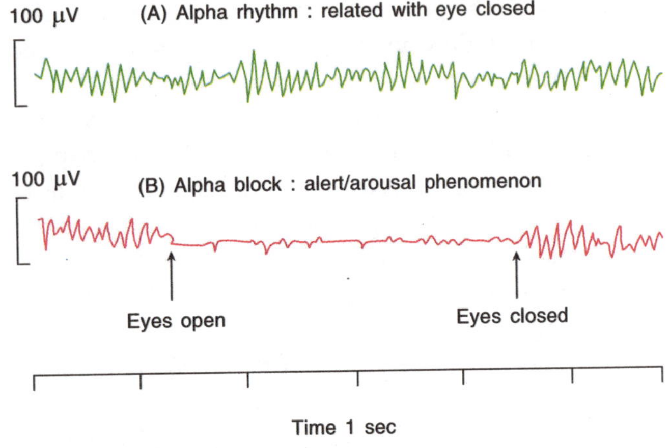

Fig. 3.24.2 Normal electroencephalogram (EEG)

Alpha Rhythm: Characteristic features

(i) They are present at rest (physical as well as mental) when the eyes are closed and form the most prominent component of the EEG.

(ii) Its frequency is

Decreased by

(a) low blood glucose level
(b) low body temperature
(c) a high arterial pCO_2
(d) low levels of adrenal glucocorticoid hormones
(e) anaesthesia or analgesia, and
(f) sleep

Increased by

(a) high blood glucose level
(b) rise in body temperature
(c) a low arterial pCO_2
(d) high levels of adrenal glucocorticoid hormones
(e) alerting states
(f) forced overbreathing which decreases arterial pCO_2

(iii) It is associated with the decreased levels of attention, and when α-rhythms are being generated, subjects commonly report that they feel relaxed and happy.

(iv) The replacement of regular α-rhythm with fast, high frequency, irregular low amplitude (voltage) activity is called ALPHA-BLOCK, or DESYNCHRONIZATION of EEG (Fig. 3.24.2). It represents a breaking up of the *synchronized* activity of the cortical neurons responsible for α-wave pattern.

A break-up of the α-pattern is also produced by any form of sensory stimulation such as the opening of the eyes or mental concentration. Because desynchronization is produced by sensory stimulation and is correlated with the aroused, alert state, it is also called the AROUSAL or ALERTING RESPONSE.

4. **Synchronizing Mehanisms**. The activity of many of the dendritic units is *synchronized* by two factors:
   (i) The synchronizing effect on each unit of activity is in its neighbours. This may be due to:
      (a) the neurons are connected to one another by inhibitory pathways and are also hyperexcitable after the inhibition. Therefore, the synaptic activity they generate tends to become synchronized; and
      (b) the effect of parallel neural processes on each other in a volume conductor. The formation of *current sinks* and *sources* in neighbouring fibres tends to synchronize current flow.
   (ii) The rhythmic discharge of impulses from the thalamus.
5. **Desynchronizing Mechanisms**. Desynchronization means the replacement of a rhythmic EEG pattern with irregular low-voltage activity. The RAS is responsible for the desynchronization of EEG following sensory stimulation.
6. **Uses of EEG**
   (i) Localization of conditions such as:
      (a) Subdural hematoma or fluid collection over cortex is associated with decreased EEG activity over this area
      (b) Lesion in the cortex cause local formation of irregular or slow waves in the EEG
   (ii) Diagnosis of Epilepsy. Epilepsy is due to the excessive discharge of cerebral neurons. Epileptic foci generate high voltage (amplitude) waves in the EEG, which can be localized.
   (iii) The diagnosis of severe organic brain disease such as brain tumour, which produces pathological δ-waves in the EEG record.

III. PROCEDURE

1. The instrument should be out of view of the subject. (Fig. 3.24.3), Make the subject comfortable either in

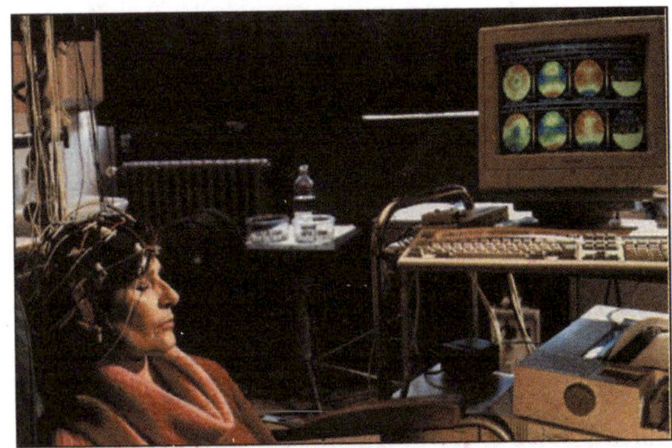

Fig. 3.24.3 Electroencephalography

sitting or lying position and apply the electrodes on his scalp with the help of EEG paste and cotton using 10-20 System (see below).

2. The electrodes from the subject head are plugged directly into the Mini electrode board (MEB), which is coded to correspond to the international as well as numerical system of electrodes placement. It connects the cerebro-electrical signals to the input of the EEG amplifier.
3. Calibrate the amplifer. How?
   (i) Use CAL position on master electrode selector.
   (ii) Select CAL signal on 'All channel controls' (50 μV).
   (iii) Depress 'push G_1 NEG' button, all channels show 7 mm pen deflection for 50 μV CAL.
4. Record for 3 minutes for each of the following procedures:
   (i) Resting record (a) open eyes and (b) closed eyes
   (ii) After hyperventilation for 2-3 minutes
   (iii) Photo stimulation at frequencies 1, 3, 5, 7, 10, 15, 20, 25 and 30/sec.
   (iv) Sleeping or drowsiness

10-20 SYSTEM

In this system electrodes are placed either 10% or 20% of the total distance between skull landmarks. It is based on proven relationship between a measured electrode site and underlying cortical structures and areas (Fig. 3.24.4).

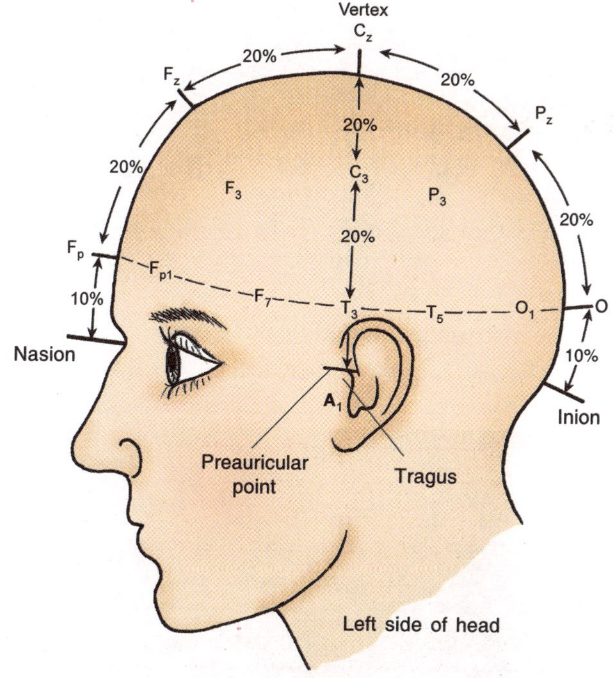

Fig. 3.24.4 10-20 system for the placement of electrodes on the scalp

Advantages

1. Uniformly followed internationally with full brain coverage
2. Uniform spacing of electrodes, placing becomes easy.
3. The comparison of records becomes easy between two individuals or in the same person during follow-up.

Landmark used

1. *Nasion:* indentation between forehead and nose
2. *Inion:* a ridge between the back of neck and skull
3. *Right and left preauricular points:* indentation just above the cartilage (tragus) which covers the external ear opening.

Electrodes placement (International system)

1. Join nasion to inion; this is taken as 100% distance. Now follow 10% or 20% rule and locate F_p, F_z, C_z, P_z and 'O' points (as marked in the figure).
2. Join right and left pre-auricular points (i.e. A_1 and A_2) through C_z (100%); follow 10% or 20% rule, and locate points T_3, C_3, C_z, C_4 and T_4.
3. Find out total head circumference by joining points F_p, T_3, 'O', T_4 and F_p (100%); follow 10% or 20% rule, locate points F_{p1}, F_7, T_3, T_5, O_1, O_2, T_6, F_8 and F_{p2}.
4. Join F_{p1} and O_1 through C_3 (100%); F_3 point is midway between F_{p1} and C_3. Similarly, P_3 point is midway between O_1 and C_3.
5. Join F_{p2} and O_2 through C_4; F_4 point is midway between F_{p2} and C_4. Similarly, P_4 point is midway between O_2 and C_4.

Final placement of electrodes

F_P - F_{p1} - F_{p2}	: Frontal pole
F_3 - F_4	: Frontal
F_7 - F_8	: Inferior frontal
T_3 - T_4	: Mid-temporal
T_5 - T_6	: Posterior temporal
C_3 - C_4	: Central
P_3 - P_4	: Parietal
O_1 - O - O_2	: Occipital
A_1 - A_2	: Auricular (non-scalp leads, for indifferent electrodes)
Z	: Zero or midline zero reference
F_z	: Mid-frontal
C_z	: Mid-central
P_z	: Mid-parietal

Conventional recording

1. In a 16-channel recording select, 1-8 channel record for right side activity, and 9-16 channels for left side activity.
2. Right-sided activity is recorded above and left-sided activity is recorded below on the paper.

Montages for usual recording

(A) *Unipolar (referential) recording*

Montage I

Channel 1 : A_2F_{p2}
Channel 2 : A_2F_8
Channel 3 : A_2T_4
Channel 4 : A_2T_6
Channel 5 : A_2O_2
Channel 6 : A_2F_4
Channel 7 : A_2C_4
Channel 8 : A_2P_4
(Right-side activity)

Montage II

Channel 9 : A_1F_{p1}
Channel 10 : A_1F_7
Channel 11 : A_1T_3
Channel 12 : A_1T_5
Channel 13 : A_1O_1
Channel 14 : A_1F_3
Channel 15 : A_1C_3
Channel 16 : A_1P_3
(Left-side activity)

(B) *Bipolar recording*

Montage I

Channel 1 : $F_{p2}F_4$
Channel 2 : F_4C_4
Channel 3 : C_4P_4
Channel 4 : P_4O_2
Channel 5 : $F_{p2}F_8$
Channel 6 : F_8T_4
Channel 7 : T_4T_6
Channel 8 : T_6O_2
(Right-side activity)

Montage II

Channel 9 : $F_{p1}F_3$
Channel 10 : F_3C_3
Channel 11 : C_3P_3
Channel 12 : P_3O_1
Channel 13 : $F_{p1}F_7$
Channel 14 : F_7T_3
Channel 15 : T_3T_5
Channel 16 : T_5O_1
(Left-side activity)

IMPORTANT VIVA-VOCE QUESTIONS

Q.1. *Give the characteristic features of EEG waves.*
Ans. Page 281.
Q.2. *What is α-block or alerting response?*
Ans. Page 282.
Q.3. *What is the source of EEG?*
Ans. Page 281.
Q.4. *What do you understand by the term desynchronization of EEG waves?*
Ans. Page 282.
Q.5. *Give the conventional speeds and amplifications used for recording EEG.*
Ans. Page 282.
Q.6. *What change is produced in EEG record when a relaxed individual closes his eyes?*
Ans. Page 282.
Q.7. *What is the effect of hyperventilation in EEG in a normal person?*
Ans. Page 282.
Q.8. *Give the clinical application of EEG.*
Ans. Page 282.
Q.9. *Give the characteristic EEG pattern in petit mal epilepsy.*
Ans. EEG shows 3 per sec doublets, each consisting of a typical spike and rounded waves.
Q.10. *What are sleep spindles?*
Ans. Sleep spindles are characteristic features of true sleep. Here EEG shows the bursts of regular waves, frequency 14-15 Hz and 50 μV amplitude of a few seconds' duration.

STUDY NOTES

RESULTS AND DISCUSSION

....

....

....

....

....

....

....

....

....

....

Date: ....

25 Autonomic Nervous System (*ANS*) Testing

I. INTRODUCTION

1. The innervation of all tissues other than skeletal muscle is by way of **Autonomic Nervous System (ANS).** It regulates the activity of smooth muscles like heart, glands of GIT, sweat glands, adrenal gland and of certain endocrine organs (Fig. 3.25.1).
2. Its main aim is to maintain the optimal internal environment (*homeostasis*) of a body. It governs the body functions which are normally carried out without conscious control. This is why ANS is also called ***vegetative*** (concerned with growth) or ***Efferent visceral*** or ***Involuntary nervous system.***
3. The ANS is divided into two divisions: **Sympathetic** and **Parasympathetic**. Functionally, the two divisions of the ANS are essentially antagonistic (Table 3.25.1) and mutual interaction between the two tends to maintain the homeostasis in the dynamics of the body.
4. The individual with the disturbances of the ANS shows complex clinical abnormalities. The diagnosis of ***autonomic neuropathy*** is often difficult to establish, since clinical symptoms generally appear late in the course of the disease and may be non-specific.
5. In **progressive autonomic failure**, there is the degeneration of both preganglionic and post-ganglionic neurons, leading to inability to maintain

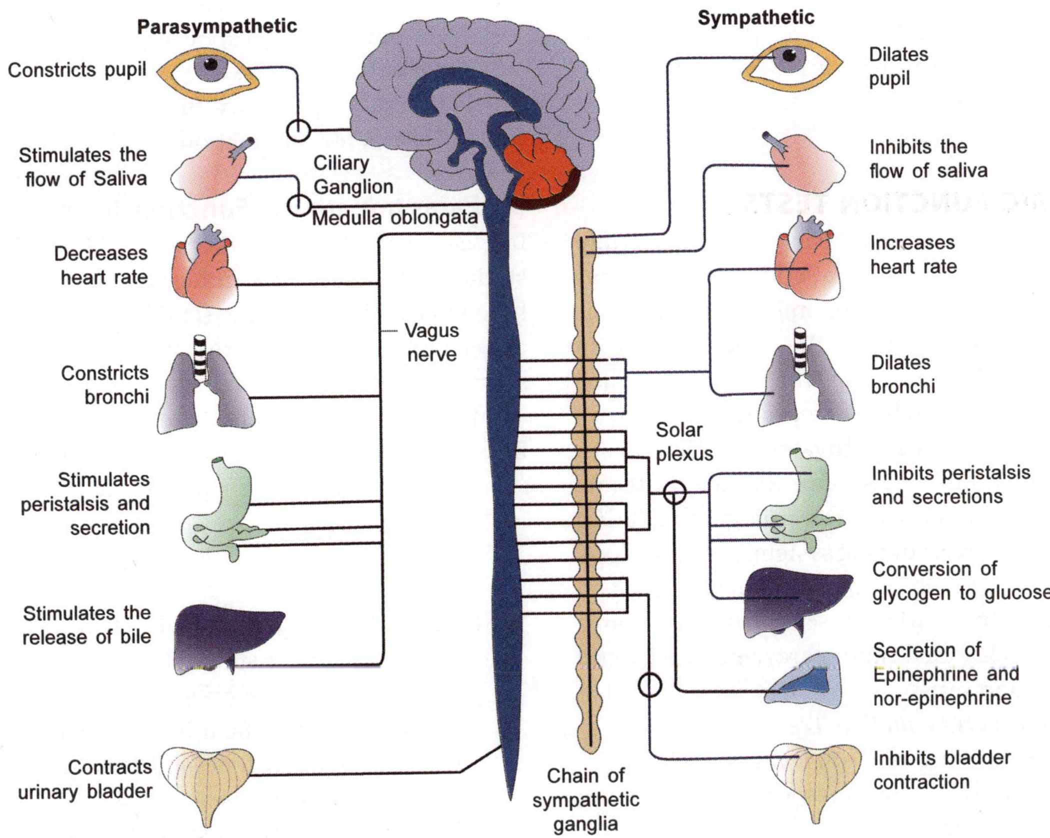

Fig. 3.25.1 Distribution of two divisions of ANS

Table 3.25.1 Functional Differences between two divisions of the ANS

Sympathetic activity	Parasympathetic activity
1. It is essentially designed to prepare the individual to cope with the emergency (*Fight or flight reactions*). For example its stimulation causes:	1. It is concerned with the vegetative aspect of day-to-day living, *i.e.* conservation and restoration of bodily resources. Its stimulation produces:
(i) relaxes accommodation and dilates the pupil (letting more light into the eyes)	(i) increases the activity of intestinal musculature and gastric secretion; and relaxes pyloric sphincters (favours digestion and absorption of food).
(ii) increases heart rate and blood pressure (providing better perfusion to vital organs and muscles).	(ii) Favours the storage of absorbed nutrients.
(iii) constricts skin blood vessels (limits bleeding from wounds).	(iii) Inhibits the heart activity.
(iv) decreases threshold in reticular formation (reinforcing alert states)	(iv) Constricts the pupil (protects the retina).
(v) increases blood glucose and FFA levels (supplying more energy)	(v) Dilates sexual erectile tissues.
(vi) skin moistened with sweat (helps in the regulation of body temperature).	
2. This division of ANS is also known as *Catabolic Nervous System.*	2. This division of ANS is also referred as *Anabolic Nervous System.*

the blood pressure in the erect position (*orthostatic or postural hypotension*), constipation, incontinence of urine, impotence, paralysis of accommodation, pupillary areflexia, disturbances of sweating and loss of lacrimation.

6. Some of the common causes of autonomic neuropathy are:
   (i) diabetic neuropathy, where post ganglionic fibres of both divisions of ANS get involved.
   (ii) uremic neuropathy
   (iii) alcoholic neuropathy

II. AUTONOMIC FUNCTION TESTS

The assessment of autonomic functions is an important part of the evaluation of peripheral and central nervous system. The diagnosis of autonomic neuropathy is indirect, often being based on the measurement of physiological variables (reflexes) which are controlled by ANS. These tests are reliable, reproducible, simple, quick to carry out and all **non-invasive.** In these tests, emphasis is placed on the measurement of the heart rate from a continuously running electrocardiographic (ECG) record (page 163) and recording of systemic arterial blood pressure (page 151). Some of the commonly employed clinical tests for the early detection of autonomic dysfunctions are classified into parasympathetic and sympathetic function tests.

(A) ***Parasympathetic Function Tests***
1. Standing to lying ratio (S/L ratio)
2. Immediate heart rate response to standing (30:15 R-R ratio)
3. Valsalva ratio
4. Tachycardia ratio; and
5. Heart rate variation with respiration: Sinus Arrhythmia.

(B) ***Sympathetic Function Tests***
1. QT/QS_2 ratio
2. Sympathetic skin response (SSR)
3. Hand Grip Test (HGT): Blood pressure response to isometric exercise
4. Cold Pressor response (CPR)

(C) ***Miscellaneous Tests***
1. Tests of pupillary functions
2. Tests for lacrimation

(A) Parasympathetic Function Tests

In general, blood pressure (B.P.) changes are studied to assess the integrity of the sympathetic functions and heart rate (H.R.) changes for those of parasympathetic functions. B.P. is recorded using standard sphygmomanometer (page 151); beat to beat H.R. can be measured from a continuous running ECG record (preferably lead II) and is calculated as:

Heart rate = 1 × 60/R-R interval
(per minute) (in sec.)

1. Standing to lying ratio: S/L Ratio

(i) Normally, when a subject lies down from a standing position, there is a brief initial rise followed by a fall in heart rate. The initial rise is due to the rapid decrease of vagal tone and later fall is because of increase in vagal tone.

(ii) This is seen in normal subjects and is more marked in young individuals. It is maximal at the 3rd or 4th beat after lying down and is followed by a decrease in heart rate beyond the resting level to reach a plateau around beats 25–30.

(iii) *Procedure*

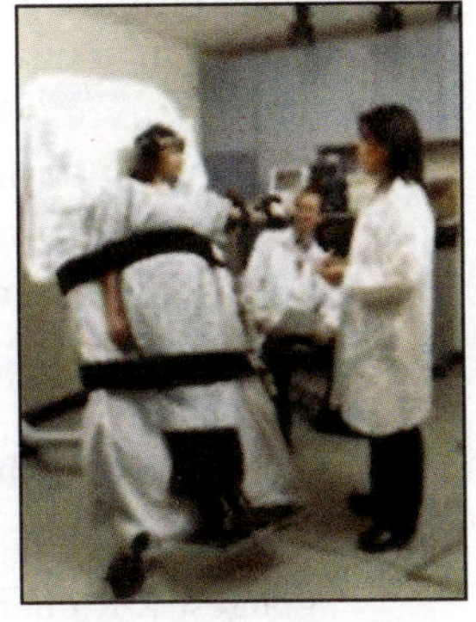

(a) Explain the test procedure to the subject and give a few trials to make him familiar with the test.

(b) Using cardic jelly apply limb leads for ECG reading, adjust lead selector knob to record activity in lead II (details page 165).

(c) Ask the subject to stand quietly and then lie down without any support.

(d) A continuous E.C.G. is recorded from 20 beats before and 60 beats after lying down. Mark the point at which the subject begin to lie down.

(e) Repeat the procedure three times with a gap of 5 minutes in between.

(iv) *Calculation of S/L ratio:* The longest R-R interval during the 5 beats before lying down to the shortest R-R interval during 10 beats after lying down is taken into the consideration.

$$\textit{S/L ratio} = \frac{\text{Longest R-R interval during 5 beats before lying down}}{\text{Shortest R-R interval during 10 beats after lying down}}$$

(v) The maximum ratio of three trials is taken; any abnormally low S/L ratio reflects parasympathetic damage.

2. Immediate heart rate response to standing: (30:15 R-R Ratio)

(i) Changing from lying to standing position produces an integrated response of CVS which includes alteration in HR and BP.

(ii) Upon standing, due to gravitational changes, the peripheral pooling of blood in dependent parts → decrease in venous return and cardiac output → fall in systolic BP upto 20mmHg → inhibit baroreceptor activity resulting in increased sympathetic tone and decreased parasympathetic tone. This produces reflex tachycardia and peripheral vasoconstriction. Thus HR increases immediately upon standing and continues to rise for the next 10–15 beats; thereafter it slows to a maximum extent at the 30th beat.

(iii) ***30:15 R-R ratio*** is the longest R-R interval (slowest HR) occurring about 30 beats after standing divided by the shortest R-R interval (fastest HR) which occurs about 15 beats after standing.

(iv) 30:15 R-R ratio is considered a measure of cardiac vagal function. It is more than 1.04 in normal subjects and less than 1.0 when there is autonomic disturbance.

(v) *Procedure*

(a) Ask the subject to lie supine quietly on a couch for 15 minutes with sphygmomanometer and E.C.G. leads attached.

(b) Record the resting ECG (lead II) and measure the baseline HR; also measure the resting BP.

(c) The subject is then asked to stand and remain motionless; a continuous ECG is recorded for 1–3 minutes. Mark a point on E.C.G. record to identify the time of standing. Also, measure the BP, 1 and 3 minutes after standing.

(d) Note the HR at the 15th and 30th beats after standing.

(e) Calculate the 30:15 R-R ratio and compare with the normal value.

(vi) *Clinical significance*

(a) The diagnosis of *orthostatic (postural) tachycardia* is based on normal (or minimally decreased BP) but sustained increase in HR of 25bpm upon standing.

(b) In *postural hypotension* (individual with autonomic dysfunction), the systolic and diastolic BP falls more than 20mmHg and 10mmHg respectively on assuming erect posture.

(c) In *vasovagal syncope,* hypotension is accompanied by paradoxical bradycardia because autonomic reflexes are overactive as opposed to autonomic failure.

Important Note: The similar responses are obtained by ***"Head-up tilt-table testing"*** in which a subject after a standard period of supine rest is positioned at an inclination of 80° from the horizontal on a tilt table and monitored for a period of 3–5 minutes.

3. Valsalva Ratio

(i) Valsalva manoeuvre (*i.e.* forced expiration against resistance) is a simple test done to assess baroreceptor integrity. Changes in the intra arterial BP have been used previously to assess the response to the valsalva manoeuvre. However, heart rate changes have also been shown to be reliable and have the advantage of being non-invasive.

(ii) ***Valsalva manoeuvre*** has 4 phases (Fig. 3.25.2)

(a) *Phase I* occurs at the onset of strain. There is transient rise in BP (without any change in HR) due to an increased intrathoracic pressure.

(b) *Phase II* occurs during straining. Initially venous return decreases resulting in fall in cardiac output and BP. This inhibits the baroreceptors producing tachycardia and peripheral vasoconstriction. As a result, BP returns towards normal. The HR increases steadily throughout the phase due to vagal withdrawl initially and increased sympathetic activity in the later stage.

(c) *Phase III* occurs following the release of strain which results in the transient decrease of BP without any change in HR. This is due to intrathoracic pressure returning to normal causing the displacement of blood to pulmonary vascular bed.

(d) *Phase IV* occurs with further cessation of strain. The BP slowly rises to reach above baseline level secondary to peripheral vasoconstriction, called *overshoot phenomenon.* This stimulates the baroreceptors producing bradycardia and drop in BP to normal levels.

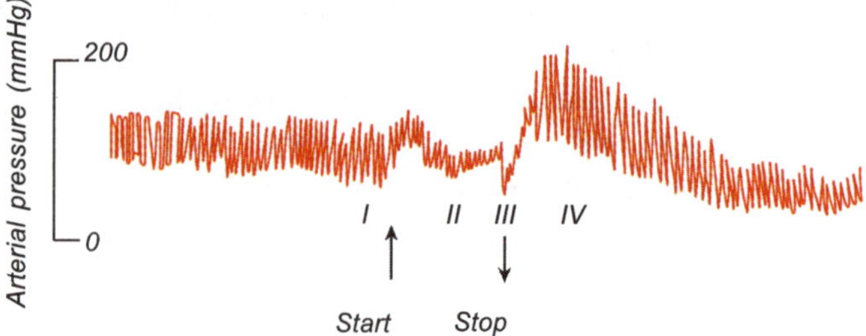

Fig. 3.25.2 Response to Valsalva manoeuvre in a normal subject. Tachycardia and peripheral vasoconstriction occurs during straining (phase II) followed by an overshoot in BP and bradycardia durig release (phase IV)

(iii) *Procedure*

(a) Explain the procedure to the subject to get maximum cooperation.

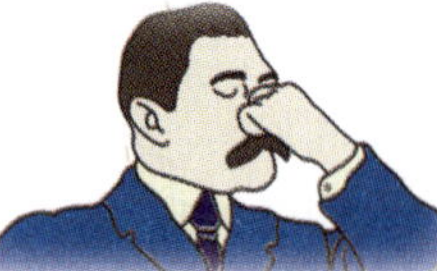

(b) The subject is made to sit comfortably in a stool with sphygmomanometer and ECG leads attached; nose is clipped with the help of a nose-clip and insert a mouth piece between the teeth and lips. Allow him to relax.

(c) Measure baseline HR and BP.

(d) Connect the other end of the mouthpiece to a mercury manometer.

(e) Ask the subject to strain by blowing against closed glottis into the mouthpiece attached to the manometer and maintaining a pressure of 40mmHg for 15 sec.

(f) A continuous ECG is recorded: 1 minute before the manoeuvre (*resting period*); during the manoeuvre (*strain period,* 15sec) and 45 seconds following strain release.

(g) Repeat the procedure three times with a gap of 5 minutes between the manoeuvre.

(iv) ***Valsalva ratio*** is taken as ratio of maximum HR during the strain (phase II) to the minimum HR after the strain (phase IV). Alternatively, it can also be calculated as:

$$= \frac{\text{Longest R-R interval after the strain (Phase IV)}}{\text{Shortest R-R interval during the strain (Phase II)}}$$

(v) The maximum valsalva ratio of three trials is taken for the autonomic activity. A ratio of greater than 1.45 is normal; 1.20 to 1.45 is borderline; and less than 1.20 is abnormal (autonomic disturbances).

(vi) *Clinical significance:* Failure of HR to increase during strain suggests a sympathetic dysfunction and failure of HR to slow during BP overshoot suggests a parasympathetic disturbance.

4. Tachycardia Ratio

(i) It is closely related to valsalva ratio and is defined as a ratio of shortest R-R interval during the valsalva manoeuvre to the longest R-R interval at rest.

(ii) It shows less variation when an individual repeats the valsalva manoeuvre as compared to valsalva ratio. Therefore, if appears to be a better index of the functioning of parasympathetic autonomic activity.

5. Heart Rate Variation with Respiration: Sinus Arrhythmia

(i) The variation of HR with respiration is called *Sinus Arrhythmia.* Inspiration increases the HR whereas expiration decreases it; this phenomenon is primarily mediated by the vagal innervation of heart, thus indicated for testing the integrity of parasympathetic functions.

(ii) *Procedure*

(a) Ask the subject to lie supine quietly on a couch with sphygmomanometer and ECG leads attached.

(b) Record the resting ECG and measure the baseline HR.

(c) Ask the subject to breathe deeply at a rate of 6 breaths per minute, allowing 5 seconds each of inspiration and expiraton.

(d) Determine the maximum and minimum HR with each respiratory cycle and mean variation.

(e) Determine the expiratory (E) to inspiratory (I) ratio as the sum of 6 longest R-R intervals, each of 6 repetitions divided by the sum of 6 shortest R-R intervals.

(f) Normal values 6 breaths/minute deep breathing expressed as average maximum to minimum variation in beats/min. is more than 18 beats/min; with autonomic disturbances the HR slows less than 10 beats/min.

(B) Sympathetic Function Tests

1. QT/QS_2 Ratio

(i) It represents a reliable index of sympathetic discharge to the heart.

(ii) QT interval is measured from the earliest point of QRS deflection to the end of T-wave.

(iii) QS_2, *i.e.* the total electromechanical systolic interval is measured from the onset of QRS complex in the ECG (ventricular depolarization) to the first major vibration of aortic component of the second heart round in phonocardiogram.

(iv) High value of QT/QS_2 ratio is indicative of greater sympathetic tone while lower values indicates reduction in sympathetic tone.

(v) *Procedure*

(a) Ask the subject to lie supine quietly on a couch with ECG lead and phonocardiograph attached.

(b) *Phonocardiogram* is recorded by placing the contact microphone over the external carotid artery on either side and precaution is taken to avoid any movement during the procedure; the speed of the paper is kept at 50mm/sec.

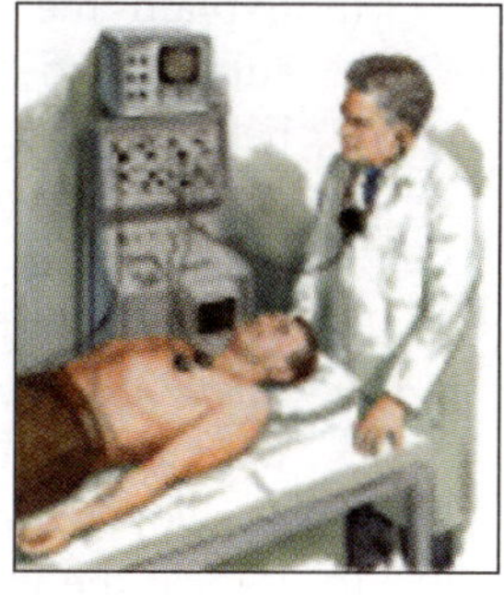

(c) Record the ECG and phonocardiogram simultaneously.

(d) Determine QT interval and QS_2 from the record and calculate the QT/QS_2 ratio; compare with the normal.

2. Sympathetic Skin Response (SSR)

(i) Sweat glands are distributed over the whole body surface. Their activity is controlled by sympathetic nervous system via post ganglionic cholinergic fibres. They are concerned with temperature regulation except those of palms and soles.

(ii) The activity of these glands can be measured electrically by passing an electric current between an electrode placed on the surface of skin and subcutaneous tissue and measuring the electrical resistance.

(iii) The stratum corneum of skin offers the greatest resistance to the passage of electricity, but is perforated by the ducts of sweat glands. The activation of sweat glands causes the duct to fill with sweat containing electrolytes thus creating conduction pathways for the passage of electric current and measurable drop in skin resistance.

(iv) Changes in skin potential in response to stimuli provoking sympathetic activity is known as ***sympathetic skin response (SSR).***

(v) The response has been measured in various conditions and is useful in studying the integrity of peripheral sympathetic cholinergic function. *The greater the sympathetic nervous system activity, the lower is the electrical resistance.*

(vi) Lack of changes in skin potential in response to stimuli provoking sympathetic activity may thus serve as an index of sympathetic insufficiency.

(vii) *Procedure*

SSR can be recorded on most EMG machines using C.R.O. as a voltage change between an indifferent area and the area of the skin under consideration. (Page 147)

(a) *Equipment set-up*

- Set pre-amplifier to GSR-AC
- Filter: low frequency at 0.1 or 0.5Hz
  high frequency at 500 to 1000Hz.
- Gain: 0.5 mV/division
- Sweep speed: 500msec/division.

(b) *Electrode placement*

- After cleaning the skin, the *active electrodes* are placed on the palm or sole and the *reference electrode* over the dorsum of the respective body part with the help of electrode paste or conducting jelly. *Ground electrode* is placed (preferably) between the recording and stimulating electrodes. (Fig. 3.25.3A)
- Connect the electrodes through pre-amplifier to EMG machine.

(c) A constant current of 5 micro-ampere is passed through the electrodes; obtain the record and calculate the latency and amplitude of response.

(d) The level of skin resistance in millivolts is calculated from the recording pen deflection. (The deflection resulting from 1mV to the amplifier is equal to a resistance change to 10 kilo-ohm).

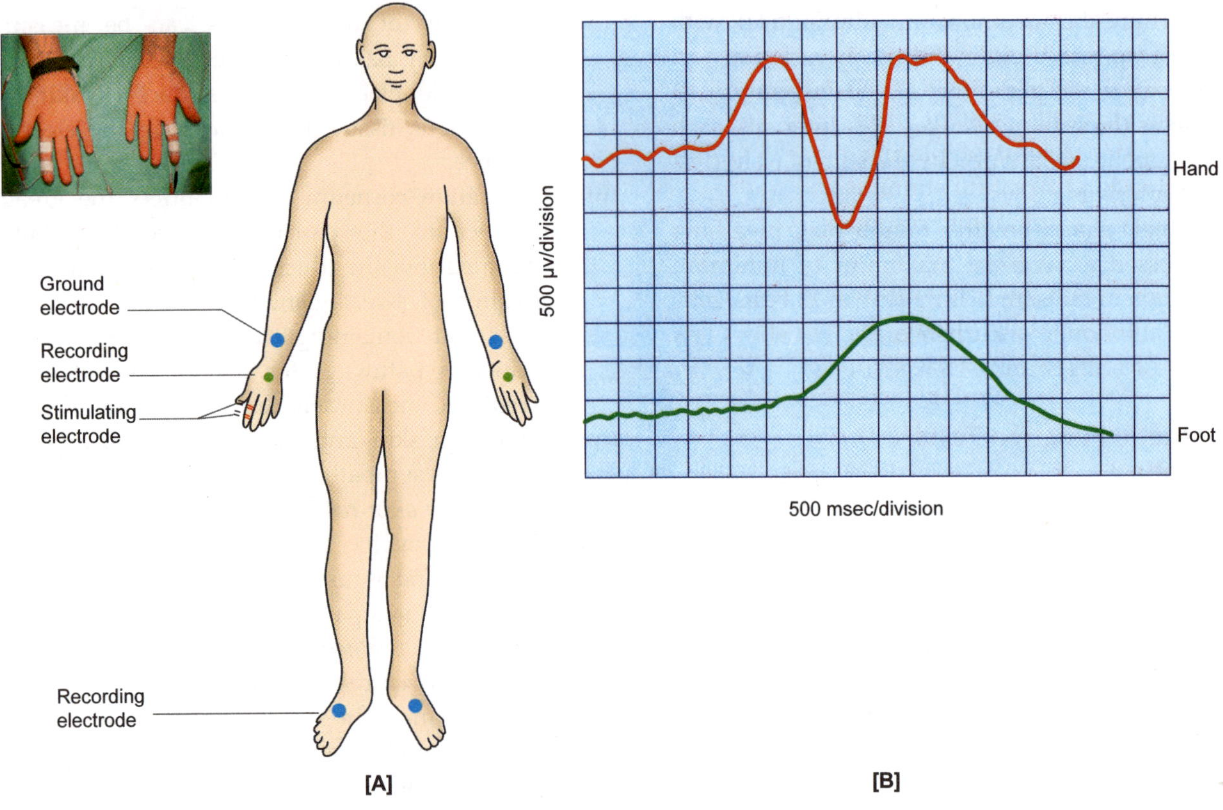

Fig. 3.25.3 (A) Electrode placement and (B) Sympathetic skin response

(viii) The SSR is mono, di or triphasic and varies from stimulus to stimulus. SSR Potentials are symmetric in homologous body regions and these have a higher amplitude (1.1–1.5mV) and a shorter latency (1.5–1.7sec) in hands compared to feet (0.7–0.9mV and 2.0–2.2sec.). (Fig. 3.25.3B)

Note: Skin cooling results in the prolongation of latency and reduction in amplitude.

(ix) *Clinical Significance:* Abnormal SSR is commonly seen in progressive autonomic dysfunction (page 285).

3. HandGrip Test (HGT): Blood pressure response to isometric exercise

(i) Isometric exercise produces a significant rise in BP and HR, a response which can easily be elicited by using sustained handgrip. The response is reflex in nature and is due to increased peripheral resistance and increased cardiac output.

(ii) The BP rises by peripheral vasoconstriction mediated by the α-adrenergic receptors of ANS. Therefore, any damage to the neurological pathways involved could lead to a diminished or an absent cardiovascular response to sustained handgrip.

(iii) The value of more than 15 mmHg rise in diastolic BP is taken as normal response; 11–15 mmHg as borderline; and 10 mmHg or less is abnormal, an indicator of sympathetic insufficiency.

(iv) *Procedure*

(a) Explain the details of test procedure to the subject and record the baseline BP with the help of sphygmomanometer.

(b) Ask the subject to hold the dynamometer (page 144) in right hand (or dominant hand) to have a full grip of it.

(c) Then instruct him to compress the hands with maximum effort. Measure the tension developed; wait for 1 minute.

(d) Repeat the whole procedure twice and take the 2nd and 3rd reading.

(e) Take mean (or highest) of three readings; this is referred as ***maximal isometric tension*** (T_{max}).

(f) Now ask the subject to maintain a pressure of 30% of T_{max} for 5 minutes.

(g) During the test procedure, record the BP every 30 seconds with the help of sphygmomanometer on the non-exercising arm.

(h) The rise in diastolic BP at the point just before the release of handgrip is taken as the index of response to handgrip test.

4. Cold Pressor Response (CPR)

(i) Under the conditions of stress of either physical or psychological origin, there is an activation of sympathetic nervous system. The cold pressor response, which consist of placing the hand into cold water, acts as a painful stimulus and has been used to study the autonomic response of different individuals.

(ii) The *afferent* fibres for this response are the pain fibres which are stimulated by placing the hand in cold water and the *efferent* fibres are sympathetic fibres.

(iii) The response of 15–20mmHg increase in systolic BP and diastolic BP by 10mmHg is considered as normal response to cold pressor test.

(iv) *Procedure:* The test is done as one of the last tests because of its slight unpleasantness (Fig. 3.25.4).

(a) Explain the nature of test to the subject and reassure that the test would not do any harm to him.

(b) Make the subject to sit comfortably in a chair and record the baseline BP.

(c) Ask the subject to immerse his hand in cold water maintained at 4–6°C; record the BP from the other arm at 30 sec intervals for a period of 2 minutes. After 2 minutes, the subject is allowed to remove the hand.

(d) Determine maximum increase in systolic and diastolic BP and compare with normal.

In any condition where there is deficient sympathetic outflow, the cold pressor test will be expected to show a smaller rise in BP.

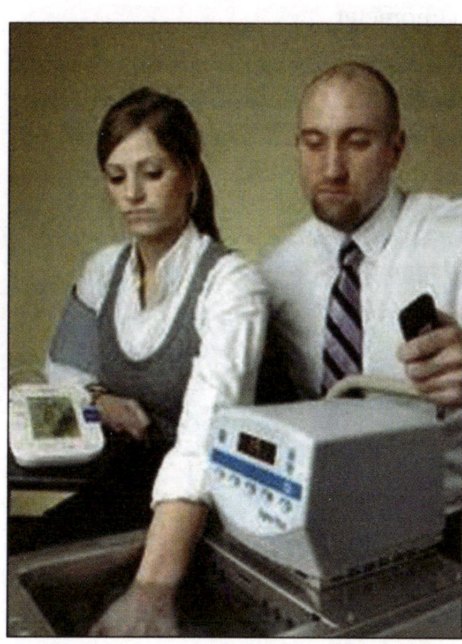

Fig. 3.25.4 Cold pressor response test

Note: The test lacks sensitivity because many normal subjects do not have a significant rise of BP on cold immersion.

(C) Miscellaneous Tests

1. Tests for pupillary functions

Sympathetic activity causes pupillary dilatation whereas parasympathetic activity causes pupillary constriction, accommodation, lacrimation and salivation.

Procedure: The topical application of pharmacological agonist is useful in establishing pupillary denervation. The basis is the phenomenon of **denervation hypersensitivity** in which an effector organ 2-3 week after the denervation becomes hypersensitive to a neurotransmitter.

(i) A dilute amount (pilocarpine 0.125%) causes minimal constriction but in the presence of parasympathetic denervation there is denervation hypersensitivity and pupil constricts.

(ii) Similarly, epinephrine in low concentration (0.1% solution, 3 drops instilled 3 times at 1 minute interval) normally produces minimal dilatation but in presence of sympathetic denervation, the pupil dilates. The size of pupil is checked at 15, 30 and 45 minutes.

2. Test for Lacrimation: Schirmer's Test

The wick end of 0.5cm wide and 25mm long thin filter paper strip is placed between the lower lid and sclera while the other end hangs over the edge of the lower lid. The length of wetting is measured at the end of 5 minutes. In normal persons, filter paper wets to an extent of 15mm. Less than 10 mm suggests parasympathetic insufficiency (Also, refer to page 249).

IMPORTANT VIVA-VOCE QUESTIONS

Q.1. *What do you understand by the term autonomic nervous system (ANS)?*

Ans. Page 285.

Q.2. *Give functional differences between the two divisions of the ANS.*

Ans. Page 286.

Q.3. *Define the anabolic and catabolic nervous system.*

Ans. Page 286.

Q.4. *Enumerate clinical symptoms due to autonomic insufficiency.*

Ans. Page 286.

Q.5. *Name the common causes of autonomic neuropathy.*

Ans. Page 286.

Q.6. *Name the test employed to assess parasympathetic and sympathetic function tests.*

Ans. Page 286.

Q.7. *What is the basis of clinical tests in assessing autonomic dysfunction?*
Ans. Page 286.
Q.8. *What is S/L ratio? How can it be determined?*
Ans. Page 286.
Q.9. *Describe the immediate cardiovascular responses to standing.*
Ans. Page 287.
Q.10. *Give the clinical significance of 30:15 R-R ratio.*
Ans. Page 287.
Q.11. *How is 'head-up tilt-table test' carried out?*
Ans. Page 287.
Q.12. *What is valsalva manoeuvre? What changes do it produce on CVS?*
Ans. Page 288.
Q.13. *How is valsalva ratio determined? Give its clinical significance.*
Ans. Page 288.
Q.14. *If heart rate fails to increase during Valsalva's manoeuvre, what does it signify?*
Ans. Page 288.
Q.15. *Define sinus arrhythmia.*
Ans. Page 288.
Q.16. *What tests would you like to perform to test the integrity of parasympathetic function?*
Ans. Handgrip test is simple, quick to carry out and reproducible.
Q.17. *What are the tests performed to assess the sympathetic nervous system functioning? Which is the most simple, reliable and reproducible?*
Ans. Page 289.
Q.18. *How is QT/QS_2 ratio determined?*
Ans. Page 289.
Q.19. *Define sympathetic skin response (SSR). How is it related with sympathetic nervous system?*
Ans. Page 289.
Q.20. *What is the effect of temperature on SSR?*
Ans. Page 289.
Q.21. *Give the common causes of progressive autonomic dysfunction.*
Ans. Pages 285 and 290.
Q.22. *Define isometric exercise. What is its effect on HR and BP?*
Ans. During isometric exercise, the muscle contracts isometrically, *i.e.*, muscle length remaining the same and tension in it develops gradually. During such exercise, a significant rise in BP and HR occurs.
Q.23. *What is maximal isometric tension (T_{max})?*
Ans. Tension that develops in a muscle during the performance of maximal isometric contraction is called T_{max}.
Q.24. *Define endurance time.*
Ans. This is the time of the onset of fatigue while performing isometric exercise on a handgrip dynamometer.
Q.25. *Describe 'hand grip test'.*
Ans. Page 290.
Q.26. *Describe briefly cold pressor response and give its significance.*
Ans. Page 290.
Q.27. *What test will you perform for lacrimation function?*
Ans. Page 291.

STUDY NOTES

RESULTS AND DISCUSSION

....

....

....

....

....

....

....

....

....

Date: ....

26 Neuro-Electro Diagnostic Techniques

I. GENERAL

1. Clinical neurophysiology has come a long way in the last 50 years and is being increasingly used in the diagnosis of various neurological disorders. The ***electrodiagnostic techniques*** involve recording, display, measurement and interpretation of action potentials arising from CNS (**Evoked potentials**), peripheral nerves (**Nerve conduction studies**) and muscles (**Electromyography**). Evoked potential includes:
   (i) *Visual Evoked Potential (VEP)*
   (ii) *Brain Stem Auditory Evoked Potential (BAEP)*
   (iii) *Somato Sensory Evoked Potential (SSEP),* and
   (iv) *Motor Evoked Potential (MEP)*

   The major components of a typical equipment used to carry out such studies are shown in the Fig. 3.26.1.
2. A constant (or steady) potential difference is observed between the inside and the outside of the normal cell at rest, called *Resting Membrane Potential.* It is due to the uniform distribution of positively charged ions outside and negatively charged ions inside the cell membrane. During the extracellular (surface) recording of action potential, *i.e.* when both the eletrodes are placed on the cell surface, the potential difference between two electrodes is zero at rest. However, during depolarization, potential difference between two electrodes occurs due to the movement of Na^+ and K^+ which is responsible for current flow along the cell membrane.

Note: The current flow is resisted by intervening tissue, called ***impedence.***

3. **Some Definitions**
   (i) The term ***voltage*** represents the difference of voltage between two points, which can be *positive* or *negative.*
   (ii) The action potentials ***amplitude*** is expressed in millivolt (mV) or microvolt (μV), ***current*** in milli ampere (mA), and ***impedence*** in kilo ohms or mega ohms.

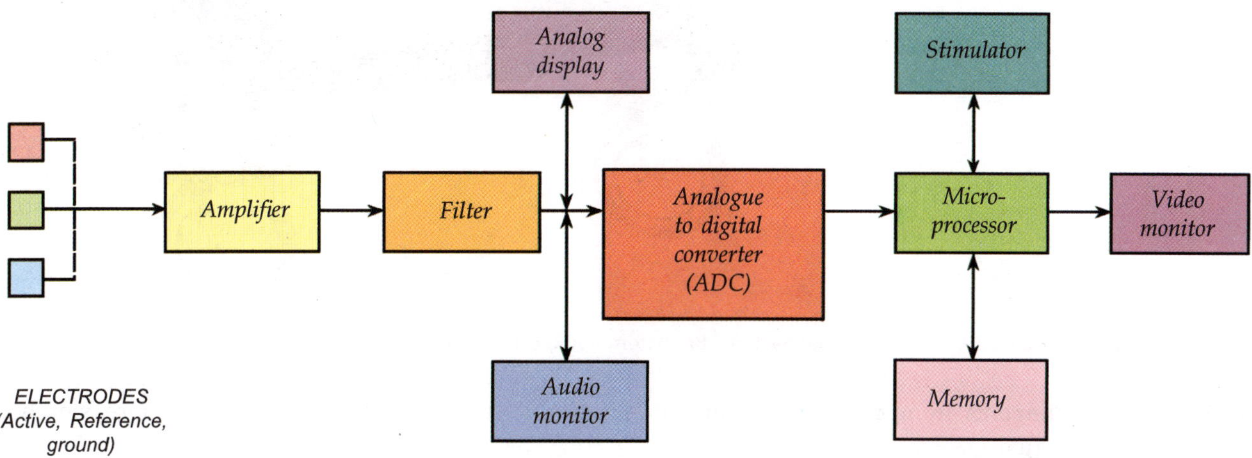

Fig. 3.26.1 Components of electrodiagnostic equipment

Note: *For the proper conduction and interpretation of electro-diagnostic studies, knowledge about the generation of action potential and factors affecting it is essential.*

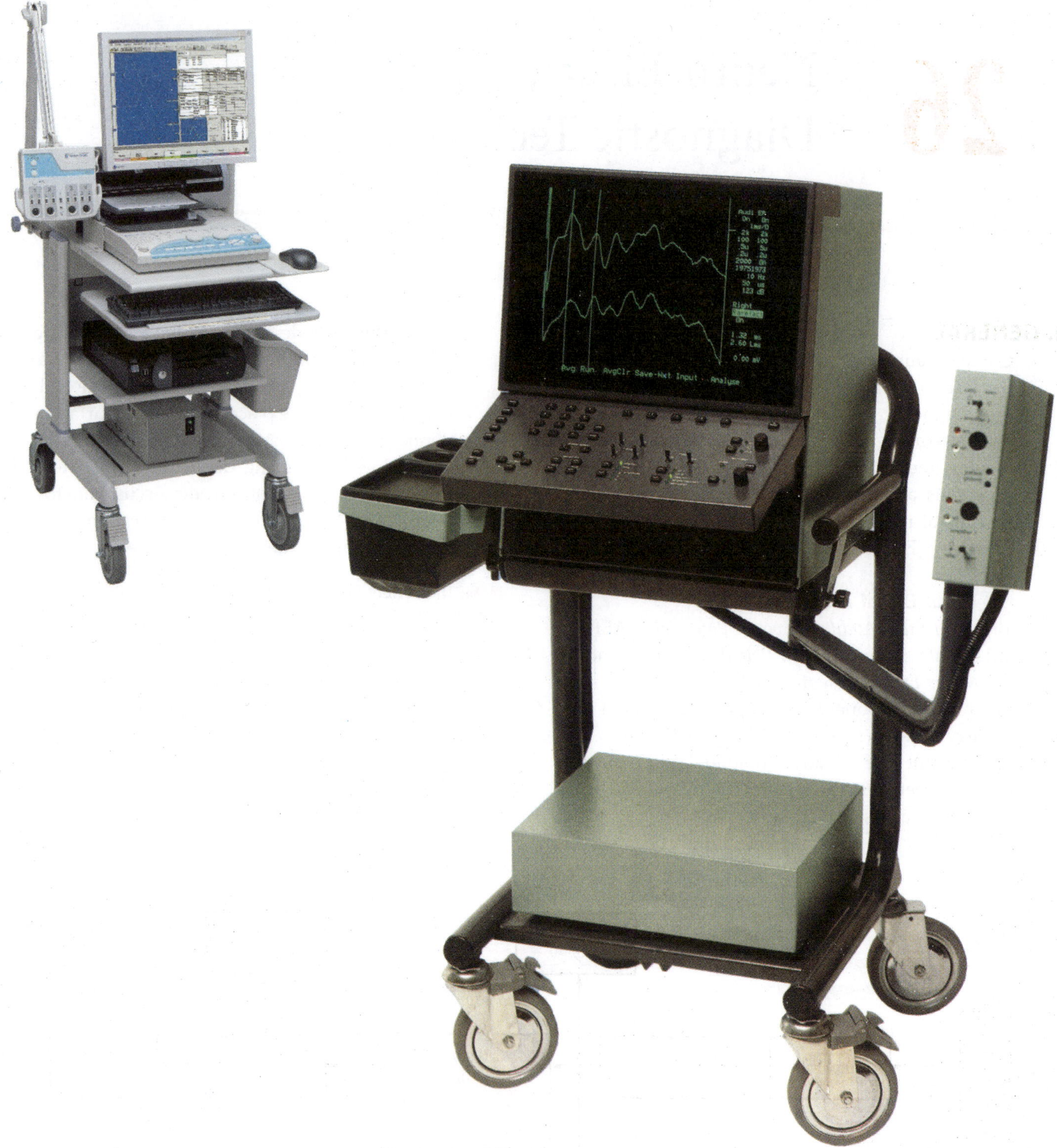

Fig. 3.26.1 (A) Computer Based Evoked Potential System (Brainstem evoked potential testing recorded)

(iii) Time measurements are in milli second (ms) or microsecond (μs).

(iv) The action potentials originating from body cells are displayed against time, called ***wave form***, in which the amplitude varies with time.

(a) Some segments change rapidly (*high frequency*); and

(b) Some segments change more slowly (*low frequency*).

Note: The ***compound muscle action potential (CMAP)*** contains mainly low-frequency components (below 1000 Hz) whereas ***sensory nerve action potential (SNAP)*** contains higher frequencies.

II. APPARATUS: *COMPONENTS OF ELECTRODIAGNOSTIC EQUIPMENT*

1. Electrodes

(i) There are *three* types of electrodes: *active*, *reference* and *ground*. The action potential is measured between active and reference electrode whereas the ground electrode serves as a '*zero*' voltage reference point.

(ii) They are made up of platinum, stainless steel, silver chloride, chromium, nickel, silver and gold. Silver or gold electrodes have the advantage of stable ***electrode polarization potentials*** (page 296) which result in noise-free recording.

(iii) In clinical practice, two varieties of electrodes are used: *surface* and *needle electrodes*. In general, surface electrode is preferred, as using the needle electrodes have a greater chance of infection.

(a) The ***surface electrodes*** are in the form of disc, cup or ring, and are used in nerve conduction and motor evoked potential recording. These electrodes are placed in position with the help of *electrode paste* or *jelly*, which is gently rubbed on the skin and then applied for proper contact.

(b) ***Needle electrode*** is commonly used for EMG study. They consist of *teflon* coated stainless steel wire which tapers to a sharp tip.

2. Amplifier

A variable degree of amplification, up to 5×10^5 folds is needed before being displayed because of the following reasons:

(i) Biological signals are very small.

(ii) Intrinsic impedence of the electrode. It varies with frequency and electrode type used. The *concentric needles* have a higher impedence.

(iii) Impedence of electrode-skin

> **Note:** Impedence results in the drop of the amplitude of action potential; amplification minimises waveform distortion and improves noise rejection.

3. Filter

It is a device that relatively allows a particular range of frequency from a signal. It is required for eliminating the noise and useful for bringing out the characteristics of the waveforms, *i.e.* optimising the recording.

(i) ***The low-frequency filters*** remove the slowly changing low-frequency (up to 100Hz) components and allow the higher frequencies to pass through. Therefore, it is also called as *high pass filter*.

(ii) ***The high-frequency filters*** remove the rapidly changing high-frequency components and allow the low frequency (up to 100Hz) to pass through; therefore, it is also called *low pass filters*.

> **Note:** The length of time during which a rapid change in potential occurs from a baseline value is called as ***rise time*** of a potential.

4. Averager

(i) It extracts very small signals which are hidden or buried in large *noise*; for example:

(a) Evoked potentials are burried in EEG noise; and

(b) Sensory nerve action potential (SNAP) in EMG noise

(ii) By averaging, the *time-locked* signals become prominent and are stored in the memory of the equipment, while the *noise* which is occurring randomly is cancelled out. Alternatively, the noise can be time-locked and can be rejected subsequently.

5. Display

Two methods of waveform display are in use:

(i) *Analogue oscilloscope display;* and

(ii) *Computer based digital video display*

(i) Analogue Oscilloscope Display

Here the action potential signals are directly displayed on cathode ray oscilloscope following amplification and filtering. It can redisplay the waveform but certain details of waveform may be lost.

(ii) Computer Based Digital Video Display

Here an *analogue to digital converter (ADC)* and *digital processing technique* are used; therefore, the signals can be redisplayed with greater sensitivity without any loss of waveform accuracy.

6. Stimulator

It is required for nerve conduction and evoked potential studies. Two types of stimulator are in use: *Electrical* and *Magnetic.*

(i) ***Electrical stimulators:*** It is of two types:

(a) *Constant current stimulator:* It delivers a constant current to the subject over a wide range of stimulating electrode impedence. Thus it is more stable and useful in repetitive nerve stimulation and evoked potential studies.

(b) *Constant voltage stimulator:* It delivers a fixed voltage between anode and cathode.

(ii) ***Magnetic stimulators:*** They are used for the non-invasive stimulation of motor cortex, spinal cord and peripheral nerves.

Important Notes

(i) Low-intensity stimulation results in current flow mostly in superficial soft tissues. As the stimulus intensity increases, more current enters at the cathode therefore, the latency shortens, amplitude and duration of action potential increases.

(ii) *Stimulus artefact* is a large amplitude spike which decays exponentially with time. It is produced as a result of:
   (a) flow of current between active and reference electrodes.
   (b) imbalance of impedence between active and reference electrodes; and
   (c) Capatitive coupling between the stimulating and recording leads

7. Sensitivity (or Gain) and Sweep Speed

The latency and duration of an action potential is influenced by *sensitivity* (*i.e.* gain) and *sweep speed* (or time).

(i) On *high sensitivity*, there is the shortening of latency due to the visualisation of smaller deflection from the base line.

(ii) Increase in *sweep speed* results in the shortening of latency.

8. Signal Trigger

It is useful for isolating and displaying the action potentials for their quantitative analysis. It can be fixed and time-locked relative to the start of sweep.

9. Delay Time

It continuously samples and stores into the memory ongoing action potential activities. The action potential when exceeds the triggering values, it is extracted from the memory and displayed.

III. PRECAUTIONS

1. Ensure that the required voltage is available at the mains.
2. The instrument should be satisfactorily earthed.
3. The subject shoud be comfortable and should not wear any magnetic/metallic articles which might interfere with the electrical signals of low voltage.
4. Reassure and relax the subject by explaining the test procedure beforehand, which is to be carried out on him.
5. All procedures should be carried out in a quiet and comfortable room.
6. The skin is cleaned and prepared by commercially available cleansing jelly. The electrode paste is gently rubbed on the skin and then applied for optimal contact.
7. Ensure all electrodes are properly placed and are in firm/good contact with the body surface.
8. Adjust the stimulus intensity and duration as per requirements.

IMPORTANT VIVA-VOCE QUESTIONS

Q.1. *What do you understand by the term 'Electrodiagnostic techniques'?*
Ans. Page 293.

Q.2. *Define evoked potential.*
Ans. Page 293.

Q.3. *Draw a well-labelled diagram showing the major components of an electrodiagnostic equipment.*
Ans. Page 293.

Q.4. *What is tissue impedence? How does it affect the recording?*
Ans. Page 293.

Q.5. *What is wave form? Give its types with suitable examples.*
Ans. Page 294.

Q.6. *Enumerate the characteristic features of electrodes used in electrodiagnostic techniques.*
Ans. Page 295.

Q.7. *What is electrode polarization potential?*
Ans. A metal electrode when interacts with an electrolyte such as sweat, electrode paste or ECF, an electrochemical reaction occurs which results in an electrode polarization potential of 100–600 mV.

Q.8. *Why is it necessary to use amplifier and filter during recording?*
Ans. Page 295.

Q.9. *Differentiate between high and low pass filter.*
Ans. Page 295.

Q.10. *How can a very small signal hidden within the large noise be extracted?*
Ans. Page 295.

Q.11. *Describe briefly the methods of waveform display in common use.*
Ans. Page 295.

Q.12. *What is ADC?*
Ans. Page 295.

Q.13. *Give the advantages of magnetic stimulator over electrical stimulator.*
Ans. Page 295.

Q.14. *What is stimulus artifact? Give its significance.*
Ans. See above.

Q.15. *Define the terms: Gain; sweep time; signal trigger and delay time.*
Ans. See above.

Q.16. *List the precautions needed to be followed while the recording of any action potential.*
Ans. See above.

(A) Nerve Conduction Study

I. APPARATUS

Subject, stimulator, stimulating electrodes, recording/surface electrodes (silver chloride cup electrodes), pre-amplifier, cathode ray oscilloscope (CRO), electrode jelly/paste, ether or spirit (for cleaning the skin)

II. THEORY

Nerve-conduction studies are most commonly used in neurophysiological laboratories not only for the understanding of normal peripheral nerve structure and function but also in relation to various diseases.

1. Based on diameter and conduction velocity, nerve fibres have been divided into A, B and C groups; 'A' group is further subdivided into α, β, γ and δ fibres (details Table 3.26.1)
2. ***Principles of Nerve Coduction Study (NCS)***

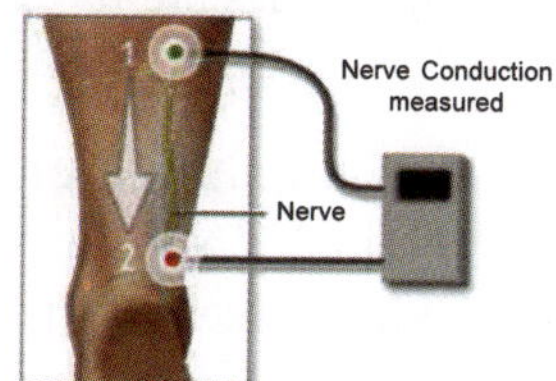

Broadly, nerve conduction study requires an external stimulation of a nerve at least at two points along its course. Nerve conduction velocity (in mt/sec) is calculated measuring the distance between two points of stimulation (in mm) which is divided by the latency difference (in msec).

The NCS involves the study of *motor* and *sensory nerve conduction.* The important nerves tested are:

(i) *in upper limb:* median, ulnar, radial nerves and brachial plexus; and

(ii) *in lower limb:* sciatic, femoral, common peroneal, tibial and sural nerves

A. Motor Nerve Conduction

(i) The motor (or mixed) nerve is stimulated separately at two points along its course; it will produce the contraction of the muscle supplied. The action potential so produced at the muscle (a ***compound muscle action potential-CMAP***) can be picked up with the help of recording electrodes suitably placed onto skin overlying the muscle. (Details page 281)

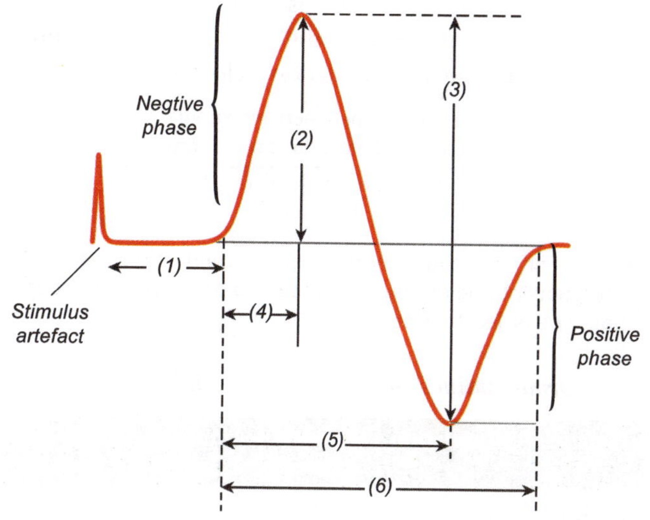

Fig. 3.26.2 Measurement of latency, amplitude and duration of CMAP

(1) onset latency; (2) base-to-peak amplitude; (3) peak-to-peak amplitude; (4) onset of negative peak; (5) onset of positive peak; (6) onset to final return to base line.

(ii) A *biphasic action potential* with initial negativity is thus recorded. (Fig. 3.26.2)

(iii) *Measurement for motor nerve conduction:* It includes the onset latency, duration and amplitude of CMAP and nerve conduction velocity.

(a) The onset latency of CMAP
- it is the time in msec from the stimulus artefact to the first negative deflection of CMAP.
- it is a measure of conduction in the fastest conducting motor fibres.
- it includes neuro-muscular transmission time and propagation time along the muscle membrane.

(b) The Amplitude of CMAP
- it is measured from baseline to the negative peak (base to peak) or between negative and positive peaks (peak to peak).

Table 3.26.1 Erlanger and Gasser's classification of nerve fibres

	Fibre type	Function	Diameter (μm)	Conduction velocity (mt/sec)
Typical Myelinated: (Motor and Sensory of spinal nerve)	Aα	Proprioception, Somatic motor	12–20	70–120
	Aβ	Touch, Pressure	5–12	30–70
	Aγ	Motor to muscle spindles	3–6	15–30
	Aδ	Pain, temperature, touch	2–5	12–30
Myelinated:	B	Preganglionic fibres of ANS	<3	3–15
Unmyelinated:	C	Dorsal root: Pain, touch, temperature,	0.4–1.2	0.5–2
		sympathetic, postgaglionic	0.3–1.3	0.7–2.3

(c) The duration of CMAP
- it is measured from the onset to the negative or positive peak or the final return of waveform to the baseline.
- it correlates with the density of small fibres.

(d) Motor nerve conduction velocity (mt/sec)

$$= \frac{\text{Distance between proximal and distal stimulation (in mm)}}{\text{Proximal latency – Distal latency (in msec)}}$$

Note: For accurate motor nerve conduction velocity measurement, the distance between two points of stimulation should be at least 10cm.

(iv) ***Normal values of motor nerve condution***

	Stimulation	Latency (msec)	Amplitude (mV)	Velocity (mt/sec)
Median nerve	wrist	3.1–3.8	4–10	52-62
	elbow	6.7–8.0	5.5–9.5	

B. Sensory Nerve Conduction

(i) The stimulation of sensory nerve will produce electrical activity, *i.e. sensory nerve action potential (SNAP)* which can be measured orthodromically or antidromically. The main differentiating features between the two are given in the table below.

(ii) The sensory nerve conduction measurements include onset latency, amplitude, duration of SNAP and nerve conduction velocity (Fig. 3.26.3)

Orthodromic Conduction	Antidromic Conduction
1. Here a distal portion of the nerve is stimulated and SNAP is recorded at a proximal point along the nerve.	1. Here, a nerve is stimulated at a proximal point and SNAP is recorded distally.
2. Ring electrodes are preferred for the stimulation of the nerve.	2. Surface-stimulating electrodes are commonly used.
3. *Latency:* Shorter	3. Longer
4. *Appearance:* Triphasic, initial a positive peak, subsequent negative peak followed by final positive peak.	4. Biphasic, initial positive peak is lacking.
5. *Amplitude:* Both base-to-peak and peak-to-peak amplitudes are lower.	5. Both amplitudes are higher because nerves are closer to recording electrode.

(iii) The *duration* of SNAP is measured from the initial positive peak to the intersection between the descending phase and the base line or to the negative or subsequent positive peak or return to the base line (Fig. 3.26.3)

(iv) In clinical practice, both orthodromic and antidromic methods provide the same information. *Amplitude* suggests the density of nerve fibres and *duration* suggests the number of slow-conducting fibres.

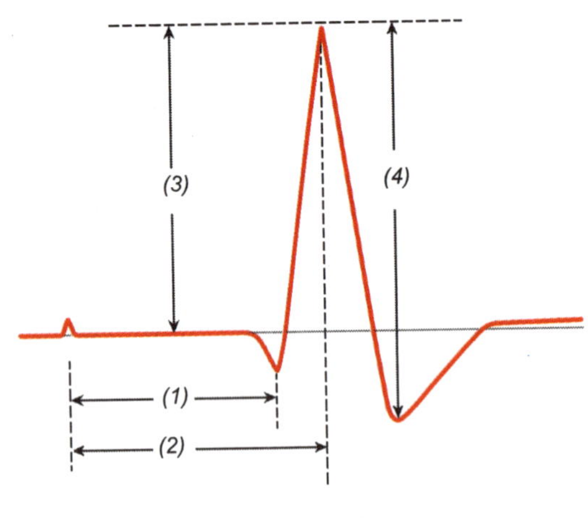

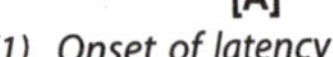

[A]
(1) Onset of latency
(2) Peak latency
(3) Base-to-peak amplitude
(4) Peak-to-peak amplitude

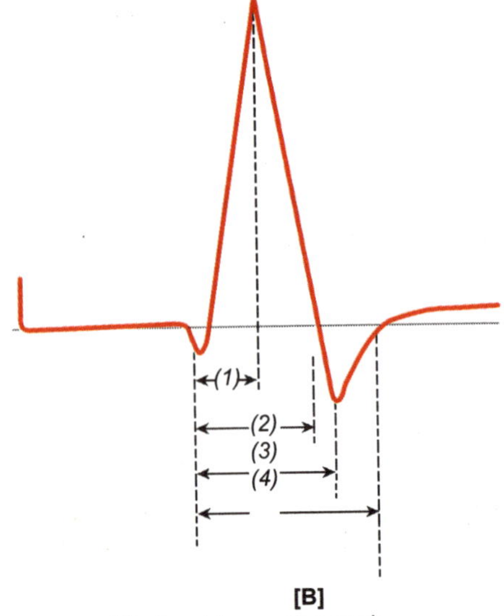

[B]
(1) Onset to negative peak
(2) Onset to intersection between descending phase and base line
(3) Onset to positive peak
(4) Onset to return to baseline

Fig. 3.26.3: Measurement of (A) latency and amplitude; and (B) duration of SNAP.

(v) Sensory nerve conduction velocity (mt/sec)

$$= \frac{\text{Distance between stimulating and recording electrodes (mm)}}{\text{Onset of latency (msec)}}$$

Note: Sensory nerve conduction velocity may be measured by stimulating at a single stimulation site because the residual latency which is comprised of neuromuscular transmission time and muscle propagation time is not applicable.

3. ***Factors affecting nerve conduction velocity***
   (i) *In general*
      (a) The greater the diameter of a given nerve fibre, the greater is its speed of conduction (because a large fibre offers less resistance to local currents).
      (b) In *myelinated fibres*, the speed of conduction is about 6 times the fibre diameter (conduction velocity varies from 6–120 mts/sec).
      (c) In *unmyelinated fibres*, the speed of conduction is proportional to the square root of the diameter; maximum conduction velocity in these fibres is 1 mt/sec.
   (ii) *Age:* At birth, nerve conduction velocity is half of the adult value (because of smaller diameter and imperfect myelination of nerve fibres). It attains adult value by 3–5 years of age to decline slowly after 30–40 years of age due to the gradual loss of larger neurons with aging.
   (iii) *Temperature:* Within physiological limits, conduction velocity varies directly with temperature. This is attributed to alteration in membrane permeability to Na^+.

Note: For each degree fall in temperature, the latency increases by 0.3 msec. Also, low temperature results in the slowing of nerve-conduction velocity.

   (iv) *Length of the nerve:* An inverse relationship exists between the length of the nerve and conduction velocity, *i.e.* the longer the nerve, the slower will be the conduction velocity. This is because of:
      (a) shorter internodal distance; and
      (b) progressive decrease in axon diameter

   This accounts for the faster conduction in the proximal nerves compared to distal; also, conduction velocity is higher in median and ulnar nerves compared to tibial and peroneal.
   (v) *Myelination:*
      (a) The length of nerve fibre covered by the myelin sheath does not conduct charges, hence the charges practically 'leap' the myelin region (*saltatory conduction*).
      (b) The nerve fibres that are myelinated early have longer internodal distance, larger diameter and wider spacing at the node of Ranvier. Hence, finally leads to faster-conduction velocity.
      (c) Myelin thickness is inversely related to internodal capacitance and conductance. Conduction velocy, therefore, increases with the increased myelin to a certain point.
   (vi) *Diameter of nerve fibre:* Refer to above.
   (vii) *Diseases:*
      (a) In *segmental demyelination* or during *demyelination*, myelin sheath is thin, internodal distance shorter, internodal conductance and capacitance increased. These result in conduction block.
      (b) In *focal compression*, conduction velocity slows down due to demyelination and decrease in fibre diameter.
4. ***Physio-Clinical significance of nerve conduction study.*** Nerve conduction study (NCS) is part of electrodiagnostic procedures that help evaluate the type and degree of abnormalities of the peripheral nerves, especially demyelination diseases and focal compression of nerves. It establishes diagnosis quite early and more accurately than other electrodiagnostic procedures because of its sensitivity to detect conduction slowing, which is an early indicator of peripheral neuropathy.

   Common neuropathies encountered in clinical practice are either due to demyelinating disorders such as diabetes mellitus, multiple sclerosis, etc. or the focal compression of the nerve during its course (due to the overuse of joints, pressure, fractures, myxoedema, tumours, etc.).

III. PROCEDURE

Note: Here procedure for **median** nerve conduction has been described.

(A) Motor Nerve Conduction

1. Keep the instrument out of view of the subject; follow general precautions (page 296).
2. Explain test procedure to the subject so as to get the maximum cooperation.
3. Allow the subject to sit comfortably on a chair in a fully relaxed state.
4. Equipment set-up:
   (i) Filter setting: Low cut (2–5Hz); high cut (10KHz).
   (ii) Sweep speed: 2–5 msec/division.
   (iii) Stimulation option: The surface stimulation of a healthy nerve requires a square wave pulse of 0.1 msec duration with an intensity of 5–40 mA. (Also, follow precautions strictly: page 301)

5. Clean the thenar area and the skin overlying the median nerve at the elbow and wrist.
6. Using conducting jelly or electrode paste, the *recording (active) cup electrode* is placed close to the motor point of abductor pollicis brevis and *reference electrode* 3cm distal to active electrode at the 1st metacarpophalangeal joint. The *ground* electrode is placed between stimulation and recording electrodes. (Fig. 3.26.4)

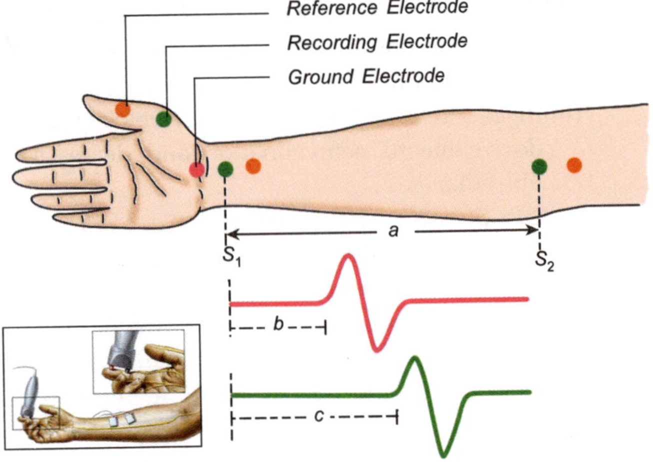

Fig. 3.26.4 Electrode placement for median motor nerve conduction (Inset : An actual placement of electrodes)

(S: stimulating electrode; a: distance between wrist and elbow points of stimulation. b and c: distal and proximal latency respectively).

7. Connect the electrodes through the pre-amplifier to the cathode ray oscilloscope (C.R.O.).
8. With the help of stimulating electrodes, a supramaximal stimulation is given first at the wrist (3 cm proximal to the distal wrist crease) and then at the elbow (near the volar crease of the brachial pulse). Observe and record the action potential on C.R.O. at each occassion.

Note: The stimulus artefact, which is due to current leak appears at the beginning of the sweep. This is useful for noting the point of stimulus.

9. The difference between two latent periods in msec (Fig. 3.26.4) gives the time taken by the impulse to travel from the elbow to the wrist.
10. Measure the distance between the wrist and the elbow points of stimulation in mm and calculate the velocity of nerve impulse conduction in the median nerve (in mt/sec) (page 298).

(B) Sensory Nerve Conduction (*orthodromically*: page 298)

1, 2, 3 steps, the same as above

4. Equipment set-up:
   (i) Filter setting: low cut (5–10Hz); high cut (2–3KHz).
   (ii) Sweep speed: 1–2 msec/division
   (iii) Gain: 1–5μV/division
   (iv) Signal enhancement with averaging is generally required. It is proportional to the square root of the number of trials (n). Therefore, change in amplitude is = $\sqrt{n}$
5. Using conducting jelly or electrode paste, place the electrodes as under: (Fig. 3.26.5)
   (i) *Recording (active) cup electrode:* 3cm proximal to the distal crease;
   (ii) *Reference electrode:* at a distance of 3cm proximal to active electrode.
   (iii) *Ground electrode:* between stimulation and recording electrodes
   (iv) For stimulation, ring electrodes are placed at the 2nd or 3rd digits (index finger). The cathode is placed at the first interphalangeal joint and anode 3 cm distal.

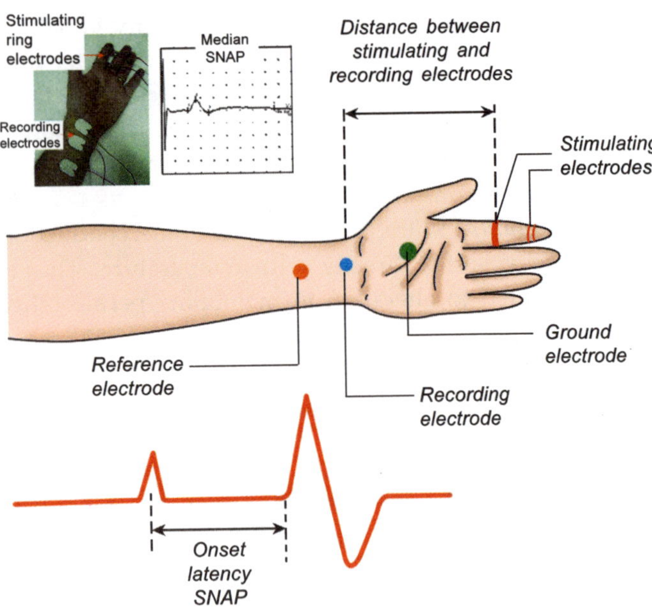

Fig. 3.26.5 Electrode placement for orthodromic sensory conduction of median nerve (SNAP: Sensory nerve action potential)

Important Note: For *antidromic conduction studies,* the location of the above-mentioned stimulating and recording electrodes are reversed. Therefore, recording is made from ring electrodes at interphalangeal joints and stimulation is given at the wrist.

6. Connect the electrodes through pre-amplifier to the C.R.O.
7. With the help of stimulating electrodes, a

supramaximal stimulation is given; observe and record action potential on C.R.O.

8. Calculate the distal latency, sensory nerve action potential (SNAP) and conduction velocity of different segments as described on page 281. Compare with normal values.

IV. PRECAUTIONS

1. Follow general precautions; refer to page 296.
2. Failure to get response may be due to defect in stimulating or recording system; this must be carefully checked before trying again.
3. Laboratory temperature should be maintained preferably between 21–23°C.

(A) Failure of stimulating system

(i) Shunting of current between anode and cathode either by sweat or bridge formation by conducting jelly
(ii) Faulty location of stimulator
(iii) Application of submaximal current during stimulation

(B) Failure of recording system

(i) Breaks in the electrode wire
(ii) Connection to a wrong pre-amplifier
(iii) incorrect oscilloscope setting of gain, sweep and filter

IMPORTANT VIVA-VOCE QUESTIONS

Q.1. *How are the nerve fibres classified? Give their functions.*
Ans. Page 297.

Q.2. *Give the principle of nerve-conduction studies.*
Ans. Page 297.

Q.3. *What does the measurement of compound muscle action potential (CMAP) include?*
Ans. Page 297.

Q.4. *Draw a well-labelled diagram depicting CMAP. Give the significance of each component.*
Ans. Page 297.

Q.5. *Give the normal velocity of conduction in human peripheral nerves.*
Ans. Average normal conduction velocity is 50–65 mt/sec.

Q.6. *What do you understand by the term SNAP? How can it be measured?*
Ans. Page 298.

Q.7. *Give differences between orthodromic and antidromic conduction.*
Ans. Page 298.

Q.8. *Draw and label SNAP.*
Ans. Page 298.

Q.9. *Enumerate the factors affecting the nerve conduction velocity.*
Ans. Page 299.

Q.10. *Give the clinical application of nerve conduction studies.*
Ans. Page 299.

Q.11. *What is the difference in the value of the normal conduction velocity of nerves in upper and lower limbs?*
Ans. Page 299.

Q.12. *If you fail to obtain a desire response to nerve conduction studies, what could be the technical errors?*
Ans. See above.

Q.13. *How is the motor and sensory velociy of nerve conduction calculated?*
Ans. Refer to pages 298 and 299.

Q.14. *Give the characterisitic features of the nerve fibres based on its diameter.*
Ans. Page 299.

Q.15. *What is saltatory conduction?*
Ans. Page 299.

Q.16. *What is multiple sclerosis?*
Ans. In this disease, there is a patchy destruction of myelin in the CNS. It is a crippling disease associated with delayed or blocked conduction in demyelinated nerve fibres.

Q.17. *What are the major causes of neuropathy?*
Ans. Page 299.

(B) Visual Evoked Potential (V.E.P.)

I. APPARATUS

Subject, cathode ray oscilloscope, pre-amplifier, ether or spirit, EEG electrodes, EEG jelly (or paste) (page 281), photostimulator

II. THEORY

1. The electrical potential differences recorded from scalp in response to visual stimuli is called **Visual Evoked Potential (V.E.P.).** It represent a resultant

response of cortical as well as subcortical areas to photostimulation.

2. A normal V.E.P. indicate the intactness of visual system. Therefore, in the localization of deficit within the visual pathway, the knowledge of physiological anatomy of the eye is essential.
3. ***Genesis of V.E.P.***
   (i) The process of visual information in retina involves a generation of electrical activity at three places:
      (a) The **first** activity is generated in photoreceptors (rods and cones) by the action of light;
      (b) The **second** in the bipolar cells; and
      (c) The **third** electrical activity is generated in the ganglion cells.

   (ii) The *retinal ganglion* cells are broadly classified into *X and Y cells;* the main differentiating features between the two are:

X-cells	Y-cells
1. These are small retinal ganglion cells with small diameter axons.	1. These are large retinal ganglion cells with large diameter axons.
2. Mediate *cone vision* with *lateral inhibition.*	2. Mediate *rod vision* without *lateral inhibition.*
3. *Receptive field:* Small	3. Large
4. *Distribution in retina: Central*	4. Peripheral
5. *Sensitivity* (a) low sensitivity to motion (b) Provide substrate for **pattern shift VEP (PSVEP)** via geniculate pathway; thus they are useful in assessing the visual acuity.	(a) High sensitivity to motion (b) Generate **flash VEP** via extra geniculate pathway; thus they determine the presence or absence of light perception.

   (iii) V.E.P. is primarily a reflection of activity originating in the central 3° to 6° of visual field which is relayed to the surface of occipital lobe.

Note: The projections arising from the peripheral retina are directed to the regions deep within the calcarine fissure, hence unrecordable on peripheral retinal stimulation.

4. ***Normal V.E.P.***
   (i) V.E.P. consists of series of waveforms of opposite polarity, the negative waveform (denoted as N) and a positive waveform (denoted as P); which is followed by the *approximate latency* in millisec. (Fig. 3.26.6)

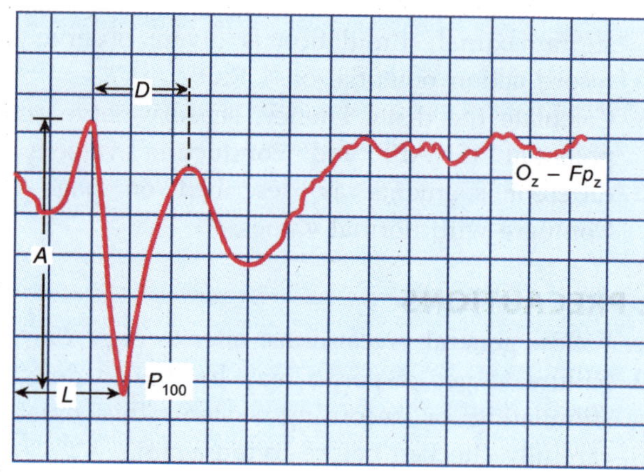

Fig. 3.26.6 V.E.P. in normal individual recording from O_z referred to Fp_z. Measurement of P_{100} is shown.

(L: latency; D: duration; A: amplitude; sweep speed 50 msec per division; sensitivity: 2μV/division)

   (ii) The commonly used waveforms are N_{70}, N_{100} and N_{135}.

Note: The subscript number denotes the time in millisec. after stimulation.

   (iii) The measurement of P_{100} peak latency, its duration and amplitude for VEP analysis is most commonly used. The P_{100} waveform of V.E.P. is generated in the occipital cortex due to the activation of primary visual cortex and also due to thalamocortical fibres discharge. (N_{25} reflects the activity of fovea and primary visual cortex while N_{135} reflects the activity of visual association areas 18 and 19).
   (iv) *Normal values* for P_{100} V.E.P. =
      (a) Latency: 100 msec.
      (b) Amplitude: 10 μV; and
      (c) Duration: 60 msec.

Important Note: For *transient V.E.P.,* the stimulation rate is 1 Hz producing the ***reversal pattern*** every 500 msec. The stimulation rate for *steady state V.E.P.* is 4–8 Hz. The *steady state* V.E.P. are repeated evoked potentials which constitute discrete frequency components and remain constant in amplitude and phase over a long period of time.

5. ***Factors affecting V.E.P. (P_{100} waveform)***

(A) Physiological factors

   (i) *Age:* In infants and young children, latency is longer and reaches the adult value by 5-6 years. (due to age related changes in the visual system). In infants, amplitude is almost the double of the adult value.
   (ii) *Sex:* Latency is larger in males compared to females due to the larger head size and low internal body temperature in males. However, amplitude is

greater in females compared to males probably due to hormonal differences.

(iii) *Hemisphere dominance:* The amplitude of V.E.P. is greater in right hemifield stimulation in right-handed individuals due to the neuro anatomic asymmetries of human striate cortex.

(iv) V.E.P. amplitude is reduced by eye movements.

(v) The latency and amplitude remain normal with visual acuity as low as 20/120; however, the amplitude decreases with a further decrease of visual acuity.

(vi) Mental activity decreases latency but increases the amplitude of V.E.P. waveform.

(B) Technical factors

Decrease in the area of retinal illumination reduces the amplitude but increases the latency of V.E.P.

Causes: (i) Decrease of luminance
(ii) Reduction of contrast between black and white squares
(iii) Constriction of pupils by miotics

6. ***V.E.P. Abnormalities***

Disturbances anywhere in the visual system can produce abnormal V.E.P. The common abnormalities are:

(A) Prolongation of Latency

The commonest cause of prolongation of P_{100} latency (without affecting the amplitude) is *demyelination in optic pathways.* This results in the delayed conduction in visual pathways.

Causes: (i) Multiple sclerosis.
(ii) Optic neuritis (alcoholism, vitamin B_{12} deficiency, tobacco).
(iii) Glaucoma

(B) Reduction in Amplitude

Ischaemic optic neuropathy resulting in the loss of axons produces normal P_{100} latency with decreased amplitude. (Latency may get affected in the later stages)

Causes: (i) Hypertension
(ii) CNS vasculitis

(C) Combined Abnormalities (A and B)

Nerve compression produces segmental demyelination. The loss of axons results in the reduced retinal illumination. Thus is produces both increase in latency and reduction in amplitude.

Causes: (i) Severe papilloedema
(ii) Pituitary tumour

(D) Shape Abnormalities

Bifid pattern of P_{100}, *i.e.* two peaks are separated by 10-50 msec, commonly seen in defects in the visual field.

Important Notes

1. As each eye projects to the occipital lobes through an optic chiasma, the unilateral V.E.P. abnormalities recorded by field monocular stimulation are due to prechiasmal lesion. If it is abnormal bilaterally; it is difficult to locate the anatomical site of conduction defect in the visual pathways.
2. The use of green-black or red-black colour increases the frequency of V.E.P. abnormalities.

7. ***Physio-clinical Significance of V.E.P.***

In a cooperative subject, the sensitivity of psychophysical tests such as visual acuity, perimetry and colour vision testing (pages 204 and 242) provide useful information for the evaluation of the visual sytem. However, in uncooperative subjects where fundus examination is not possible V.E.P. testing is necessary.

(i) A normal V.E.P. is usually associated with normal visual examination; however, an abnormal V.E.P. study may or may not be associated with abnormal clinical findings.

(ii) V.E.P. provides an objective and sensitive information of abnormalities in visual system (especially anterior to optic chiasma).

Important Notes

1. V.E.P. abnormalities are non-specific and are not characteristic of any specific aetiology.
2. V.E.P. has not been found to be very useful in establishing the diagnosis or prognosis in individuals with cortical blindness because of dissociation between V.E.P. and vision.
3. It is of great value in individuals with *hysterical blindness.* V.E.P. remains normal with vision as low as 20/120.

III. PROCEDURE

(A) Prerequisites:

Follow general precautions: page 296

1. Avoid hair spray or oil after hair wash.
2. The usual glasses if any should be put on during the test.
3. Review finding regarding ophthalmological examination such as visual acuity, field of vision and colour vision.
4. Avoid any miotic or mydriatic drugs 12 hours before the test.
5. As the visual field defects, alter the potential field distribution of P_{100}, the lateral placement of electrode is also necessary.

(B) Equipment Set-up for V.E.P. Study as recommended by International Federation of Clinical Neurophysiology (IFCN) committee

Suggested Montage

Two channels (As per 10–20 international system of EEG electrode placement, page 283)

1. Channel 1: O_z–Fp_z } Reference electrode
2. Channel 2: O_z–A_1A_2 (linked ear) } Reference electrode
3. Ground electrode position at: C_z

Recording Conditions

1. Filter: (i) low-filter cut: 1–3Hz
   (ii) high-filter cut: 100–300Hz
2. Amplification between 20,000 and 1,00,000
3. Sweep duration between: 250 and 500 msec.
4. Number of epochs: At least 100 are averaged.
5. Electrode impedence should be kept below 5 kilo-ohms.

Stimulation Options

1. Black-and-white checker board or vertical grating
2. Distance between subject and screen: 70–100cm
3. Contrast between: 50–80%
4. Fixation point for full field size greater than 8°
5. Size of pattern element: 14 × 16 minute
6. Rate of stimulation
   (i) For transient V.E.P.: 1Hz.
   (ii) For steady state V.E.P.: 4–8Hz.
7. Mean luminance of the central field: 50cd/m^2; background luminance 20–40cd/m^2. (The difference of luminance between the centre and periphery of field should not exceed 20%)
8. The subject is instructed to fix gaze at the centre of screen.

Note: In children, only 1 electrode, approximately 1cm anterior to Oz, is preferred.

(C) Steps

Note: One eye should be tested at a time and the instrument should be out of view of the subject.

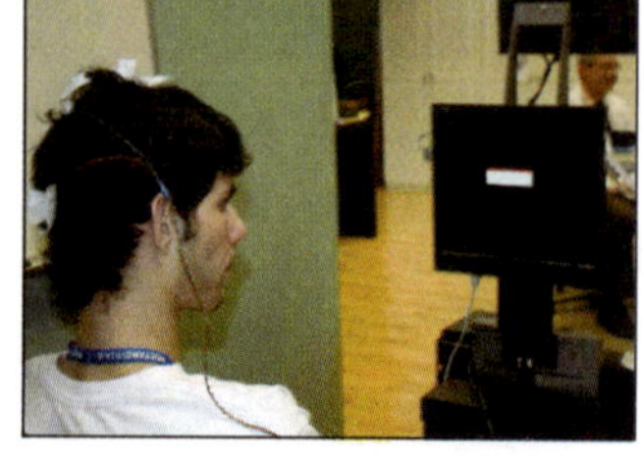

1. Allow the subject to sit comfortably in a chair in a fully relaxed state.
2. The skin at the point of the placement of electrodes is cleared with ether or spirit.
3. Using electrode paste or conducting jelly, the *recording electrode* is placed at Oz as per 10–20 international system of EEG electrode placement (page 283); the *reference electrode* is placed at Fpz or 12cm above the nasion. Linked ear reference is also used as non-cephalic reference. The *ground electrode* is placed at the vertex, *i.e.* at Cz. (Fig.3.26.7)

Note: Standard disc EEG electrodes are used. Needle electrodes are *not* used because of the possibility of infection and being unsuitable for long-term monitoring.

4. Check the equipment set-up as described above.
5. The electrodes are connected through the preamplifier to the cathode ray oscilloscope (CRO).

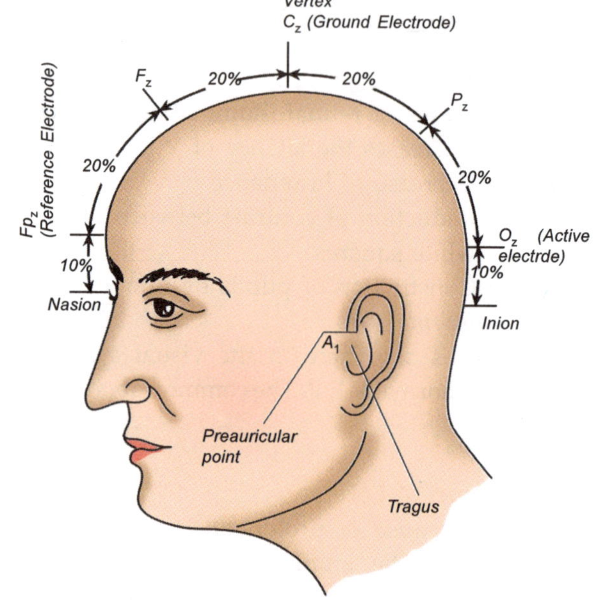

Fig. 3.26.7 Electrode placement for visual evoked potential (two channel)

6. Instruct the subject to fix the gaze at the centre of the screen.
7. The visual stimulus is delivered by *photostimulator*; white flashes should be given at frequencies 1, 3, 6, 10 and 20 flashes/sec.
8. Obtain the response: the peak latency and the peak-to-peak amplitude of these waves are measured and compared with the normal.

IV. PRECAUTIONS

1. Follow general precautions, refer to page 296.
2. Strictly follow all the prerequisites; refer to page 303.
3. Instruct the subject beforehand not to sleep during the test procedure.
4. Instruct the subject to fix his gaze at the centre of screen.
5. In persons with visual field defects, besides the midline electrode, the lateral placement of electrode is also necessary.

IMPORTANT VIVA-VOCE QUESTIONS

Q.1. *Define visual evoked potential (V.E.P.). What does it signify?*
Ans. Page 301.

Q.2. *What is the physiological basis of V.E.P.?*
Ans. Page 302.

Q.3. *What do you understand by the term visual information?*
Ans. Visual images have different characteristics such as colour, form, depth, movement and texture; each processed simultaneously by a separate channel in the visual system, called **parallel processing of visual information.**

Q.4. *Give the major differences between the two main types of retinal ganglion cells.*
Ans. Page 302.

Q.5. *Define: Receptive field and lateral inhibition.*
Ans. **Receptive field** is the area of body surface that when stimulated, leads to activity in the neuron and is called the receptive field for that neuron.
Lateral (or afferent) inhibition is a form of inhibition in which the activation of a particular neural unit is associated with the inhibition of the activity of surrounding units. This helps to sharpen the edges of a stimulus and improve discrimination.

Q.6. *What is pattern shift V.E.P. and flash V.E.P.?*
Ans. Page 302.

Q.7. *Draw a well-labelled V.E.P. in a normal individual. What is P_{100} V.E.P.? Give its normal values.*
Ans. Page 302.

Q.8. *What is transient V.E.Ps.? How does it differ from steady-state V.E.Ps.?*
Ans. Page 302.

Q.9. *Enumerate the factors influencing the P_{100} waveform of V.E.P.*
Ans. Page 302.

Q.10. *Mention the abnormalities associated with the P_{100} waveform of V.E.P.*
Ans. Page 303.

Q.11. *Give the clinical application of V.E.P.*
Ans. Page 303.

Q.12. *What is the limitation to V.E.P.?*
Ans. Page 303.

Q.13. *What is hysterical blindness?*
Ans. Page 303.

Q.14. *How far is V.E.P. study useful in the person with cortical blindness?*
Ans. Page 303.

Q.15. *Enlist the prerequisites/precautions needed during the record of V.E.P.*
Ans. Page 304.

Q.16. *Name the physiological conditions in which V.E.P. waveform gets altered.*
Ans. Page 302.

(C) Brainstem Auditory Evoked Potentials (B.A.E.P.)

I. APPARATUS

Subject, cathode ray oscilloscope, pre-amplifier, ether or spirit, EEG electrodes, EEG jelly (or paste), earphone

II. THEORY

1. The potentials recorded from the ear and vertex in response to a brief auditory stimulation are called **Brainstem Auditory Evoked Potentials (B.A.E.P.).** These are produced within 10 msec. by a brief click stimulus. A series of potentials are generated corresponding to the sequential activation of peripheral, pontomedullary, pontine and midbrain portion of auditory pathway. It helps to assess:
   (i) Conduction through the auditory pathway upto midbrain
   (ii) Severity of hearing deficits; and
   (iii) middle portion of brainstem functions
2. ***Normal BAEP***
   The acoustic nerve and brainstem auditory potentials are volume conduction to surface recording electrodes. At the vertex and ear lobe, these form vertex positive and vertex negative potentials. It consists of 5 or more distinct waveforms (*vertex positive peaks*) labelled with Roman numerals, I to V. (Table 3.26.2 Fig. 3.26.8 A and B)
3. ***Analysis of BAEPs*** (Fig. 3.26.8 B)
   (i) *Absolute latency:* It is measured in msec. from the peak of the respective waves.
   (ii) *Absolute amplitude:* It is measured in μV from the peak of the wave to the bottom of the trough of the wave.
   (iii) *Interpeak latency (IPL):* Commonest used IPLs in clinical practice are: I-V, I-III and III-V.
      (a) **I-V** *IPL, i.e.* latency difference between wave V and I.
      It is a measure of conduction from proximal VIII nerve through pons to midbrain;
      - Normal: 4.0 msec.

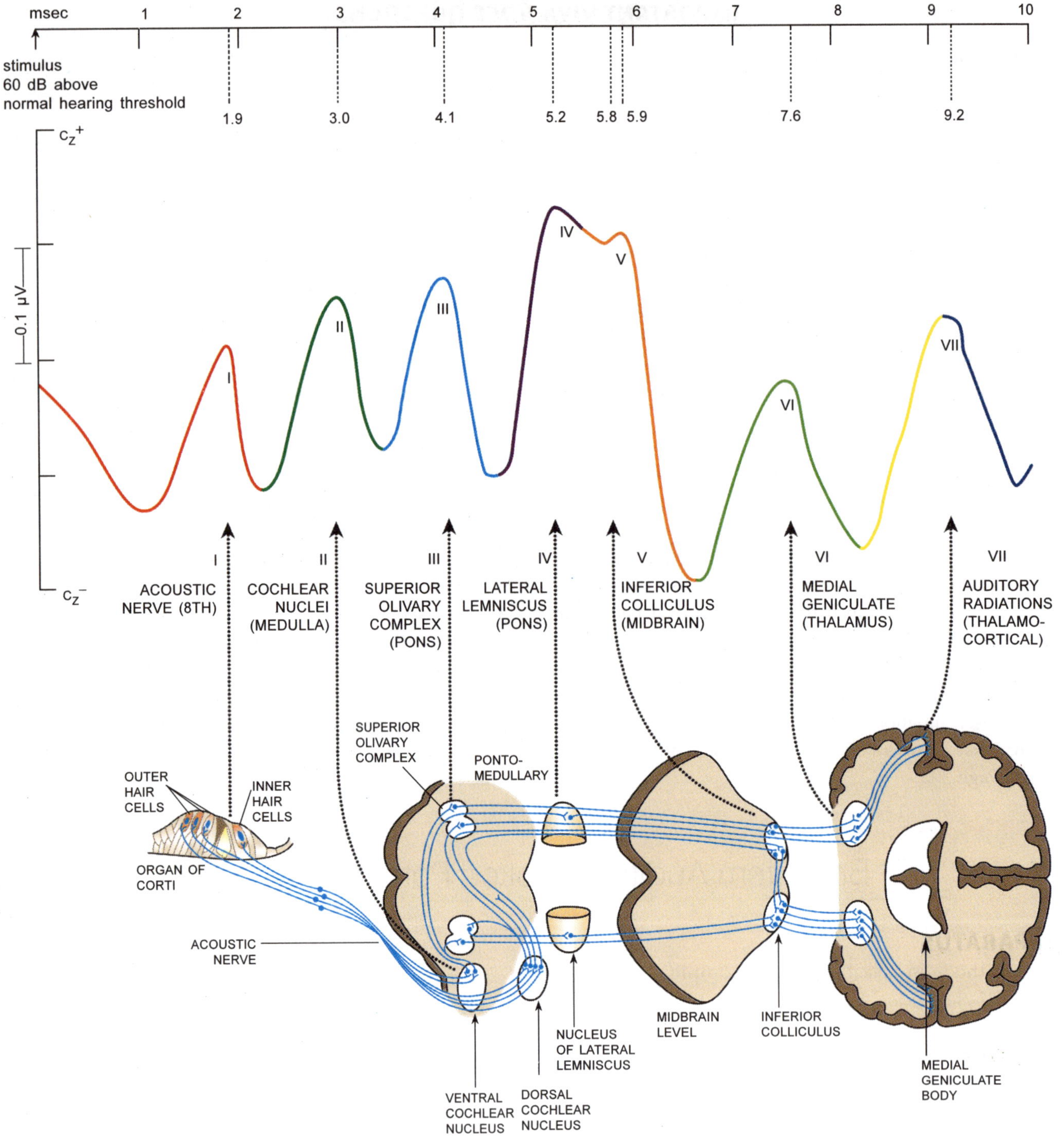

Fig. 3.26.8 (A) Physio-Anatomical correlation of Brainstem auditory evoked potential (BAEP) waveforms (For details, refer to the text).

- It is slightly shorter in young women and longer in older men.
- Normal right-to-left asymmetry should not exceed 0.5 msec.
- If gets prolonged, *causes* are:
  - demyelination
  - ischaemia
  - tumours
  - brain damage due to hypoxia.

(b) **I-III** *IPL, i.e.* latency difference between wave I and III. It is a measure of conduction from the VIII nerve across subarachnoid space.

- Normal: 2.1msec.
- Right-to-left asymmetry: less than 0.5msec.

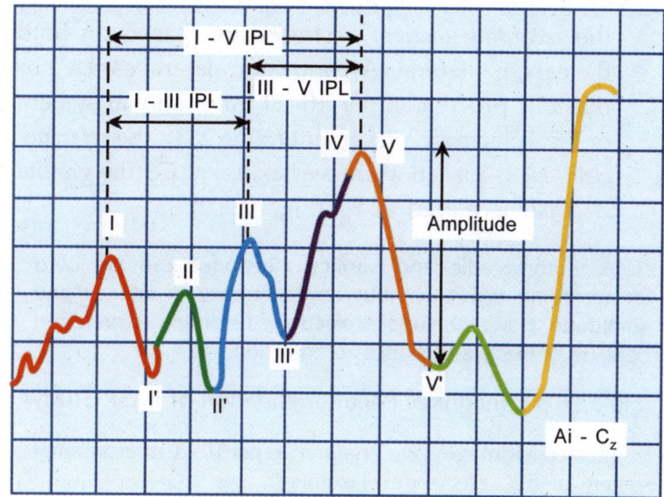

Fig. 3.26.8 B Brainstem auditory evoked potential (BAEP) in a normal individual (IPL: Inter Peak Latency)

- Prolongation is seen in: tumour or inflammation affecting the proximal portion of the VIII nerve.

(c) **III-V** *IPL*

- It measures conduction from lower pons to midbrain
- Normal: 1.9msec and right-to-left asymmetry up to 0.5msec.

(iv) *Amplitude ratio of wave V/I:* Since wave I is generated outside the CNS and wave V inside, therefore, these can be compared to determine the relationship of the expected signal amplitude. *Normal ratio* is between 50% and 300%.

(a) If ratio is lower than 50%, it suggests a *central hearing impairment* such as:
- multiple sclerosis; and
- hydrocephalus

(b) Ratio higher than 300%, suggests *peripheral hearing impairment.*

4. ***Factors affecting BAEP waveforms***

(i) *Age:*

(a) I-V **inter peak latency (IPL)** is longer in adults as compared to young children.

(b) Females have shorter latency and higher amplitude (due to higher internal body temperature and shorter length of brainstem auditory pathway).

(ii) *Body temperature:* The absolute latency and IPL are prolonged on lowering body temperature. This is why wave V is slightly prolonged in the individual addicted to alcohol or barbiturate because these agents produce hypothermia.

(iii) *Hearing status:* The impairment of hearing

Table 3.26.2 Brainstem auditory evoked potentials

Waveform	Genesis (origin)	Characteristic feature	Wave latency	Clinical Significance
Wave I	Peripheral portion of the VIII nerve	1. It is a prominent initial negative peak confined to ipsilateral ear and is absent from contralateral ear recording channel. 2. Its trough is designated as 'I'	1.5 msec.	Absent in the patients in peripheral hearing impairment. *Causes:* (i) large tumour damaging the VIII nerve (ii) VIII nerve ischaemia
Wave II	Cochlear nucleus	1. It appears as a small peak. 2. More prominent in contralateral channel recording	2.8 msec.	Absent in cochlear nucleus lesion
Wave III	Superior olivary nucleus	1. Seen as a prominent peak and followed by a prominent trough 2. In contralateral channel recording it appears smaller and earlier than the ipsilateral ear.	4 msec.	Absent in superior olivary nucleus lesion
Wave IV	Lateral lemniscus	Appears as a very small wave in the upgoing slope of wave V	5.1 msec.	Absent in lateral lemniscus lesion
Wave V	Inferior colliculus	1. It starts above the baseline and its trough is maximum below the baseline. 2. In ipsilateral recording channel it may fuse with wave IV forming *IV-V complex.* However, in contralateral recording, the IV and V waves separate out.	5.5 msec.	Absent in inferior colliculus lesions

can alter the BAEPs, therefore, audiometry and hearing tests should be evaluated before conducting BAEP study.

5. ***Physio-clinical significance of BAEPs***
   Although the changes in BAEPs are non-specific yet they provide information about the function of corresponding auditory pathways. It helps to assess:
   (i) Conduction through the auditory pathway upto midbrain.
   (ii) Severity of hearing deficits; and
   (iii) Middle portion of brainstem functions.
   It is important to realise that BAEP is not really a test of hearing; there may be an individual with disturbed hearing who has normal BAEP. Similarly, there may also be individuals with apparently normal hearing but have abnormality on BAEP study.
   The *major role* of BAEP in neurology is:
   (i) Identification, characterisation and quantification of hearing loss in children who are uncooperative for audiometry.
   (ii) Confirmation and localization of brainstem dysfunction
6. ***Abnormal BAEPs***
   BAEPs abnormalities include:
   (i) *Absence of wave I:* It is seen in:
      (a) Large tumour damaging the VIII nerve
      (b) VIII nerve ischaemia
   (ii) *Absence of waves beyond wave I:*
      Causes: (a) acoustic neuroma
      (b) meningioma
      (c) demyelinating disorders
   (iii) *Absence of waves IV and V:*
      Causes: (a) multiple sclerosis
      (b) hydrocephalus
   (iv) The right-to-left latency asymmetry exceeding 0.5msec is seen in acoustic neuroma.

Also, refer to page 307 for more abnormalities.

III. PROCEDURE

(A) Equipment Set-Up (Refer to Table 3.26.3)

(B) Steps

1. Keep the instrument out of view of the subject.
2. Allow the subject to sit comfortably on a chair in a fully relaxed state.
3. The skin at the point of the placement of electrodes is cleaned with ether or spirit.
4. Using electrode paste or conducting jelly, the *recording (active) electrodes* are placed on both the ears, ipsilateral (Ai) and contralateral ear (A_c) or mastoid process as per 10–20 international system of EEG electrode placement (page 283); the *reference electrode* is placed at the vertex, *i.e.* at C_z; the *ground electrode* is placed at F_z. (Fig. 3.26.9)

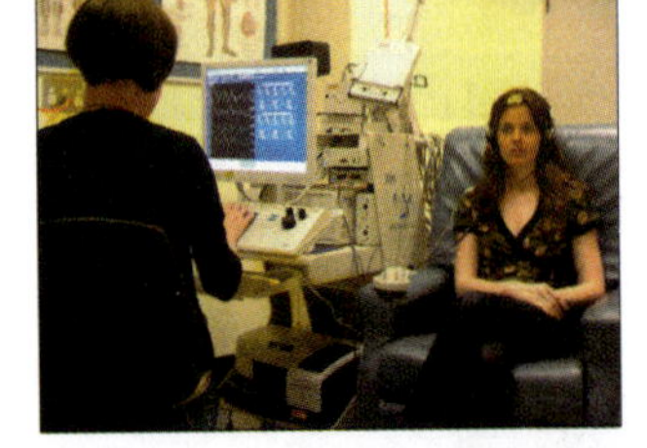

Note: Both needle and surface electrodes can be used for recording BAEPs without any difference in latency and amplitude. However, surface electrode recording is preferred because of the lesser chances of infection.

Table 3.26.3 Technical Recommendation of BAEP Study

Suggested Montage: Two-channel (as per 10–20 international system of EEG electrode placement, page 283).

1. Channel 1	: A_i–C_z	*Active (recording) electrodes*
2. Channel 2	: A_c–C_z	*Ipsilateral ear (A_i), Contralateral ear (A_c) or mastoid process*
3. Ground	: F_z	*Reference electrode:* C_z, *i.e.* at vertex (it is regarded as a suitable location as waves II-V have a good amplitude at the vertex.)

Recording conditions
1. Filter
   (i) Low-filter cut: 10-100Hz
   (ii) High-filter cut: 3000Hz.
2. Amplification between 2,00,000–5,00,000
3. Sweep speed: 1msec/division
4. Number of epochs: at least 100
5. Electrode impedence should be kept below 5 kilo-ohms.

Stimulation Options
1. Sensitivity: 0.3μv/division
2. 60 db sensory level, *i.e.* point at which the individual can barely appreciate the stimulus.

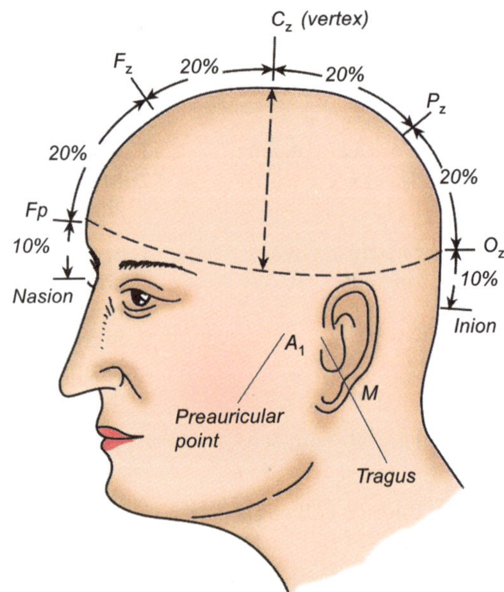

Fig. 3.26.9 Electrode placement for Brainstem auditory evoked potential (two channels) A_i: ipsilateral ear (active/recording electrode); M: Mastoid process; C_z (vertex): reference electrode; F_z: ground electrode.

5. Check the equipment set-up as per-technical recommendation of BAEP study (Table 3.26.3).
6. The electrodes are connected through the preamplifier to the cathode ray oscilloscope (C.R.O.)
7. Give a brief click stimulus which is usually a square wave pulse of 0.1 msec duration. A click rate of 11–31Hz is most commonly used in clinical practice.

Notes

(i) The pulse wave can move the *earphone* diaphragm either towards or away from the ear, called *condensation* or *rarefaction stimulus* respectively. Wave I amplitude tends to be greater with rarefaction compared to condensation stimulus. Therefore, rarefaction click polarity is usually employed.

(ii) The click **not** only stimulates the ipsilateral ear but also travels by bone and air conduction to stimulate the contralateral ear at an intensity of 40–50db lower than the ipsilateral ear.

8. Observe the effect of click intensity on BAEP. Analyse the BAEPs wave form and compare with the normal (page 305).

IV. PRECAUTIONS

1. Follow the general precautions; refer to page 296.
2. Auditory hearing tests should be reviewed before conducting BAEP (as hearing impairment can alter the BAEPs waveforms).
3. The room should be quiet and comfortable.

IMPORTANT VIVA-VOCE QUESTIONS

Q.1. *Define brainstem auditory evoked potential (BAEP). Give its physiological basis.*
Ans. Page 305.
Q.2. *Give the potential field distribution, waveform recognition and normal values of BAEP.*
Ans. Page 305.
Q.3. *Draw a well-labelled BAEP in a normal person.*
Ans. Page 307.
Q.4. *List the factors influencing BAEP waveform.*
Ans. Page 307.
Q.5. *Give the basis of the analysis of BAEPs waveform.*
Ans. Page 305.
Q.6. *Name the commonest used interpeak latency (IPL) in clinical practice. Give their characteristic features.*
Ans. Page 305.
Q.7. *Give the clinical significance of BAEPs.*
Ans. Page 308.
Q.8. *Give the abnormalities and their cause in BAEPs waveform.*
Ans. Page 308.
Q.9. *Give the technical recommendation of BAEP study.*
Ans. Page 308.
Q.10. *Why is BAEP recording with surface electrode preferred over needle electrode?*
Ans. Page 308.
Q.11. *Explain condensation and rarefaction stimulus.*
Ans. See above.
Q.12. *Does a click stimulus applied to one ear activate both the ears at the same intensity?*
Ans. See above.
Q.13. *List the precautions to be observed while recording BAEPs.*
Ans. See above.

(D) Somatosensory Evoked Potentials (S.E.P.)

I. APPARATUS

Subject, cathode ray oscilloscope, pre-amplifier, ether or spirit, EEG electrodes, EEG jelly (or paste)

II. THEORY

1. The electrical potential generated mainly by the *large diameter* sensory fibres in the peripheral and central portion of the nervous system in response to a stimulus are called **Somatosensory Evoked Potentials (S.E.P.)**.

Note: Since large sensory axons (12–20 mm diameter) are concerned mainly with proprioceptive sensation and smaller sensory axons (<12mm diameter) are concerned with pain and temperature sensations, therefore, *somatosensory evoked potential* studies evaluate the proprioceptive pathways, *i.e.* pathways that carry information about changes in body position in space especially the joints or tension of muscle at any given moment.

2. ***Genesis of S.E.P.***
The SEPs can be recorded by stimulating any large peripheral nerve. However, in clinical practice, SEPs are commonly recorded from median nerve (**Median SEP**) and posterior tibial nerve (**Tibial SEP**).

3. *Neural pathway for proprioception*

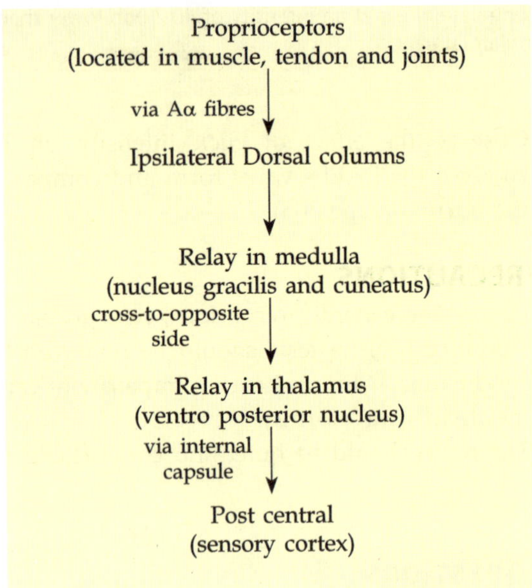

4. *Normal Median SEP*

(i) It consists of the series of the *waveform* of opposite polarity: N and P (Page 279). The commonly used waveforms are: N_9, N_{11}, N_{13}, P_{14}, N_{18} and N_{20}. The genesis (origin) of these waveforms are:

Waveforms	Genesis (origin)
N_9	Brachial plexus
N_{11}	Posterior column of 5th cervical spinal segment
N_{13}	Rostral cervical spinal cord from dorsal horn
P_{14}	Medial lemniscus or its brainstem collaterals
N_{18}	Rostral brainstem nuclei, thalamus
N_{20}	Primary sensory cortex, ventro posterior nucleus of thalamus

(ii) Waveforms (Fig. 3.26.10)

(a) N_9 *(Erb's potential)* is seen as a principal negative peak in EP_i–EP_c channel.
Erb's point (2–3cm above midclavicular point) electrodes are designated as EP_i and EP_c, *i.e.* ipsilateral and contralateral to stimulation respectively.

(b) N_{11} *(spinal potential)* is a negative peak recorded at spinous process of the 5th cervical vertebra referred to EP_c. In some normal individuals, N_{11} is inconspicuous or absent.

(c) N_{13} *potential* is a subsequent negative wave of higher amplitude than N_{11}.

(d) P_{14} *potential* is a positive peak widely distributed over scalp. It usually occurs 1msec. after N_{13}.

(e) N_{18} *potential* is a negative peak widely distributed over the scalp and is prominent in C_c-EP_c channel.

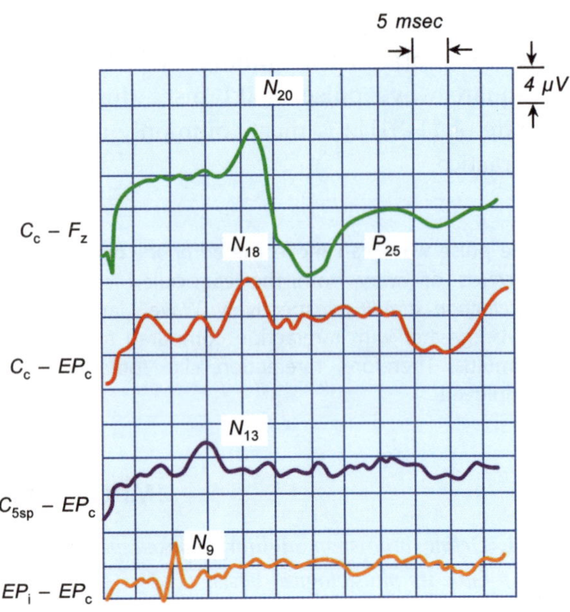

Fig. 3.26.10 Normal Median S.E.P.

(f) N_{20} *potential* is a negative waveform in C_c-F_z channel, and is just preceding the sharp drop off towards the successive cortical positive peak P_{25}.

(iii) Waveform analysis

(a) N_9 *potential*
- Latency is measured from stimulus artefact to its peak. Normal: 9.8msec.
- Amplitude is measured from the peak to the succeeding positive deflection. Normal: 4.8μV.

(b) *Inter peak latency (IPL)* from brachial plexus to spinal cord (N_9–N_{13}) is 3.5msec.

(c) *IPL* from brachial plexus to cortex (N_9–N_{20}) is 9.3 msec.

(d) *Central sensory conduction time* (N_{13}–N_{20}) is 5.7 msec.

(e) N_{20} *potential amplitude* measured from peak to the trough of P_{25} is 3.2 μV.

Note: The amplitudes of waveforms are quite variable and are less important in clinical practice compared to IPLs.

5. *Normal Tibial SEP*

(i) Like median SEP, it also consists of N and P waveforms (see above). The commonly used waveforms are N_8, N_{22}, N_{28} and P_{37}. The genesis of these waveforms is:

Waveforms	Genesis (origin)
N_8	Tibial or Sciatic nerve
N_{22}	Dorsal grey matter of lumbar spinal cord
N_{28}	Cervical spinal cord
P_{37}	Primary sensory cortex

(ii) *Waveforms* (Fig. 3.26.11)

(a) *N_8 potential* is the principal negative peak in PF-K channel (see below);
Normal latency: 8.5 msec.

(b) *N_{22} potential* is the main negative peak, most prominent in L_1 and T_{12} recording.
Normal latency: 22 msec.

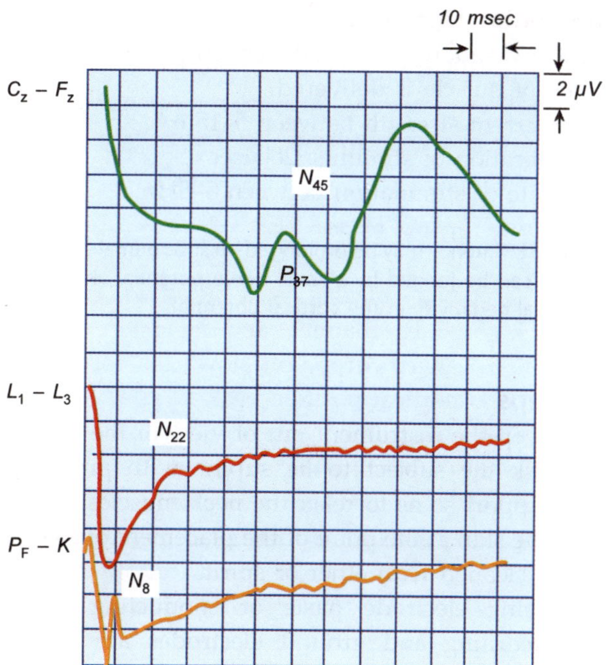

Fig. 3.26.11 Normal waveforms of tibial SEP

(c) *P_{37} potential* is the major initial positive peak in the Cz-Fz channel. It may be preceeded by a small negative potential and followed by a prominent negative peak N_{45}. *Normal latency:* 37.5 msec.

(d) *Inter peak latency (IPL)* of N_{22}-P_{37} gives central sensory conduction time of entire sensory pathway. *Normal:* 15.5 msec.

6. ***Factors affecting SEPs***

(i) *Age:*

(a) In children, N_9 and N_{13} potentials of median SEP occur quite early, while the central conduction is relatively slow.

(b) In old individuals, most of the latencies are longer with increase in N_{13}-N_{19} inter peak latency. The prolongation of latencies is due to peripheral and central changes.

(c) Interpeak latencies are decreased with increase in age.

(ii) *Sex:* Females have a shorter central conduction time compared to males.

(iii) *Drugs:* SEPs are resistant to tranquilizers and sedatives; therefore, sedation can be used for better recording in uncooperative persons.

(iv) *Sleep:* It may change the SEP latency by increasing the amplitude of the peak component compared to awake state.

(v) *Temperature:* There exists a linear correlation between temperature and latency; with temperature changes, the peripheral conduction is affected more than the central. The amplitude of waveform has poor correlation with temperature.

7. ***Clinical Significance of SEP***

(i) The short latency potentials which lie within 50msec after the stimulus are of clinical value because of their uniformity and consistency. Since the sensory pathways are vulnerable to a number of diseases because of their length; therefore, SEP helps evaluate these long sensory pathways (especially proprioceptive) from peripheral nerve to spinal cord and cerebral cortex.

(ii) SEPs play an important role in detecting subclinical sensory abnormalities. In general, *latency abnormalities* are more pronounced in demyelinating (multiple sclerosis) and *amplitude* in ischaemic lesions. A combination of both latency and amplitude abnormalities are found in compressive lesions.

(iii) *Multiple sclerosis* manifests with delay in cortical and subcortical potentials resulting in abnormal interpeak latency with normal peripheral potentials.

(iv) In acute *spinal cord injury,* SEP waveforms are normal below and abnormal at or above the site of lesion.

Note: SEPs are normal if the posterior column is spared.

(v) *In stroke,* SEP recordings are useful for the objective documentation of sensory defitcit. A thalamic haemorrhage is associated with persistant unrecordable median SEP.

Important Note: The changes in SEP are non-specific and not diagnostic of any specific pathology.

III. PROCEDURE

(A) Prerequisites

1. Follow general precautions (page 296)
2. Avoid any stimulant in the breakfast.
3. Obtain the information about sensory symptoms, signs and peripheral nerve injury.
4. In uncooperative subjects or children, mild sedative hypnotics may be used for obtaining an optimal recording.

(B) Equipment set-up for SEP Study as recommended by International Federation of Clinical Neurophysiology (IFCN) Committee.

Suggested Montage for Median SEP

1. Channel 1 : C_c-F_z (cephalic reference)
2. Channel 2 : C_c-EP_c (non-cephalic reference)
3. Channel 3 : C_5S_p-EP_c
4. Channel 4 : EP_i-EP_c
5. Ground electrode position: between stimulating and recording site

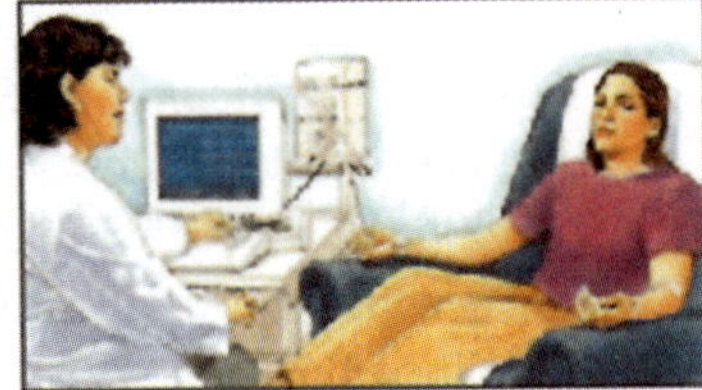

Placement of recording electrodes

(i) Erb's point (EP: 2-3cm above midclavicular point): Left and right EP electrodes are designated as EP_1 and EP_2 respectively or EP_c (contralateral to stimulation) and EP_i. (ipsilateral to stimulation)

(ii) Spinal electrode: At spinous process of the 5th cervical vertebrae (C_5S_p)

(iii) Scalp electrode: 2cm posterior to C_3 and C_4 of 10–20 international system of EEG placement (page 283).

C_4 or C_c: contralateral to stimulation. F_z electrode or ear lobe is used as reference.

Suggested Montage for Tibial SEP

1. Channel 1 : C_z-F_z
2. Channel 2 : T_{12}-T_{10}
3. Channel 3 : L_1-L_3
4. Channel 4 : PF-K
5. Ground electrode position: between stimulating and recording site.

Placement of recording electrodes

(i) At the popliteal fossa (PF) 4–6cm above the popliteal crease, midway between semitendinosus and biceps femoris.,

(ii) Reference electrode: On the medial surface of knee (K)

(iii) Spinal electrode: Over the first lumbar vertebrae (L_1) referred to the third lumbar (L_3); and the tenth thoracic vertebrae (T_{10}) referred to T_{12} or iliac crest.

(iv) Scalp electrode: 2 cm posterior to C_z referred to F_z (page 304)

Recording conditions

1. Filter
   (i) low-filter cut: 5–20Hz
   (ii) High-filter cut: 1–2KHz
2. Amplification of potential between 10,000 and 5,00,000.
3. Sweep duration between 50–60msec.
4. Number of epochs: 1000–2000 responses should be twice averaged. (Since the SEPs are very small).
5. Electrode impedence should be kept below 5 kilo-ohms.

Stimulation Options

A 200 mV square pulse sufficient to produce a painless twitch of muscle is delivered.

1. Current strength between 5–15mA
2. Duration of stimulus: 200μsec
3. Rate of stimulation between 3–8Hz

Note: SEP latency may be prolonged on suboptimal stimulation which can be judged by a small nerve potential and absence of initial negativity in the cortical potential.

(C) Steps

1. Keep the instrument out of view of the subject.
2. Ask the subject to lie supine with proper head support so as to relax the neck muscles.
3. The skin at the point of the placement of electrodes is cleaned with ether or spirit.
4. Using electrode paste or conducting jelly, the recording and ground electrodes are placed as described above (Fig. 3.26.12).

Note: surface electrodes are preferred because of the lesser chances of infection and better stability compared to needle electrodes; also there is no significant difference between surface and needle SEP recording.

5. Check the equipment set-up as described above.
6. The electrodes are connected through the pre-amplifier to the cathode ray oscilloscope.
7. (i) ***For Median SEP recording***
   Stimulation is applied (see above) to median nerve at the wrist keeping the cathode 2 cm proximal to the wrist crease.
   (ii) ***For Tibial SEP recording***
   The stimulus is delivered to the posterior tibial nerve at the ankle. The cathode is placed at the mid-point between tendon achilles and medial malleolus, and the anode 3cm distal to the cathode.

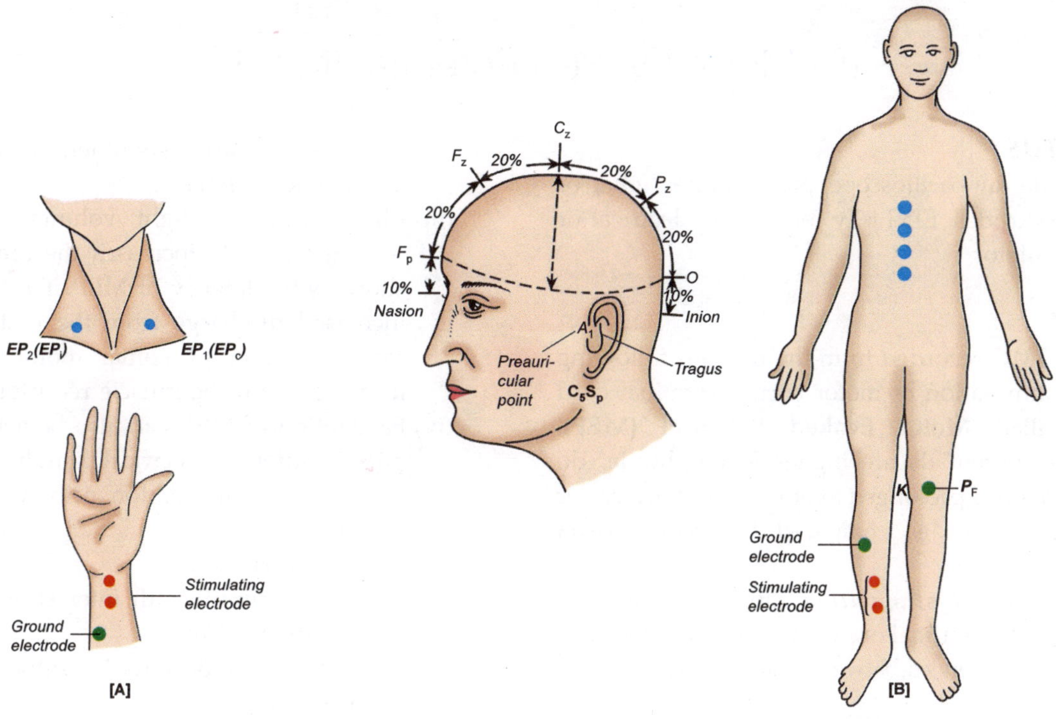

Fig. 3.26.12 Electrode palcement for (A) Median SEP and (B) Tibial SEP. (For abbreviations and details, refer to the text page 294)

> **Important Notes**
> (i) The electrode closest to the generator site gives the optimal recording.
> (ii) Avoid high rate stimulation as it is painful and results in decrease in amplitude and latency.

8. Obtain the response, analyse the SEP waveform for latency, amplitude and interpeak latency; and compare with the normal (Page 310).

III. PRECAUTIONS

1. Follow general precautions; refer to page 296.
2. Follow all the pretest instructions strictly, page 312.
3. The stimulation should not be applied over or adjacent to catheters or wires going to heart or great vessels.
4. Avoid high rate stimulation because it is painful and results in the progressive loss of amplitude and decrease in latency.
5. The recording should be twice averaged to check for reproducibility.
6. There should be no bridge of current between the two limbs of the stimulator due to the seepage of conducting jelly. This may reduce the strength of the current.

IMPORTANT VIVA-VOCE QUESTIONS

Q.1. *Define somatosensory evoked potentials (SEPs).*
Ans. Page 309.

Q.2. *Differentiate between large and small sensory axons.*
Ans. Page 309.

Q.3. *Give the neural pathways for proprioception.*
Ans. Page 310.

Q.4. *What is the genesis of SEPs?*
Ans. Page 310.

Q.5. *Name the commonly used waveform of median SEP. Give the origin, latency and amplitude of each potential.*
Ans. Page 310.

Q.6. *Draw and label a normal median SEP.*
Ans. Page 310.

Q.7. *Describe the normal tibial SEPs.*
Ans. Page 310.

Q.8. *Mention the factors influencing SEPs.*
Ans. Page 311.

Q.9. *Give the clinical application of SEP.*
Ans. Page 311.

Q.10. *What condition needs to be fulfilled prior to SEP study?*
Ans. Page 312.

Q.11. *Give the electrode placement sites for recording median and tibial SEPs.*
Ans. Page 312.

Q.12. *Enumerate the precautions to be followed during SEP study.*
Ans. See above.

(E) Motor Evoked Potential (M.E.P)

I. APPARATUS

Subject, cathode ray oscilloscope, pre-amplifier, ether or spirit, EEG electrodes, EEG jelly (or paste), Electrical or magnetic stimulator

II. THEORY

1. The EMG recorded from the muscles following the stimulation of motor cortex or spinal cord is called **Motor Evoked Potential (MEP).** These potentials are higher in amplitude, do not require prolonged averaging and are easier to carry out as compared to other evoked potentials.
2. ***Transcranial stimulation*** can be carried out either by electrical or magnetic stimulation. The main differences between the two are given in table 3.26.3.

Table 3.26.3 Electrical and magnetic stimulation compared

Electrical stimulation	Magnetic stimulation
1. It is carried out either by a bipolar or unipolar montage; the latter has the advantage of locality, greater penetration to stimulate the underlying brain structures and achieving the stimulation	1. It activates the pyramidal axons directly and more efficiently due to more repetitive discharges produced. It is able to stimulate the deep structures also. at lower current strength.
2. It is painful.	2. It is painless.
3. Unipolar stimulation is carried out by anode which is placed on the motor area and cathode along the head circumference.	3. Magnetic stimulator delivers two types of pulses: *monophasic* and *biphasic* (or *polyphasic*) stimulus induced current. There is no difference in the latency of MEP by two types of magnetic stimulators.
4. *MEP latency:* shorter.	4. Longer
5. *Cost:* low	5. High

3. ***Factors affecting MEP***
   (i) *Intensity of transcranial stimulation:* On increasing the current strength, the greater area of cerebral cortex is stimulated and MEP can be recorded from a number of muscles with an increasing amplitude, a shorter latency and longer duration.
   (ii) *Type of the muscle:* The hand muscles have the lowest threshold followed by wrist extensors, wrist flexors, arm, shoulder, trunk, leg, foot, and pelvic muscles.
   (iii) *Muscle tone:* A slight voluntary contraction of target muscle increases the amplitude and shortens the latency of MEP. This is due to an increased discharge from the motor area and the facilitation of spinal motor neurons by impulses from the muscle receptors.
   (iv) Facilitation of MEP can also be achieved by:
      (a) Conditioning electrical stimulus to the target muscle or its tendon prior to transcranial stimulus.
      (b) Painful stimuli.
      (c) Paired stimuli with inter stimulus interval less than 0.5 msec.
      (d) Contraction of muscles other than target muscles.

Note: MEPs are restricted to the muscles contralateral to the side of cortical stimulation. The direct (or uncrossed) corticospinal fibres are too less to cause motor response on the ipsilateral side.

4. ***Central Motor Conduction Time (CMCT)***
   (i) The differece in the latencies between cortical and spinal stimulation is known as CMCT. It includes:
      (a) True time for central motor conduction
      (b) Time taken for at least one synaptic delay; and
      (c) The conduction time in proximal root
   (ii) The *normal values of* CMCT (in msec) for diferent muscles are:

Muscle	Latency (msec)	Right-to-left asymmetry (msec)	CMCT (msec)
(a) Deltoid	10.6	0.5	4.9
(b) Biceps	11.6	0.4	4.9
(c) Thenar group of muscles	20.1	0.4	6.4
(d) Tibialis anterior	26.7	0.7	13.2
(e) Abductor hallucis	35.9	0.6	12.9

   (iii) CMCT latency value decreases with increasing age and reaches the adult value by adolescence due to the myelination of pyramidal tracts.
5. ***Clinical Significance of MEP***
   Like other evoked potential, changes in MEP

studies are non-specific and not diagnostic of any specific pathology. It may reveal two major types of abnormalities: prolongation of CMCT and inexcitabillity of motor pathways:

(i) *Prolongation of CMCT:* It indicates slowing in central pathways. This is seen in demyelinating condition like multiple sclerosis.

(ii) *Inexcitability of motor pathways:* This occurs in degeneration or damage to corticospinal tracts due to motor neuron disease, infarction, trauma, etc. It manifests either as absence of any response or a small amplitude and short duration MEP.

Note: Since the amplitude in normal subjects has a wide range of variations, amplitude changes are not very useful clinically.

III. PROCEDURE

(A) Prerequisites

1. The subject's and the examiner's magnetic belongings (watch, ring, chain, credit cards) should be removed and kept at least 50cm away from the stimulator.

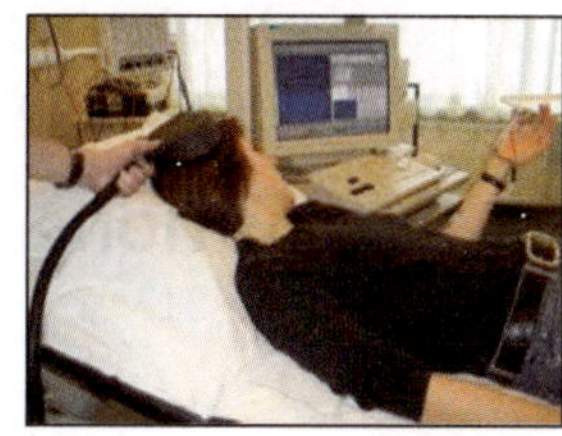

2. The MEP studies are contraindicated in patients with cardiac pacemaker, cochlear device and intracranial clipping or wiring, as stimulation test can dislodge them.
3. Transcranial stimulation should be avoided in the patients with uncontrolled seizures.
4. MEP studies are not advisable in the patients taking hypnotics, tranquilizer, anticonvulsants and antispastic drugs, as these drugs may affect the excitability threshold.
5. Follow general instructions (page 296).

(B) Steps

1. Keep the instrument out of view of the subject.
2. Explain the test procedure to the subject so as to get the maximum cooperation.
3. Ask the subject to lie supine with proper head support so as to relax the neck muscles.
4. ***Equipment set-up***
   (i) Keep electrode impedence below 5 kilo-ohms.
   (ii) Set filter band width between 20–2000Hz, *i.e.* (low cut: 20Hz, high cut: 2000Hz).
   (iii) Duration of post stimulus analysis time:
      (a) for upper limb: 50 msec.
      (b) for lower limb: 100 msec.
5. Using electrode paste or conducting jelly the electrodes are placed in proper position as described below:

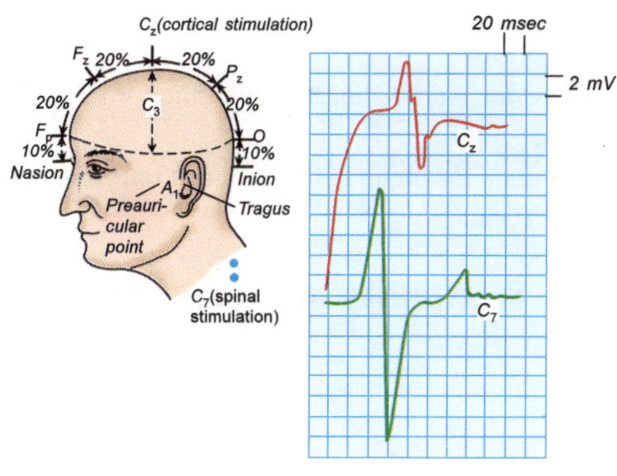

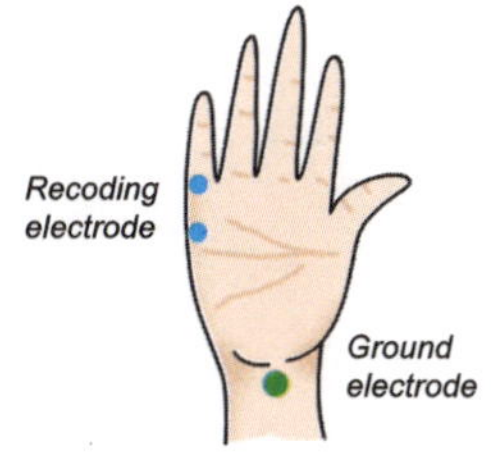

(A)

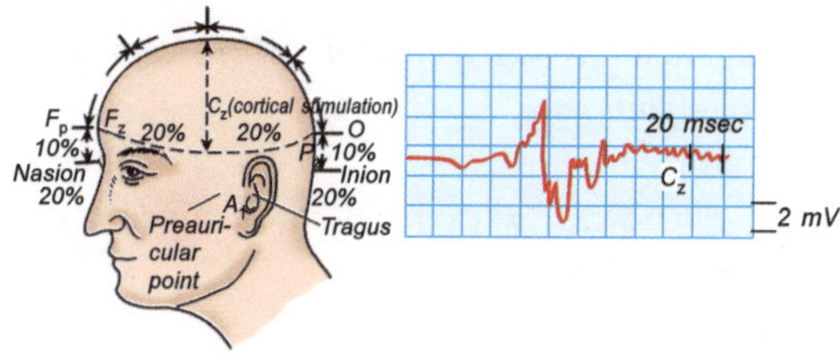

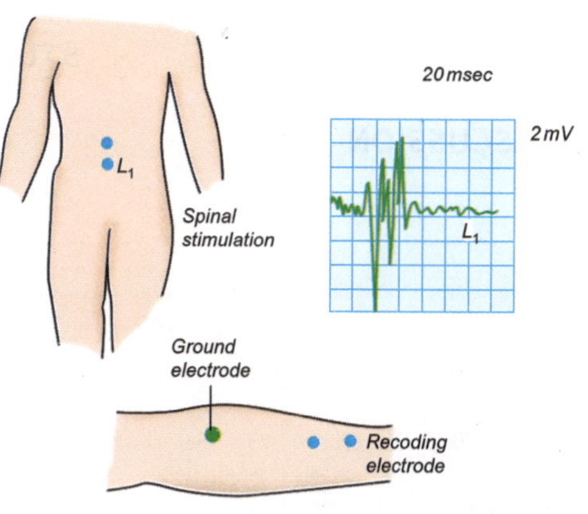

(B)

Fig. 3.26.13 Electrode placement for electrical stimulation and recording of MEPs to abductor (A) digiti minimi and (B) tibialis anterior.

Electrode placement for electrical stimulation (Fig. 3.26.13)

Important Note: The MEPs are commonly recorded from the contralateral upper or lower limb muscles. The common recording sites are:
- *In upper limb:* biceps, abductor digiti minimi and abductor pollicis brevis
- *In lower limb:* Tibialis anterior and extensor digitorum brevis

Cortical Stimulation	Spinal Stimulation
1. *For upper limb*	
Anode is placed 5–7cm lateral and 2cm anterior to interaural line; and cathode 7cm away from the anode over the vertex.	Cathode is placed over the cervical spine and the anode proximally.
2. *For lower limb*	
Anode is placed 2cm anterior to C_z in 10–20 international electrode placement system (page 283); and cathode is placed 7cm posterior to C_z.	Cathode is placed on the 1st lumbar spine and the anode proximally.

Note: For *magnetic stimulation*, the magnetic coil should be centred on the anodal position as described for electrical stimulation.

6. For recording MEPs from the target muscles, the surface EMG electrodes are placed over the muscle. (refer to page 147).
7. The electrodes area connected through the pre-amplifiers to the cathode ray oscilloscope.
8. The stimulator is placed on the vertex and ***cortical stimulation*** is performed. The stimulator output is gradually increased in steps of 10–20%. The patient is asked to contract the target muscle slightly (for the optimal facilitaion of MEP) and then to relax it immediately after the stimulus is felt.
9. On getting a satisfactory recording, three repetitions are carried out at an interval of at least 5 secs.
10. Measure the shortest latency and maximum base to peak or peak-to-peak amplitudes.
11. Perform the ***Spinal Stimulation*** in the similar manner but the patient is asked to relax the target muscle during the procedure.
12. Calculate the difference in the latencies between cortical and spinal stimulation; this gives a measure of central motor conduction time (CMCT).

IV. PRECAUTIONS

Refer to page 313.

IMPORTANT VIVA-VOCE QUESTIONS

Q.1. *Define Motor evoked potential (MEP) and give its clinical significance.*
Ans. Page 314.
Q.2. *Give differences between electrical and magnetic transcranial stimulation.*
Ans. Page 314.
Q.3. *Enumerate the factors affecting MEP.*
Ans. Page 314.
Q.4. *What do you understand by 'central motor conduction time' (CMCT)?*
Ans. Page 314.
Q.5. *Give the physio-clinical significance of CMCT.*
Ans. Page 315.
Q.6. *Mention the preset instruction and contraindication for MEP studies.*
Ans. Page 315.
Q.7. *List the precautions associated with MEP studies.*
Ans. Page 313.

STUDY NOTES

RESULTS AND DISCUSSION

....

....

....

....

....

....

Unit IV
Mammalian Experiments (Dog/Rabbit)

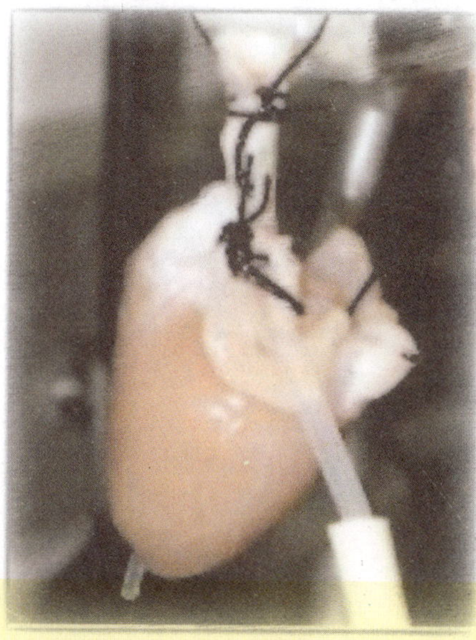

Date: ....

1 Recording of the Movements of Isolated Rabbit's Intestine and Effect of Drugs and Ions

I. APPARATUS

Dales organ bath, Tyrode's solution, thread and needle, petridish, frontal writing lever, aerator, scissors, thermometer

Dales Organ Bath

This apparatus consists of: (Fig. 4.1.1)

1. Large **perspex rectangular bath** meant for keeping water at appropriate body temperature (37°C) with the help of a **heating element** and a **thermostat** and a **stirrer**
2. A **central glass organ bath** of 20 ml capacity and provided with an outlet
3. A **hollow bent glass tube**, curved at the lower end for fixing intestine. This tube can be inserted in the centre of the organ bath and is also used for passing air (or O_2) through the solution.
4. A **frontal writing lever** can be attached to the assembly for recording the movements of the isolated intestine on the drum.

Tyrode's solution: composition and function

Glucose	: 0.1 gm/dL	Provides nutrition
NaCl	: 0.8 gm/dL	(i) Helps to maintain iso-tonicity
KCl	: 0.02 gm/dL	(ii) Provides optimal electric condition
$CaCl_2$	: 0.02 gm/dL	

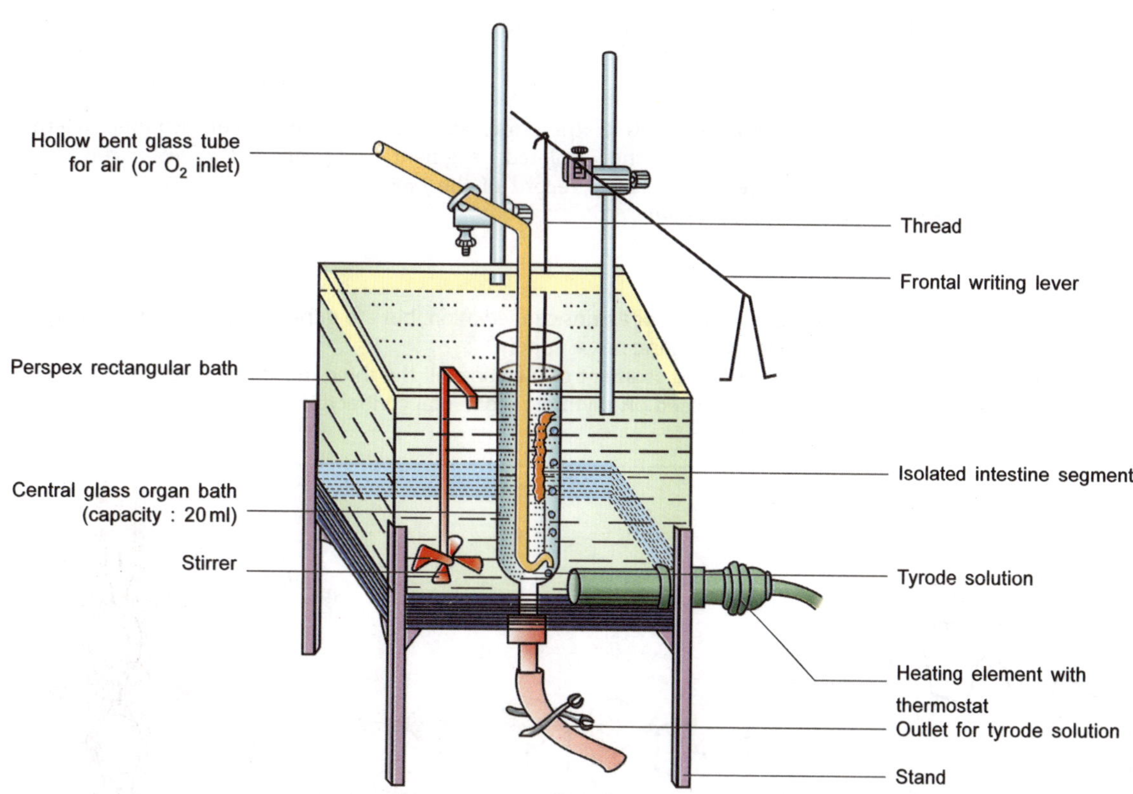

Fig. 4.1.1 Dales organ bath: set-up to record the movements of isolated rabbit's intestine

$MgCl_2$: 0.01 gm/dL Helps to regulate intestinal motility by competing with Ca^{2+}; in fact, it decreases contraction. However, this gets compensated by stretching the segment.

$NaHCO_3$: 0.01 gm/dL
NaH_2PO_4 : 0.005 gm/dL } Helps maintain pH between 7.4 to 7.6

Add water to make 100 ml.

II. THEORY

1. The movements of the intestine are due to the rhythmic contractions affecting both coats (the circular and longitudinal), causing alteration in the lumen as well as varying curvature of different coils.
2. An isolated segment of small intestine continues to contract and responds to various stimuli, if kept in a suitable medium and at optimum temperature.

Three kinds of intestinal movements are generally observed: (Refer to Table 4.1.1 and Fig. 4.1.2)

III. PROCEDURE

1. Keep a petridish containing Tyrode's solution and threaded needle ready. Fill the organ bath with Tyrode's solution and outer bath with water at 37°C.
2. Stun a rabbit; open the abdomen through a

Table 4.1.1 Different types of movements of the small intestine (Fig. 4.1.2)

A. Muscle tones (or tonus)	B. Rhythmic Segmental or pendular contractions	C. Peristaltic contractions
(i) These are irregular (asynchronous) continuous contractions which are myogenic in origin, *i.e.* inherent property of the smooth muscle.	(i) These are regular rhythmic contractions and pacemaker is responsible for their initiation which is located in the second part of duodenum in longitudinal muscle layer *(that is why this segment is preferred* for study purpose).	(i) These are regular rhythmic slow contractions due to the inherent property of the smooth muscle, and depend on the integrity of myenteric plexus.
(ii) Increase or decrease in muscle tone is recorded as the shifting of baseline record up or down respectively.	(ii) Occurs in several regions of GIT with varying frequencies (duodenum: 12/min; ileum: 9/min).	(ii) These contractions propagate @ 2.25 cm/sec; increased by lumen distension; therefore, obstruction to lumen causes them to disappear.
	(iii) Stretch-sensitive; therefore, slightly stretching the isolated segment provides a better record of the *rate of movements.*	(iii) These contractions determine the *amplitude of movements.*

Important Notes:

(i) All these intestinal movements can occur in the absence of extrinsic innervation, but are dependent on the integrity of myenteric plexus. However, their activity can be modified by extrinsic nerve supply.

(ii) During the recording of the contractions of an isolated segment of intestine, all the three movements get recorded; *tone* mainly forms baseline with peristaltic movements superimposed on rhythmic segmental contractions.

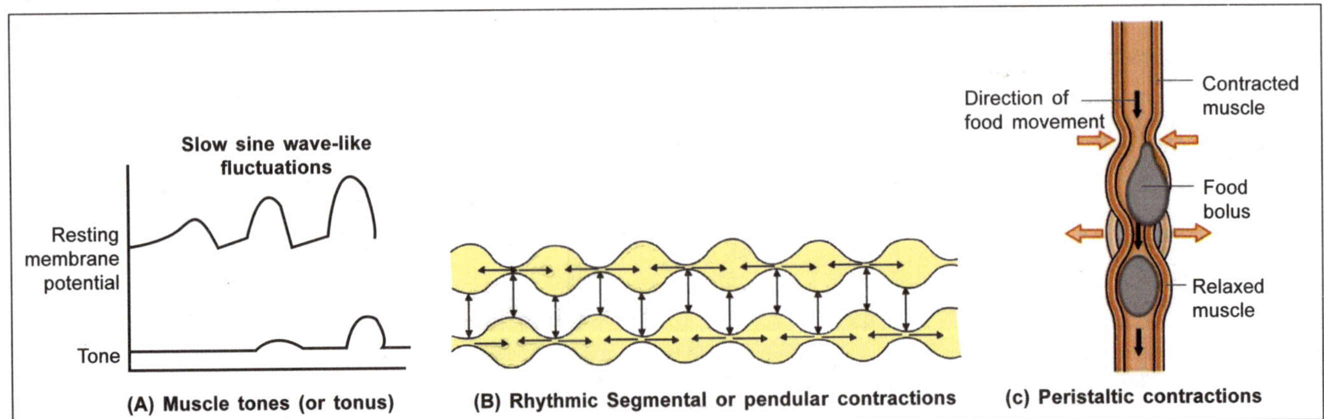

Fig. 4.1.2 Movements of small intestine

midline incision and remove 5 or 6 small segments (each about 2-3 cm) of jejunum, close to the duodenum.

3. Rinse the intestinal lumen with Tyrode's solution with the help of pipette or by pushing gently the solution from a syringe. Place the segment in well-aerated (or oxygenated) Tyrode's solution in a petridish.
4. Pass the threaded needle through the segment's wall about 3 mm from one of its cut ends; remove the needle and make a loop from the thread. Repeat the same at the other end but tie a long thread for attaching to the lever.
5. Mount the segment in the organ bath filled with Tyrode's solution by securing the thread loop to the curved end of the glass tube. Maintain aeration/oxygenation of the Tyrode solution.
6. Set the drum revolving at its slowest speed (2.5 mm/sec); keep a watch of *intestinal movements;* it should show wormlike movements. The beat occur @ 10-20 times/minute; the tone of the muscle improves with aeration/oxygenation as indicated by the level of the lever.
7. Maintain aeration (or oxygenation) by allowing it to pass through Tyrode's solution at slow rate of about 2-3 bubbles/sec; keep the temperature of the water at 37°C.
8. Attach the isolated intestine segment to the frontal writing lever and record movements on a slow moving drum.
9. For recording the effect of drugs/ions, add 0.5 to 1 ml of drug or ions by a pipette or syringe and mix. Mark the point of adding drug on the graph. After recording the effect, drain off the organ bath and fill it with fresh Tyrode's solution. Wait for 5-10 minutes. Study the action of other drugs after intestine has shown normal movements.
10. Use the following drugs in the given order:
    (i) Acetyl choline - 1:100,000 (i.e. 10 μgm/ml); add 1 ml.
    (ii) Eserine (physostigmine); add 0.2 ml.
    (iii) Adrenaline - 1:100,000 (i.e. 10 μg/ml); add 0.5 ml.
    (iv) Atropine - 0.01% (i.e. 100 μg/ml); add 1 ml.
    (v) Repeat acetyl choline after atropinisation.
    (vi) Histamine - 50 μg/ml; add 1 ml.
    (vii) 1% KCl solution - add 1 ml.
    (viii) 1% $CaCl_2$ solution - add 1 ml.
    (ix) 1% barium chloride solution - add a few drops.

IV. PRECAUTIONS

1. Use only freshly prepared Tyrode solution.
2. Do not mishandle the preparation, else it will be ruined
3. Tyrode solution should be at proper temperature (37°C) and well aerated or oxygenated.
4. Isolate either the duodenal or jejunal segments; these two work well.
5. Do not apply excessive stretch.
6. Ensure that lumen is patent while fixing the preparation.

IMPORTANT VIVA-VOCE QUESTIONS

Q.1. *Give the composition and functions of Tyrode's solution.*

Ans. Page 319.

Q.2. *Give the capacity of central glass organ bath.*

Ans. 20 ml.

Q.3. *What will happen if the lumen of the intestinal segment is obstructed?*

Ans. Lumen obstruction results in peristaltic contractions to disappear; then only rhythmic segmental contraction will be recorded.

Q.4. *What is the effect of varying the length of isolated intestinal segment on the movements?*

Ans. The longitudinal stretching of the isolated segment increase the tone and amplitude of contractions. However, there is an optimal length at which these responses are maximum; stretching beyond this point produces opposite effect.

Q.5. *What is the clinical significance of this experiment?*

Ans. This demonstration provides a useful information about:
(i) atonic constipation;
(ii) intestinal spasm resulting in colic pain;
(iii) how to preserve intestine movements during surgical handling.

Q.6. *Describe the effects and mechanism of the action of various agents which influence the movements of an isolated intestinal segment.*

Ans. See Table 4.1.2 and Fig. 4.1.3.

Q.7. *Describe the various types of movements of the small intestine. Can you tell which type of movements you are recording?*

Ans. Three major types of intestinal movements occur in an isolated intestinal preparation provided optimal temperature and pH of the medium is maintained (Table 4.1.1):

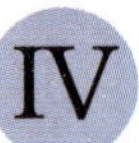

Table 4.1.2 Effect and mechanism of the action of various agents on the movements of isolated rabbit's intestine

Agent	Effect (Fig. 4.1.3)	Mechanism of action
(A) STIMULANTS		
1. Parasympathomimetics (i) Acetyl-choline 1:100,000 (10μg/ml) (ii) Carbachol	Increase in tone, frequency and height of contraction	(i) By increasing Na^+ and Ca^{2+} influx, increases RMP (depolarizes the membrane) (ii) Increases spike frequency (A-ch action is brief whereas carbachol action is longer and more stable).
(iii) Anticholinesterase (a) Eserine (physostigmine) (b) Neostigmine	Potentiates the effect of A-ch, thus a larger contraction is obtained	Inhibits acetyl-cholinesterase which destroys the A-ch (used in treatment of atonic constipation)
2. Sympatholytics (α and β adrenergic blockers).	No role in isolated preparation	Blocks the action of adrenaline in vivo
3. Cold saline; stretch	Increases the tone and height of contraction	Stimulates cholinergic nerve endings to cause release of A-ch
4. 1% $CaCl_2$	Increases the height of contraction	Increases spontaneous contraction due to Na^+ influx
5. 1% $BaCl_2$	Marked increase in frequency and force of contraction	Directly stimulant to smooth muscle producing violent colicky pain; hence used as rat poison
6. Histamine	Increases the frequency of contraction.	(i) Direct stimulant of GIT muscle. (ii) Facilitates the action of A-ch.
(B) DEPRESSANTS		
1. Sympathomimetics Adrenaline 1:100,000 (10 μgm/ml)	Decreases the tone, frequency and height of contraction	(i) By decreasing RMP (hyperpolarization of the membrane) (ii) Decreases spike frequency (β-effect mediated through cAMP which increases intracellular binding of Ca^{2+}; α-effect leads to increase Ca^{2+} efflux.)
2. Parasympatholytic e.g. Atropine (0.01%) - 100 μg/ml.	-do- (more effective in vivo)	Abolishes the action of A-ch by competitive inhibition; therefore, blocks extrinsic control only, thereby arresting the spasm but not the normal peristalsis
3. Warm saline	Decreases the tone and height of contraction	Opposite to the action of cold saline
4. NaCl	No effect	Spontaneous activity in smooth muscle is not affected by Na^+ influx
5. Papaverine	Decreases the tone and height of contraction.	Direct action, producing relaxation of smooth muscle

Table 4.1.3 Effect of drugs and ions on isolated rabbit's intestine

Agent	Effect on intestinal movement			Remarks
	Tone (or tonus)	Rate	Amplitude (or height) (in cm)	
1. Acetyl choline (A-ch)–1 : 100,000 (1 ml)				
2. Eserine (physostigmine)–0.2 ml				
3. Adrenaline–1 : 100,000 (0.5 ml)				
4. Atropine–0.01% (1 ml)				
5. A-ch after atropinisation				
6. Histamine–1 ml (50μgm/ml)				
7. 1% KCl–1 ml				
8. 1% $CaCl_2$–1 ml				
9. 1% $BaCl_2$–Few drops				

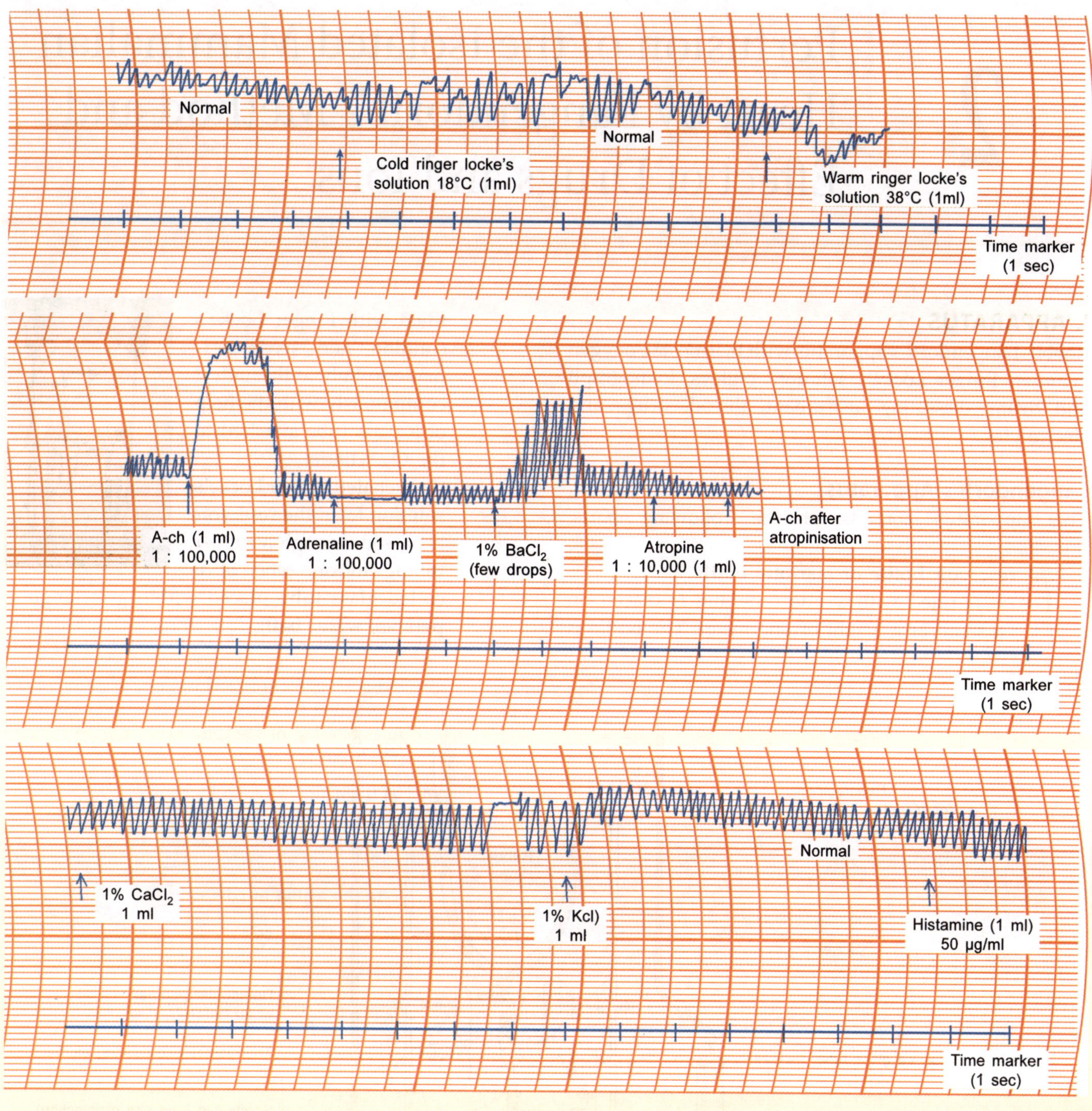

Fig. 4.1.3 Effect of various agents on the movements of isolated rabbit's intestine

STUDY NOTES

RESULTS AND DISCUSSION

....

....

....

....

Date: ....

2 Perfusion of the Isolated Mammalian Heart by Langendorff's Method and Effect of Drugs and Ions

I. APPARATUS

Rabbit, Langendorff's apparatus with thermostat, oxygen cylinder, Ringer Locke's solution, pulleys, kymograph and drum, dissecting instrument, thread, drugs and electrolytes

Langendorff's Apparatus

This apparatus consists of the following parts: (Fig. 4.2.1)

1. **A reservoir bottle or mariotte bottle**
   (i) It is fitted with a side tube and is placed on a stand at a height of one meter. The bottle is filled with Ringer Locke's solution and oxygen is made to bubble through it continuously with the help of a glass tube attached to the O_2 cylinder.

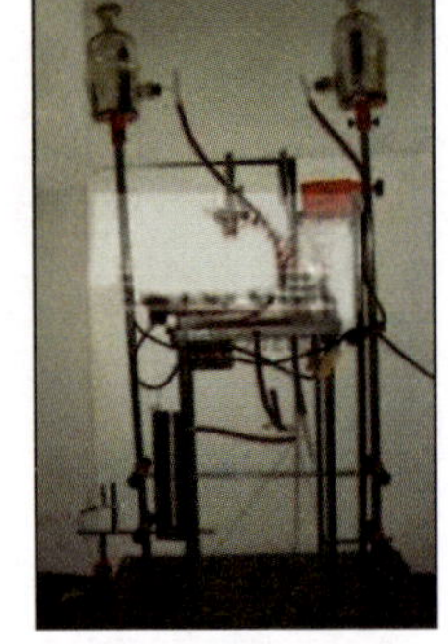

   (ii) Oxygenated Ringer Locke's solution from the reservoir is passed through a rubber tubing to one end of a **coiled glass tube placed** within a rectangular **perspex water bath.**

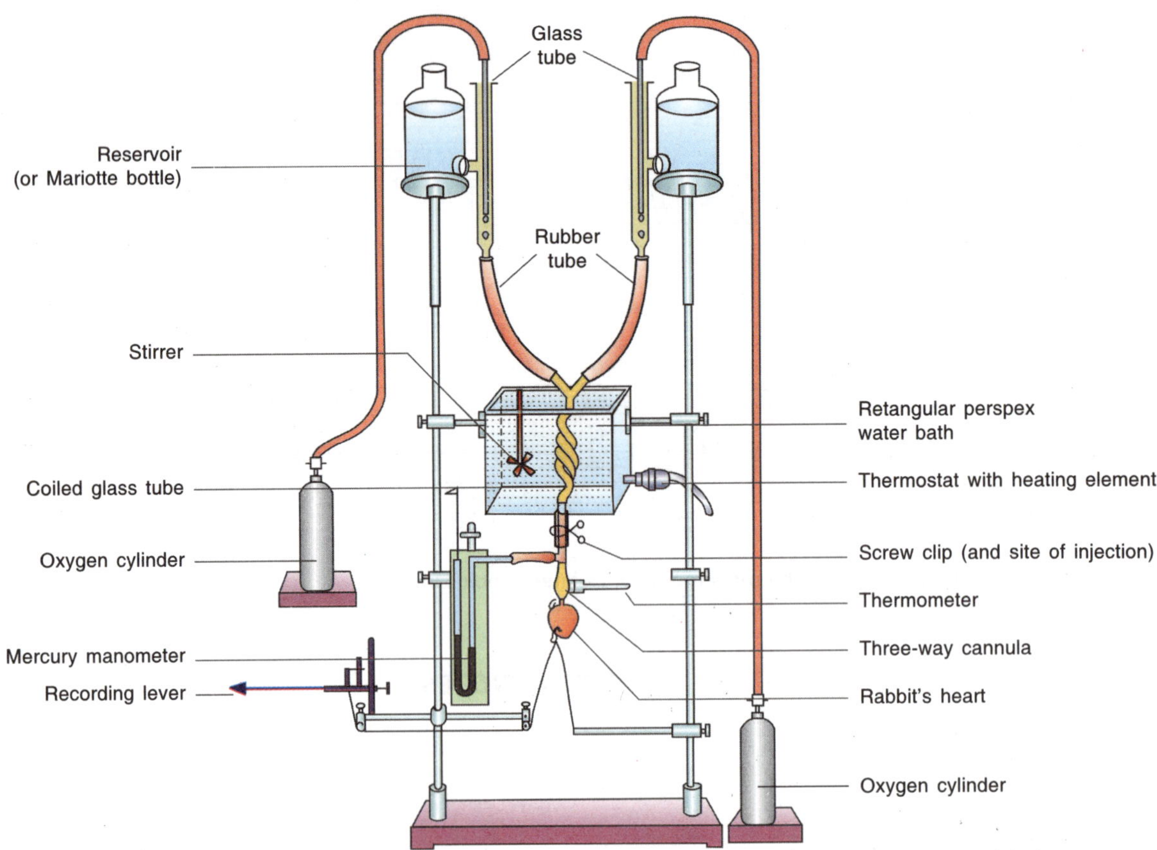

Fig. 4.2.1 Langendorff's apparatus: Assembly for the perfusion of the isolated mammalian heart

2. The water bath is fitted with **a heating element, a thermostat** and **an electric stirrer**. All these help to maintain the temperature of water in the bath at 37°C.
3. The other end of the coiled tube is connected through a rubber tubing to a **cannula** having a central bulb, two-side arms and a nozzle:
   (i) One of the *side arms* is used to accommodate the thermometer and the other side arm is connected to a mercury manometer for recording perfusion pressure.
   (ii) The nozzle is directed downwards which is to be inserted into the aorta of an isolated heart preparation.
4. The apparatus is also fitted with **two pulleys** and a **lever** for the transmission of the contractions of the heart to the kymograph.

Ringer Locke's Solution: Composition and functions

NaCl	: 0.9 gm/dL	(i) To maintain isotonicity
KCl	: 0.042 gm/dL	(ii) Ca^{2+} keeps the heart ready in a state of spontaneous contraction
$CaCl_2$	: 0.024 gm/dL	
$NaHCO_3$	: 0.015 gm/dL	To maintain the pH between 7.1 to 7.6
Glucose	: 0.1 gm/dL	To provide nutrition

Aqua to add to make 100 ml.

Important Note: *Glucose should be added on the same day; if added earlier, it gets fermented and alters the pH of the solution.*

II. PRINCIPLE

To maintain a mammalian heart beating outside the body, the heart must be placed in adequate optimal conditions as regards oxygen supply, temperature and composition of the perfusion fluid. The Ringer Locke's solution with continuous bubbling of pure O_2 through the fluid makes it suitable for the mammalian heart; the rabbit heart is most suitable for this experiment.

III. PROCEDURE

1. Fill the reservoir bottle with Ringer Locke's solution; adjust the reducing valve on the O_2 cylinder so that a good stream of O_2 bubbles may continuously pass through it.
2. Fill the rectangular perspex bath water; connect it to the mains; adjust the thermostat so that the temperature of the Ringer Locke's solution coming out from the cannula may be maintained at 37°C.
3. The rabbit is then stunned by a hard blow on its head; quickly expose the heart by cutting the thorax; and separate the pericardium.
4. Hold the heart up and cut through the roots of the lungs, the venae cavae and aorta. At least 1 cm of the aorta should be left attached to the heart.
5. Rapidly transfer the excised heart into the oxygenated Ringer Locke's chilled solution contained in a petri-dish. Squeeze out the blood clots.
6. Make a short cut in the wall of the pulmonary artery to facilitate the passage of the outflow fluid.
7. Identify the ascending aorta, slide it on to the nozzle of the cannula, taking care that the nozzle does not penetrate the aortic valve. Ligate the aorta securely around the cannula. (Fig. 4.2.2)

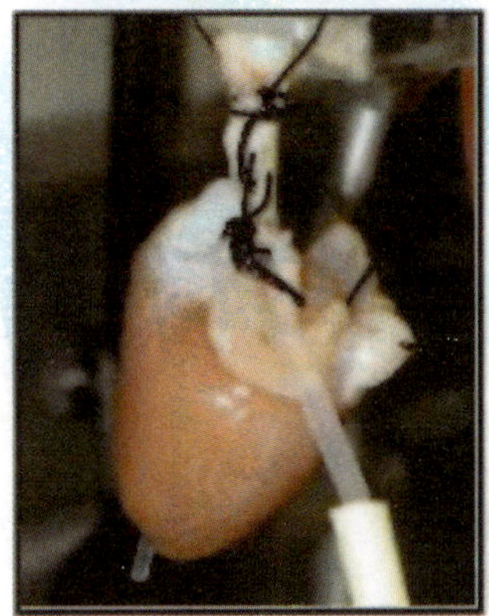
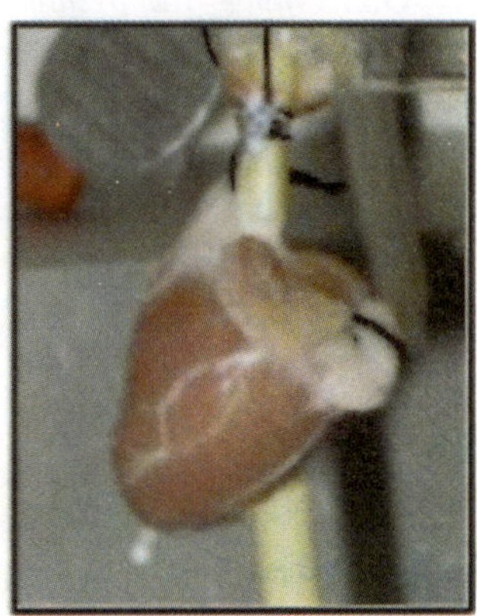

Fig. 4.2.2 Cannulation of aorta

8. The flow of Ringer Locke's solution is now increased by opening the screw clip. The perfusion pressure should be fixed around 60-80 mmHg; the warm oxygenated Ringer Locke's fluid will soon revive the heart.
9. Now pass a pin attached with a thread through the apex of the ventricle and take the thread over a system of pulleys and rod to connect to the recording lever. Record a normal cardiogram on a slow-moving drum (speed 2.5 mm/sec.).
10. After taking a normal cardiogram, study the effect of the following agents in the order given by injecting through the side rubber tube with the help of a syringe using hypodermic needle:
    (i) Adrenaline 1:100,000 (10 μgm/ml); inject 1 ml.
    (ii) Acetylcholine 1:100,000 (10 μg/ml); inject 0.5 ml.
    (iii) Atropine sulphate 1:2000 (0.5 mg/ml); inject 1 ml.

(iv) Effect of A-ch after atropinisation.
(v) 1% $CaCl_2$ solution; inject 1 ml.
(vi) 1% NaCl solution; inject 1 ml.
(vii) 1% KCl solution; inject 1 ml.
(viii) *Effect of anoxaemia.* When the heart beat has once more returned to normal, the O_2 supply to the Ringer Locke's solution is stopped. The heart continues to beat normally for some time, but soon the contractions become weaker; the heart stops in diastole if the supply of O_2 is not restored in time.

Important Notes

1. Wash out each drug and wait for the heart beats to become normal before proceeding to the next.
2. Study the effect of drugs by injecting alternately with stimulators and depressors; this allows the preparation to work longer.

IV. PRECAUTIONS

1. The heart after removal from the animal body should be transferred as quickly as possible into cold oxygenated Ringer Locke's fluid.
2. The end of the cannula should lie well above the coronary arteries.

IMPORTANT VIVA-VOCE QUESTIONS

Q.1. *Give the composition and function of Ringer Locke's solution.*

Ans. Page 325.

Q.2. *Why is the freshly prepared Ringer Locke's solution preferred/ideal for the experiment?*

Ans. Page 325.

Q.3. *How will you check the pH of Ringer Locke's solution?*

Ans. By using the litmus paper; pH being alkaline turns the red litmus paper blue.

Q.4. *If pH of Ringer Locke's solution is less or more, how can it be adjusted to normal?*

Ans. (i)Less pH means acidic pH, add alkali to the solution such as $NaHCO_3$.

(ii)More pH means alkaline pH, add acid to the solution e.g. NaH_2PO_4.

Q.5. *Give the path of perfusate.*

Ans. The perfusate enters retrogradely through the **aorta** into the coronary arteries (right and left), perfuses the **myocardial tissues** and returns through the **coronary veins** (superficial and deep system) mainly to the **right atrium** from where it is thrown to the **exterior** via inferior and superior venae cavas. The part of the fluid which returns directly to the left ventricle via thebesian vein gets recirculated due to the contraction of ventricles into the aorta.

Q.6. *What will happen if coronaries are tied along with the aorta to the cannula?*

Ans. In this situation, whole of the perfusate enters the left ventricle resulting in the enlargement of the heart; the overstretching of left ventricle makes the preparation non-functional.

Q.7. *What will happen to the preparation if the aortic valves are incompetent?*

Ans. See answer 6.

Q.8. *The isolated heart preparation tends to become oedematous after some time. Explain why.*

Ans. Since the perfusate fluid does not contain any colloid substance which can counteract the oncotic pressure of the tissue fluid, therefore, it loses its fluid to the tissues.

Q.9. *What is the effect of altering the perfusion pressure?*

Ans. Normal perfusion pressure should be maintained between 60-80 mmHg; if it increases, perfusate enters the left ventricle resulting in the enlargement of the heart (see question 6). If perfusion pressure falls below 60 mmHg, insufficient tissue perfusion results in the failure of the preparation after some time.

Q.10. *Give the relevance of perfusion pressure to medical physiology.*

Ans. The incidence of myocardial infarction is more in the early morning hours of sleep, as the perfusion pressure is minimum at this time. Moreover, the over-correction of systemic BP in hypertensive individuals may precipitate the myocardial infarction.

Q.11. *Is it possible to demonstrate the Starling Law of the heart with this preparation?*

Ans. Yes, it is possible by modifying this preparation to Starling heart-lung preparation.

Q.12. *Describe the effects and mechanism of the action of various agents on the isolated mammalian heart.*

Ans. Refer to Table 4.2.1 and Fig. 4.2.3.

Table 4.2.1 Effect and mechanism of the action of variables on the perfused isolated rabbit's heart

Agent	Effect (Fig. 4.2.3)	Mechanism of action
(A) STIMULANTS		
1. Sympathomimetics (i) Adrenaline 1:100,000 (10 μg/ml) - inject 1 ml (ii) Nor-Adrenaline	Marked increase in heart rate and force of contraction (via β-receptors) Greater effect as it potentiates the effect of adrenaline by inhibiting MAO enzyme which destroys adrenaline.	(i) Increases Na^+ influx and decreases the K^+ efflux of nodal tissues. (ii) Activates cAMP to cause increased Ca^{2+} influx in both atria and ventricular fibres.
2. Parasympatholytic: Atropine sulphate 1:2000 (0.5 mg/ml) - 1 ml	Increases heart rate and force of contraction	Acts peripherally by blocking the muscarinic action of A-ch (however, it cannot prevent the formation of A-ch).
3. Warm saline	Increases the heart rate and initially slight increase in the force of contraction by decreasing the viscosity.	Increases the permeability of nodal tissue to Na^+ (mainly).
4. $CaCl_2$ (1%) - 1 ml	Increases HR and the force of contraction; finally heart stops in systole (***calcium rigor***).	(i) Decreases the threshold potential of SAN. (ii) Directly activates contractile process; in large doses, heart relaxes less in diastole to stop in systole finally.
5. Nicotine 2% - 0.5 ml	Increases HR.	Paralysis of synapse in the ganglia
6. Digitalis (few drops)	Increases the force of contraction.	Direct stimulator; in large doses, diastole duration decreases and heart stops in systole.
(B) DEPRESSANTS		
1. Parasympathomimetics (i) A-ch (1:100,000) 10 μg/ml - 0.5 ml.	Decreases HR and the force of contraction; acts via muscarinic receptors.	(i) Increases the K^+ efflux of nodal tissues (hyperpolarization)
(ii) Pilocarpine	-do-	(ii) Decreases the Ca^{2+} influx of the myocardium.
(iii) Anticholinesterase; Eserine (physostigmine) - 0.5 ml.	-do-	Inhibits enzyme acetyl cholinesterase which destroys A-ch, thus potentiates the action of A-ch.
2. Sympatholytic: α and β blockers	No effect in vitro.	–
3. 1% NaCl - 1 ml	Decreases HR and the force of contraction.	(i) Increases the threshold potential of nodal tissue. (ii) Na^+ competes with Ca^{2+} in contractile process thus decreasing Ca^{2+} influx.
4. 1% KCl - 1 ml	-do- Heart finally stops in diastole.	(i) Decreases RMP; therefore, depolarization is not followed by repolarization. (ii) Decreases the magnitude of action potential.
5. Cold saline	Decreases HR	Mechanism opposite of warm saline.
6. 1% Nicotine - 1 ml	Decreases HR	Stimulates peripheral ganglia.

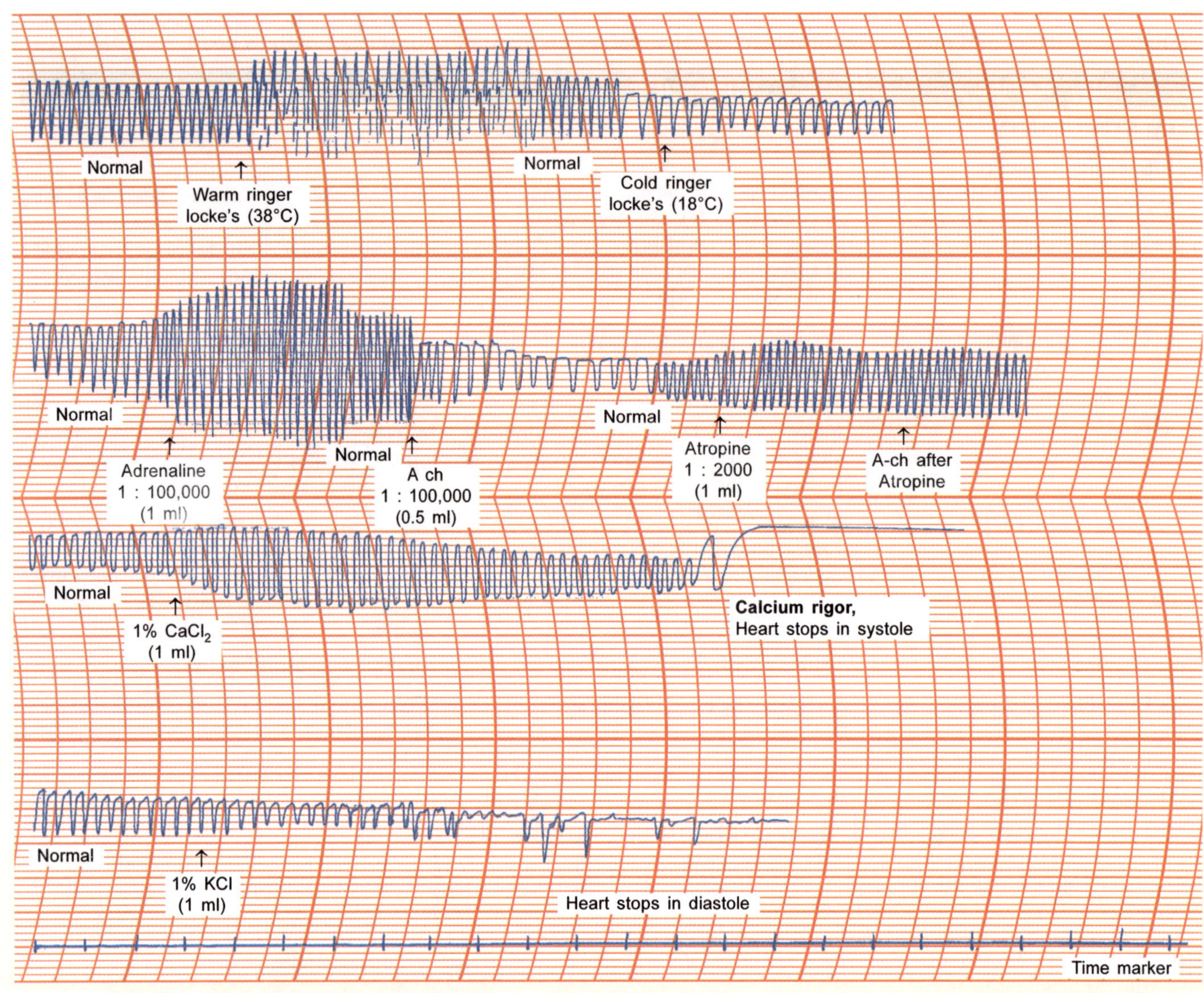

Fig. 4.2.3: Effect of variables on the perfused isolated rabbit's heart

STUDY NOTES

RESULTS

Table 4.2.2: Effect of drugs and ions on the isolated mammalian heart

Agent	Effect on			
	Heart rate (bpm)		Force of contraction (in cm)	
	Before	After	Before	After
1. Effect of change in perfusion pressure				
(i) Increase in pressure				
(ii) Decrease in pressure				
2. Adrenaline—1 : 100,000 (1 ml)				
3. Acetyl choline—1 : 100,000 (0.5 ml)				
4. Atropine—1 : 2000 (1 ml)				

Agent	Effect on			
	Heart rate (bpm)		Force of contraction (in cm)	
	Before	After	Before	After
5. Effect of A-ch after atropinisation				
6. 1% $CaCl_2$−1 ml				
7. 1% NaCl−1 ml				
8. 1% KCl−1 ml				
9. Anoxaemia				

COMMENTS AND DISCUSSION

....

....

....

....

....

....

....

....

....

....

....

....

Date: ....

3 Recording of Blood Pressure and Respiration in Dog/Rabbit and Effect of Variables on It

I. APPARATUS

For the recording of systemic arterial blood pressure (by direct method) and respiration in dog/rabbit, a special set of apparatus is required as described below (Fig. 4.3.1).

1. **Kymograph**. It consists of two cylinders, a large and a small.
   - (i) **Large cylinder**. There is a power-driven axle which carries a recording cylinder (the same as used in nerve muscle experiments); the driving mechanism has different gears giving various speeds.
   - (ii) **Small cylinder**. It is mounted on another axle which rolls passively; it is fixed onto a sliding bed and can be clamped at any position.

   A suitable length of smoked paper is mounted on the two cylinders to roll smoothly as the driving cylinder moves.
2. **Time recorder**. It provides time marking at pre-fixed intervals.
3. **Signal marker: Induction coil**. Refer to page 77
4. **Manometer** *for direct recording of systemic arterial B.P.* It is a 'U' shaped glass tube mounted on an adjustable stand with the inner and outer limbs.
   - (i) The **inner limb** carries a **float recorder** which has a solid base made up of mercury repellant material, and a light and thin metal alloy wire to which a **writing point** is attached. A **thread with a plumb** hanging from it keeps the writing point in contact with the smoked paper.
   - (ii) The **outer limb**. It has the following connections:
     - (a) Through a side opening connected to the **pressure bottle** containing 3.8% sodium citrate solution (*isotonic and anticoagulant*). The pressure bottle is corked tightly and a pressure as high as 240-300 mmHg can be raised into the system with the help of the sphygmomanometer pump attached to it.
     - (b) Through a top opening connected via pressure rubber tubing and **arterial cannula** to the artery of the animal.

   The manometer carries a **movable scale** with markings from zero to 24 (or 30); each mark on the scale denotes 10 mmHg pressure in the system. Zero mark is set when mercury column occupies the same height in the two limbs of the manometer.
5. **Marey's tambour**. Refer to page 171. It records the respiration (rate and depth) of the animal.
6. **The respiratory pump (or Respirator)**. This provides artificial respiration during emergencies. The stroke of the pump is adjusted beforehand to give the correct tidal volume (dogs: 200 ml; cat: 100 ml; rabbit: 50 ml).
7. **Operation table**. This is used to strap the dog and hold its legs and mouth in position. The dissection of the dog and all experimental procedures are carried out on it (Fig. 4.3.1).
8. **Arterial cannula**. It is a three-way glass cannula with a central bulb; one limb is meant for the manometer, the other to remove air bubble or blood clots and the third (the nozzle) to be inserted into the artery of the animal.
9. **Venous cannula**. It is a simple glass tube with a nozzle to be inserted into a vein (Fig. 4.3.1).
10. **Dissection instruments** like a pair of scissors, scalpel, aneurysm needle, bull dog clamps, forceps, retractor, cotton, thread, kidney tray, beaker, syringe, etc.
11. **Drugs and other chemicals**. Adrenaline, nor-adrenaline, A-ch, anaesthetic agents (see below), heparin, 3.8% sodium citrate, etc.

Note: Alternatively, BP and respiration can also be recorded with the help of electronic equipment, the **polyrite** or **student physiograph** and appropriate transducers (for details, refer to page 81.

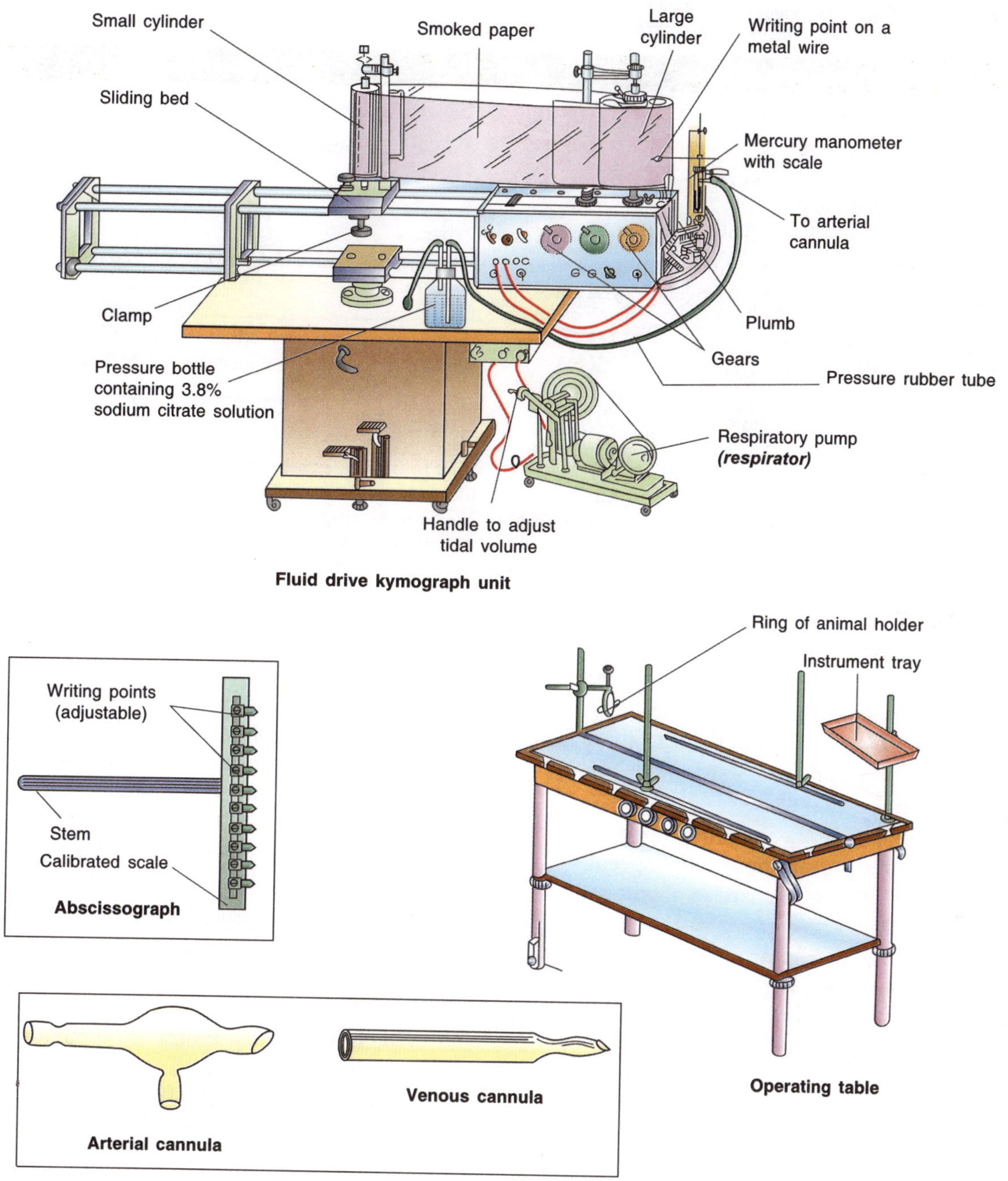

Fig. 4.3.1 Experiment set-up for the recording of systemic arterial BP and respiration in dog/rabbit

II. ANAESTHESIA

To perform a successful physiological experiment, it is important to have the animal properly anaesthetised. **No experiment is reliable if the animal feels pain.** Anaesthesia is best performed on the fasting healthy animal.

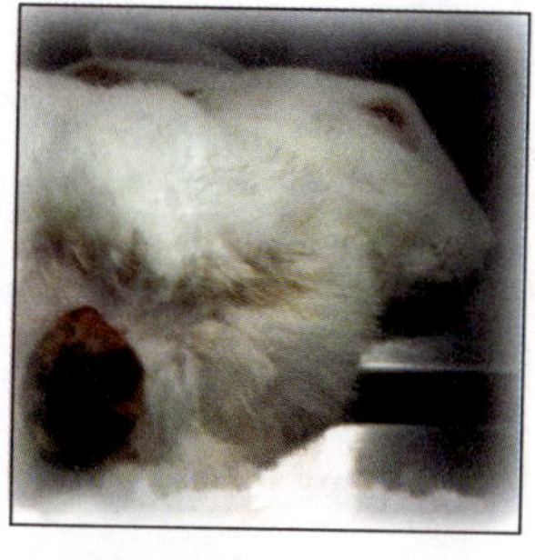

Broadly, two groups of anaesthetic agents are used for mammalian experiments: *Barbiturate* and *Chloralose group* (Table 4.3.1).

When the animal is completely anaesthetized:

1. Its respiration becomes deep and regular;
2. Voluntary movements disappear;
3. Muscular tone greatly decreases;
4. The corneal reflex is lost or becomes sluggish; and
5. Loss of reaction to cutaneous stimuli

An anaesthetised animal has the appearance of being in a deep sleep.

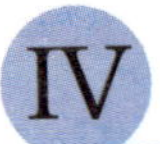

Table 4.3.1 Barbiturate and chloralose anaesthetic agents compared

(A) Barbiturate group	(B) Chloralose group
1. **Onset of action**: Almost immediate	1. Slow: 15-30 minutes
2. **Duration of action**: Variable. (i) Phenobarbitone (gardenal/luminal) : 2 hours (ii) Pentobarbitone (nembutal) : 1 hour (iii) Sodium thiopentone (pentothal) : 15 minutes	2. Longer: 2-6 hours
3. **Dosage:** 30 mg/kg body weight. I.V. or *intraperitoneally* (I/p) (I/p-induction is slow and maintenance dose cannot be regulated). **How to prepare** 100 mg powder dissolved in 5 ml N-saline provides a concentration of 20 mg/ml.	3. 100 mg/kg body weight. I.V. or I/p with equally good results 1 gm powder dissolved in 10 ml propylglycol by slight warming provides a concentration of 100 mg/ml.
4. **Maintenance dose**: 1/4th of original dose; difficult to regulate	4. Regulation of maintenance dose possible with routes (I.V. and I/p).
5. **Advantages** (i) Produces a good amount of light anaesthesia. (ii) Autonomic functions are not affected even during surgery.	(i) Produces a good amount of light anaesthesia. (ii) Autonomic functions are not affected initially; however, later during surgical procedures, it may cause an increase in B.P. and dehydration.

III. PROCEDURE

(A) Arrangement of experimental set-up

Before starting the experiment, arrange for the experimental set-up and check the following:

1. The working of kymograph (a polyrite and various transducers), time marker, signal marker and Marey's tambour.
2. Proper mounting of the recording paper on the kymograph and set it at the desired speed.
3. The various writing points are in alignment.
4. Any leak in the B.P. recording system.
5. Working of the respiratory pump; set the rate (12-14/min) and volume (200 ml in dog; 50 ml in rabbit) according to the animal's requirement.
6. All surgical items and chemicals are available.

(B) Calibration

1. **Of the kymograph paper**. Bring the manometer pressure at 'zero' mmHg and run the paper to draw a zero line (base line). Each 5 mm vertical distance from this line indicates 10 mmHg pressure; or alternatively, raise the manometer pressure with the help of rubber pump by 10 mmHg each time and take the corresponding points on the recording paper.
2. **Of the polyrite/physiograph**
   (i) Connect an arterial cathether having a three-way cannula to a pressure transducer which, in turn, is connected to one channel of the **polyrite/physiograph** recording instrument.
   (ii) Connect the second limb of the three-way cannula to mercury manometer; and the third limb to a 10 ml syringe filled with heparinized saline.
   (iii) Fill the entire system with heparinized saline; bring the manometer pressure to zero mmHg; manipulate balance position on the recording instrument to make the pen position central.
   (iv) Press the plunger of the syringe to increase the pressure inside the transducer which is measured directly by the mercury manometer; calibrate the simultaneous deflection in the writing lever of the recording instrument accordingly.
   (v) Repeat the procedure by raising the pressure in steps of 10 mmHg each time.

(C) Anaesthesia

1. Weigh the animal to nearest 50 gm and administer appropriate anaesthesia after taking into account all the factors (page 331).
2. Ensure that the animal is completely anaesthetized.

(D) Fixing the animal

1. Place the animal supine on the operating table.
2. The head of the animal is fastened by means of a metal holder and the legs are tied to the table with a string.
   Care should be taken while fixing the animal's head in the holder to have the animal's tongue pulled out of the mouth. If this is not done, the tongue slips backwards and blocks the larynx so that the animal may be unable to breathe.
3. Insert a chemical thermometer into the rectum through the anus of the animal, keep it there and make a note of temperature.

(E) Dissection to record BP and respiration

Dissection to expose trachea, carotid artery and vagus nerve

1. Give a midline incision on the ventral surface of neck extending 2-3 cm below the larynx up to the manubrium sterni; cut through the skin and subcutaneous tissues and retract the sternohyoid and sternothyroid muscles laterally to expose the trachea.

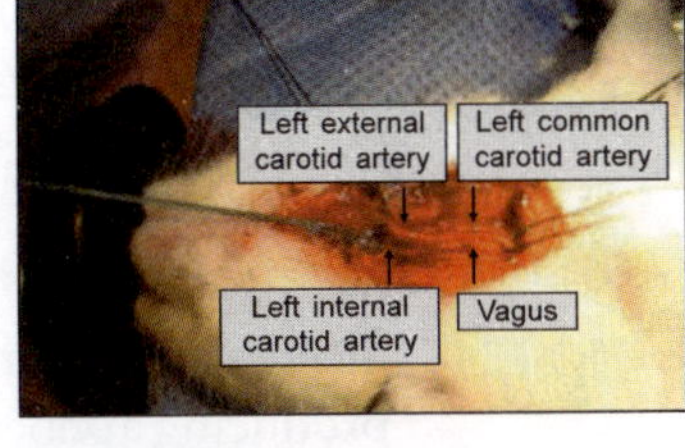

2. Select a proper-sized tracheal cannula and accordingly cut the second or third tracheal ring transversely in the centre to introduce it; tie a tight ligature to secure it in position.
3. Connect the open end of cannula to a Y-shaped glass cannula; one limb of this is connected to Marey's tambour for recording respiration, and the other limb is connected through a rubber tubing to the respiratory pump. This is selectively clamped.
4. Identify carotid sheath lying on either side of trachea, feel for carotid pulsations, dissect bluntly and expose carotid artery and vagus nerve on both the sides. Pass separate ligatures around each structure.
   Whole of the dissection is covered with cotton gauze soaked in Ringer solution.

Dissection for femoral artery and vein

(Femoral artery for the purpose of recording the systemic arterial BP and femoral vein for the injection of drugs and saline)

1. Stretch the leg, feel and locate the femoral artery, give a 8-10 cm long incision parallel to the artery, starting from mid inguinal point; separate the skin, subcutaneous tissue and deep fascia by blunt dissection using artery forceps only. This exposes the femoral vessels and nerve, identify them separately (femoral vein, artery and nerve from medial to lateral, in that order).
2. Clean about 5 cm of the femoral vein having no branch, pass two ligatures round it; place two bulldog clamps at either end of the segment, first at the proximal end to allow segment to be filled with blood. Give a V-shape incision on the segment, insert *venous cannula,* directing its tip proximally, fix it by tying the ligature; remove the first proximal clamp and then the distal clamp after tying the ligature.
3. ***Recording of B.P.***
   (i) Check the manometer system is in working order; see both rubber tubings on the outer limb of manometer are filled with air free 3.8% sodium citrate solution and are clamped. Remove the clamp from tubing connecting to the pressure bottle and raise the pressure in the system just above the expected systolic B.P. (150 mmHg), then clamp this tube permanently.
   (ii) Femoral artery is cannulated with arterial cannula in similar fashion as femoral vein has been cannulated earlier.
   (iii) Remove the clamp over the rubber tubing connecting artery to the manometer; a junction of blood and citrate fluid will form in the bulb of the cannula, and float recorder will start oscillating freely with pressure changes in the artery. Record the tracing on the kymograph.

> **Important Note:** If the manometer pressure is high, citrate will start entering the artery, and if femoral artery pressure is high, blood will gush forcibly into the cannula and try to enter the rubber tubing of the manometer.

4. *How to remove the blood clot from the arterial cannula*
   Apply a bulldog clamp on the femoral artery proximal to cannula, take out the cannula from the artery. Remove the clamp from tubing connecting the pressure bottle with the mercury manometer; raise the pressure in the pressure bottle to about 180-200 mmHg, clot will be flushed out. Further more, raise the pressure, if necessary. Reapply the arterial cannula in position after adjusting the pressure in the manometer. Do not forget to clamp the tube connecting the pressure bottle to the manometer.

IV. OBSERVATIONS AND RESULTS

(A) Recording of normal BP and respiration

1. The **BP record** shows small waves synchronous with the pulse, upstroke indicates systole and downstroke diastole (Fig. 4.3.2). The difference between systolic and diastolic BP record is small (15-20 mmHg), while actual difference is 30-50 mmHg. This is due to the fact that mercury possesses the inertia of high degree.
2. The **Respiration record** shows expiration as an upstroke and inspiration as downstroke. Respiratory rate : Heart rate :: 1 : 5-6, therefore, each respiratory cycle is associated with 5-6 cardiac cycles.
3. **Relationship between BP and Respiration.** Usually BP increases with inspiration and falls with expiration. This cyclical fluctuation in BP waves caused by respiration is called ***Traube Hering Waves*** (Fig. 4.3.2).
   Inspiratory rise of BP is due to:
   (i) irradiation of impulses to vasomotor centre (VMC) from inspiratory centre, and

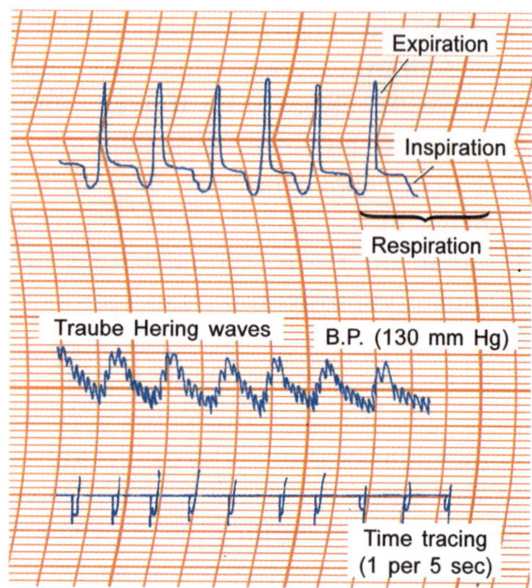

Fig. 4.3.2 Record of normal BP and respiration

(ii) fall in intrathoracic pressure decreases the pressure over great veins; this results in an increase in venous return, to cause BP to rise.

(iii) rise in the cardiac output caused by an increase in heart rate during inspiration

Important Note : In a normal healthy human being, usually there occurs a fall of BP during early inspiration followed by a rise in the late inspiration and during expiration.

(B) Effect of drugs

1. ***Adrenaline.*** Dose: 2 μgm/kg body weight; inject 0.5 ml of 1 : 10,000 adrenaline I.V. (= 50 μgm).
   (i) *On the BP* (Fig. 4.3.3)
   (a) via direct effect on heart, increases the HR and force of contraction;
   (b) produces generalised peripheral vasoconstriction, to cause BP to rise.

   Net effect, rise in BP. This, however, stimulates the sino-aortic nerves, so inhibits the rise in BP.

   (ii) *On the respiration* (Fig. 4.3.3)
   (a) In a small dose, it stimulates the respiration by the stimulation of peripheral baroreceptors.
   (b) In high doses, it causes marked rise in the BP which, in turn, via sino-aortic mechanism, inhibits the respiration producing apnoea, called ***Adrenaline Apnoea*** (*reflex effect*).

Note: The administration of adrenaline *after vagotomy,* the BP rise is marked because sino-aortic nerves fail to regulate the rise in BP and adrenaline apnoea will also disappear.

2. ***Nor-adrenaline.*** Dose: 2 μg/kg body weight. Inject 0.5 ml of 1 : 10,000 I.V. (= 50 μg). The effect on BP and respiration is the same as with the adrenaline but it is more pronounced (Fig. 4.3.3).
3. ***Acetyl choline (A-ch).*** Dose: 2 μg/kg body weight; inject 0.5 ml of 1 : 10,000 A-ch (= 50 μg).
   (i) *On BP* (Fig. 4.3.4)
   (a) via direct action on heart, decreases the HR and force of contraction;
   (b) produces peripheral vasodilatation.

   Net effect, fall in the BP. The effect is temporary and degree of fall in BP is directly related to the dose used.

   (ii) *On respiration* (Fig. 4.3.4). The reflex stimulation of respiration may occur due to indirect effect, secondary to fall in the BP via baro and chemoreceptors.
4. ***Atropine.*** Dose: 2 ml of 1 : 1000 atropine, I.V. (= 2 mg). It acts by blocking the action of vagus on CVS, therefore, the extent of rise in HR and BP

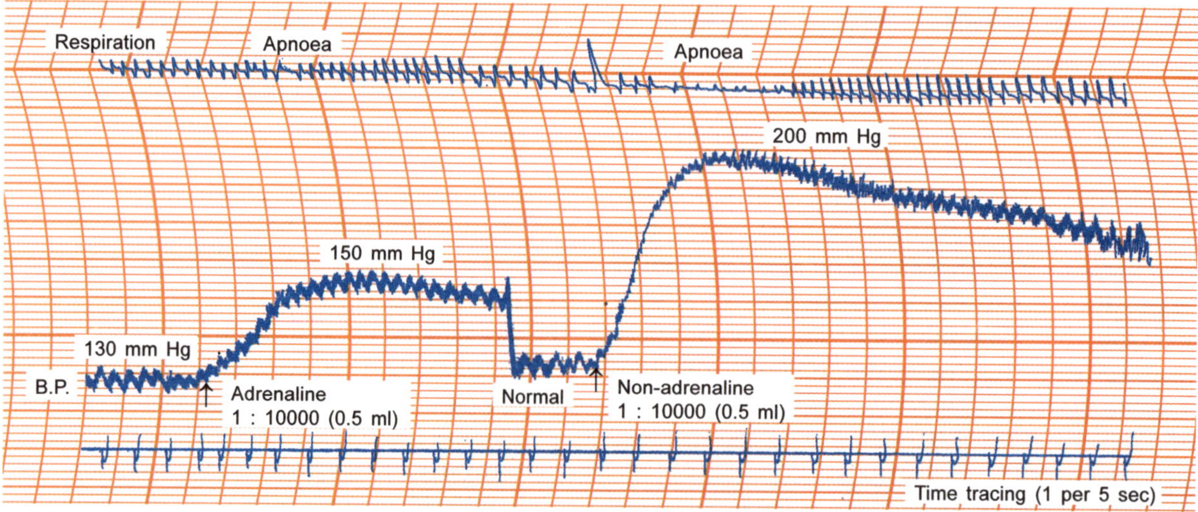

Fig. 4.3.3 Effect of adrenaline and nor-adrenaline on BP and respiration

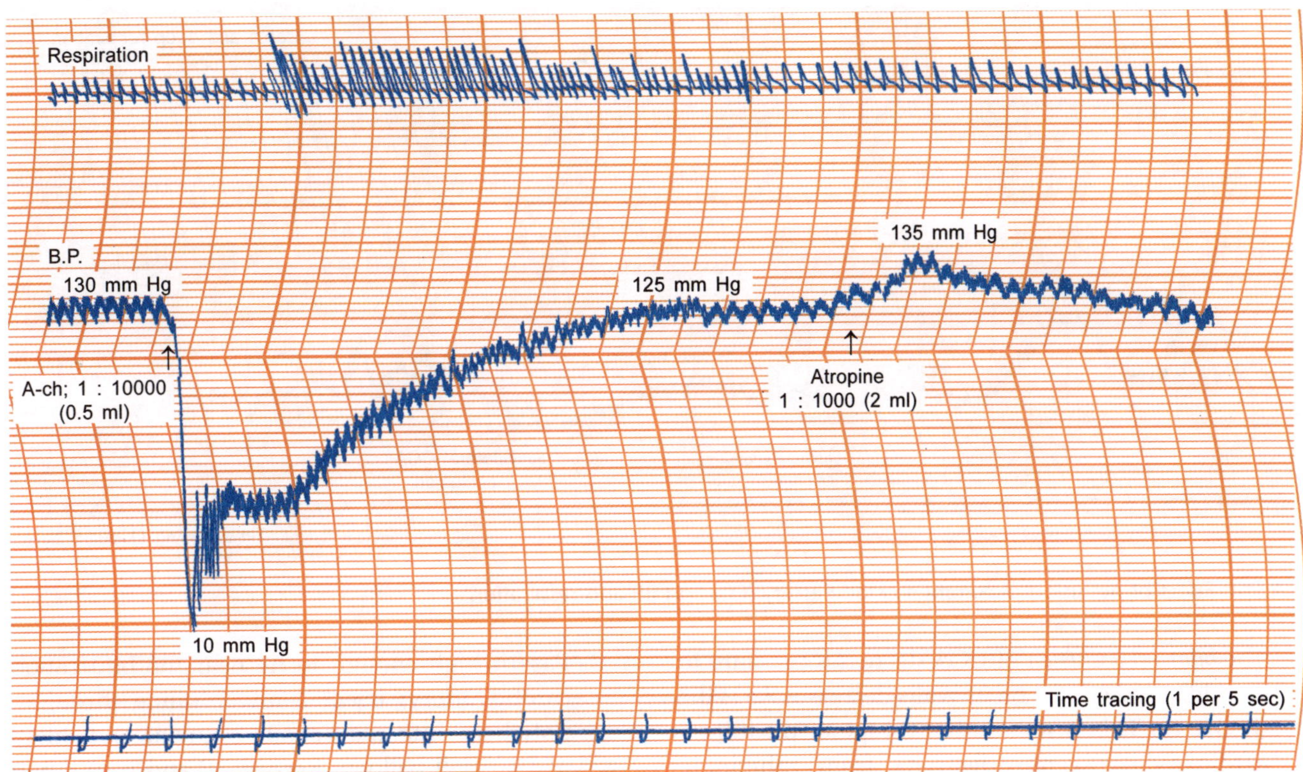

Fig. 4.3.4 Effect of acetyl-choline (A-ch) and atropine on BP and respiration

depends on the degree of vagal tone present in the animal (Fig. 4.3.4)

(C) Effect of asphyxia

To produce asphyxia, occlude either the tracheal cannula or the tube connecting the Marey's tambour with the trachea. This produces hypoxia (decrease in arterial pO_2) and hypercapnia (increase in arterial pCO_2).

1. *Initial effect* (Fig. 4.3.5)
   (i) The gradual rise in BP and HR occurs due to the stimulation of VMC via sino-aortic mechanism.
   (ii) Marked stimulation of respiration causing rapid, deep respiration
2. *Late effect.* This is seen after 2-3 minutes, when CO_2 increases alone to a certain level with severe hypoxia, causing the stimulation of cardiac vagal centre and inhibition of VMC. Thus BP begins to fall with HR and respiration.

Important Note: If asphyxia is removed as soon as there is fall in BP, the animal can recover. Asphyxia, **after vagotomy**, increase in BP will be more marked. This reflexely produces apnoea (as adrenaline apnoea occurs, see page 334.

(D) Effect of occlusion of common carotid artery (CCA)

Clamp the CCA temporarily using a bull dog clamp, first on one side and then on both sides. Note the effect on BP and respiration. Release after 15 sec.

1. The *unilateral occlusion* of CCA causes only a slight rise in BP, HR and respiration (Fig. 4.3.6) (*Mechanism*, see below).

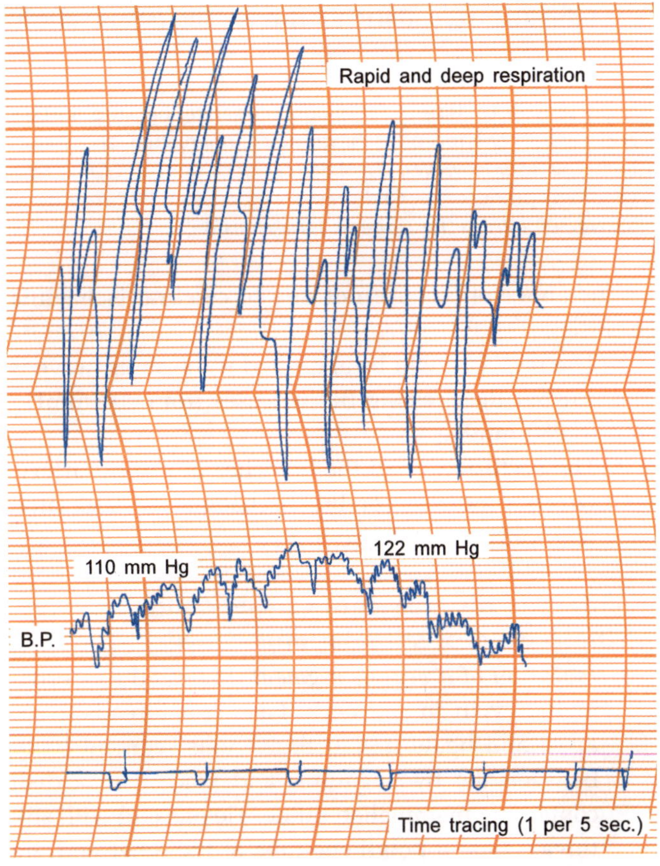

Fig. 4.3.5 Effect of asphyxia (for 30 sec) on BP and respiration

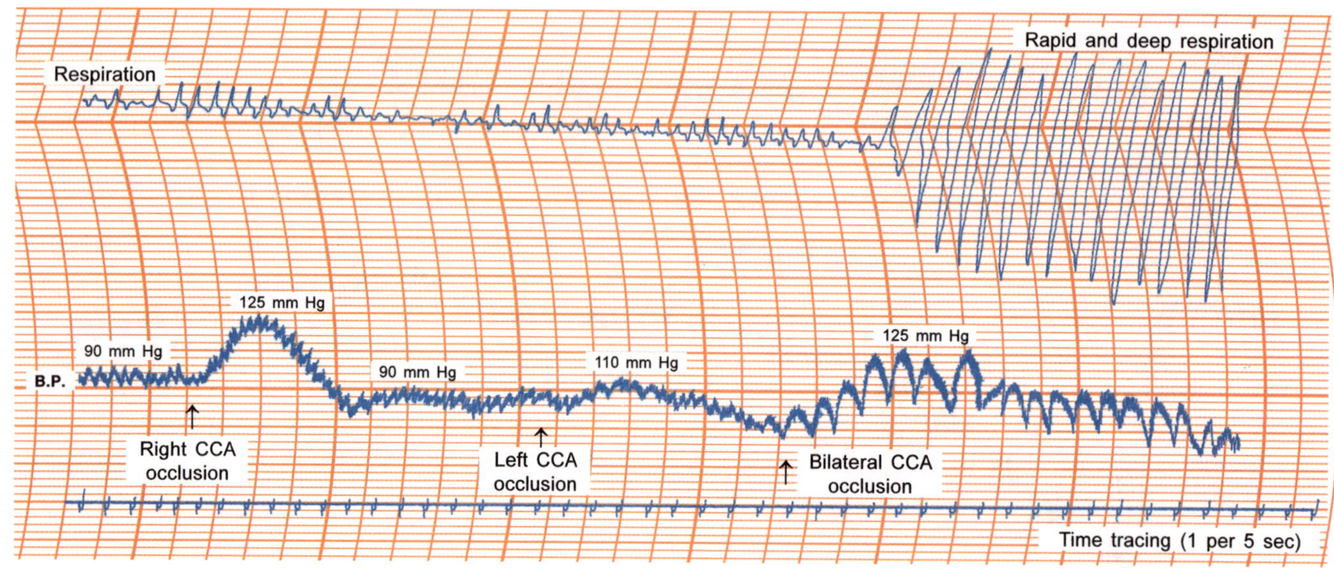

Fig. 4.3.6 Effect of occlusion of common carotid artery (CCA) on BP and respiration

2. The *bilateral occlusion* of CCA decreases pressure in carotid sinus; stretch on its walls decreases, so is the discharge. This results in the escape of medullary cardiovascular centre neurons from inhibition. Consequently, increased sympathetic drive increases BP and HR. The respiration gets reflexely inhibited secondary to rise in BP (slight effect) (Fig. 4.3.6).

> **Important Note:** Rise in BP is only moderate, because aortic and cardiac baroreceptors have intact innervation and they limit the rise. However, the bilateral occlusion of CCA *after vagotomy* produces marked pressor response and BP may rise above 300 mmHg (***Neurogenic Hypertension***).

The above effects **are not due to cerebral ischaemia** because:

1. The response will be abolished if the sinus nerve is cut but then resting BP increases from 200 mmHg to 280 mmHg.
2. The occlusion of all the branches of carotid artery, which produces cerebral ischaemia is associated with only a slight rise in BP.

(E) Effect of distension of carotid sinus (baroreceptor stimulation)

1. ***Isolation of a venous segment.*** Expose the external jugular vein in the neck. Pass two threads 2 cm apart and ligate it. Cut the venous segment lying between the two ligatures and place it in a dish containing mammalian saline. Tie one end with silk thread, pass a polythene tube at the other end, tie it and keep it.
2. Clamp the CCA. Make a nick on the artery distal to the clamp. Introduce the isolated venous segment into the collapsed artery.
3. Pass it high enough to tie near the bifurcation of carotid artery; inject 2 ml of saline through the polythene into the venous segment and inflate it like a small balloon. Record BP and respiration.
4. If necessary, repeat the whole procedure on the other side as well.

The stimulation of the carotid sinus mechanically by stretching its walls by pressure from within produces a combined reflex of cardiac inhibition and a fall of BP (Fig. 4.3.7).

(F) Effect of stimulation of carotid sinus nerve

Follow the CCA upwards and clear the underlying tissues with a blunt forceps to expose the bifurcation of CCA. Identify carotid sinus (as dilated initial part of internal carotid artery). Separate very gently the sinus nerve fibres at the back of the sinus with a fine forceps. Connect the electrodes to the induction coil, place the electrodes under the sinus nerve, stimulate it at different strength and frequencies, and observe the effect as above (Fig. 4.3.7).

> Note: This procedure is not an ideal way to study the functioning of the carotid sinus nerve.

(G) Effect of stimulation of peripheral somatic nerve (sciatic nerve)

1. Let loose one of the hind limbs and place it over the other limb. Feel for the ischial tuberosity and greater trochanter. Give an incision 8-10 cm long midway between these bony prominences.
2. Clean the fascia and separate the underlying muscles by introducing a closed artery forceps between them and opening it. Identify a white cord of nerve, the sciatic nerve. Pass an aneurysm needle with two threads under it and tie two ligatures at

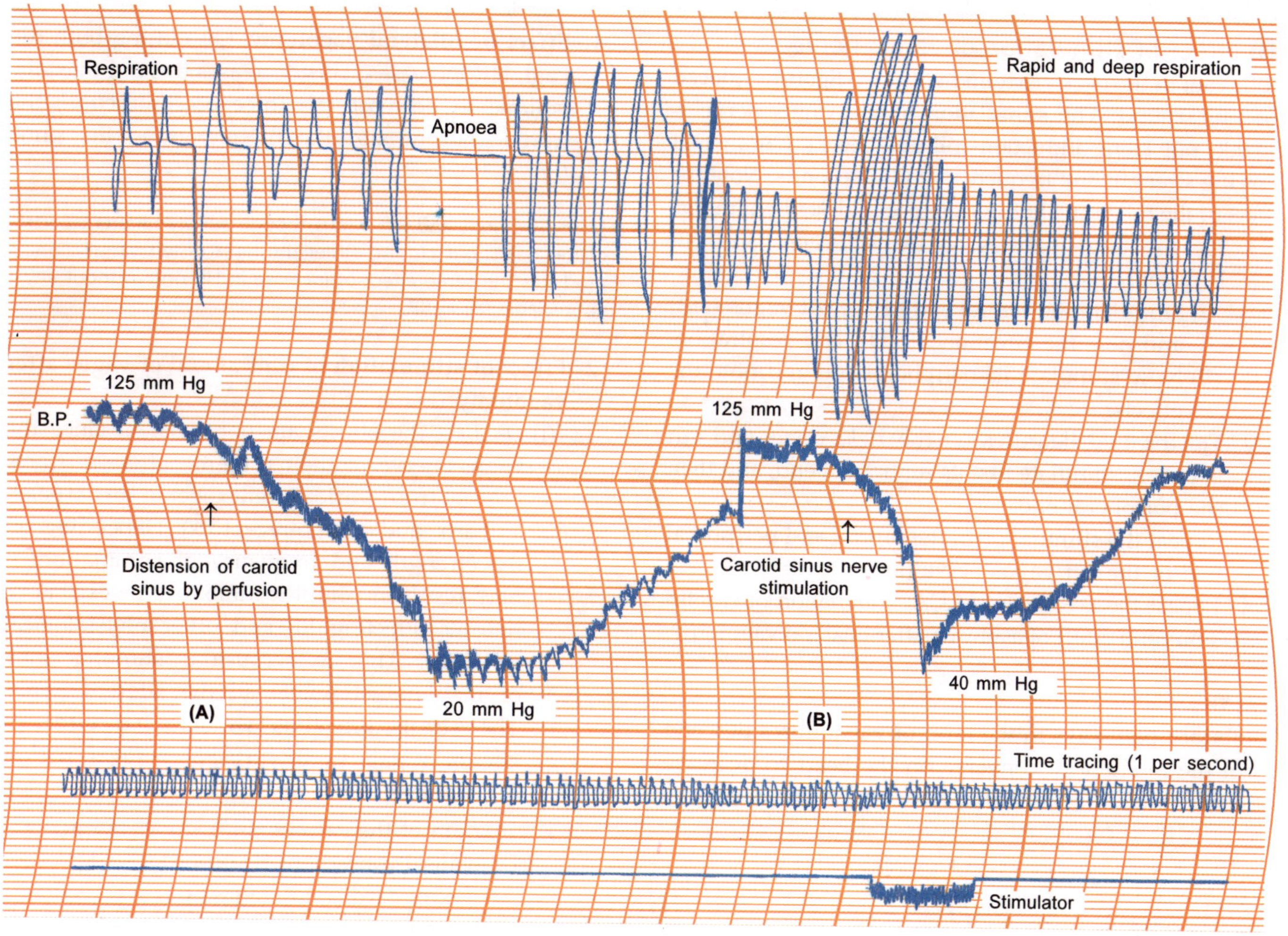

Fig. 4.3.7 Effect of the distension of carotid sinus (A) and stimulation of carotid sinus nerve (B) on BP and respiration

a distance of 2 cm around the nerve. Cut the nerve between the ligatures.

3. Place the proximal end over the stimulating electrodes and stimulate it with varying strength and frequencies of current and observe the effect. Note the rise in BP and HR due to reflex vasoconstriction. It may produce a slight depressor effect on respiration secondary to rise in B.P. (Fig. 4.3.8).

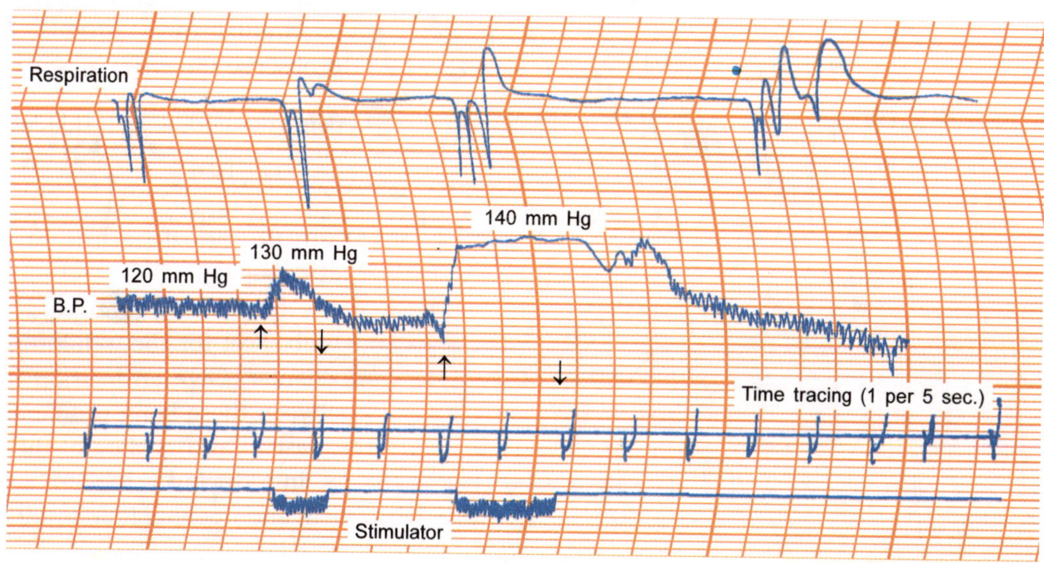

Fig. 4.3.8 Effect of the stimulation of the sciatic nerve (central end) at two different frequencies on BP and respiration

(H) Effect of stimulation of vagus nerve

Both vagi in the neck are found with two ligatures placed loosely around. The stimulation of the vagus nerve is carried out using induction coil and Neef's hammer at varying strength and frequencies for 10 seconds. Note the effect of the following in the sequence as described under:

1. Tie the two ligatures on the *left vagus* and cut between:
   (i) Stimulate the central end of the cut vagus (left) and note the effect on BP, HR and respiration.
   (ii) Now stimulate its peripheral end and note the effects.
2. Tie the two ligatures on the *right vagus* and cut between; stimulate first its central cut end, and then the peripheral end.
3. Repeat the stimulation of the central and peripheral end of the cut vagus nerve (left).
4. Repeat the occlusion of CCA, stimulation of carotid sinus and effect of asphyxia after bilateral vagotomy.

Results

Inhibitory pathways in the form of vagal fibres descend from the medulla to converge on the heart to decrease HR and force of contraction.

1. **Effect of bilateral vagotomy**. On cutting both the vagi, HR increases. This decreases the end diastolic volume to decrease the force of contraction; the cardiac output and the BP remaining the same (Fig. 4.3.9).

Note: The right and left vagus though supply different parts of the heart, but cutting either the right or left vagus alone produces the same effect of increase in HR only without any appreciable fall in BP.

2. **Effect of stimulation of central end of vagus after vagotomy** (Fig. 4.3.9)
   (i) *On BP*. The effects are not constant since the vagus nerve contains many afferent fibres arising from various reflexogenic areas (such as baro- and chemo-receptors). Depending on the strength and frequency of stimulation, it may result in complex inhibitory or excitatory reflexes affecting BP and other physiological activities. This is because a stimulus may or may not stimulate all the afferent fibres. The effects are thus variable, *i.e.* either a rise or a fall in BP (*usually a slight rise in BP is seen*).

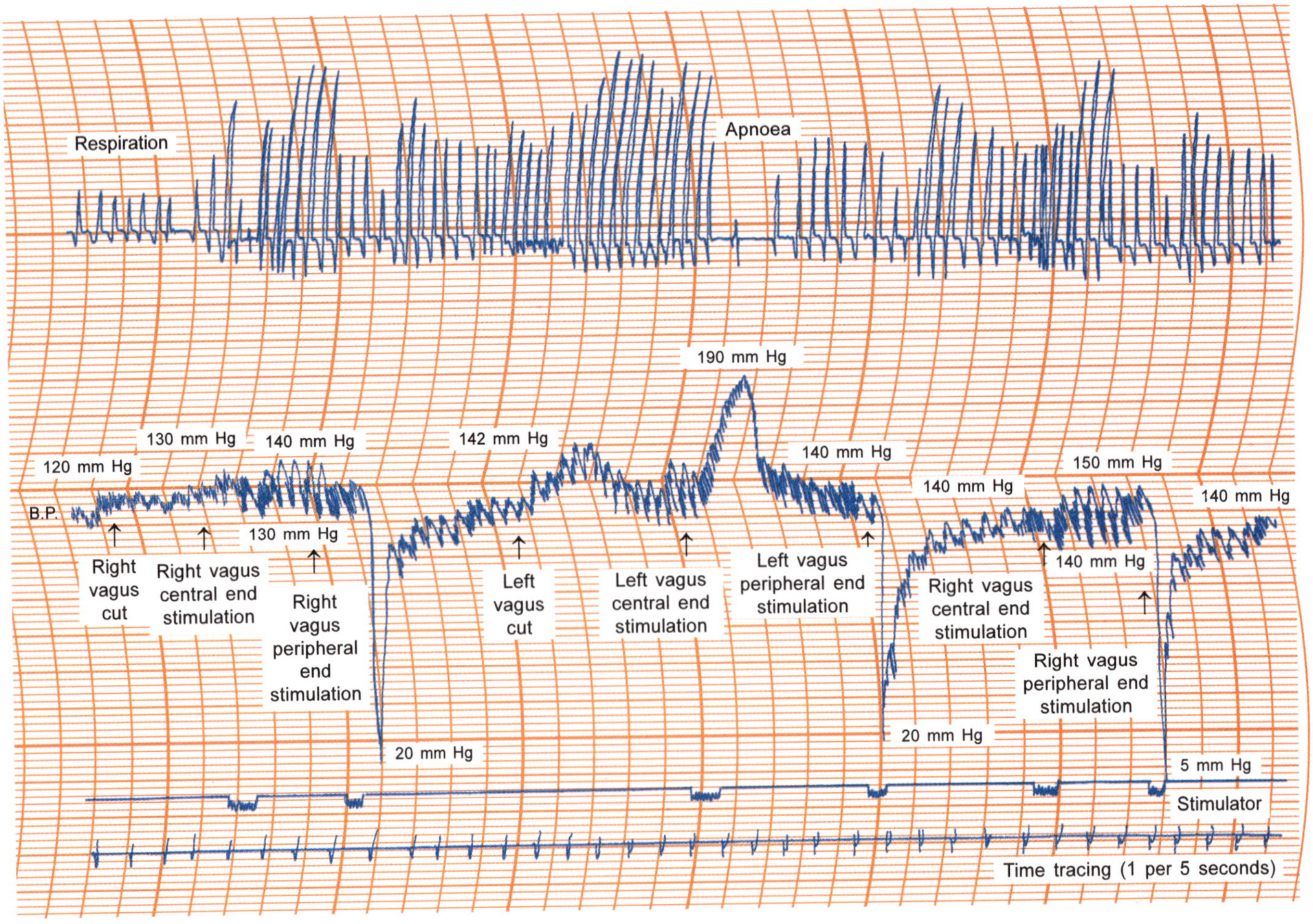

Fig. 4.3.9 Effect of the stimulation of the vagus nerve on BP and respiration

(ii) *On respiration.* The afferent impulses of Hering-Breuer reflex travel along vagi. The effects are thus due to the stimulation of these fibres directly and reflexely secondary to fall in the BP. The respiratory responses are never constant as they depend on the number and type of fibres stimulated, strength and nature of respiratory activity existing at the time of stimulation. Usually, they depend on the type of breathing present prior to stimulation:

(a) *if breathing is normal* in rate and depth, stimulation produces no effect;

(b) *if breathing is slow,* rate may increase even at the cost of amplitude;

(c) *if breathing is fast and jerky,* it becomes slow and deep.

All these changes last only during the period of stimulation. As soon as the stimulus is stopped, reflex fall in the BP, increases the respiratory rate but its depth decreases (*i.e.* respiration becomes rapid and shallow); with the BP becoming normal, respiration also returns back to normal.

3. **Effect of stimulation of peripheral end of vagus after vagotomy** (Fig. 4.3.9)

(i) *On BP*

(a) A sudden fall in BP is seen which may even reach zero level (due to temporary inhibition which varies with the strength of stimulation).

(b) On the stoppage of stimulation, rapid recovery occurs (not so quick as the fall). BP after recovery may reach a higher level than the previous one (*Reactionary Rise in BP*). This depends on the site of cutting the vagus nerve.

Causes of reactionary rise in BP

- The stagnation of blood during the period of inhibition increases the cardiac output resulting from an increased venous return.
- A sudden fall in the BP increases the activity of the VMC.

(ii) *On Respiration.* No direct effect is seen on respiration; however, a fall in BP may reflexely stimulate the respiration via the carotid bodies.

4. **Effect of occlusion of CCA, stimulation of carotid sinus nerve and effect of asphyxia after bilateral vagotomy**. Refer to page 335.

(I) Effect of stimulation of splanchnic nerve

1. Place the animal in lateral position, give an incision 10 cm long parallel to the last rib, divide the connective tissues to expose the sheath of erector spinae, open the sheath and retract the muscle laterally with metal retractor, separating it from the anterior layer of the sheath.
2. Open this sheath by inserting the two forefingers to expose the kidney. Press it downwards and outwards, the adrenal gland comes into view, with a vein lying superficial to it.
3. Behind the vein, running from the adrenal gland to the crus of the diaphragm, is the *splanchnic nerve.*
4. Stimulate the intact nerve by placing electrodes for 10 seconds; note the effect.

Result

BP rises in two stages: (Fig. 4.3.10)

(i) the first rise is immediate due to vaso-constriction caused by the stimulation of the splanchnic nerve (**resistance effect**); and

(ii) the second rise is due to the liberation of adrenaline from the adrenal medulla. It has to reach the heart through the blood flow before it can stimulate and cause a rise in B.P. (**capacity or capacitance effect**). HR increases during this second rise of B.P.

(J) Effect of bleeding and perfusion

Theory

1. The effect of haemorrhage on BP and respiration depends upon the rate and amount of blood lost relative to the total blood volume.
2. Total blood volume is 75-80 ml/kg body weight (or 8% of body weight). Accordingly, haemorrhage can be classified as:

(i) **Mild haemorrhage**, loss up to 10% of total blood volume. Usually, there is a slight fall in BP but it will quickly come back to normal without infusion due to compensatory mechanisms. No change in respiration.

(ii) **Moderate haemorrhage**, loss up to 10-30% of the total blood volume.

(iii) **Severe haemorrhage**, loss up to 40% of the total blood volume.

In **moderate to severe haemorrhage**, as the blood loss increases, a progressive decrease in BP with the stimulation of respiration is observed (Fig. 4.3.11). But if blood volume is made up with adequate transfusion (either blood or normal saline), BP and respiration returns to normal over a period of 20-30 minutes. This is called **Reversible Shock**.

(iv) Blood loss of more than 40% of total blood volume, precipitates **Irreversible Shock** and no amount of transfusion (blood or normal saline)

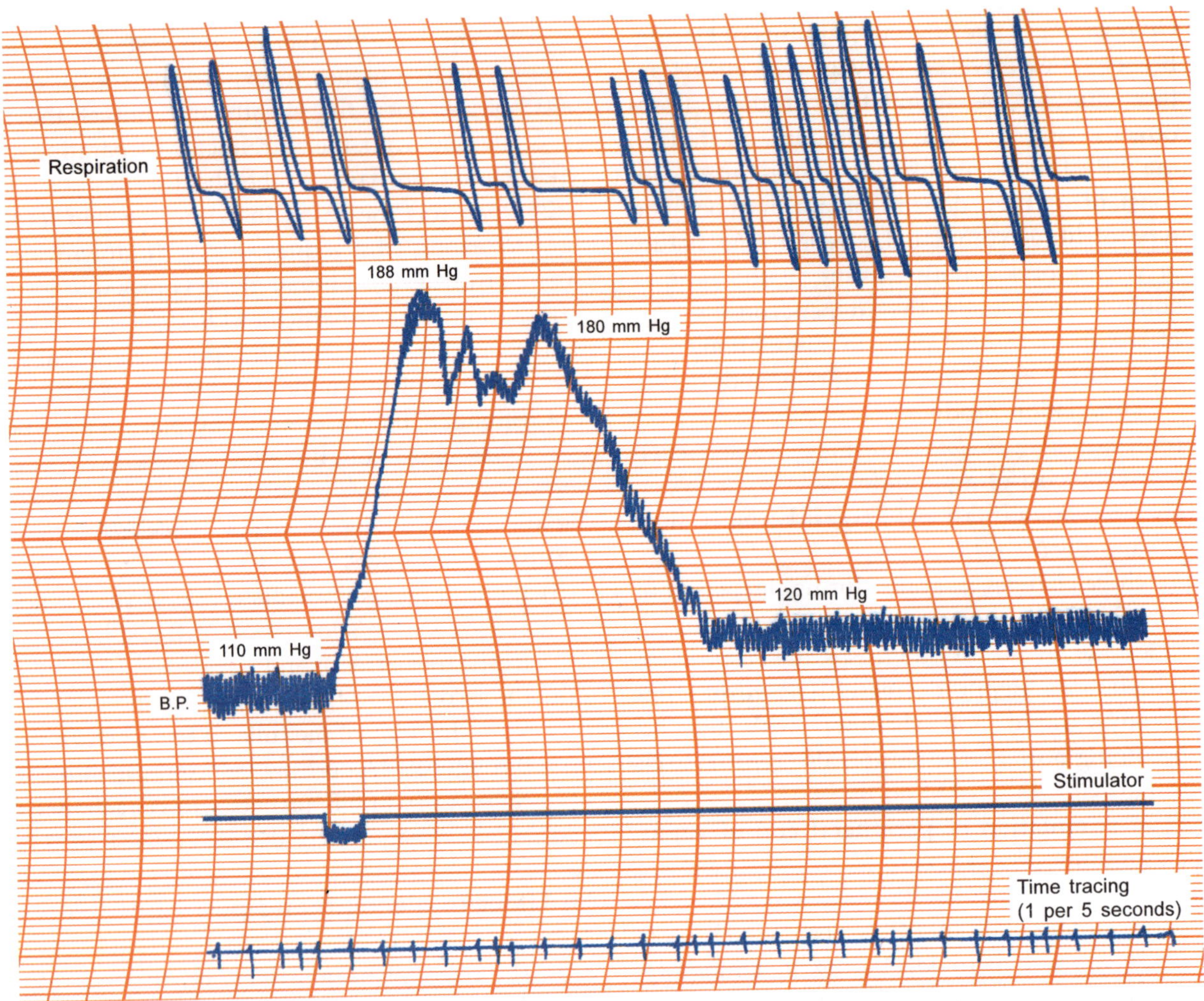

Fig. 4.3.10 Effect of the stimulation of splanchnic nerve on BP and respiration

can save the animal. This is due to the setting up of various *positive feedback mechanisms* which tend to worsen the situation.

> **Important Note:** If the animal is injected with a warm normal saline, say about 30 ml at a time, BP increases at each injection.The rise does not remain, however, for long, the salt solution being inadequate to restore BP for more than a short period of time. However, if the warm blood is injected into the animal, BP rises and stays at the new level for much longer time.

Procedure

1. **For mild haemorrhage**, about 10% of the total blood volume is taken out from the femoral artery by opening the cannula into a measuring jar containing anticoagulant (heparin). Note the effect produced on BP and respiration.
2. Wait for a few minutes for resting parameters to come back to normal.
3. **For moderate to severe haemorrhage**, 10-40% of the total blood volume is taken out at gradual intervals. About 25-30 ml is let out at a time. Once bleeding is stopped, both BP and respiration will return to normal due to various compensatory mechanisms over a period of 20-30 minutes (Fig. 4.3.11). To speed up the process, the infusion of blood or normal saline should be given simultaneously.
4. Wait till BP and respiration return back to almost resting values.
5. **Now produce very severe haemorrhage** in the similar fashion as in step (3). Bleed the animal rapidly to about 40% of the total blood volume. Note the marked fall in BP (below 40 mmHg) with the subsequent appearance of ***Mayer's Waves*** and tremendous stimulation of the respiration (Fig. 4.3.11). These changes fail to come back to normal by transfusing any amount of blood, thus indicating the precipitation of **Irreversible Shock**.

What are Mayer's Waves and how are they produced?

The threshold of baroreceptor discharge is 60 mmHg;

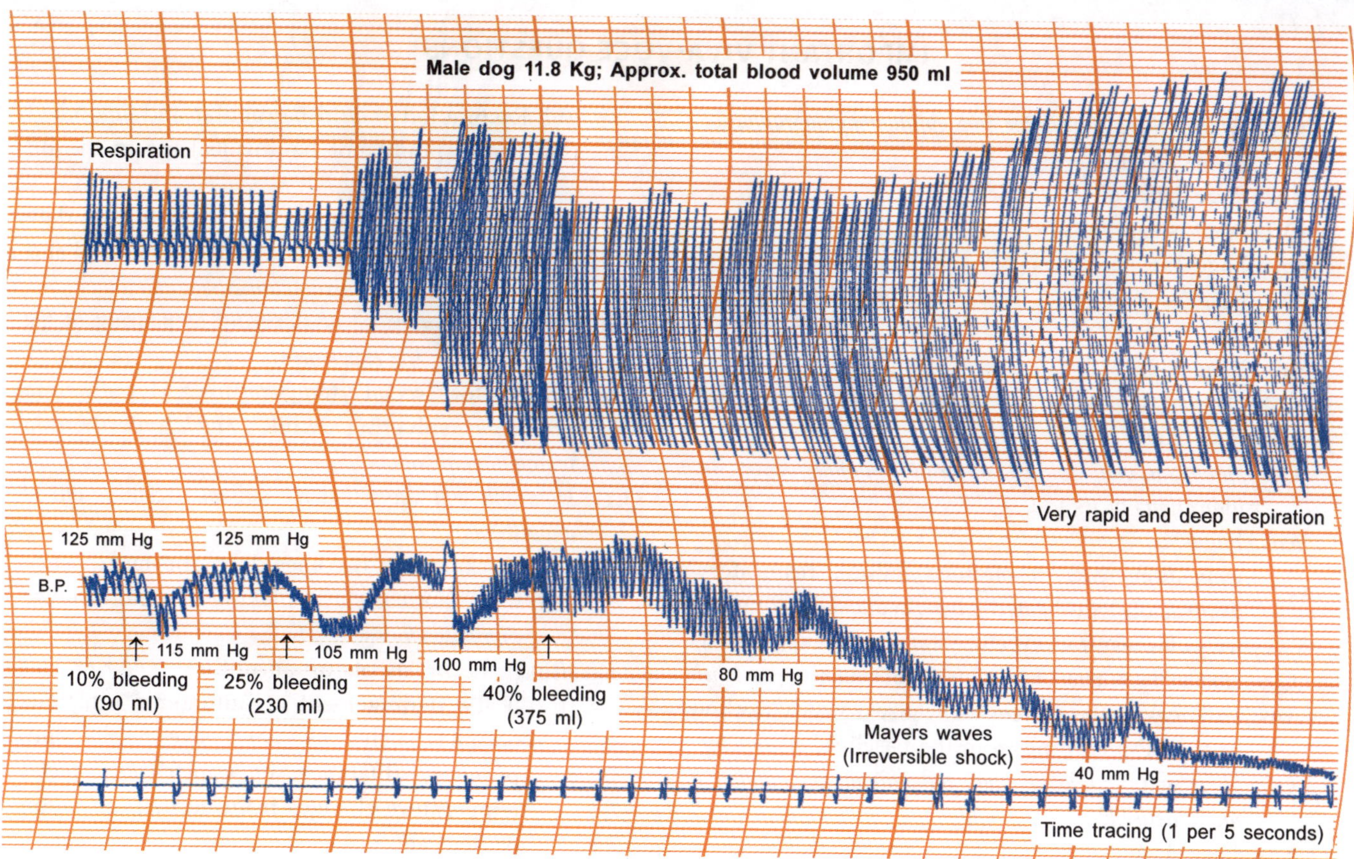

Fig. 4.3.11 Effect of bleeding and perfusion on BP and respiration

therefore, when BP falls below this value, chemoreceptors stimulate the VMC and BP rises. Any rise in BP above 60 mmHg causes baroreceptors to fire to produce reflex inhibition of the VMC. However, haemorrhage being continued, BP falls again. Thus the whole cycle is repeated every 20-40 seconds giving rise to an alternate rise and fall in BP. These waves which appear at a *frequency of 2-3 per minute* are called **Mayer's Waves**. These are characterized by *small amplitude* but are of long duration. Each crest or trough of the wave includes 3 to 4 respiratory cycles. The waves are, therefore, *attributed to the rhythmic fluctuating excitability of the VMC.*

Important points to remember before coming to any conclusion:

1. Look at the record carefully and make a note of the following:
   (a) HR
   (b) BP
   (c) Pulse pressure
   (d) Inspiratory and expiratory phases of respiration
   (e) Relationship between HR and respiration rate
   (f) Fluctuation in the BP waves caused by respiration
2. To comment on the effect of any variable, try to explain from the actual record obtained and not from what is expected of it.
3. Proper signals should be used to make the beginning and end of each procedure.
4. Wait for a minimum of 30 seconds before proceeding to the next procedure or till the resting BP and respiration is restored.

IMPORTANT VIVA-VOCE QUESTIONS

Q.1. *Why is there a need for two cylinder kymographs for the record purposes?*

Ans. Page 330.

Q.2. *What is end pressure?*

Ans. Page 151.

Q.3. *How is kymograph paper calibrated for recording BP?*

Ans. Page 332.

Q.4. *How is 'zero' of the scale adjusted in the manometer?*

Ans. Page 330.

Q.5. *How can one use the respiratory pump? Give the indications of its use.*

Ans. Page 330.

Indications are: respiratory failure, respiratory depression (indicated by cyanosed tongue), irregular respiration before starting the experiment.

Q.6. *How will you detect any leak in the BP recording system?*

Ans. Any leak in the system will cause a steady decline in the BP recording from the baseline.

Q.7. *How will you know that the animal is completely anaesthetised?*

Ans. Page 331.

Q.8. *Give the merits and demerits of commonly used anaesthetic agents for this experiment.*

Ans. Page 332.

Q.9. *List the requirements which should be fulfilled before the start of this experiment.*

Ans. (i) Ensure the animal is under complete anaesthesia.

(ii) The tongue should be pink.

(iii) The pupils should not be dilated.

(iv) The rectal temperature should be normal (in dogs it is 39-40°C due to high BMR).

(v) There should not be excessive salivation. If present, this indicates the derangement of the autonomic functions.

(vi) Respiration should be regular and smooth.

(vii) There should not be any leakage in the BP recording system.

(viii) Make a note of the animal's weight, sex, date and time of experiment, anaesthesia used and its mode of administration.

Q.10. *Give the major cause of shivering or panting of the animal during the experiment.*

Ans. Check for rectal temperature. Hypothermia produces shivering while the hyperthermia induces panting.

Q.11. *How will you know that the animal is coming out of anaesthesia?*

Ans. (i) If respiration becomes deep and fast.

(ii) If the animal starts making a peculiar noise of restlessness.

(iii) If the BP shoots up abruptly.

(iv) If the derangement of autonomic functions occurs such as excessive salivation, pupillary dilatation or constriction, rectal temperature changes from normal, urination or defecation.

Q.12. *How will you manage if the animal starts coming out of anaesthesia?*

Ans. Administer the maintenance dose of anaesthesia (page 332).

Q.13. *Give the normal values of the following in dogs and rabbits: heart rate, respiratory rate, mean blood pressure, tidal volume.*

Ans.

Feature	Dog	Rabbit
(i) Heart rate:	120 bpm.	100 bpm
(ii) Respiratory rate:	18-20 breaths/min	12-14 breaths/min
(iii) Mean BP:	130-140 mmHg	70-80 mmHg
(iv) Tidal volume	200 ml	50 ml

STUDY NOTES

RESULTS AND DISCUSSION

....

....

....

....

....

....

APPENDIX I

SPOTTING (Frequently Asked SPOTS in the Examination)

1.	A compound Microscope	(Refer to page 3)
2.	RBC pipette	(Refer to page 10)
3.	WBC pipette	(Refer to page 11)
4.	Improved Neubauer's counting chamber	(Refer to page 11)
5.	Sahli's Haemoglobinometer	(Refer to page 14)
6.	Graduated haemoglobinometer tube	(Refer to page 14)
7.	Haemoglobinometer pipette	(Refer to page 14)
8.	WBC Diluting fluid/Turk's fluid	(Refer to page 27)
9.	Focussing of different types of WBCs in a peripheral smear	(Refer to page 33)
10.	Capillary tube	(Refer to page 41)
11.	Wintrobe's Haematocrit tube	(Refer to page 50)
12.	Westergren's pipette	(Refer to page 50)
13.	Westergren's Stand	(Refer to page 50)
14.	Peripheral smear showing a reticulocyte	(Refer to page 59)
15.	Peripheral smear showing clumps of platelets	(Refer to pae 31)
16.	Simple/Primary key	(Refer to page 75)
17.	Short circuiting key or secondary key	(Refer to page 75)
18.	Reversing key	(Refer to page 76)
19.	Tap key	(Refer to page 76)
20.	Induction coil	(Refer to page 76)
21.	Variable interruptor	(Refer to page 77)
22.	Time marker/Signal marker	(Refer to page 77)
23.	Kymograph	(Refer to page 77)
24.	Myograph board	(Refer to page 78)
25.	Lucas chamber or muscle trough	(Refer to page 78)
26.	Isotonic muscle lever	(Refer to page 78)
27.	Hooks and Weights	(Refer to page 78)
28.	Starling heart lever	(Refer to page 79)
29.	Tuning Fork	(Refer to page 79)
30.	Student Physiograph	(Refer to page 81)
31.	Mosso's Ergograph	(Refer to page 141)
32.	Hand grip spring dynamometer	(Refer to page 142)
33.	Mercury sphygmomanometer	(Reger page 152)
34.	An Electrocardiograph	(Refer to page 163)
35.	A Stethograph	(Refer to page 171)
36.	A Vitalometer	(Refer to page 176)
37.	A Spirometer	(Refer to page 179)
38.	Wright's peak flow meter	(Refer to page 182)
39.	A Perimeter	(Refer to page 204)
40.	A Stethoscope	(Refer to page 218)
41.	Snellen's Chart	(Refer to page 241)
42.	Ishihara"s plates	(Refer to page 243)
43.	A patellar/knee hammer	(Refer to page 262)
44.	A aethesiometer	(Refer to page 270)
45.	Arterial Canula	(Refer to page 330)
46.	Venous Canula	(Refer to page 330)

APPENDIX

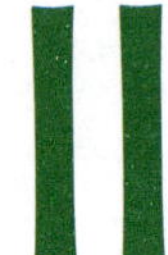

Routine Haematological Values for Normal Individuals

1. Haemoglobin

(i) At birth: 23 gm/dL
(ii) At the end of 3 months: 10.5 gm/dL
(iii) Adults – (a) males: 14-18 gm/dL (average: 15.5 gm/dL)
(b) females: 12-15.5 gm/dL (average: 14 gm/dL)

2. RBC Count

(i) At birth: 6-7 million/μL
(ii) Adults – (a) males: 5-6 million/μL (average: 5.5 million/μL)
(b) females: 4.5-5.5 million/μL (average: 4.8 million/μL)

3. WBC Count (TLC)

(i) At birth: 20000/μL
(ii) Adults: 4000-11000/μL

4. RBC Indices or Blood Standards

(i) Mean Corpuscular Volume (MCV): 78-94 μm^3 (86 ± 8 μm^3)
(ii) Mean Corpuscular Haemoglobin (MCH): 28-32 pg (29.5 ± 2.5 pg)
(iii) Mean Corpuscular Haemoglobin Concentration (MCHC): 32-38% (35 ± 3%)
(iv) Colour Index (CI): 0.85 - 1.15 (1.0 ± 0.15)

5. Differential Leucocyte Count (DLC)

	Absolute count
(i) Neutrophils: 50-70%	(3000-6000/μL)
(ii) Eosinophils: 1-4%	(150-300/μL)
(iii) Basophils: <1%	(10-100/μL)
(iv) Lymphocytes: 20-40%	(1500-2700/μL)
(v) Monocytes: 2-8%	(300-600/μL)

Note: In children, lymphocytes are 60% and neutrophils are 40%, a condition called **Relative Lymphocytosis**.

6. Arneth Count

(i) One lobed neutrophils – N_1 : 5%
(ii) Two lobed neutrophils – N_2 : 30%
(iii) Three lobed neutrophils – N_3 : 45%
(iv) Four lobed neutrophils – N_4 : 18%
(v) Five or more lobed neutrophils – N_5 : 2%

7. Bleeding Time (BT)

(i) Duke's method: 2-6 minutes
(ii) Ivy's method: 3-7 minutes

8. Clotting Time (CT)

(i) Capillary glass tube method: 2-8 minutes
(ii) Lee and White method (a) in glass tube: 6-12 minutes
(b) in silicon tube: 20-60 minutes

9. Frequency of Distribution of Blood Groups in India

	Blood group	Percentage
(i)	A	21
(ii)	B	39
(iii)	AB	9
(iv)	O	31
(v)	Rh positive	94-95
(vi)	Rh negative	5-6

10. Specific Gravity

(i) Of blood : 1.048 - 1.066
(ii) Of RBC : 1.092 - 1.095
(iii) Of plasma : 1.026 - 1.035

11. Erythrocyte Sedimentation Rate (ESR)

(i) Wintrobe's method
 (a) males: 0-9 mm 1st hour
 (b) females: 0-20 mm 1st hour
(ii) Westergren's method
 (a) males: 3-5 mm 1st hour
 (b) females: 4-7 mm 1st hour

12. Packed Cell Volume (PCV): Haematocrit

(i) Males: 45% (40-50%)
(ii) Females: 42% (37-42%)

13. Osmotic Fragility of RBCs

(i) Begins in 0.48% NaCl solution
(ii) Ends in 0.34% NaCl solution

14. Platelet Count

1.5-4 lacs/μL (average 2.59 lacs/μL)

15. Reticulocyte Count

(i) Adults and children: 0.2-2% (average 1%)
 Absolute count: 24000-84000/μL
(ii) Infants: 2-6%
(iii) New borns: 30-50%; decreases to 2% in 1st week of life.

16. Bone Marrow Examination

(i) Haemopoietic cells : 50-80%
(ii) Myeloid : erythroid ratio :: 2.5-15 : 1
(iii) Leuco : erythrogenic ratio :: 0.56-2.67 : 1
(iv) Myeloid : lymphoid ratio :: 1-1.7 : 1
(v) Lymphoid : erythroid ratio :: 0.2-4.0 : 1

17. Plasma Volume

40-50 ml/kg body weight (2.8-3.5 L)

18. Total Blood Volume

60-80 ml/kg body weight (5-6 L) or 8% of body weight

19. RBCs Volume

(i) Males: 30 ml/kg body weight
(ii) Females: 25 ml/kg body weight

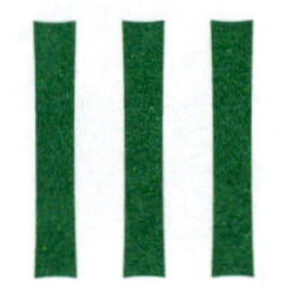

APPENDIX III

Composition and function of Stains, Diluting Fluids and Solutions used in Physiology Experiments

RBC Diluting Fluid (*Hayem's fluid*)

Each 100 ml of fluid contains:

1. Sodium sulphate (Na_2SO_4) : 2.5 gm (prevents rouleaux formation)
2. Sodium chloride NaCl) : 0.5 gm (maintains isotonicity)
3. Mercuric chloride ($HgCl_2$) : 0.25 gm (preservative, antibacterial, antifungal)
4. Distilled water : 100 ml (solvent)

WBC Diluting Fluid (*Turk's fluid*)

Each 100 ml of fluid contains:

1. Glacial acetic acid : 3 ml (lyses membrane of red blood cells)
2. Gentian violet (1%) : 1 ml (stains WBCs nuclei)
3. Distilled water to make 100 ml (solvent)

Leishman's Stain

1. Leishman powder 0.15 gm
   (i) Eosin : An acidic dye (negatively charged)
   (ii) Methylene blue : A basic dye (positively charged)
2. Acetone free methyl alcohol (fixative) : 100 ml

{**How to prepare?** Take 0.15 gm of Leishman powder in a beaker, add 100 ml of acetone free methyl alcohol, warm the mixture to 50°C, allow it to cool to 20°C and shake several times; after standing for 24 hours, filter the solution.}

Procedure for preparation of $CuSO_4$ of specific gravity (SG) ranging from 1.050 to 1.066
(*for determination of SG of blood*)

Test Tube Number	1	2	3	4	5	6	7	8	9
$CuSO_4$ solution (ml)	4.9	5.1	5.3	5.5	5.7	5.9	6.1	6.3	6.5
Distilled water (ml)	5.1	4.9	4.7	4.5	4.3	4.1	3.9	3.7	3.5
SG of solution	1.050	1.052	1.054	1.056	1.058	1.060	1.062	1.064	1.066

Procedure for preparation of increasing hypotonicity of NaCl solution
(for determination of osmotic fragility of RBCs)

Test Tube Number	1	2	3	4	5	6	7	8	9	10	11	12
Number of drops of distilled water	3	9	10	11	12	13	14	15	16	17	18	25
Number of drops of 1% NaCl	22	16	15	14	13	12	11	10	9	8	7	0
% saline solution	0.88	0.64	0.60	0.56	0.52	0.48	0.44	0.40	0.36	0.32	0.28	0

Important Note: Use the same dropper (after thorough rinsing) for saline and distilled water so that the volume of drops is equal for all test tubes.

Platelets Diluting Fluid

1% Ammonium oxalate (anticoagulant, preserves the platelets and destroys the RBCs)

or

Rees-Ecker diluting fluid: Each 100 ml contains:

1. Sodium citrate : 3.8 gm (anticoagulant)
2. Brilliant cresyl blue : 0.1 gm (for staining purposes)
3. Formalin or formaldehyde : 2 ml (fixative for stain and lysis the RBCs)
4. Distilled water to make 100 ml (solvent)

Vital Stains for Reticulocytes

1% brilliant cresyl blue in isotonic saline or methyl alcohol.

or

1 gm of methylene blue dissolved in 100 ml of citrate saline solution {i.e. 3 gm/L sodium citrate plus 9 gm/L NaCl) (anticoagulant, isotonic) and bicarbonate buffer, pH 7.4}.

or

1 gm of new methylene blue dissolved in 100 ml of iso-osmotic phosphate buffer, pH 7.4 (i.e. 24.3 gm/l of NaH_2PO_4 and 21.3 gm/l of Na_2HPO_4 for iso-osmotic buffer).

Note: It is superior to above two solutions.

Pilot's fluid for Absolute Eosinophil Count

Each 100 ml of solution contains:

1. Pholoxine : 10 ml (stains only eosinophilic granules)
2. Propylene glycol : 50 ml (solvent for stain and lyses RBCs)
3. Sodium carbonate (1%) : 1 ml (lyses all WBCs except eosinophils)
4. Heparin : 100 units (anticoagulant)
5. Distilled water to make 100 ml (solvent)

Amphibian Ringer Solution

1. 0.6% NaCl : Isotonic with amphibian plasma.
2. 0.14% KCl : Helps maintaining the membrane potential.
3. 0.012 $CaCl_2$: Helps maintaining the muscle excitability and stimulates ATPase activity.
4. 0.02% $NaHCO_3$: Provides optimal pH.

Ringer Locke's Solution

(For perfusion of isolated mammalian heart)

1. NaCl : 0.9 gm/dL
2. KCl : 0.042 gm/dL
3. $CaCl_2$: 0.024 gm/dL

} (isotonic; Ca^{2+} keeps the heart ready in a state of spontaneous contraction)

4. $NaHCO_3$: 0.015 gm/dL (maintains the pH between 7.1 to 7.6)
5. Glucose : 0.1 gm/dL (provides nutrition)
6. Distilled water to make 100 ml (solvent)

Tyrode's Solution

(For isolated rabbit's intestine)

1. Glucose : 0.1 gm/dL (provides nutrition)
2. NaCl : 0.8 gm/dL
3. KCl : 0.02 gm/dL (isotonic, provides optimal electric condition)
4. $CaCl_2$: 0.02 gm/dL
5. $MgCl_2$: 0.01 gm/dL (regulates intenstinal motility)
6. $NaHCO_3$: 0.01 gm/dL
7. NaH_2PO_4 : 0.005 gm/dL (helps maintaining pH between 7.4 to 7.6)
8. Distilled water to make 100 ml (solvent).

INDEX

Q

R